Lymphedema

Arin K. Greene • Sumner A. Slavin
Håkan Brorson

Editors

Lymphedema

Presentation, Diagnosis, and Treatment

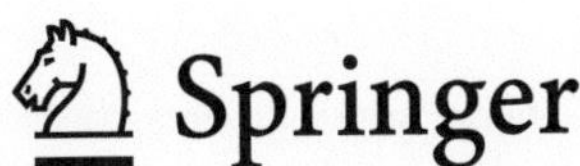 Springer

Editors
Arin K. Greene, M.D., M.M.Sc.
Department of Plastic and Oral Surgery
Boston Children's Hospital
Co-Director Lymphedema Program
Associate Professor of Surgery
Harvard Medical School
Boston, MA, USA

Sumner A. Slavin, M.D.
Division of Plastic Surgery
Beth Israel Deaconess Medical Center
Co-Director Lymphedema Program
Associate Professor of Surgery
Harvard Medical School
Boston, MA, USA

Håkan Brorson, M.D., Ph.D.
Senior Consultant, Associate Professor
Director, The Lymphedema Unit
Department of Clinical Sciences
Lund University
Plastic and Reconstructive Surgery
Skåne University Hospital
Malmö, Sweden

Professor
Esculera de Graduasos
Asociación Médica Argentina
Buenos Aires, Argentina

ISBN 978-3-319-38269-2   ISBN 978-3-319-14493-1   (eBook)
DOI 10.1007/978-3-319-14493-1

Springer Cham Heidelberg New York Dordrecht London
© Springer International Publishing Switzerland 2015
Softcover reprint of the hardcover 1st edition 2015

Springer International Publishing AG Switzerland is part of Springer Science+Business Media (www.springer.com)

This book is dedicated to patients with lymphedema—we hope that it improves their quality of life and translates into improved therapies.

Preface

Although lymphedema affects millions of people around the world, the pathophysiology of the disease is poorly understood and the condition remains incurable. Lymphedema is associated with many myths; patients often are misdiagnosed and receive incorrect treatment. Individuals with lymphedema typically are medical nomads being transferred from physician to physician until they find someone who understands their disease. The goal of this book is to improve the lives of patients with lymphedema by providing an evidence-based resource for health-care providers.

The editors of the book direct Lymphedema Programs and share many principles related to the management of lymphedema. Experts from around the world were recruited to author chapters on his/her expertise. The book was designed to be clinically oriented, rather than focused on history or research; references were limited to no more than 30 for each chapter. The book was written to be an easy-to-read resource that highlights principles by including an abstract, conclusion, and list of key points. The text also can be used for more in-depth study of a subject, teaching, or research. Hopefully, the book will stimulate readers to improve their understanding of lymphedema and to develop better treatments.

Boston, MA, USA
Boston, MA, USA
Malmö, Sweden

Arin K. Greene
Sumner A. Slavin
Håkan Brorson

Acknowledgments

<hr>

The Editors

We thank all of the contributing authors who have shared their expertise to improve the care of patients with lymphedema. We also thank Springer Publishing, and particularly Elektra McDermott, who have done an outstanding job editing and helping us put the book together.

<hr>

Arin Greene

My interest in lymphedema began when I was exposed to children with primary disease in the Vascular Anomalies Center at Boston Children's Hospital. I was troubled by the significant morbidity that lymphedema could cause, the lack of understanding regarding its pathogenesis, and the often less-than-satisfactory treatments. My passion for the condition was further stimulated by Sumner Slavin who exposed me to patients with secondary lymphedema in the Lymphedema Program at the Beth Israel Deaconess Medical Center.

I would like to thank Sumner Slavin and Håkan Brorson who have been my biggest influences in the field of lymphedema. I am also grateful to Steven Fishman and John Mulliken who not only first exposed me to primary lymphedema but also have encouraged my interest in lymphedema and recommended that patients with primary lymphedema be managed in our dedicated Lymphedema Program rather than the Vascular Anomalies Center. I would like to acknowledge John Meara who has encouraged my interest in lymphedema and given me tremendous professional support. Dr. Meara also supported moving the Lymphedema Program from the Beth Israel Deaconess Medical Center to the Department of Plastic and Oral Surgery at Boston Children's Hospital. Since relocating the center to our department several years ago, we have been able to manage both children and adults with the disease. In addition, we have learned from our high volume of patients, which has translated into innovation and improved care.

Our multidisciplinary management of patients with lymphedema would not be possible without the work of Jennifer Jagielski and Susan Rajotte who attend our Lymphedema Clinics and provide static and pneumatic compression, respectively. I am grateful for our other team members, Elizabeth Hunter, Ashley D'Eon, and Reid Maclellan, who provide outstanding patient care and administration. I would like to thank our close colleagues in the

Nuclear Medicine Department, Frederick Grant and Stephan Voss, who perform lymphoscintigraphy on our patients and collaborate with us through research as well.

Finally, I want to acknowledge my family. I am not sure I would be a plastic surgeon today without my grandparents, Albert and Ruth, who had a profound influence on my life. Most importantly, I want to thank my wife, Sarah, and three boys, Albert, Mac, and Henry, who encourage and support the passion I have for my "job."

Contents

Editors and Authors

List of Editors

Håkan Brorson, M.D., Ph.D. The Lymphedema Unit, Department of Clinical Sciences, Lund University, Plastic and Reconstructive Surgery, Skåne University Hospital, Malmö, Sweden

Arin K. Greene, M.D., M.M.Sc. Department of Plastic and Oral Surgery, Boston Children's Hospital, Harvard Medical School, Boston, MA, USA

Sumner A. Slavin, M.D. Division of Plastic Surgery, Beth Israel Deaconess Medical Center, Harvard Medical School, Boston, MA, USA

List of Authors

Ahmad I. Alomari, M.D., M.Sc., F.S.I.R. Department of Vascular and Interventional Radiology, Boston Children's Hospital, Harvard Medical School, Boston, MA, USA

Sigrid Bairdain, M.D., M.P.H. Department of Pediatric Surgery, Boston Children's Hospital, Boston, MA, USA

Ruediger G.H. Baumeister, Prof. Dr. Dr. med. Habil. Plastic-, Hand-, Microsurgery Department of Surgery, Ludwig Maximilians University Munich, Muenchen, Germany

Laurence M. Boon, M.D., Ph.D. Center for Vascular Anomalies, Cliniques universitaires Saint-Luc, Universite Catholique de Louvain, Brussels, Belgium

Pierre Bourgeois, M.D., Ph.D. Service of Nuclear Medicine, Clinic of Lymphology, Institute Jules Bordet, Université Libre de Bruxelles, Brussels, Belgium

Pascal Brouillard, Ph.D. Laboratory of Human Molecular Genetics, De Duve Institute, Universite catholique de Louvain, Brussels, Belgium

Gulraiz Chaudry, M.B.Ch.B. Department of Vascular and Interventional Radiology, Boston Children's Hospital, Harvard Medical School, Boston, MA, USA

Hung-Chi Chen, M.D., Ph.D., F.A.C.S. Department of Plastic Surgery, China Medical University Hospital, Taichung, Taiwan

Shih-Heng Chen Department of Plastic Surgery, China Medical University Hospital, Taichung, Taiwan

Neil R. Feins, M.D. Department of Surgery, Boston Children's Hospital, Harvard Medical School, Boston, MA, USA

Steven J. Fishman, M.D. Department of Pediatric Surgery, Boston Children's Hospital, Boston, MA, USA

Pradeep Goyal, M.D. Department of Vascular and Interventional Radiology, Boston Children's Hospital, Harvard Medical School, Boston, MA, USA

Geoffrey E. Hespe, B.S. Department of Surgery, Memorial Sloan Kettering Cancer Center, New York, NY, USA

Jung-Ju Huang, M.D. Plastic and Reconstructive Microsurgery, Chang Gung Memorial Hospital, Taoyuan County, Taiwan

Heli Kavola, M.D., Ph.D. Department of Plastic Surgery, Helsinki University Hospital, Helsinki, Finland

Reid A. Maclellan, M.D., M.M.Sc. Department of Plastic and Oral Surgery, Boston Children's Hospital, Harvard Medical School, Boston, MA, USA

Jiro Maegawa, M.D., Ph.D. Department of Plastic and Reconstructive Surgery, Yokohama City University Hospital, Yokohama, Japan

Michele Maruccia, M.D. Department of Plastic Surgery, China Medical University Hospital, Taichung, Taiwan

Harvey N. Mayrovitz, Ph.D. Department of Physiology, College of Medical Sciences, Nova Southeastern University, Fort Lauderdale, FL, USA

Babak J. Mehrara, M.D., F.A.C.S. Department of Surgery, Memorial Sloan Kettering Cancer Center, New York, NY, USA

Rudy Murillo, M.D. Department of Surgery, Boston Children's Hospital, Boston, MA, USA

Matthew D. Nitti, B.A. Department of Surgery, Memorial Sloan Kettering Cancer Center, New York, NY, USA

Karin Ohlin, B.S., O.T. The Lymphedema Unit, Department of Clinical Sciences, Lund University, Plastic and Reconstructive Surgery, Skåne University Hospital, Malmö, Sweden

Anne Saarikko, M.D. Department of Plastic Surgery, Töölö Hospital, Helsinki, Finland

Matthieu J. Schlögel, M.Sc. Laboratory of Human Molecular Genetics, De Duve Institute, Universite Catholique de Louvain, Brussels, Belgium

Sinikka Suominen, M.D., Ph.D. Department of Plastic Surgery, Helsinki University, Helsinki, Finland

Barbro Svensson, B.S., P.T., L.T. The Lymphedema Unit, Department of Clinical Sciences, Lund University, Plastic and Reconstructive Surgery, Skåne University Hospital, Malmö, Sweden

Stéphane Vignes, M.D. Department of Lymphology, Hopital Cognacq-Jay, Paris, France

Miikka Vikkula, M.D., Ph.D. Laboratory of Human Molecular Genetics, De Duve Institute, Universite Catholique de Louvain, Brussels, Belgium

Walloon Excellence in Life Sciences and Biotechnology (WELBIO), Brussels, Belgium

Leigh C. Ward, B.Sc. (Hons), Ph.D., R.N.U.T.R. School of Chemistry and Molecular Biosciences, The University of Queensland, Brisbane, QLD, Australia

Part I

Overview of Lymphedema

The Lymphatic System

Reid A. Maclellan

Key Points
- The lymphatic system travels parallel to the cardiovascular system.
- In the extremities there are both superficial and deep lymphatics.
- The thoracic duct is the main lymphatic collecting vessel; it obtains lymph fluid from the entire body except the upper right quadrant.

Introduction

The lymphatic system parallels the cardiovascular system. It consists of lymphatic vessels and secondary lymphoid organs. It returns lymph fluid to the circulation via a one-way system [1]. Lymphatic vessels were first described as "white blood" by Hippocrates who coined the term "chyle" from the Greek *chylos,* meaning juice [1, 2]. Gaspar Aselli first illustrated the lymphatic system in 1622. As he was studying the abdomen of a well-fed dog, he noted a large number of mesentery cords that were very white and extremely thin. A white milk-like substance discharged from the vessels as he dissected them. *De lactius sive lacteis venis* was the first color-printed medical publication [1, 3]. An

additional 300 years passed before it was discovered that the lymph system is responsible for returning protein molecules from tissues back to the central circulation. It also was determined that blocking lymphatic vessels led to lymphedema [4].

The lymphatic system is an open, linear structure. In the extremities it consists of an epifascial and a subfascial arrangement. It begins by collecting lymph fluid in tissue, delivers the fluid to filtering nodes through many small afferent vessels, exits the nodes via large efferent channels, and ends at the lymph–vein connection of the thoracic duct [5]. The lymphatics are absent in the brain, spinal cord, retina, bone, and cartilage [1].

Lymphatic Anatomy

Vasculature

Lymphatic capillaries are designed to obtain drained lymph fluid. They only have a single layer of overlapping lymphatic endothelial cells that are attached by filament bundles. In comparison to blood capillaries, they are not lined by a basement membrane or smooth-muscle like pericytes. This allows them to be highly permeable to interstitial fluid and macromolecules [6, 7]. Lymphatic capillaries normally are collapsed because they do not have the type of hemodynamic pressure that blood capillaries have that forces them to stay open [1, 8, 9]. An increase in interstitial pressure leads

The author has no disclosures.

R.A. Maclellan, M.D., M.M.Sc. (⊠)
Department of Plastic and Oral Surgery,
Lymphedema Program, Boston Children's Hospital,
Harvard Medical School, 300 Longwood Avenue,
Boston, MA 02115, USA
e-mail: reid.maclellan@childrens.harvard.edu

A.K. Greene et al. (eds.), *Lymphedema: Presentation, Diagnosis, and Treatment,*
DOI 10.1007/978-3-319-14493-1_1, © Springer International Publishing Switzerland 2015

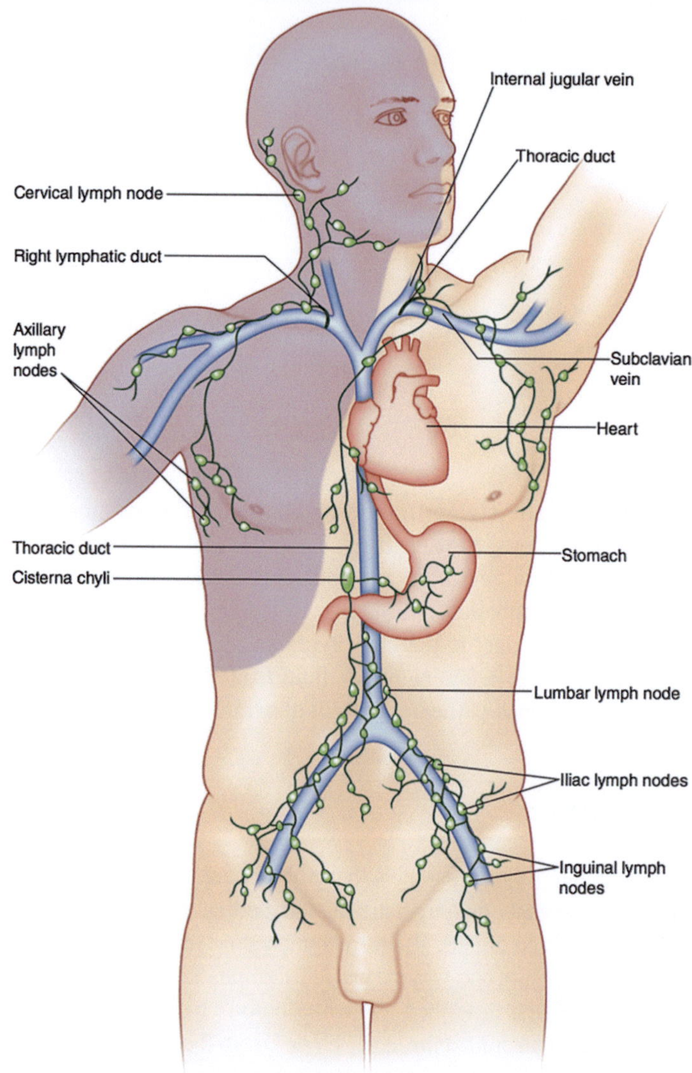

Fig. 1.1 Schematic of the lymphatic collection system. The right lymphatic duct obtains lymph fluid from the *shaded area*, while the thoracic duct accumulates lymph from the *non-shaded region*

to the anchoring filaments pulling the lymphatic endothelial cells apart and opening the capillaries. Lymph fluid then drains into the lymphatic capillaries [7, 10]. These capillaries are connected to precollecting lymphatic vessels, which eventually merge into secondary lymphatic collecting vessels.

Unlike lymphatic capillaries, lymphatic collecting vessels are constructed to return drained fluid into the circulation. They have lymphatic endothelial cells that are surrounded by a continuous basement membrane and pericytes. These endothelial cells tightly line up side by side [1, 11]. The collecting vessels possess valves that inhibit retrograde lymph flow. Muscle contraction propels lymph fluid through the collecting vessels [1].

Thoracic Duct

The thoracic duct is the main lymphatic collecting vessel of the body. It obtains lymph fluid from the entire body except the right head and neck, right hemithorax, and right upper extremity (Fig. 1.1).

It measures approximately 45 cm in length and 5 mm in width [12]. The thoracic duct is divided into three parts: abdominal, thoracic, and cervical. The duct originates with the abdominal portion at the cisterna chyli and ascends upward to form the thoracic portion as it traverses the aortic hiatus of the diaphragm into the posterior mediastinum [13]. The duct continues posteriorly along the esophagus until it reaches the fifth thoracic vertebra where it ascends on the left of the esophagus. The cervical segment of the duct begins when it descends across the subclavian artery at the seventh cervical vertebra [13]. The cervical thoracic duct is the widest of the three parts and has the greatest amount of variability between patients. There also are move valves in the "cervical" region than any other portion of the duct [14].

Several researchers have studied the termination of the thoracic duct. One anatomist reviewed over 500 patients and cadavers and determined 36 % of ducts end in the internal jugular vein, 34 % terminated in the junction of the internal jugular and subclavian veins, 21 % had multiple closures, and 17 % concluded in the subclavian vein [15]. Another group found the most common location of cessation was the venous angle (38 %) followed by the external jugular vein (28 %) and internal jugular vein (27 %) [16]. They noted 7 % of patients had a complex configuration. These individuals had a higher likelihood of metastasis in the cervical region [16]. Surgeons should take extra caution when dissecting in the vicinity of the thoracic duct because of its highly variable anatomy.

Right Lymphatic Duct

The right lymphatic duct drains the upper right body including the right head and neck, right upper extremity, right diaphragm, right lung, lower left lung, most of the heart, and part of the right lobe of the liver [13]. It is formed by the joining together of the right jugular, right subclavian, and right bronchomediastinal lymphatic trunks and measures 2 cm in length, respectively. The right bronchomediastinal trunk is the

vestigial portion of the embryologic right thoracic duct [13]. The right lymphatic duct mainly terminates in the junction of the right subclavian and right internal jugular veins; however, it has numerous variations like the thoracic duct [13].

Cisterna Chyli

The cisterna chyli is a 2–5 cm elongated sac located retroperitoneally approximately at the second lumbar vertebra. It is the beginning of the thoracic duct. It drains lymph from the right and left lumbar trunks, the intestinal trunk, and the lowest intercostal vessels. These vessels either form a single sac or multiple sacculations. The union of the individual vessels may occur in the thoracic region instead of the abdomen [14]. The lumbar trunks obtain lymph from the pelvis, kidneys, adrenal glands, and area of the abdominal wall below the umbilicus. The intestinal trunk drains lymph from the celiac and superior mesenteric arteries [13].

Lymphatics of the Extremity

In the extremities there is an epifascial and a subfascial lymphatic system. The epidermal valveless lymphatics drain toward the subdermal valved lymphatics which then flow to collecting vessels above the fascia. The subdermal lymphatics are responsible for draining the integument and normally follow along with the veins. The epifascial and subfascial lymphatics communicate via perforators. The deep lymphatics flow below the deep fascia and course parallel with the main vascular structures [5]. In both the superficial and deep lymphatic system several small afferent lymphatic vessels lead lymph fluid to lymph node sinuses. The fluid exits the lymph node hilum via large efferent channels on its return to the cardiovascular system [5, 17]. The epifascial lymph nodes interconnect into four central draining chains: the paired axillary and inguinal lymph node systems [5].

The superficial lymphatic system of the upper extremity is divided into an ulnar bundle and a radial bundle. The ulnar bundle drains the medial arm and follows the basilic vein to the axillary lymph nodes [5]. Part of the ulnar bundle branches at the hiatus basilicus and connects with the deep lymphatic system of the upper extremity via perforators. The radial bundle obtains lymph from the lateral arm and accompanies the cephalic vein until it joins the axillary lymph nodes at the lower margin of the pectoralis major muscle [5]. Lymph will then drain from the axillary lymph nodes to either the supraclavicular and/or infraclavicular lymph node and then to either the thoracic duct (left upper extremity) or the right lymphatic duct (right upper extremity) [5].

The epifascial system of the lower extremity collects lymph from the skin and subcutaneous layers and is divided into two bundles: ventromedial and dorsolateral bundles [5]. The dorsolateral bundle parallels the lesser saphenous vein, passes through the popliteal nodes, continues as the subfascial lymphatics of the thigh, and ends either in the deep inguinal or anterior iliac nodes. The ventromedial bundle runs with the greater saphenous vein but has greater variability in how it terminates [5]. The subfascial system accompanies the anterior and posterior tibial vasculature until they join with the dorsolateral bundle at the popliteal nodes. These collector vessels drain the muscles and fascia of the lower extremity [5].

Lymphatic Function

The lymphatic vasculature recycles interstitial fluids from veins back to the circulatory system, contributes to the immune response, and participates in the digestive tract [1, 5, 18]. Fifty to 100 % of plasma exits into the interstitium daily and provides nourishment to surrounding tissues [19, 20]. Ninety percent is recycled via venous capillaries; however, the remaining fluid has a molecular weight that is too large to pass through these vessels [5, 19, 20]. The differences in hydrostatic pressure and colloidal pressure in surrounding tissues and the lymphatic vasculature force the high molecular weight plasma through collecting lymphatics [5]. The lymph is then transported back to the cardiovascular system. The lymphatics also function in the immune system both by activating inflammatory responses in lymphatic endothelial cells and trafficking lymphocytes and antigen-presenting cells to lymph nodes [1, 21]. The lymphatics final purpose is to assist in the digestive tract. Lacteals are specialized lymphatic vessels located in the intestines. They carry fats and lipids in the form of chylomicrons [1, 22].

Conclusion

The lymphatic system runs one-way. The extremities have an epifascial and a subfascial system for collecting lymph. Lymph fluid drains from capillaries to afferent collecting vessels to lymph nodes to efferent lymphatic vessels to either the thoracic duct or the right lymphatic duct and back to the cardiovascular system.

References

1. Choi I, Lee S, Hong YK. The new era of the lymphatic system: no longer secondary to the blood vascular system. Cold Spring Harb Perspect Med. 2012;2:a006445.
2. Grotte G. The discovery of the lymphatic circulation. Acta Physiol Scand Suppl. 1979;463:9–10.
3. Aselli G. De lactibus sive lacteis venis. Milan: Mediolani; 1627
4. Drinker CK, Field ME, Ward HK. The filtering capacity of lymph nodes. J Exp Med. 1934;59:393–405.
5. Clodius L. Lymphedema. In: McCarthy J, editor. Plastic surgery, vol. 6. Philadelphia: WB Saunders Company; 1990.
6. Tammela T, Alitalo K. Lymphangiogenesis: molecular mechanisms and future promise. Cell. 2010;140: 460–76.
7. Leak LV, Burke JF. Fine structure of the lymphatic capillary and the adjoining connective tissue area. Am J Anat. 1966;118:785–809.
8. Alitalo K. Growth factors controlling angiogenesis and lymphangiogenesis. Ugeskr Laeger. 2002;164: 3170–2.
9. Alitalo K, Carmeliet P. Molecular mechanisms of lymphangiogenesis in health and disease. Cancer Cell. 2002;1:219–27.
10. Leak LV, Burke JF. Ultrastructural studies on the lymphatic anchoring filaments. J Cell Biol. 1968;36: 129–49.

11. Baluk P, Fuxe J, Hashizume H, Romano T, Lashnits E, Butz S, Vestweber D, Corada M, Molendini C, Dejana E, McDonald DM. Functionally specialized junctions between endothelial cells of lymphatic vessels. J Exp Med. 2007;204:2349–62.
12. Langford RJ. Valves in the subsidiary lymph trunks in the neck. J Craniomaxillofac Surg. 2002;30:121–4.
13. Skandalakis JE, Skandalakis LJ, Skandalakis PN. Anatomy of the lymphatics. Surg Oncol Clin N Am. 2007;16:1–16.
14. Jacobsson S. Clinical anatomy and pathology of the thoracic duct: an investigation of 122 cases. Stockholm, Sweden: Almqvist & Wiksell; 1972.
15. Kinnaert P. Anatomical variations of the cervical portion of the thoracic duct in man. J Anat. 1973; 115(Pt 1):45–52.
16. Shimada K, Sato I. Morphological and histological analysis of the thoracic duct at the jugulo-subclavian junction in Japanese cadavers. Clin Anat. 1997;10: 163–72.
17. Olszewski W. Anatomy of the lymphatic system and its disorders. In: Lee B, Bergan J, Rockson SG, editors. Lymphedema: a concise compendium of theory and practice. New York: Springer; 2011.
18. Hussain MM. A proposed model for the assembly of chylomicrons. Atherosclerosis. 2000;148:1–15.
19. Casley-Smith JR. The functioning and interrelationships of blood capillaries and lymphatics. Experientia. 1976;32:1–12.
20. Foldi-Borcsok E, Foldi M. Lymphedema and vitamins. Am J Clin Nutr. 1973;26(2):185–90.
21. Kang S, Lee SP, Kim KE, Kim HZ, Memet S, Koh GY. Toll-like receptor 4 in lymphatic endothelial cells contributes to LPS-induced lymphangiogenesis by chemotactic recruitment of macrophages. Blood. 2009;113:2605–13.
22. Rosen ED. The molecular control of adipogenesis, with special reference to lymphatic pathology. Ann N Y Acad Sci. 2002;979:143–58. discussion 88–96.

Geoffrey E. Hespe, Matthew D. Nitti, and Babak J. Mehrara

Key Points

- Lymphedema is a pathophysiologic process resulting from injury, infection, obstruction, or congenital defects in the lymphatic system.
- Primary lymphedemas occur as a result of genetic or developmental abnormalities in the lymphatic system; secondary lymphedemas are caused by secondary insults to the lymphatic system
- The histological hallmarks of lymphedema are lymphatic fluid stasis, chronic inflammation, fibroadipose tissue deposition, and hyperkeratosis.
- Risk factors for development of lymphedema include genetic abnormalities, obesity, radiation, and infection.
- Cellular mechanisms of lymphedema are unknown; however, recent studies have demonstrated a critical role for CD4+ cells in the regulation of fibrosis in animal models and correlative clinical studies.

G.E. Hespe, B.S. • M.D. Nitti, B.A.
B.J. Mehrara, M.D., F.A.C.S. (⊠)
Department of Surgery, Memorial Sloan Kettering Cancer Center, 1275 York Avenue, Suite MRI 1005, New York, NY 10065, USA
e-mail: mehrarab@mskcc.org

Introduction

The lymphatic system is an essential component of the circulatory system whose main roles are maintaining fluid homeostasis, acting as a conduit for migration and transport of immune cells, regulation of inflammatory responses, and enabling dietary absorption of fat. Networks of lymphatic vessels begin as blind-ended lymphatic capillaries and transport interstitial fluid unidirectionally back to the heart. Disruption of lymphatic vasculature secondary to chronic parasitic infections, during the course of cancer treatment, after trauma, or as a consequence of genetic mutations results in stasis of protein rich interstitial fluid and chronic inflammation. These pathologic changes, over time, lead to lymphedema; a progressive disease characterized by adipose deposition and tissue fibrosis. It is well established that patients with lymphedema have significant impairments in quality of life, recurrent infections, and in some cases deadly secondary tumors.

Broadly speaking, lymphedema can be categorized as either primary or secondary. Primary lymphedema, as the name implies, is caused by abnormal development of the lymphatic system or pathological changes intrinsic to the lymphatic vasculature. These developmental abnormalities may be related to genetic defects that either directly or indirectly regulate lymphatic differentiation and function. In contrast, secondary lymphedemas occur as a consequence of postnatal iatrogenic, infectious, or traumatic insults to the

A.K. Greene et al. (eds.), *Lymphedema: Presentation, Diagnosis, and Treatment*, DOI 10.1007/978-3-319-14493-1_2, © Springer International Publishing Switzerland 2015

lymphatic system. Although both primary and secondary lymphedemas share similar pathologic features including chronic swelling, inflammation, adipose deposition, and fibrosis, there important pathologic distinctions remain between patient responses, disease course, and response to treatments. In addition, although recent studies have improved our understanding of the pathology of lymphedema in general, the mechanisms that regulate these disease specific responses remain unknown and are an important area of research.

Classification of Lymphedema

Primary Lymphedema

Primary lymphedemas can be classified either by the timing of presentation, mode of inheritance (genetic linked or sporadic), or region of pathology (e.g., systemic or visceral). Traditionally, the timing of presentation has been used most commonly to categorize patients as having congenital lymphedema (i.e., present at birth), developing lymphedema around the time of puberty (lymphedema praecox), or presenting in adults older than 35 years (lymphedema tarda). The vast majority of patients present with either congenital lymphedema or lymphedema praecox; lymphedema tarda is diagnosed in less than 10 % of patients [1].

Classification of lymphedema based on timing of presentation is not particularly useful since there is no reference to the pathological causes. More recently, Connell et al. published a classification system and diagnostic algorithm that subcategorizes congenital lymphedemas as syndromic, systemic/visceral, disturbed growth, congenital onset, and late onset [2]. This classification system is helpful because it takes a more functional approach to lymphatic development and will likely aid in identifying genetic mutations due to its more inclusive nature.

Primary lymphedemas, in general, affect females twice as often as males and tend to more frequently involve the lower extremities. It is estimated that nearly 30 % of patients with primary lymphedema have an identifiable genetic mutation (often in the signaling pathway for vascular endothelial growth factor-C (VEGF-C)). The most studied example of this scenario is **Milroy's disease**, a form of congenital primary lymphedema that is caused by a heterozygous inactivating mutation of FLT4, the gene that encodes for the receptor for VEGF-C (Vascular Endothelial Growth Factor Receptor-3 (VEGFR-3). Milroy's disease is a familial, sexlinked condition and accounts for approximately 2 % of all lymphedemas. These patients most commonly have bilateral lower extremity lymphedema that is, in some cases, accompanied by hydroceles. Another common genetic cause of lymphedema is an autosomal dominant condition known as *lymphedema–distichiasis syndrome.* These patients have an autosomal dominant mutation in the FOXC2 gene, resulting in a combination of lower extremity lymphedema and an extra row of eyelashes.

Sporadic (i.e., not familial) cases are the most common causes of primary lymphedema accounting for ~60 % of all patients with lymphedema. The most common form of sporadic primary lymphedema is **Meige's disease**. Patients with this disorder present with symptoms usually around the time of puberty with a female to male ratio of 4:1. These facts have led some authors to suggest that female sex hormones may play a role in the development of lymphedema.

Secondary Lymphedema

Secondary lymphedema is the most common cause of lymphedema and develops secondary to either direct or indirect injury to the lymphatic system. The most common form of secondary lymphedema worldwide is filariasis, a condition in which parasitic roundworms *Wuchereria bancrofti* occupy the lymphatic vasculature, thereby blocking the flow of lymph from the extremity. Although the true incidence of filariasis remains unknown, estimates ranging between 140 and 200 million are commonly cited among patients residing primarily in third world countries [3]. In contrast, this form of lymphedema is very rare in developed countries.

In developed countries secondary lymphedema occurs most commonly as a complication of cancer treatment with breast cancer being the most common cause. It is estimated that nearly one in three patients who undergo axillary lymph node dissection for staging or treatment of breast cancer go on to develop lymphedema. Lymphedema, however, is not limited to breast cancer survivors, as a recent study demonstrated that nearly one in six patients who undergo treatment for other solid tumors such as melanoma, sarcoma, and gynecological malignancies also go on to develop lymphedema [4]. Even relatively minor disruption of the lymphatic system with sentinel lymph node biopsy, a procedure in which only a few lymph nodes are sampled for cancer staging, can result in lymphedema in 5–7 % of patients [5]. Lymphedema can also develop in patients who do not have lymph node biopsy but rather wide skin excisions (for example during the course of treatment for sarcoma or melanoma) particularly when these procedures are combined with radiation therapy suggesting that extensive injury of either the deep (i.e., lymph nodes) or superficial (i.e., dermal) lymphatic system can result in lymphedema development.

Importantly, the development of lymphedema after lymphatic injury usually occurs in a delayed fashion. Thus, although virtually all patients experience minor swelling immediately following surgery, in the vast majority of cases the swelling resolves within the first 4–6 weeks. However, a subset of patients develop recurrent swelling at a later point, typically 6–12 months postoperatively (77 % within the first 3 years) that does not resolve. In these cases, the diagnosis of lymphedema can be made when other causes of swelling (e.g., recurrent disease, deep venous thrombosis, systemic fluid overload,) are ruled out. This diagnosis is often confirmed with physiologic studies such as lymphoscintigraphy or indocyanine green near infrared angiography demonstrating diminished lymphatic transport capacity, dermal back flow, and dysfunctional lymphatic vessels. Lymphedema may even develop after very prolonged periods of time in at-risk patients with the longest reported case occurring 30 years after the initial surgery.

In these cases, often an inciting event such as an infection or additional injury precedes the development of progressive limb swelling and lymphedema.

Recent studies have suggested that progression of lymphedema may be retarded during its early stages through the use of conservative measures such as compression garments or manual lymphatic massage therapy. Although there is some debate regarding the efficacy or timing of these treatments in preventing lymphedema development, the fact that measures aiming to decrease interstitial fluid stasis can alter disease progression/development is interesting and suggests that lymph stasis (rather than lymphatic injury alone) is necessary for development of lymphedema. However, once lymphedema develops it is usually progressive and chronic in nature although there is wide variability in the rate at which pathologic changes occur. Thus, in some cases lymphedema has a smoldering course with relatively mild changes in limb volume or tissue changes over very long periods of time (often years), while in other cases there is rapid progression of disease with disabling swelling and physiologic changes.

Risk Factors for Lymphedema

A large number of epidemiologic studies have analyzed genetic and comorbid factors that increase the risk of developing lymphedema. A clear understanding of these risk factors is important in preoperative surgical consultation and can be used as a means of tailoring surgical procedures to individual patients in an effort to decrease the risk of lymphedema development.

Genetics

The discovery of lymphatic markers and mechanisms that regulate lymphangiogenesis has led to an attempt by numerous researchers to test the hypothesis that mutations in the coding or noncoding regions of these genes increase the risk of developing primary or secondary lymphedema.

The majority of these studies have been performed in patients with primary lymphedema; however, recent studies have also targeted genetic risk factors for secondary lymphedema. The study of genetic risk factors for development of secondary lymphedema is interesting and based at least partially on the observation that some patients with breast cancer-related lymphedema exhibit abnormalities in lymphatic transport even in their unaffected normal extremity.

An interesting report by Mendola and colleagues from the lymphedema research group analyzed genetic mutations in 78 patients with familial (i.e., inherited) and 149 patients with sporadic primary lymphedemas. The investigators found that mutations in seven genes encoding molecules regulating VEGFR3 and its downstream pathways were responsible for 36 % of inheritable forms of primary lymphedema. In contrast, only 8 % of patients with sporadic primary lymphedema exhibited these mutations [6]. These findings are important and demonstrate that complex pathways regulate development of hereditary lymphedema. More importantly, these studies highlight the need for additional study since the majority of hereditary and sporadic primary lymphedema patients did not exhibit known genetic mutations.

Recent studies provide support for the theory that genetic mutations may also increase the risk of secondary lymphedema after surgery. For example, Feingold et al. sequenced the coding and flanking noncoding regions of the hepatocyte growth factor (HGF) and its high affinity receptor MET in 59 women with breast cancer-related upper extremity lymphedema, and 159 unrelated matched controls. This analysis was based on previous studies demonstrating that this signaling pathway is an important regulator of lymphangiogenesis in a number of physiologic settings [7]. Interestingly, the authors identified an increased rate of mutations in HGF/MET pathways in patients with lymphedema suggesting that impairments in lymphatic regeneration after injury due to dysfunctional HGF/MET signaling contributes to an increased risk of developing lymphedema. In a follow-up case–control study (80 patients with breast cancer-related lymphedema compared with 108 breast cancer controls), Feingold and colleagues found mutations in CJC2 (encoding connexin 47), a gap junction protein that is thought to regulate dermal lymphatic transfer, in four patients with lymphedema but not in any of the controls. Similar mutations have been observed in cohorts of patients with primary lymphedema [8]. Interestingly, in contrast to their previous report the authors identified only one patient with a MET mutation, suggesting that larger samples of patients are needed for these studies.

Newman and colleagues used a nested case–control approach to study genetic changes in 22 patients who developed breast cancer-related lymphedema within 18 months of surgery (case) as compared to 98 patients who did not develop lymphedema. The authors reported that single nucleotide polymorphisms (SNPs) within VEGFR2, VEGFR3, and RORC were associated with development of lymphedema [9]. SNPs are variations in DNA sequence that occur normally in the general population. These variations can occur in both coding and noncoding regions of the DNA and although gene function may be normal under physiologic conditions, some SNPs may lead to gene function changes that increase the risk of pathology. Future studies in this arena should focus on identifying the functional gene changes that occur in patients with SNPs that increase the risk of lymphedema after breast surgery.

Obesity

The increased risk of developing lymphedema in obese patients is well described in previous epidemiologic studies. In a seminal study in 1957, Treves followed over 1,000 patients after treatment for breast cancer and found that obese patients were at significantly increased risk of developing lymphedema [10]. This observation has been confirmed in numerous subsequent studies. For example, Werner et al. reviewed 282 patients with upper extremity lymphedema after treatment for breast cancer and showed that patients with a higher body mass index (BMI) also had a higher incidence of lymphedema. Another prospective study examined the risk of developing lymphedema in the upper extremity in 137 patients with breast cancer and showed that patients with a BMI >30 had a threefold greater risk than patients with a BMI <25 [11]. The best supporting evidence is a randomized controlled trial in which patients with upper arm lymphedema underwent 12 weeks of dieting and nutritional counseling as compared with patients who did not. The results showed that patients who lost weight had significant reductions in arm volumes and upper arm lymphedema when compared to the control patients who did not diet [12]. These results suggest that lymphatic impairment in obesity is reversible. More importantly, these studies show that obesity and lymphedema are intricately linked. This is not surprising since a defining feature of chronic lymphedema is progressive adipose tissue deposition. This observation has led some authors to conclude that lymphedema may be a form of "regional" obesity in which tissues are more prone for depositing fat in the setting of caloric excess. This hypothesis is supported by the fact that lymphatic fluid has been shown to increase adipocyte proliferation and differentiation and by other studies demonstrating that even mild lymphatic injury activates expression of genes necessary for adipocyte activation.

Obesity, independent of surgery, has been shown to decrease lymphatic function. For example, previous studies have shown that obese patients have decreased clearance of macromolecules from the skin and subcutaneous tissues as compared with lean individuals [13, 14]. In addition, Greene and colleagues have shown that morbidly obese patients (BMI >59) develop primary lower extremity lymphedema (i.e., without antecedent trauma or injury) characterized by decreased lymphatic transport and dermal back flow on lymphoscintigraphy [13]. Interestingly, the upper extremity seems to be less susceptible to obesity-induced lymphedema as the obese patients in Greene's series who developed upper extremity lymphedema tended to be significantly more obese (BMI >65) than those who had just lower extremity lymphedema.

In order to study the molecular mechanisms that regulate obesity induced lymphatic function, Weitman et al. and Blum and colleagues have used a mouse model of diet induced obesity and have found that increasing obesity results in impaired transport of interstitial fluid, decreased migration of immune cells, decreased pumping capacity of collecting lymphatics, and abnormal lymph node architecture [15, 16]. Further investigation with this model showed that obese mice have heightened inflammatory responses following lymphatic injury and that these promoted increased adipose deposition and fibrosis.

Radiation

Radiation therapy is frequently used as an adjunct to the treatment of a variety of cancers. Although these treatments are highly effective in some settings, they also are known to cause significant tissue damage and fibrosis. Not surprisingly, numerous studies have shown that radiation therapy delivered to lymph node basins is a significant contributor to the development of lymphedema particularly when radiation follows surgical injury. Thus, radiation in isolation is rarely associated with development of lymphedema; however, the combination of surgery and radiation significantly increases risks. For example, Hinrich et al. analyzed 105 patients who received postmastectomy radiotherapy and found that total dose, posterior axillary boost, and overlapping techniques were significantly associated with development of lymphedema [17]. Other studies have suggested that radiation increases the risk of lymphedema by as much as tenfold.

Although the precise mechanisms by which radiation increases the risk of lymphedema remain unknown, preclinical studies suggest that radiation-induced fibrosis is a major contributor. For example, using a mouse tail model of radiation injury, Avraham and colleagues demonstrated that lymphatic endothelial cells are sensitive to radiation and that this injury can induce apoptosis and subclinical lymphatic dysfunction [18]. These findings were corroborated by a clinical study demonstrating that radiation treatment decreases the density of small vessel lymphatics [19]. Interestingly, however, in the mouse studies protection of lymphatic endothelial cells from apoptotic death did not decrease lymphatic dysfunction even though the lymphatic architecture was largely preserved. In contrast, inhibition of radiation induced fibrosis markedly improved lymphatic function suggesting that changes in the extracellular matrix independently regulate lymphatic function. Therefore, clinical strategies that decrease fibrosis after radiation treatment may be a novel means of decreasing the risk of lymphedema in cancer survivors.

Infection

Patients who undergo lymph node dissection are at increased risk for infections. Unfortunately, infections often precede the development of lymphedema and may cause progressive damage to the lymphatic system. This concept is supported by numerous studies examining the association between cellulitis and development of lymphedema after treatment for gynecological or breast malignancies. For example, Gould et al. assessed complications associated with inguinal lymphadenectomy in vulvar cancer and found that patients who developed early cellulitis were at a significantly increased risk for the development of subsequent lymphedema [20]. Another cross sectional study evaluating 807 patients with lymphedema secondary to breast cancer treatment found that a past history of cellulitis was a significant factor associated with increased upper extremity volume [21]. This finding led the authors to conclude that avoidance of cellulitis through meticulous skin care is an effective means of preventing development or progression of lymphedema.

Lymphedema Staging

Clinical Staging

Whether it is primary or secondary lymphedema, the timeline by which symptoms present themselves is highly variable and difficult to predict. Likewise, staging systems for lymphedema are numerous and inconsistent. Many traditional classifications rely on clinical findings and physical exam to diagnose lymphedema. The most commonly used staging system is The International Society of Lymphology staging system that divides lymphedema into four stages. Briefly, a patient is classified as having **Stage 0**, or *latent*, lymphedema when their lymphatic vasculature has been damaged but they have no clinically measurable swelling or edema. These patients may present with subjective symptoms of heaviness, discomfort, or early fatigue in the affected extremity with activity. **Stage I** lymphedema, or *spontaneously reversible lymphedema*, occurs when measureable swelling starts to occur and is manifested by pitting edema. Patients with stage I lymphedema primarily have accumulation of interstitial fluid in the limb, and as a result, may have an excellent response to conservative treatments such as compression or complete decongestive therapy. **Stage II** lymphedema, or *spontaneously irreversible lymphedema*, is described as non-pitting swelling of the limb. At this point, adipose deposition and fibrosis prevent conservative therapies from being highly effective (hence the lack of pitting) and, as a result, patients have relatively modest improvements secondary to compression. The most advanced stage of lymphedema, **Stage III** lymphedema, is also known as lymphostatic elephantiasis, which is characterized by significant non-pitting swelling, fibroadipose deposition, hyperkeratosis, and acanthosis. These patients, in general, do not respond to conservative measures and typically have progression of disease.

Campisi et al. have proposed another alternative, albeit less commonly used staging system for lymphedema; stage I is defined as initial or irregular edema, stage II is persistent lymphedema, stage III is persistent lymphedema with lymphangitis, stage IV is fibrolymphedema ("column" limb), and stage V is elephantiasis [22].

Other studies have classified lymphedema based on circumference measurements or changes in excess volume relative to the contralateral normal limb (or preoperative) measures [23]. A change in circumference of less than 2 cm is considered to be mild lymphedema, a change in 2–4 cm is considered to be moderate lymphedema, and a change in circumference of over 4 cm is considered to be severe lymphedema. One problem with this method is that it does not take into account differences in relative size of the upper and lower limb (for example, a 2 cm change in an arm is much more significant than a 2 cm change in a leg) or the effect of BMI (a given change in circumference is more severe in a thin person than an obese person). Other studies measure differences in limb volume either by water displacement or the use of the truncated cone formula and multiple measurements. In these studies an excess volume of 200 cm^3 is typically used to make the diagnosis of lymphedema. These measurements may be more accurate than circumference measurements; however, a complete classification systems using changes in volume has not been proposed.

Functional/Physiological Staging

While most staging methods have used physical measurements to categorize and diagnose lymphedema, more recently developed methods have advocated the use physiological studies for diagnosis and staging. These systems quantify and analyze lymphatic function using imaging techniques with compounds that are selectively taken up by the lymphatic system. For example, in a study of 72 consecutive patients with lower limb lymphedema secondary to treatment for gynecological malignancies, a prolific group from Japan published an interesting study subclassifying patients into 12 subtypes based on patterns of indocyanine green lymphangiography (ICG) flow in the superficial and collecting system. However, while this work is interesting and worthy of further pursuit, the classification system is complicated and requires refinement [24]. More importantly, future studies should address the implications of these findings on surgical or medical treatment options

Finally, recent efforts have proposed the use of histological methods to classify lymphedema. For example, in an interesting study by Mihara et al. published in 2012, the authors reviewed macroscopic and microscopic findings in 114

lymphatic collector histological specimens from 37 patients who had lower limb lymphedema after treatment for gynecological malignancies [25]. Based on their detailed histological analysis demonstrating progressive fibrosis and obliteration of the lymphatic vessels, the authors defined lymphedematous changes as normal, ectasis, contraction, and sclerosis types (NECST) and attempted to correlate clinical/pathological degrees of lymphedema staging with these outcomes. Although these histological classification schemes are invasive and therefore less likely to be useful clinically, the implications of these findings on the pathology of lymphedema are extremely important and worthy of additional future study (see below).

Pathologic Changes in Lymphedema

Numerous studies have analyzed histologic changes in lymphedema and have shown that characteristic features of this disease include fibrosis, hyperkeratosis, chronic inflammation, and adipose deposition. Although the cellular and molecular mechanisms that regulate these responses remain unknown, this area has been a focus of intense study in recent years and important advancements have been made both clinically and in animal models of lymphedema. For purposes of discussion, it is helpful to think of lymphedema as a progression from a disease of interstitial fluid accumulation to a disease of fibroadipose tissue deposition. This model of lymphedema pathophysiology is reflected in the current clinical staging systems of lymphedema. For example, **stage 0** (latent lymphedema) reflects symptomatic changes related to lymphatic injury and impaired drainage; **stage I** (spontaneously reversible) reflects *initial accumulation of interstitial fluid*; **stage II** (spontaneously irreversible) patients have *progressed from fluid accumulation to fibroadipose deposition*; **Stage III** (elephantiasis) is the end stage of disease with *massive fibroadipose deposition*. Clearly this is somewhat simplistic and there are likely to be important clinical parameters that regulate the progression of disease, however, this model serves as a simple starting point for studies aiming to elucidate the pathological mechanisms of lymphedema.

Interstitial Fluid Accumulation

A major function of the lymphatic system is to transport protein rich interstitial fluid. Conservative estimates suggest that the venous system is responsible for absorbing more than 90 % of extracellular fluid produced as a consequence of cellular metabolism and capillary perfusion. The remaining 10 % is transported by the lymphatic system. Ordinarily, the lymphatic system has a large reserve for fluid transport and mild disturbances in function (or baseline variability between individuals) do not result in noticeable fluid accumulation. However, when the system is damaged or overloaded, then interstitial fluid accumulation can occur and manifest as pitting edema. This fluid can have major effects on the cellular behavior of the affected limb, resulting in activation of inflammatory cascades and adipose cell differentiation. Chronic fluid accumulation, as can occur in patients with early stage lymphedema, leads to progressive inflammation. These changes are important because recent studies have shown that inflammatory reactions play a major role in the pathology of lymphedema. In addition, recent studies have shown that control of interstitial fluid accumulation by complete decongestive therapy significantly decreases inflammatory reactions lending support to the concept that early intervention with compression and prevention of fluid accumulation can prevent progressive lymphatic injury and development of overt lymphedema.

Chronic Inflammation and Fibrosis

Chronic inflammation and fibrosis are histological hallmarks of lymphedema. For example, Koshima et al. biopsied lymphatics in patients with lymphedema and found lymphatic vessels became progressively fibrosed and occluded due to proliferation of surrounding smooth muscle cells [26]. Similarly, Suami et al. studied lymphatic vessels in a cadaver that had undergone unilateral axillary lymph node dissection and found that this treatment was associated with chronic inflammation and collagen deposition around collecting lymphatic vessels [27]. More recent studies have shown that although a variety of inflammatory cells are present in lymphedematous tissues, the vast majority of these cells (>70 %) express the cell surface receptor CD4. CD4+ cells constitute a large number of different mature cell types but can be broadly categorized as T-helper cells, natural killer cells, and T-regulatory cells. T helper, in turn can be subclassified into T helper type 1 (TH1), T helper type 2 (Th2), among others. Th1 reactions occur in response to acute inflammation and help defend against bacterial pathogens by producing cytokines such as interferon gamma. In contrast, Th2 responses play an important role in responses to parasites and have been shown to promote tissue fibrosis in other organ systems by producing profibrotic cytokines such as interleukin 4 (IL4), interleukin 13 (IL13), and transforming growth factor beta-1 (TGF-B1).

Interestingly, comparison of normal and lymphedematous tissues obtained from patients with lymphedema has shown that the degree of CD4+ cell infiltration correlates positively with the severity or stage of lymphedema. In addition, these tissues demonstrate a mixed Th1/Th2 inflammatory response. This finding is important since fibrosis is a major pathological component of lymphedema and suggests that CD4+ cell responses contribute to this end result. In fact, preclinical studies in mice have shown that depletion of CD4+ cells in general, or inhibition of IL4, IL13, or TGF-B1 in particular potently decreases fibrosis after lymphatic injury and this response is associated with improved lymphatic function. More importantly, these preclinical studies have shown that these approaches can successfully treat established lymphedema and may therefore represent a novel means of treating lymphedema. Thus, these approaches may be used to prevent the development of lymphedema in high-risk patients, treat patients with early stage lymphedema, or be used in conjunction with surgical management to improve outcomes. This is an exciting development and a paradigm shift in the treatment of lymphedema away from the use of conservative measures or experimental interventions that aim to increase lymphatic repair/regeneration.

Adipose Deposition

The cellular and molecular mechanisms that regulate adipose deposition in lymphedema remain unknown. However, recent studies have begun to decipher these pathways and shed light into this area. For example, using mouse models of lymphedema and axillary lymph node dissection, Zampell et al. have shown that lymphatic injury and interstitial fluid stasis rapidly and significantly activates differentiation of local adipocytes [28]. Similarly, Harvey et al. have shown that lymphatic fluid in culture is a potent activator of adipocyte differentiation and lipid storage [29]. In addition, these authors found that mice bearing a heterozygous inactivating mutation of Prox-1, a transcription factor that is required for differentiation of lymphatic, were prone to development of adult onset obesity suggesting that impaired lymphatic function and chronic leakage of lymphatic fluid may regulate differentiation of preadipocytes and be a predisposing factor to the development of obesity.

Adipose deposition after lymphatic injury requires activation and accumulation of CD4+ cells since depletion of these cells or inhibition of Th2 differentiation potently decreases adipose deposition after lymphatic injury. In addition, recent studies have suggested that inflammatory responses can indirectly contribute to adipose deposition by regulating adipocyte breakdown/ turnover. For example, Cuzzone et al. found that expression of interleukin 6 (IL6) is significantly increased in the tissues and serum of patients with lymphedema. IL6 is known to be produced by adipose tissues and is an important regulator of adipose cell metabolism. Interestingly, these authors found that inhibition of IL6 paradoxically increased adipose deposition in lymphedema suggesting that the expression of this cytokine may play a homeostatic role in lymphedema aiming to decrease adipose deposition. This hypothesis is supported by previous studies demonstrating that IL6 may play a lipolytic role depending on its source and pattern of expression [30].

Summary

The lymphatic system plays an essential role in fluid homeostasis in the body. Disruption of the lymphatic system can occur as a result of a number of causes including inherited or sporadic genetic mutations, surgical injury, or chronic infection. These pathologic states result in progressive interstitial fluid accumulation, chronic inflammation, fibrosis, and adipose deposition. The progression from a disease of fluid accumulation to fibroadipose deposition limits the potential for conservative treatments to improve lymphedema clinically since fibroadipose tissues are not compressible.

Although the cellular and molecular mechanisms that regulate pathological changes in lymphedema remain unknown, recent studies suggest that infiltration of lymphedematous tissues by CD4+ cells and differentiation along the Th2 lineage plays a key role in this process. These cells are thought to regulate fibrosis by producing profibrotic cytokines and either directly or indirectly regulate adipose deposition. Inhibition of these responses may therefore represent a novel means of preventing or treating lymphedema. It is hoped that advances in the understanding of the pathophysiology of lymphedema will help identify future diagnostic tests and therapies in a previously neglected field.

References

1. Segal J, Turner AF. Lymphedema tarda. JAMA. 1976;235(18):1996–7.
2. Connell FC, Gordon K, Brice G, Keeley V, Jeffery S, Mortimer PS, et al. The classification and diagnostic algorithm for primary lymphatic dysplasia: an update from 2010 to include molecular findings. Clin Genet. 2013;84(4):303–14.

3. Babu S, Nutman TB. Immunopathogenesis of lymphatic filarial disease. Semin Immunopathol. 2012; 34(6):847–61.

4. Cormier JN, Askew RL, Mungovan KS, Xing Y, Ross MI, Armer JM. Lymphedema beyond breast cancer: a systematic review and meta-analysis of cancer-related secondary lymphedema. Cancer. 2010;116(22): 5138–49.

5. McLaughlin SA, Wright MJ, Morris KT, Sampson MR, Brockway JP, Hurley KE, et al. Prevalence of lymphedema in women with breast cancer 5 years after sentinel lymph node biopsy or axillary dissection: patient perceptions and precautionary behaviors. J Clin Oncol. 2008;26(32):5220–6.

6. Mendola A, Schlogel MJ, Ghalamkarpour A, Irrthum A, Nguyen HL, Fastre E, et al. Mutations in the VEGFR3 signaling pathway explain 36% of familial lymphedema. Mol Syndromol. 2013;4(6):257–66.

7. Finegold DN, Schacht V, Kimak MA, Lawrence EC, Foeldi E, Karlsson JM, et al. HGF and MET mutations in primary and secondary lymphedema. Lymphat Res Biol. 2008;6(2):65–8.

8. Ferrell RE, Baty CJ, Kimak MA, Karlsson JM, Lawrence EC, Franke-Snyder M, et al. GJC2 missense mutations cause human lymphedema. Am J Hum Genet. 2010;86(6):943–8.

9. Newman B, Lose F, Kedda MA, Francois M, Ferguson K, Janda M, et al. Possible genetic predisposition to lymphedema after breast cancer. Lymphat Res Biol. 2012;10(1):2–13.

10. Treves N. An evaluation of the etiological factors of lymphedema following radical mastectomy; an analysis of 1,007 cases. Cancer. 1957;10(3):444–59.

11. Helyer LK, Varnic M, Le LW, Leong W, McCready D. Obesity is a risk factor for developing postoperative lymphedema in breast cancer patients. Breast J. 2010;16(1):48–54.

12. Shaw C, Mortimer P, Judd PA. A randomized controlled trial of weight reduction as a treatment for breast cancer-related lymphedema. Cancer. 2007;110(8):1868–74.

13. Greene AK, Grant FD, Slavin SA. Lower-extremity lymphedema and elevated body-mass index. N Engl J Med. 2012;366(22):2136–7.

14. Arngrim N, Simonsen L, Holst JJ, Bulow J. Reduced adipose tissue lymphatic drainage of macromolecules in obese subjects: a possible link between obesity and local tissue inflammation? Int J Obes (Lond). 2013;37(5):748–50.

15. Weitman ES, Aschen SZ, Farias-Eisner G, Albano N, Cuzzone DA, Ghanta S, et al. Obesity impairs lymphatic fluid transport and dendritic cell migration to lymph nodes. PLoS One. 2013;8(8):e70703.

16. Blum KS, Karaman S, Proulx ST, Ochsenbein AM, Luciani P, Leroux JC, et al. Chronic high-fat diet impairs collecting lymphatic vessel function in mice. PLoS One. 2014;9(4):e94713.

17. Hinrichs CS, Watroba NL, Rezaishiraz H, Giese W, Hurd T, Fassl KA, et al. Lymphedema secondary to postmastectomy radiation: incidence and risk factors. Ann Surg Oncol. 2004;11(6):573–80.

18. Avraham T, Yan A, Zampell JC, Daluvoy SV, Haimovitz-Friedman A, Cordeiro AP, et al. Radiation therapy causes loss of dermal lymphatic vessels and interferes with lymphatic function by TGF-beta1-mediated tissue fibrosis. Am J Physiol Cell Physiol. 2010;299(3):C589–605.

19. Jackowski S, Janusch M, Fiedler E, Marsch WC, Ulbrich EJ, Gaisbauer G, et al. Radiogenic lymphangiogenesis in the skin. Am J Pathol. 2007;171(1):338–48.

20. Gould N, Kamelle S, Tillmanns T, Scribner D, Gold M, Walker J, et al. Predictors of complications after inguinal lymphadenectomy. Gynecol Oncol. 2001; 82(2):329–32.

21. Vignes S, Arrault M, Dupuy A. Factors associated with increased breast cancer-related lymphedema volume. Acta Oncol. 2007;46(8):1138–42.

22. Campisi C, Campisi C, Accogli S, Campisi C, Boccardo F. Lymphedema staging and surgical indications in geriatric age. BMC Geriatr. 2010;10 Suppl 1:2.

23. Tiwari P, Coriddi M, Salani R, Povoski SP. Breast and gynecologic cancer-related extremity lymphedema: a review of diagnostic modalities and management options. World J Surg Oncol. 2013;11:237.

24. Mihara M, Hayashi Y, Hara H, Iida T, Narushima M, Yamamoto T, et al. High-accuracy diagnosis and regional classification of lymphedema using indocyanine green fluorescent lymphography after gynecologic cancer treatment. Ann Plast Surg. 2014;72(2):204–8.

25. Mihara M, Hara H, Hayashi Y, Narushima M, Yamamoto T, Todokoro T, et al. Pathological steps of cancer-related lymphedema: histological changes in the collecting lymphatic vessels after lymphadenectomy. PLoS One. 2012;7(7):e41126.

26. Koshima I, Kawada S, Moriguchi T, Kajiwara Y. Ultrastructural observations of lymphatic vessels in lymphedema in human extremities. Plast Reconstr Surg. 1996;97(2):397–405. discussion 6–7.

27. Suami H, Pan WR, Taylor GI. Changes in the lymph structure of the upper limb after axillary dissection: radiographic and anatomical study in a human cadaver. Plast Reconstr Surg. 2007;120(4):982–91.

28. Zampell JC, Aschen S, Weitman ES, Yan A, Elhadad S, De Brot M, et al. Regulation of adipogenesis by lymphatic fluid stasis: Part I. Adipogenesis, fibrosis, and inflammation. Plast Reconstr Surg. 2012;29(4):825–34.

29. Harvey NL, Srinivasan RS, Dillard ME, Johnson NC, Witte MH, Boyd K, et al. Lymphatic vascular defects promoted by Prox1 haploinsufficiency cause adult-onset obesity. Nat Genet. 2005;37(10):1072–81.

30. Cuzzone DA, Weitman ES, Albano NJ, Ghanta S, Savetsky IL, Gardenier JC, et al. IL-6 regulates adipose deposition and homeostasis in lymphedema. Am J Physiol Heart Circ Physiol. 2014;306(10):H1426–34.

Genetic Causes of Lymphedema

Matthieu J. Schlögel, Pascal Brouillard,
Laurence M. Boon, and Miikka Vikkula

Key Points
- Careful patient examination for all signs and symptoms is important for precise clinical diagnosis.
- Primary lymphedema has a high underlying genetic heterogeneity. Currently, 20 genes are implicated.
- Neonatal edema, including non-immune hydrops fetalis, can also be caused by mutations in some of these genes.
- Genetic predisposing factors are unknown for a large fraction of patients.
- There is large variability in clinical expressivity and often incomplete penetrance for all signs and symptoms.

- Panel-based targeted next-generation sequencing is the most efficient approach for diagnostic screens.
- Secondary lymphedema may be influenced by genetic predisposition.

Introduction

Lymphedema is known since the middle of the nineteenth century, yet the first genes associated with this condition have been discovered only in the twenty-first century. Since then, more than 20 genes have been linked to the development of primary lymphedema. Originally discovered using linkage analysis in large families or animal models, the more recent approach using Next-Generation Sequencing (NGS) has allowed to discover genes using smaller families and even sporadic cases. In parallel, detailed in vitro and in vivo studies on molecular and cellular mechanisms involved in lymphangiogenesis have unraveled numerous novel functional candidate genes.

Primary lymphedema can be present as an inherited or a sporadic trait. It can be dominant, recessive (with consanguinity or not), or linked to the X-chromosome. There is important heterogeneity in the clinical appearance of lymphedema. Primary lymphedema can be the unique sign, affect different parts of the body (limb(s), arms, hands, head and neck, abdomen, etc.), be unilateral or bilateral, and appear at different ages at onset. It can also be part of a complex syndrome,

M.J. Schlögel, M.Sc. • P. Brouillard, Ph.D.
Laboratory of Human Molecular Genetics,
de Duve Institute, Université catholique
de Louvain, Brussels, Belgium

L.M. Boon, M.D., Ph.D.
Cliniques universitaires Saint-Luc, Center
for Vascular Anomalies, Universite catholique
de Louvain, Brussels, Belgium

M. Vikkula, M.D., Ph.D. (✉)
Laboratory of Human Molecular Genetics,
de Duve Institute, Université catholique
de Louvain, Brussels, Belgium

Walloon Excellence in Lifesciences
and Biotechnology (WELBIO), Brussels, Belgium
e-mail: miikka.vikkula@uclouvain.be

A.K. Greene et al. (eds.), *Lymphedema: Presentation, Diagnosis, and Treatment*,
DOI 10.1007/978-3-319-14493-1_3, © Springer International Publishing Switzerland 2015

some of which are very rare, with only few cases reported.

Our current knowledge on the environmental and genetic variability as the cause of primary lymphedema is limited. Most of the Mendelian mutations have been identified in a limited number of patients or even only few families used in the original linkage study, several of the genes have been identified very recently limiting the time they have been used in clinical setting for diagnostic screening, the number of patients screened in reports is often very limited, and most screens have been done on gene-by-gene basis. Moreover, some of the clinical signs may be missed, and thus, the clinical classification is not necessarily correct. This renders it difficult to have a representative and a comprehensive overview of the current state of the art.

In this chapter, we make an extensive review of the medical literature. Clinical data was collected for all patients with a proven mutation, taking into account each mentioned sign and symptom. In the presentation, we divide the genes (and associated lymphedemas) into two groups. The first category includes the genes that cause lymphedema as the major sign, which is also the reason for medical consultation (Table 3.1). The second group contains the genes that are related to a usually well-known syndrome and for which lymphedema is minor sign (Table 3.2). Only a quarter of all cases are explained by mutations within the 20 genes. It appears that the historical classification based on the age of onset, i.e., congenital (at birth or early in life), praecox (teenage years), and tarda (late in life) is becoming irrelevant, as this does not correlate with the genetic background. Instead, the clinical presentation of the signs and symptoms can be helpful to associate the primary lymphedema to the most likely causative gene.

Lymphedema as a Major Sign

Phenotype of Patients

Lymphedema is the major sign for 14 of the genes currently known to cause primary lymph-

edema when mutated. The penetrance of lymphedema is though often incomplete, i.e., even though an individual carries a familial mutation, (s)he does not necessarily have lymphedema. This is also true for the other associated signs and symptoms listed in Table 3.1.

The cardiovascular system is often affected; varicose veins are not infrequent. Hydrocele can be present in at least four of the entities (Table 3.1). In the nervous system, symptoms range from hearing loss to learning difficulties and macrocephaly. Cutaneous and subcutaneous symptoms are frequent, including infection, papillomas, and cellulitis, many of which are considered secondary. Yet there are subtype-specific differences in prevalence (Table 3.1). In the musculoskeletal system, syndactyly or camptodactyly is observed. Mutations in GATA2 affect the respiratory system, generating pulmonary alveolar proteinosis. Mutations in GATA2, as well as IKBKG, also predispose to severe infections. Involvement of the digestive system is relatively rare (GJC2 and IKBKG), and renal abnormalities have been reported only in some cases (VEGFR3, FOXC2, and SOX18). Patients with a GATA2 mutation have a susceptibility to hematologic malignancies.

Genetic Differential Diagnosis: Which Gene to Screen?

The unraveled high genetic heterogeneity in primary lymphedema has resulted in a high number of clinical subcategories. Currently 21 genetically defined subgroups, as well as the subgroup of undefined ones, exist. Moreover, the latter mostly likely involves several genes. Some of the genetically defined 21 subgroups have typical signs, the presence of which can help in clinical diagnosis. In addition, familial history (Table 3.3) is an important factor in determining candidate genes for diagnostic screens.

The "unique" signs, i.e., those specific to one or two genes, are variable. Isolated lower limb lymphedema present at birth (the classic presentation of Milroy disease) suggests a FLT4/ VEGFR3 (FMS-like tyrosine kinase 4/vascular

Table 3.1 Signs and symptoms by mutated gene; lymphedema a cardinal sign

System	Sign	FLT4	VEGFC	FOXC2	PTPN14	GJC2	GJA1	KIF11	CCBE	FAT4	GATA2	SOX18	IKBKG	HGF	ITGA9
		(139)	(10)	(120)	(7)	(12)	(5)	(75)	(13)	(9)	(110)	(6)	(70)	(4)	(12)
Cardiovascular	Lymphedema	81 %	8/8	71 %	5/7	100 %	1/5	51 %	100 %	9/9	15 %	5/6	13 %	3/4	0/4
	Hydrops (fetalis)	¶	–	1/6	–	–	–	–	23 %	–	–	1/6	–	–	42 %
	Lymphangiectasia	–	–	–	–	–	–	–	100 %	7/9	–	–	–	1/4	
	Lymphatic anomaly	36 %	–	¶	–	–	–	–	–	–	–	¶	–	–	100 %
	Varicose veins	7 %	–	49 %	–	42 %	–	–	–	–	–	–	–	–	–
	Vascular anomaly	28 %	4/7	–	–	25 %	1/5	–	23 %	–	25 %	¶	–	–	–
	Hemangioma	¶	–	–	–	–	–	–	–	–	–	–	–	–	–
	Hydrocoele	35 %	2/4	1 %	–	–	–	–	–	–	–	3/3	–	–	–
	Telangiectasia	–	–	–	–	–	–	–	–	–	–	3/5	1/2	–	–
	Heart defect	–	–	7 %	1/7	–	–	9 %	15 %	–	–	–	–	–	–
Nervous	Intellectual disability	5 %	–	3 %	–	–	–	69 %	69 %	7/9	–	¶	–	–	–
	Neurologic defect	–	–	¶	–	–	–	19 %	8 %	1/8	–	–	–	–	–
	Microcephaly	–	–	–	–	–	–	91 %	46 %	1/9	–	–	–	–	–
	Macrocephaly	–	–	–	–	–	–	–	–	–	–	–	–	–	–
	Ptosis	–	–	59 %	–	17 %	–	–	–	–	7 %	–	–	–	–
	Ophthalmologic problem	13 %	–	74 %	–	–	¶	69 %	–	–	–	¶	–	–	–
	Hearing loss	–	–	–	–	–	–	–	–	2/9	7 %	–	–	–	–
Integumentary	Papilloma (papule)	10 %	20 %	–	–	–	–	–	–	–	–	1/5	–	–	–
	Skin infection	–	–	¶	–	33 %	–	–	–	–	–	–	–	–	–
	Cellulitis	19 %	30 %	¶	–	50 %	–	–	–	–	–	–	–	–	–
	Eczema	–	–	–	–	8 %	–	–	–	–	–	1/5	1/2	–	–
	Skin problem	10 %	2/7	–	–	–	–	–	–	–	¶	3/5	78 %	–	–
	Hair problem	–	–	–	–	–	–	–	–	–	–	5/5	–	–	–
	Nail or toe anomaly	28 %	3/3	12 %	–	–	–	–	–	–	–	–	–	–	–
	Distichiasis	–	–	86 %	–	–	–	–	–	–	–	–	–	–	–
	Dental anomaly	–	–	–	–	–	¶	–	–	–	–	–	–	–	–

(continued)

Table 3.1 (continued)

System	Sign	FLT4 (139)	VEGFC (10)	FOXC2 (120)	PTPN14 (7)	GJC2 (12)	GJA1 (5)	KIF11 (75)	CCBE (13)	FAT4 (9)	GATA2 (110)	SOX18 (6)	IKBKG (70)	HGF (4)	ITGA9 (12)
Musculoskeletal	Reduced growth	–	–	–	–	–	–	–	69 %	5/9	–	–	–	–	–
	Cleft lip and Palate	–	–	21 %	¶	–	–	–	–	–	7 %	–	–	–	–
	Dysmorphic face	4/5	–	¶	–	–	¶	40 %	100 %	9/9	¶	1/5	–	–	–
	Thoracic/vertebral	–	–	7 %	¶	–	–	–	–	–	–	¶	–	–	–
	Joint	¶	–	–	–	–	–	–	–	–	–	–	–	–	–
	Syndactyly	–	–	–	–	–	4/5	27 %	31 %	2/8	–	–	–	–	–
	Choanal atresia	–	–	–	7/7	–	–	–	–	–	–	–	–	–	–
	Bone	–	–	–	–	–	–	–	38 %	6/9	–	–	10 %	–	–
Respiratory	Pulmonary	–	–	–	–	–	–	–	–	–	24 %	–		–	–
Immunitary	Infection	–	–	–	–	–	–	–	–	–	56 %	–	98 %	–	–
	Warts	2 %	–	–	–	–	–	–	–	–	53 %	–		–	–
	Hematological dysfunction	–	–	–	–	–	–	–	–	–	86 %	–	24 %	–	–
Digestive	Gastrointestinal	–	–	–	–	8 %	–	–	–	–	–	–	2/2	–	–
Urogenital	Genitourinary	4 %	–	3 %	–	–	–	–	–	–	–	¶	–	–	–
	Kidney	2 %	–	7 %	–	–	–	–	–	–	–	2/5	–	–	–
	M:F>2:1	–	–	¶	–	–	–	–	–	–	–	–	–	–	–
Malignancy	Tumor	–	–	1 %	–	8 %	–	–	–	–	73 %	–	–	–	–

The frequency of observation is translated in percentage when the number of examined patients was above 10. Number of patient studied is in parentheses. ¶ represents symptoms mentioned occasionally

Table 3.2 Signs and symptoms by mutated gene; lymphedema a non-cardinal sign

System	Signs	TSC1 (>100)	TSC2 (>100)	PTPN11 (31)	SOS1 (56)	KRAS (26)	Monosomy X (>500)	RASA1 (314)
Cardiovascular	Lymphedema	4 %	4 %	16 %	30 %	¶	36 %	¶
	Hydrops (fetalis)	–	–	–	–	–		0.60 %
	Lymphangiectasia	–	–	–	–	–	–	¶
	Lymphatic anomaly	–	–	–	–	–	¶	¶
	Vascular anomaly	71 %	82 %	–	–	–	–	97 %
	Heart defect	–	–	90 %	77 %	¶	53 %	0.60 %
Nervous	Intellectual disability	49 %	83 %	27 %	10 %	92 %	11 %	0.60 %
	Neurological defect	91 %	91 %	23 %	–	–	¶	¶
	Macrocephaly	–	–	–	59 %	79 %	–	–
	Ptosis	–	–	69 %	7/8	–	–	–
	Ophthalmologic problem	10 %	37 %	31 %	3/8	3/5	–	0.60 %
	Hearing loss	–	–	19 %	–	–	–	–
Integumentary	Papilloma (papule)	–	–	–	–	–	–	–
	Skin problem	93 %	99 %	–	82 %	–	–	¶
	Nail or toe anomaly	45 %	34 %	–	–	–	–	–
	Dental anomaly	53 %	50 %	–	–	–	–	–
Musculoskeletal	Reduced growth	–	–	56 %	29 %	83 %	69 %	–
	Fetal macrosomia	–	–	–	31 %	–	–	–
	Dysmorphic face	–	–	63 %	82 %	60 %	–	–
	Thoracic/vertebral	–	–	38 %	44 %	4/5	–	–
	Limb defect	–	–	–	–	–	–	–
Respiratory	Pulmonary	–	–	–	–	–	–	–
Immune	Warts	–	–	–	–	–	–	–
	Hematological dysfunction	–	–	48 %	4/8	–	–	–
Digestive	Gatrointestinal	–	–	38 %	5/8	–	–	–
Urogenital	Genitourinary anomaly	–	–	27 %	3/6	2/3	22 %	–
	Renal defect	7 %	0.5 %	–	–	–	40 %	–
Malignancy	Tumor	42 %	42 %	¶	–	–	–	¶

The frequency of observation is translated in percentage when the number of examined patients was above 10. Number of patients studied is in parentheses. ¶ represents symptoms mentioned occasionally

Table 3.3 Diseases and genes associated with primary lymphedema

Diseases	Genes (proteins)	OMIM diseases	Inheritances	Lymphatic anomalies	Types of mutations	Patients[a]
Primary congenital lymphedema/Nonne–Milroy lymphedema	FLT4 (VEGFR3)	153,100	AD, AR, de novo	Bilateral congenital LE	Inactivating	139
Milroy-like disease	VEGFC	–	AD	Bilateral congenital LE	LOF	10
Lymphedema–distichiasis syndrome (LD)	FOXC2	153,400	AD, de novo	Late-onset LE	LOF	120
Choanal atresia/lymphedema syndrome	PTPN14	613,611	AR	LE	LOF	7
Hereditary lymphedema IC (Meige disease)	GJC2 (CX47)	613,480	–	4-limbs late-onset LE	Missense	12
Oculodentodigital dysplasia/lymphedema syndrome	GJA1 (CX43)	164,200	AD	LE	Missense	5
Microcephaly Chorioretinopathy Lymphedema Mental Retardation syndrome (MCLMR)	KIF11 (EG5)	152,950	AD, de novo	Lower-limbs LE	LOF	75
Hennekam lymphangiectasia–lymphedema syndrome	CCBE1	235,510	AR, de novo	4-limbs LE	LOF	13
Hennekam lymphangiectasia–lymphedema syndrome	FAT4	235,510	AR	4-limbs LE	LOF	9
Primary lymphedema with myelodysplasia (Emberger syndrome)	GATA2	614,038	AD, de novo	LE	LOF	110
Hypotrichosis–lymphedema–telangiectasia (renal defect) syndrome (HLTR)	SOX18	607,823	AD, AR	LE	LOF/D-N	6
Ectodermal dysplasia, anhidrotic, with immunodeficiency, osteopetrosis, and lymphedema (OLEDAID)	IKBKG	300,301	X-linked	LE	Hypomorphic	70
Lymphedema–lymphangiectasia	HGF	–	AD?	LE	LOF?	4
Fetal chylothorax	ITGA9	–	AR, de novo	Hydrops fetalis	Missense	12
Tuberous sclerosis-1 (TSC1)	TSC1	191,100	AD, de novo	LE	LOF	>100
Tuberous sclerosis-2 (TSC2)	TSC2	613,254	AD, de novo	LE	LOF	>100
Noonan syndrome 1 (NS)	PTPN11 (SHP2)	163,950	AD	Nuchal edema	GOF	31
Noonan syndrome 4 (NS)	SOS1	610,733	AD	Nuchal edema	GOF	56
Noonan syndrome 3 (NS)	KRAS	609,942	AD	Nuchal edema	GOF	26
Turner syndrome	Monosomy X	–	X-linked	Edema	–	>500
Capillary malformation—arteriovenous malformation (CM-AVM), including Parkes Weber syndrome	RASA1	608,354	AD	LE	LOF	314

AD autosomal dominant, *AR* autosomal recessive, *LOF* loss-of-function, *D-N* dominant-negative, *GOF* gain-of-function, *LE* lymphedema

Question marks indicate that mutation type and/or inheritance is unclear

[a]Number of patients studied

endothelial growth factor receptor 3) or VEGFC (vascular endothelial growth factor C) mutation. For VEGFR3, the intracellular part is most frequently mutated and should be sequenced first (exons 17–25), whereas any part of the VEGFC coding sequence can be mutated. Functional aplasia of the lymphatic vessels (failure of initial lymphatic absorption) in lymphoscintigraphy underscores the clinical diagnosis of VEGFR3 mutation. Patients with a mutation in VEGFC have reduced uptake with tortuous lymphatic tracts and evidence of rerouting [1–3].

When a patient has distichiasis (double rows of eyelashes, which is not always easy to notice) and lower limb lymphedema, the likely candidate is FOXC2 (forkhead box C2). The lymphedema is often of late onset, even if some patients with congenital lymphedema or hydrops fetalis have been described [4]. The presence of a cleft lip and/or palate also guide towards this gene. Individuals with FOXC2 mutation demonstrate reflux of lymph within the lower limbs as a result of valve failure within the hyperplastic lymphatic vessels [3].

Patients with lymphedema on all four extremities, whether early or late onset, evoke GJC2 (gap junction protein gamma-2) [5]. In lymphoscintigraphy, lymphatic tracts appear normal, but with a significant reduction in absorption by peripheral lymphatics in all four limbs [3]. Mutations in another gap junction protein GJA1 (gap junction protein alpha-1) have been found in patients with lymphedema and, among other signs, microdontia; a syndrome known as oculodentodigital dysplasia. The patient had clear lower limb lymphedema and subclinical upper limb lymphedema by lymphoscintigraphy [6].

Microcephaly can be helpful as a sign for differential diagnosis. Within the genetically defined groups, it is described, as a major sign, in patients with a mutation in KIF11 (kinesin family member 11). This phenotype combines microcephaly with or without chorioretinopathy, lymphedema, and intellectual disability into a syndrome, abbreviated as MCLMR. Microcephaly is present in 91 % (68/75) of the patients and two other major signs, intellec-

tual disability and eye anomalies, both in 69 % of the patients (MJ Schlögel, Submitted). As for VEGFR3, failure of initial lymphatic absorption is observed in lymphoscintigraphy [3].

Facing a patient with microcephaly, 4-limb lymphedema and "unusual face" suggests CCBE1 (collagen and calcium-binding EGF domain-containing protein 1) and FAT4 (homolog of drosophila FAT tumor suppressor 4) as the mutated gene. This entity is known as the lymphedema–intestinal lymphangiectasia–intellectual disability syndrome or the Hennekam syndrome. There is no family history, or history is suggestive of recessive inheritance. The patient can be homozygous or compound heterozygous for the mutation(s) [7]. In one patient with a mutation in CCBE1, abnormal drainage in the upper and lower limbs, and the thoracic duct, was observed in lymphoscintigraphy [3].

GATA2 (gata-binding protein 2) and IKBKG (inhibitor of kappa light polypeptide gene enhancer in B-cells, kinase gamma) are associated with severe immunological problems. Patients with a GATA2 mutation develop warts, and viral and/or bacterial infections [8]. Lymphoscintigraphy reveals hypoplasia of lymphatics within the affected lower limbs [3]. Similar features, as well as ectodermal dysplasia, are seen in patients mutated for IKBKG [9]. It is important to note that GATA2 predisposes to several cancers. This syndrome is known as primary lymphedema with myelodysplasia or Emberger syndrome.

There are some additional rare associations. In one family, lymphedema was associated with choanal atresia, and the affected individuals had a partial deletion (exons 7) in *PTPN14* (protein-tyrosine phosphatase nonreceptor-type 14) [10]. Another rare syndrome combines lymphedema with hypotrichosis and telangiectasias (HLT = Hypotrichosis–lymphedema–telangiectasia). It is caused by dominant or recessive mutations in SOX18 (SRY-Box 18) [11]. A particular stop codon in this gene causes severe glomerulonephritis leading to end-stage renal disease necessitating renal transplantation [12].

Lymphedema as a Minor Sign

In some well-known syndromes, such as tuberous sclerosis, Noonan syndrome and Turner syndrome, lymphedema can be present, although the diagnosis is made on the basis of other signs and symptoms. In some syndromes, such as in capillary malformation–arteriovenous malformation or CM-AVM, presence of lymphedema is only rarely reported, and/or it is subclinical, and thus not systematically looked for. Therefore, prevalence figures are only weak estimates. These genes are presented in Table 3.2.

Tuberous Sclerosis 1 and 2

Tuberous sclerosis (TSC) is an autosomal dominant disease characterized by hamartomas in different organ systems (skin, brain, heart, etc.). TSC affects between 1/6.000 and 1/10.000 individuals [13]. Compared to patients with a TSC1 mutation, those with a TSC2 mutation are more likely to have partial epilepsy, complex partial seizures, infantile spasms, subependymal giant-cell astrocytomas, and intellectual disability. Dental pits are often noted (Table 3.2). Primary lymphedema is present in less than 10 % of the cases.

Noonan Syndrome

Noonan syndrome (NS) is usually considered as a clinical diagnosis on the basis of the "typical face," including a broad forehead, hypertelorism, down-slanting palpebral fissures, ptosis, a high-arched palate, and low-set and posteriorly rotated ears. Cardiac anomalies and cryptorchidism can also be present. Mutations in PTPN11, SOS1, RAF1, KRAS, NRAS, SHOC2, or CBL cause this syndrome [14]. The overall incidence of lymphatic manifestations among NS is estimated to be ~20 % [15]. Lymphedema has only been reported in patients with a mutation in PTPN11, SOS1, or KRAS; thus, only these subtypes are

included in Table 3.2. With enlarged screens it may become evident that the other genetic subtypes can also be associated with lymphedema. Patients with RAF1 (Raf-1 proto-oncogene, serine/threonine kinase) mutation have been reported with lymphangiectasia or microkystic lymphatic malformation. The Costello syndrome, caused by KRAS (Kirsten rat sarcoma viral oncogene homolog) mutations, shares many features with Noonan syndrome and patients can also present lymphatic anomalies. Patients with a PTPN11 (protein tyrosine phosphatase, non-receptor type 11) mutation could have thrombocytopenia, while mutations in SOS1 (son of sevenless homolog 1) or KRAS seem to commonly cause macrocephaly.

Turner Syndrome

Turner syndrome occurs in 1/2.500–1/3.000 live-born girls. About 50 % have monosomy X (45,X), and 5–10 % have a duplication of the long arm of one X (46,X,i(Xq)). Most of the rest are mosaic for 45,X [16]. The main signs are mental retardation, cardiac disease, renal malformation, short stature, and edema (puffy hands and feet, and redundant nuchal skin). Most cases of Turner syndrome are diagnosed prenatally, by the presence of edema. Karyotype can easily reveal the genetic defect in most cases.

Capillary Malformation– Arteriovenous Malformation Syndrome

Heterozygous mutations in *RASA1* (RAS p21 protein activator 1) cause multiple capillary malformations (CM) associated with fast-flow vascular malformations (CM-AVM). There is high intrafamilial phenotypic variability. Almost all patients with a RASA1 mutation have one or more capillary malformations (97 %) and 23 % have also a fast-flow lesion [17]. In a few patients with Parkes Weber syndrome and a RASA1 mutation, primary lymphedema is also present [18]. As for the other syndromes in this subclass, the signs of CM-AVM lead to the correct differential diagnosis.

Approach for Genetic Screening

Most diagnostic genetic tests have relied on Sanger sequencing of the exonic parts of a given candidate gene. When more than one possible candidate gene exists, a sequential approach has classically been used, starting with the gene that most often is mutated in the given clinical subtype. The high genetic heterogeneity within patients with primary lymphedema (so far 20 "candidate" genes) renders this approach time-consuming and labor intense. Only precise clinical diagnosis can help target the correct gene. Yet the incomplete penetrance of the associated signs and symptoms, and the high frequency of de novo cases for some of the genes may make differential diagnosis impossible. Targeted high-throughput sequencing now allows to screen several genes at a time using panels. This is replacing the sequential method. The panel approach allows the clinician to obtain results for multiple genes at once, which in turn helps in clinical diagnosis, even in the absence of associated symptoms.

Prenatal Testing

Many signs and symptoms associated with a mutation in the 20 genes and monosomy X are detectable only after birth. Thus, differential diagnosis is even more difficult in the prenatal period. Fetal edema may appear as nuchal edema, ascites, pleural effusion, chylothorax, pericardial effusion, cutaneous edema, or hydrops fetalis. These can be caused by mutations in VEGFR3, FOXC2, CCBE1, RASA1, PTPN11, and SOS1, and Monosomy X. In families at risk for lymphedema, detailed morphological ultrasound should be carried out paying attention to the signs in Tables 3.1 and 3.2. It is also important to search for familial history of the various signs, as they could help establish the correct differential diagnosis. The usefulness of the novel panel approach is particularly appreciated for prenatal genetic testing due to its completeness and rapidity.

Genetic Counseling

Diagnostic Genetic Testing

The identification of a mutation in one of the known genes allows more precise structure of the follow-up for the patient, especially regarding the signs and symptoms that develop with time. For example, myelodysplasia is not present at birth and necessitates a careful monitoring in patients with a GATA2 mutation (Table 3.1). Genetic counseling for risk calculation and prenatal genetic testing also become possible via the identification of the causative genetic mutation.

Despite an increased number of genes involved in lymphangiogenesis and/or in the etiology of primary lymphedema, a large proportion of lymphedema patients still remain unexplained after diagnostic genetic testing. Based on the analysis of more than 400 index patients, mutations in the known genes only explain about one third of the patients [19]. It could be that some of the mutations in these genes go undetected, as they are not in the parts that are classically screened (i.e., the exons) or they are not detected by the methods used. These could be intronic or promoter mutations, or large deletions or insertions. They would likely not explain the majority of the unexplained patients. Thus, additional genes should exist.

Genetic diagnosis is important to advance our knowledge on primary lymphedema. Precise sub-classification on the basis of genetic data is needed to better define the patient groups for genotype–phenotype correlations. Prognosis may also differ between the subgroups. Moreover, targeted therapies are best developed on detailed comprehension on the underlying pathophysiological mechanisms.

Next-Generation Sequencing and the Usefulness of a Panel-Based Approach

During the past few years, Next-Generation Sequencing (NGS) has opened a new era for mutation screens. Whole-exome sequencing (WES) allows to screen all the coding exons of the human genome in one experiment. However, not all genes are equally well covered. This may be due to for example inequalities in exome capture and difficulty in amplifying areas rich in G and C nucleotides. Moreover, the cost and ethical issues limit the WES approach in clinical settings.

Another interesting approach is targeted next-generation sequencing. This is based on capture or amplification of a certain, much more limited, number of exons from the human genome. For example, the 20 known "lymphedema genes" cover a total target size of around 117 kb. With a specifically designed panel, they can be analyzed in one experiment for a given patient often for a similar prize as a single gene screen using Sanger sequencing. For the Noonan syndrome, a study shows a sixfold reduction in cost using a RASopathy panel with a target area of 30 kb [20]. Therefore, it can be used as a primary genetic screen, which does not need a finalized, detailed clinical diagnosis to be efficient. The value of this technique also lies in its rapidity. Thus, genetic results do not only confirm a clinical diagnosis but help, in a timely manner, to establish it.

How to Identify the Causative Variant?

The Sanger-sequencing-based monogenic screens often reveal one probably pathogenic variant in one gene. If no such variant is identified, screening of a second gene is started. When a "causative mutation" is identified, screens are stopped. This differs fundamentally from the targeted NGS approach, which renders data available on all targeted genes at once. Thus, hundreds of variants can be analyzed at the same time, not limited to a single gene only. This allows to study possible interacting variants between the screened genes. However, software in diagnostic routine cannot address this question. Moreover, identifi-

cation of even the monogenic disease-causing mutation(s) is not without caveats, as it is often difficult to make the distinction between an amino acid changing polymorphism and a disease-causing mutation.

Co-segregation analysis of the identified changes within the family can give further proof for the implication of a given nucleotide change. This can be done using classic Sanger sequencing. Alternatively, several family members may be sequenced in parallel using a panel approach.

To predict the impact of a mutation at the protein level, different tools based on evolutionary conservation, structural constraints, or chemical qualities of the protein with the changed and unchanged amino acids have been developed. Moreover, databases, such as dbSNP (http://www.ncbi.nlm.nih.gov/projects/SNP/), 1000Genomes (http://browser.1000genomes.org/index.html), and GoNL (http://www.nlgenome.nl/search/), collect reference sequence variants (most of which are polymorphisms) from different populations. These can be used to filter out known polymorphisms. In contrast, the absence, or a low allele frequency indicates that the variant is rare and may have a deleterious impact on the protein function. Other databases, such as HGMD (www.hgmd.org), regroup the known mutations in most genes, including small changes (Single Nucleotide Changes, Multiple Nucleotide Changes, insertions, and deletions) and larger structural variations, such as chromosomal deletions, insertions, or amplifications.

Even with these tools, many identified variants are reported as having "an unknown significance." For these, tests for in vitro and in vivo functional analysis would need to be developed. This is time-consuming and out of scope for routine diagnostic laboratories.

The Lymphedema-Causing Proteins

The genes that harbor mutations causing primary lymphedema and especially the proteins they encode can be grouped around the VEGFC–VEGFR3 ligand–receptor signaling complex and the downstream signaling pathways via PI3Kinase-AKT and MAPK [21].

VEGFC–VEGFR3 Axis

VEGFR3 was the first protein found to be mutated in primary lymphedema patients and the VEGFC–VEGFR3 signaling pathway is a major regulator of lymphangiogenesis. VEGFC and PTPN14 interact directly with VEGFR3. CCBE1 increases the capacity of VEGFC to activate VEGFR3 phosphorylation. Downstream of this complex, activation of the transcription factor FOXC2 ensues. GATA2 also regulates the expression of FOXC2, which plays a major role in the development of valves in lymphatic vessels by regulating the expression of connexin CX47/GJC2. Connexin, CX43/GJA1 is enriched on the upstream side of the lymphatic valves. Phosphorylation of FOXC2 is also linked to the expression of KIF11 [22]. The transcription factor SOX18 regulates PROX1 (prospero homeobox 1), a main factor for lymphangiogenesis, which regulates ITGA9, another valvular protein. So far, there is no clear link between VEGFR3 and FAT4, but the latter is regulated by the miRNA MIR31, linked to lymphangiogenesis [23].

Ras/MAPK Axis

Another major signaling pathway associated with lymphedema is the RAS-MAPK pathway. Mutations in this family of proteins can cause RASopathies. Mutations in each component of the pathway cause a distinct disease, but all the RASopathies share common features, such as craniofacial dysmorphology and cardiac malformations [14]. The pathway is involved in cell cycle, cellular growth, differentiation and senescence. The activation of the pathway can come from a membrane receptor that upon activation binds adaptors (PTPN11/SHP2, SOS1, and RASA1), which increase the proportion of the active form of a RAS protein (KRAS, HRAS). The activated RAS is able to activate the MAPK (RAF1) signaling cascade. The MAPK phosphorylates, among others, TSC1 and TSC2, and inhibits their function [24].

Therapeutic Targets

To date, no curative treatment exists for primary lymphedema. Symptomatic alleviation can be achieved by lymphatic drainage, elastic compression, and debulking surgery. The risk of infection is not negligible and should also be adequately managed. The numerous associated clinical features require their specific management.

Alternative treatments are being developed. Sorafenib, a tyrosine kinase inhibitor used in selected cancers, decreases vascular permeability by suppressing VEGFRs, and it is in a clinical trial for secondary lymphedema [25]. Another ongoing trial combines autologous lymph node grafts with adenoviral expression of VEGF-C [26]. It seems to improve the connectivity of the graft with the lymphatic system. Animal models are also developed and used to test inventive therapies. Plasmid-based expression of Hepatocyte growth factor (HGF) in rat-tail or in mice with induced upper limb edema inhibits the growth of swelling and lymphangiogenesis [27]. As there is high genetic heterogeneity within the causes of primary lymphedema, it would be interesting to identify if there is any common pathologic molecular alteration. This would allow a more general, targeted therapy, to be developed. For example, if the RAS/MAPK pathway would be altered in various patients in similar fashion independent of the underlying causative gene, molecules developed to treat cancer could be used for RASopathies and primary lymphedema [14].

Secondary Lymphedema

Secondary lymphedema is the most common form of lymphedema. It may be caused for example by infection, surgery, radiation, or injury. Secondary lymphedema occurs in approximately 30 % of breast cancer patients who undergo surgery or irradiation. Risk factors include the extent of surgery and irradiation, disease related factors (stage at diagnosis, pathological nodal status, and number of dissected lymph node), and patient-related factors (age at diagnosis, body mass index, and presence of a sedentary lifestyle). A study suggests a link between germline mutations in CX47/GJC2 and the occurrence of secondary lymphedema [28]. Another study genotyped 155 patients and 387 controls without lymphedema for 17 candidate genes (including FOXC2, HGF, VEGFC, and VEGFR3, but not GJC2) [29]. A significant association was found with LCP2 (lymphocyte cytosolic protein 2), NRP2 (neuropilin 2), SYK (spleen tyrosine kinase), VCAM1 (vascular cell adhesion molecule 1), FOXC2, and VEGFC. However, other studies are needed to confirm the significance of these associations and to identify the nucleotide changes that are causative for the predisposition.

Conclusion

Although more than 20 genes have been found to be mutated in patients with primary lymphedema, they explain less than a third of all cases. However, all the 20 genes have never been exhaustively screened for any patient cohort, and the respective prevalences are likely underestimated. Moreover, detailed genotype–phenotype correlation studies have not been exhaustive, especially when lymphedema was not the major feature of the disease/syndrome. Although it remains important to look for all additional signs to orient diagnosis, the targeted panel approach, which allows to obtain results for all known genes at ones, will greatly help primary diagnosis and genotype–phenotype correlation studies.

References

1. Balboa-Beltran E, Fernandez-Seara MJ, Perez-Munuzuri A, Lago R, Garcia-Magan C, Couce ML, et al. A novel stop mutation in the vascular endothelial growth factor-C gene (VEGFC) results in Milroy-like disease. J Med Genet. 2014;51(7):475–8.

2. Gordon K, Spiden SL, Connell FC, Brice G, Cottrell S, Short J, et al. FLT4/VEGFR3 and Milroy disease: novel mutations, a review of published variants and database update. Hum Mutat. 2013;34(1):23–31.

3. Connell F, Brice G, Jeffery S, Keeley V, Mortimer P, Mansour S. A new classification system for primary lymphatic dysplasias based on phenotype. Clin Genet. 2010;77(5):438–52.

4. Finegold DN, Kimak MA, Lawrence EC, Levinson KL, Cherniske EM, Pober BR, et al. Truncating mutations in FOXC2 cause multiple lymphedema syndromes. Hum Mol Genet. 2001;10(11):1185–9.

5. Ferrell RE, Baty CJ, Kimak MA, Karlsson JM, Lawrence EC, Franke-Snyder M, et al. GJC2 missense mutations cause human lymphedema. Am J Hum Genet. 2010;86(6):943–8.

6. Brice G, Ostergaard P, Jeffery S, Gordon K, Mortimer PS, Mansour S. A novel mutation in GJA1 causing oculodentodigital syndrome and primary lymphoedema in a three generation family. Clin Genet. 2013;84(4):378–81.

7. Alders M, Al-Gazali L, Cordeiro I, Dallapiccola B, Garavelli L, Tuysuz B, et al. Hennekam syndrome can be caused by FAT4 mutations and be allelic to Van Malder gem syndrome. Hum Genet. 2014;133(9):1161–7.

8. Spinner MA, Sanchez LA, Hsu AP, Shaw PA, Zerbe CS, Calvo KR, et al. GATA2 deficiency: a protean disorder of hematopoiesis, lymphatics, and immunity. Blood. 2014;123(6):809–21.

9. Kawai T, Nishikomori R, Heike T. Diagnosis and treatment in anhidrotic ectodermal dysplasia with immunodeficiency. Allergol Int. 2012;61(2):207–17.

10. Au AC, Hernandez PA, Lieber E, Nadroo AM, Shen YM, Kelley KA, et al. Protein tyrosine phosphatase PTPN14 is a regulator of lymphatic function and choanal development in humans. Am J Hum Genet. 2010;87(3):436–44.

11. Irrthum A, Devriendt K, Chitayat D, Matthijs G, Glade C, Steijlen PM, et al. Mutations in the transcription factor gene SOX18 underlie recessive and dominant forms of hypotrichosis-lymphedema-telangiectasia. Am J Hum Genet. 2003;72(6):1470–8.

12. Moalem S, Brouillard P, Kuypers D, Legius E, Harvey E, Taylor G, et al. Hypotrichosis-lymphedema-telangiectasia-renal defect associated with a truncating mutation in the SOX18 gene. Clin Genet. 2014. Article first published online: 16 APR 2014, DOI: 10.1111/cge.12388.

13. Geffrey AL, Shinnick JE, Staley BA, Boronat S, Thiele EA. Lymphedema in tuberous sclerosis complex. Am J Med Genet A. 2014;164A(6):1438–42.

14. Rauen KA. The RASopathies. Annu Rev Genomics Hum Genet. 2013;14:355–69.

15. Romano AA, Allanson JE, Dahlgren J, Gelb BD, Hall B, Pierpont ME, et al. Noonan syndrome: clinical features, diagnosis, and management guidelines. Pediatrics. 2010;126(4):746–59.

16. Sybert VP, McCauley E. Turner's syndrome. N Engl J Med. 2004;351(12):1227–38.

17. Revencu N, Boon LM, Mendola A, Cordisco MR, Dubois J, Clapuyt P, et al. RASA1 mutations and associated phenotypes in 68 families with capillary malformation-arteriovenous malformation. Hum Mutat. 2013;34(12):1632–41.

18. Burrows PE, Gonzalez-Garay ML, Rasmussen JC, Aldrich MB, Guilliod R, Maus EA, et al. Lymphatic abnormalities are associated with RASA1 gene mutations in mouse and man. Proc Natl Acad Sci U S A. 2013;110(21):8621–6.
19. Mendola A, Schlogel MJ, Ghalamkarpour A, Irrthum A, Nguyen HL, Fastre E, et al. Mutations in the VEGFR3 signaling pathway explain 36% of familial lymphedema. Mol Syndromol. 2013;4(6):257–66.
20. Lepri FR, Scavelli R, Digilio MC, Gnazzo M, Grotta S, Dentici ML, et al. Diagnosis of Noonan syndrome and related disorders using target next generation sequencing. BMC Med Genet. 2014;15:14.
21. Brouillard P, Boon L, Vikkula M. Genetics of lymphatic anomalies. J Clin Invest. 2014;124(3):898–904.
22. Ivanov KI, Agalarov Y, Valmu L, Samuilova O, Liebl J, Houhou N, et al. Phosphorylation regulates FOXC2-mediated transcription in lymphatic endothelial cells. Mol Cell Biol. 2013;33(19):3749–61.
23. Wu YH, Hu TF, Chen YC, Tsai YN, Tsai YH, Cheng CC, et al. The manipulation of miRNA-gene regulatory networks by KSHV induces endothelial cell motility. Blood. 2011;118(10):2896–905.
24. Sevick-Muraca EM, King PD. Lymphatic vessel abnormalities arising from disorders of Ras signal transduction. Trends Cardiovasc Med. 2014;24(3):121–7.
25. Moncrieff M, Shannon K, Hong A, Hersey P, Thompson J. Dramatic reduction of chronic lymphoedema of the lower limb with sorafenib therapy. Melanoma Res. 2008;18(2):161–2.
26. Honkonen KM, Visuri MT, Tervala TV, Halonen PJ, Koivisto M, Lahteenvuo MT, et al. Lymph node transfer and perinodal lymphatic growth factor treatment for lymphedema. Ann Surg. 2013;257(5):961–7.
27. Saito Y, Nakagami H, Morishita R, Takami Y, Kikuchi Y, Hayashi H, et al. Transfection of human hepatocyte growth factor gene ameliorates secondary lymphedema via promotion of lymphangiogenesis. Circulation. 2006;114(11):1177–84.
28. Finegold DN, Baty CJ, Knickelbein KZ, Perschke S, Noon SE, Campbell D, et al. Connexin 47 mutations increase risk for secondary lymphedema following breast cancer treatment. Clin Cancer Res. 2012;18(8):2382–90.
29. Miaskowski C, Dodd M, Paul SM, West C, Hamolsky D, Abrams G, et al. Lymphatic and angiogenic candidate genes predict the development of secondary lymphedema following breast cancer surgery. PLoS One. 2013;8(4):e60164.

Epidemiology and Morbidity of Lymphedema

4

Arin K. Greene

Key Points

- Lymphedema is common, affecting approximately 140–250 million persons worldwide and 1/1,000 Americans.
- 99 % of patients with lymphedema develop the condition following axillary/inguinal radiation and/or lymphadenectomy or from a parasitic infection.
- Patients with lymphedema may have minimal morbidity from the disease.
- The most common problem from lymphedema is that it can lower a patient's self-esteem because the disease causes a deformity of their limb or genitalia.
- Other complications of lymphedema include: infection, decreased ability to use the affected area, and rarely malignant degeneration.

Introduction

Lymphedema is a common condition, although the exact prevalence is unknown. The disease is a major burden to the health care system because it is chronic and incurable. Although lymphedema can cause major morbidity, many patients have minimal problems if they are compliant with conservative treatments. In some individuals,

A.K. Greene, M.D., M.M.Sc. (✉)
Department of Plastic and Oral Surgery,
Boston Children's Hospital, Harvard Medical School,
300 Longwood Avenue, Boston, MA 02115, USA
e-mail: arin.greene@childrens.harvard.edu

however, the condition can be significantly progressive and life-threatening. In general, patients with primary (idiopathic) lymphedema have less morbidity compared to individuals with secondary disease from injury to a normally functioning lymphatic system [1]. Patients born with an anomalous system may compensate better for lymphatic dysfunction compared to individuals who had a normal lymphatic system that was disrupted by trauma.

Epidemiology

Overview

Lymphedema is a common condition, and may affect as many as 140–250 million persons worldwide [2]. Two population studies have estimated the prevalence of lymphedema to be between 1.33 and 1.44 per 1,000 persons in two European countries [3, 4]. The true rate of lymphedema is unknown, but is likely underestimated because patients with latent or mild disease may not seek treatment. Approximately 99 % of individuals with lymphedema have secondary disease; primary lymphedema is rare (Table 4.1). In developed countries the most common cause of lymphedema is lymphadenectomy and/or radiation for cancer treatment. In third-world nations lymphedema most frequently arises because of a parasitic infection. At least 90 % of patients with lymphedema worldwide have lower extremity

A.K. Greene et al. (eds.), *Lymphedema: Presentation, Diagnosis, and Treatment*,
DOI 10.1007/978-3-319-14493-1_4, © Springer International Publishing Switzerland 2015

Table 4.1 Epidemiology of lymphedema (listed from most common to least common)

Primary (prevalence 1/1,00,000 persons)	Secondary (prevalence 1/1,000 persons)
Infant-onset	Filariasis
Adolescent-onset	Axillary/inguinal lymphadenectomy
Childhood-onset	Axillary/inguinal radiation
Adult-onset	Obesity

disease because of (in order): filariasis, inguinal radiation/lymphadenectomy, obesity, or primary lymphedema. Nine percent of patients with lymphedema have upper extremity disease; most are women who have been treated for breast cancer. Isolated genital lymphedema is the third most common site of disease (~1 %) and usually results from inguinal radiation/lymphadenectomy, obesity, or primary lymphedema. Genital lymphedema typically is associated with lower extremity disease.

Primary Lymphedema

Primary lymphedema is rare, affecting approximately 1/100,000 children [5]. In the pediatric population onset occurs in infancy (49.2 %), childhood (9.5 %), or adolescence (41.3 %) [1]. Primary lymphedema develops during adulthood in 19 % of patients [6]. Males are more likely to present in infancy (68 %), while females most commonly develop the disease during adolescence (55 %) [1]. The lower extremities are affected in 91.7 % of patients; 50 % have unilateral lymphedema and 50 % have bilateral disease [1]. Bilateral lower extremity lymphedema is more common in patients presenting in infancy (63 %), compared to adolescence (30 %) [1]. Eighteen percent of children with primary lymphedema have genital disease, which is usually associated with lower extremity lymphedema. Four percent of patients with primary lymphedema have isolated genital involvement. Sixteen percent of children with idiopathic lymphedema have upper extremity disease [1].

Rarely, a child can have lymphedema affecting the legs, genitalia, and/or arms.

Secondary Lymphedema

Cancer-Related Treatment

Injury to the lymphatic system is responsible for approximately 99 % of adult cases and 3 % of pediatric disease [1]. The overall risk of lymphedema following treatment for malignancy is 15 %; the two variables that most importantly predict if a patient develops the condition is if he/she underwent lymphadenectomy or radiation [7]. The overall risk of lymphedema after treatment for the following cancers (including patients who did and did not have lymphadenectomy or radiation) has been estimated to be: head/neck (4 %), genitourinary (10 %), melanoma 16 % (arm 5 %, leg 28 %), gynecologic (20 %), sarcoma (30 %) [7].

Upper extremity lymphedema from breast cancer treatment is the most common etiology of the disease in the USA. One-third of women who have axillary lymphadenopathy and radiation develop the condition [8]. Edema typically begins 12 months following the injury to lymph vessels [9]. Three-fourths of patients develop swelling within 3 years after the injury and the risk of lymphedema is 1 % each year thereafter [10]. Advanced disease, the extent of resection, and number of lymph nodes removed increases the risk of lymphedema [11]. Modified radical mastectomy has a greater chance of causing lymphedema compared to partial mastectomy; removal of more than 15 axillary lymph nodes increases the rate of lymphedema tenfold, compared to excising less than 5 nodes [12]. Sentinel lymph node biopsy reduces the rate of lymphedema (0.5 %) compared to axillary lymph node dissection [13]. Radiation is a major risk factor for breast cancer-related lymphedema; when the axilla is included in the radiation field the risk of lymphedema doubles, compared to radiation of the breast and supraclavicular nodes only [14]. In patients who have undergone lymphadenectomy and/or radiation, the most significant variable that will increase their risk of lymphedema is obesity [15].

Pelvic or abdominal malignancy is the most frequent reason for lower extremity lymphedema. The rate of lymphedema following lymphadenectomy and/or radiation for the following malignancies has been estimated to be: prostate (13 %), uterine (18 %), melanoma (25 %), vulvar (28 %), sarcoma (25 %). penile (30 %), cervical (42 %) [4]. Lower-extremity and genital lymphedema rates decrease when inguinal sentinel lymph node biopsy is performed (1.9 %) instead of lymphadenectomy [16].

Filariasis

A parasitic infection is the most common etiology of lymphedema in the world; 90 % of cases are cause by *W. bancrofti* [2]. Eighty-three countries are endemic to the disease; 70 % of cases are in Bangladesh, India, Indonesia, and Nigeria [2]. Other affected areas include Africa (central), Brazil, Burma, China (southern), Dominican Republic, Guiana, Guyana, Haiti, Malaysia, Nile delta, Pacific Islands, Pakistan, Sri Lanka, Surinam, and Thailand [2]. It is estimated that although 120 million people are infected with a lymphedema-causing parasite, 40 million persons exhibit lymphedema clinically [2]. Patients at risk for filariasis live in tropical/subtropical environments because these habitats are humid which is necessary for the parasites to survive [2]. Most individuals with filariasis live in rural locations that have poor sanitation [2]. The most common location for lymphedema caused by filariasis is the lower extremity and/or genitalia, but the upper extremity and breast can be affected as well.

Obesity

Obesity affects one-third of the US population, and 6 % have a body mass index (BMI) >40 [17]. The proportion of the population that is obese is increasing at a rate of 2–4 % every 10 years [17]. Patients with a BMI > 50 are at risk for developing obesity-induced lower extremity lymphedema, and individuals with a BMI > 60 are very likely to have the disease. Although the percent of the US population with a BMI > 60 is unknown,

using a conservative estimate of 0.5 % then the number of Americans (population 315 million) with obesity-induced lymphedema would be 1.575 million.

Morbidity

Some patients with lymphedema do not have problems, while others can have significant complications (Table 4.2). Generally, individuals who are compliant with intervention have less disability than patients who are noncompliant (Fig. 4.1). Individuals with an active lifestyle have fewer problems than patients who are sedentary. Exercise likely improves proximal lymphatic flow by muscle contraction and helps the individual maintain a normal BMI. Obese individuals have more complications from lymphedema compared to normal-weighted persons because obesity adversely affects lymphatic function [15, 18]. Morbidity from lymphedema is described below from the most common problem, to the least frequent complication.

Progression

Almost all patients with lymphedema have progression of their disease. Over time the high-protein interstitial fluid causes subcutaneous adipose deposition [19]. Consequently, the circumference of the limb or genitalia gradually enlarges. Fat in an extremity can increase by 73 % [19]. As the lymphedematous area becomes larger, the patient's ability to use the area decreases.

Table 4.2 Morbidity from lymphedema (listed from most common to least common)

Progression of disease
Lowered self-esteem
Infection
Fitting clothing
Difficulty using the extremity
Skin changes
Massive localized lymphedema
Discomfort
Malignant transformation

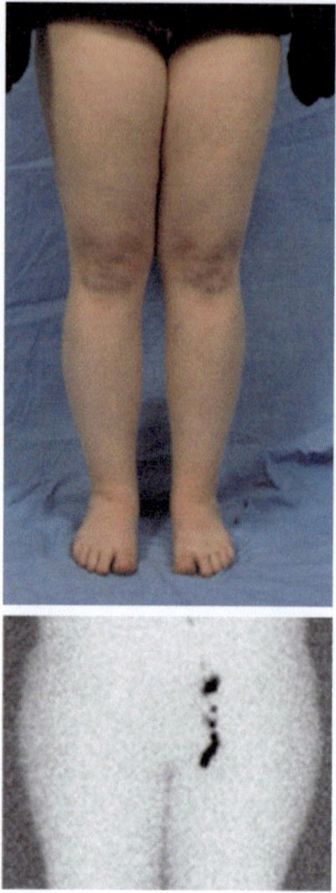

Fig. 4.1 Asymptomatic lymphedema. 19-year-old female with recent swelling of the right lower extremity. Lymphoscintigram shows absent transit of tracer to the right inguinal nodes 2 h following injection. The patient does not have any complaints and the appearance of her legs is similar

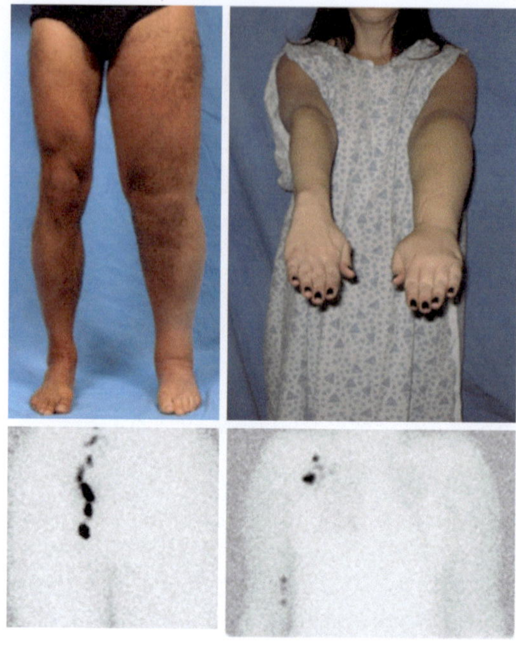

Fig. 4.2 Psychosocial morbidity caused by lymphedema. (*Left*) 50-year-old male with adult-onset left-lower extremity lymphedema. (*Right*) 40-year-old female with left upper extremity lymphedema following breast cancer treatment. Both patients had lowered self-esteem because they were unhappy with the appearance of their diseased limb

Psychosocial

Lymphedema negatively impacts a patient's social well-being, body image, and sexuality [20]. The most common problem expressed by patients with lymphedema is that they are unhappy with the appearance of their limb or genitalia. Patients have lowered self-esteem because the involved area does not look normal (Fig. 4.2). The more severe the disease, the greater the loss of self-esteem and negative impact on quality of life. Unilateral limb involvement can be more distressing than bilateral disease because the asymmetry is more noticeable. Individuals may not feel comfortable wearing clothing that exposes their diseased limb. Patients may avoid changing clothes in front of their peers or refrain from swimming. Lymphedema can impede the establishment of new relationships and genital disease can negatively impact an individual's sexual activity.

Patients with secondary lymphedema from cancer treatment often state that although they are cured of their malignancy, lymphedema is a daily reminder of their cancer. Children with primary disease often feel that they are "different" than their peers; the emotional aspect of their condition worsens during adolescence. Many patients believe that wearing a compression garment is a worse deformity than the appearance of their lymphedematous extremity. The most common reason for individuals to seek surgical intervention is to improve the appearance of the area affected by lymphedema. Patients with psychosocial distress can be helped with counseling. Conservative compression strategies, as well as excision of excess subcutaneous fat using liposuction, can improve a patient's asymmetry as well as their self-esteem.

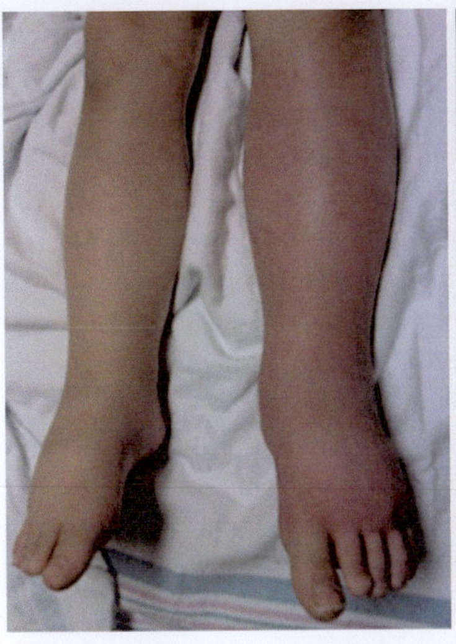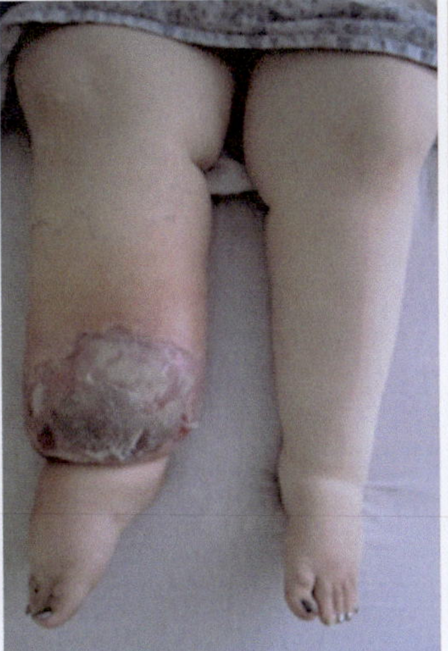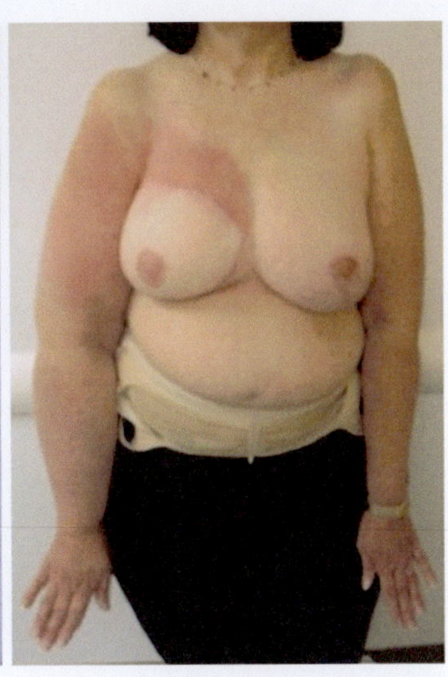

Fig. 4.3 Lymphedematous areas are at increased risk for infection. (*Left*) 4-year-old male with primary lymphedema developed left leg cellulitis requiring hospital admission. (*Center*) 18-year-old female with primary lymphedema had right lower extremity infection necessitating intravenous antibiotics; note skin epidermolysis and blistering. (*Right*) 64-year-old female with cellulitis complicating secondary lymphedema of the right arm following breast cancer treatment

Infection

The most frequent "functional" problem caused by lymphedema is infection. A lymphedematous extremity has a significantly increased risk of cellulitis compared to the non-affected limb (Fig. 4.3). Lymph stagnation increases the risk of infection after minor trauma because of: (1) impaired immunosurveillance (lymphatics function as an immunologic defense), (2) decreased oxygen delivery to the skin, and (3) a proteinaceous environment favorable for bacterial growth. In one community study of both primary and secondary lymphedema, 29 % of patients had an infection over the previous 12 months, and one-fourth required hospitalization for intravenous antibiotics [3]. In another study of patients with primary lymphedema, 19 % have a history of cellulitis, 13 % have been hospitalized, and 7 % have >3 attacks each year [1].

Infections in a lymphedematous area typically do not spontaneously occur, but result from a break in the skin. The most common etiology is incidental trauma; the patient is unaware of a cut or scrape. Less frequently, the source of an infection can be a problem with a finger/toe nail.

Rarely, a systemic infection can secondarily infect a lymphedematous extremity.

Cutaneous infection in patients with lymphedema can spread more quickly compared to individuals without the disease. A superficial cellulitis may develop rapidly into sepsis. Patients are counseled to seek medical attention quickly if they suspect an infection in a lymphedematous area. Often, individuals will carry oral antibiotics with them and administer the medication during the onset of the infection. Patients who have ≥3 episodes of cellulitis/year are placed on chronic suppressive antibiotic therapy following infectious disease consultation. The most frequent organism responsible for cellulitis is *Streptococcus* (*S. Pyogenes*), and patients are usually treated with penicillin or cephalexin.

Fitting Clothing

A common complaint from patients with lymphedema is that they have difficulty fitting clothing (Fig. 4.4). Symptoms are exacerbated when the individual has unilateral disease because of the asymmetry between the limbs.

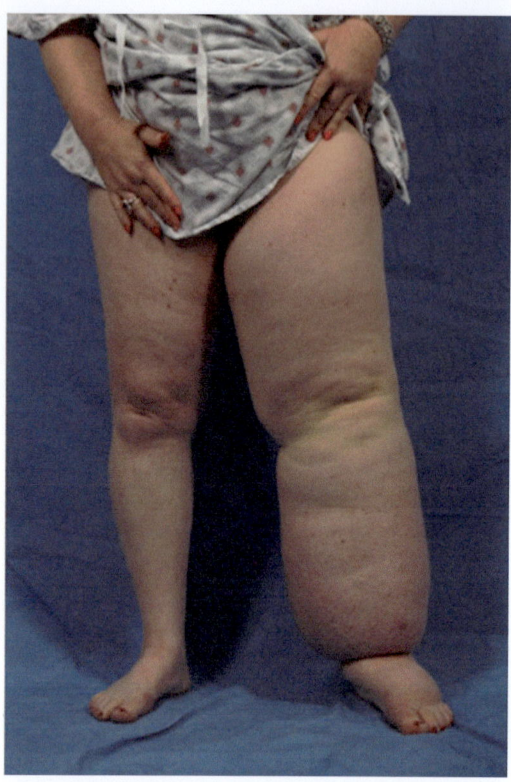

Fig. 4.4 Patients with lymphedema can have difficulty fitting clothing. 55-year-old female with secondary lower extremity lymphedema has problems wearing pants because her left leg is significantly larger than her unaffected extremity

The most problematic location is the feet: (1) individuals may have to wear two different sized shoes and/or (2) patients have problems with pressure from the shoe and need to wear sandals or other open footwear. Individuals with significant lower extremity lymphedema have difficulty fitting jeans or slacks and often need to wear oversized sweat pants. Patients with severe upper extremity lymphedema may not be able to wear tight-fitting long sleeve shirts and instead use short sleeves and/or oversized shirts. Individuals with upper extremity disease may need to have the size of their rings and wrist jewelry increased.

Orthopedic

Lymphedema is confined to the skin and subcutaneous tissue and does not directly involve muscles, bones, or joints. The disease, however, can secondarily affect the musculoskeletal system because of circumferential overgrowth of the skin and subcutaneous tissue. Because lymphedema does not affect bone, children are not at risk for vertical limb overgrowth and do not need to be monitored for a leg-length discrepancy.

Patients with lymphedema can have reduced ability to use an extremity (particularly an arm) because of weakness and/or heaviness. The ability to use the limb for daily activities can be further impeded by operative or radiation fibrosis which may affect joint mobility. In early disease controlled compression therapy using custom compression garments can improve the use of the limb for activities of daily living.

As the lymphedematous extremity enlarges, the ability to use the limb for routine activities decreases. Muscle mass increases in an extremity with lymphedema because the added subcutaneous adipose tissue acts as a "weight" that builds muscle strength [19]. For example, secondary upper extremity lymphedema increases the amount of subcutaneous adipose (73 %), muscle (47 %), and bone (7 %) [19]. Hypertrophied muscles enable the patient to use the lymphedematous limb with minimal morbidity initially. However, added muscle mass cannot compensate for severely affected limbs and patients can have decreased function. For example, individuals with significant upper extremity disease may have difficulty lifting their arm over their head which can impede getting dressed (Fig. 4.5). Patients with severe lower extremity disease can have problems ambulating because of the weight of the extremity (Fig. 4.6). As the size of a limb increases, patients can have discomfort from stress on their joints.

Musculoskeletal manifestations of lymphedema typically occur with severe disease following fibroadipose deposition. Consequently, conservative interventions (e.g., compression garments, pneumatic compression, massage) are unlikely to significantly alleviate symptoms. Morbidity can be improved with an excisional operative procedure to reduce the amount of subcutaneous tissue which facilitates the use of the extremity. I prefer suction-assisted lipectomy because it can significantly improve extremity volume, has predictable and long-lasting results,

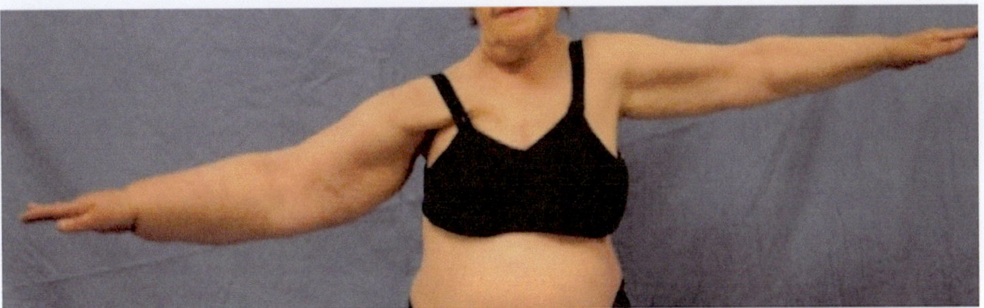

Fig. 4.5 Upper extremity lymphedema can negatively affect arm function. 86-year-old female with secondary upper extremity lymphedema following breast cancer treatment. Note her inability to fully raise her right arm

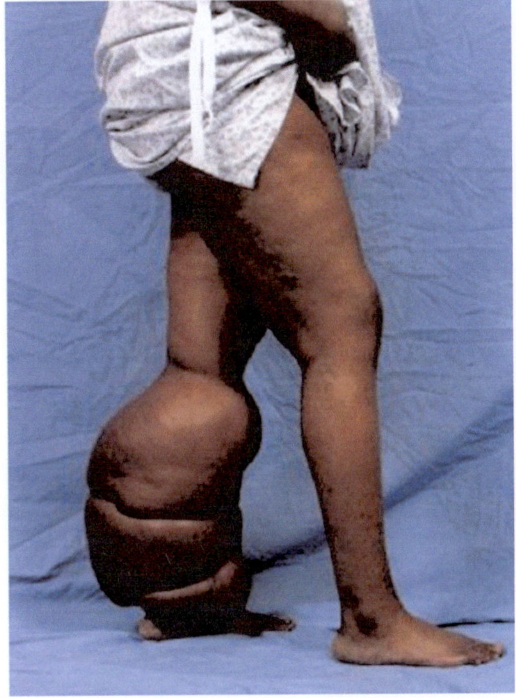

Fig. 4.6 Lower extremity lymphedema can limit ambulation. 40-year-old female with adolescent-onset primary lymphedema. She has difficulty ambulating because of the weight of her left extremity

and is safe. Other options to reduce the excess tissue of the extremity is staged skin/subcutaneous excision or the Charles procedure.

Skin Changes

Patients with lymphedema generally have normal appearing skin. However, individuals with lymphedema can develop cutaneous lymphatic vesicles that may cause: (1) a "cosmetic" deformity, (2) bleeding, (3) or leakage of fluid (lymphorrhea) (Fig. 4.7). The skin also may become hyperkeratotic (Fig. 4.8) [1]. Ulceration rarely affects patients with lymphedema because their arterial and venous circulations are intact. Vesicles and hyperkeratosis most frequently involves the distal lower extremity, particularly the feet and toes. The penis and scrotum also can exhibit lymphatic vesicles. A lymphedematous upper extremity is less frequently complicated by cutaneous pathology.

The appearance of lymphatic vesicles and hyperkeratosis can lower a patient's self-esteem. Lymphatic vesicles also are a portal of entry for bacteria and can significantly increase the risk of infection. Typically, patients who have repeated episodes of cellulitis also have numerous lymphatic vesicles involving their skin. When vesicles bleed or leak lymph fluid the patient's clothing becomes saturated which causes distress. In addition, leaking vesicles are typically malodorous which further creates psychosocial morbidity.

Vesicles can be treated with sclerotherapy, carbon dioxide laser, or resection. Excision usually is not performed because the area of vesicles is large and the distal extremity is an unfavorable location for the removal of skin. Injecting vesicles with a scleroscent causes scarring which effectively reduces leakage; I prefer sodium tetradecyl sulfate. Carbon dioxide laser also causes fibrosis of the vesicles and gives favorable results. Localized vesicles can be treated with sclerotherapy in the office, but large areas are best managed with carbon dioxide laser under general anesthesia.

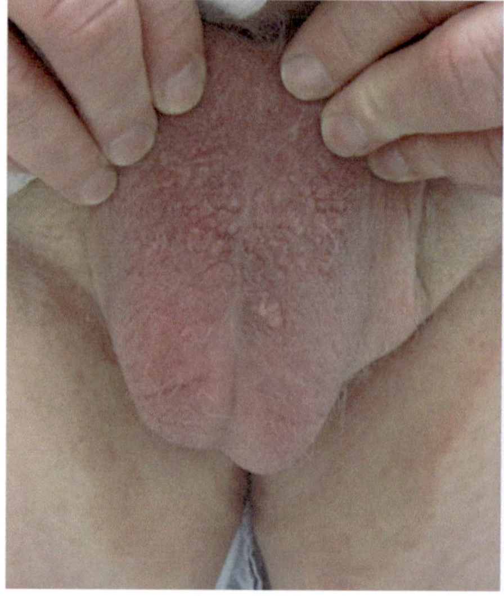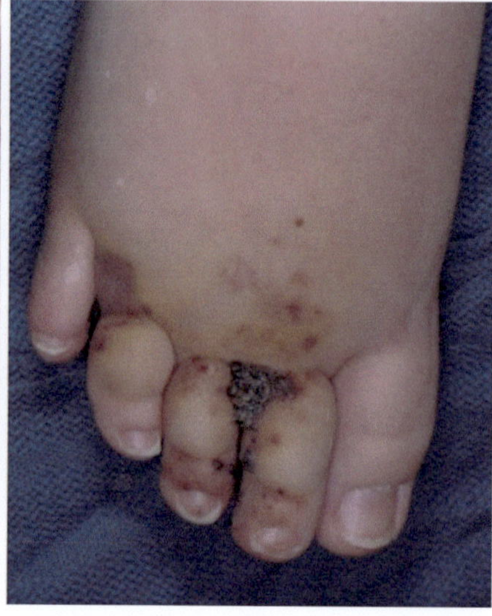

Fig. 4.7 Vesicles can develop in lymphedematous areas. (*Left*) 51-year-old with secondary lower extremity and genital lymphedema has scrotal vesicles leaking lymph fluid (lymphorrhea). (*Right*) 11-year-old male with primary lower extremity lymphedema has vesicles of his feet causing bleeding and multiple infections

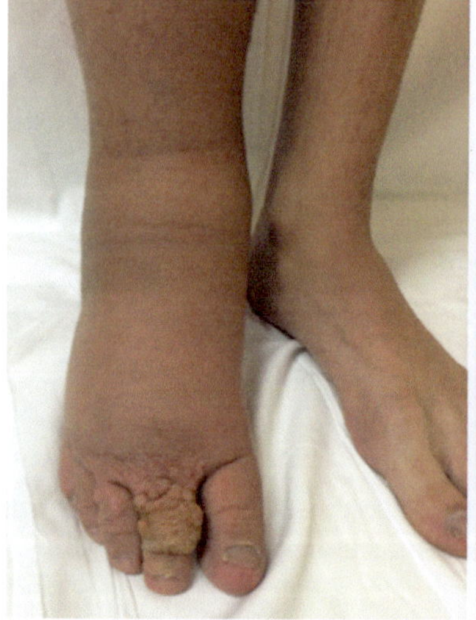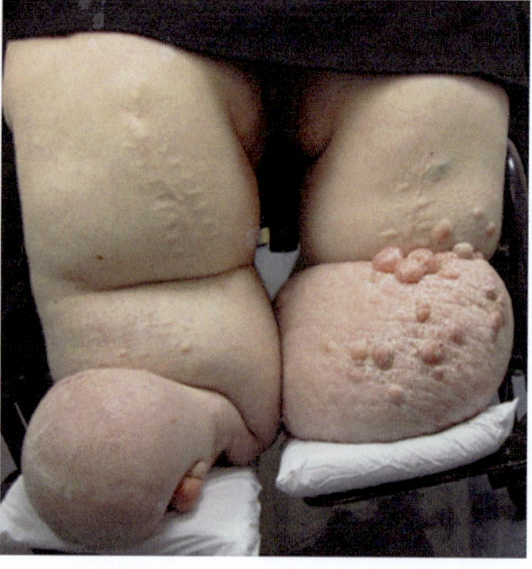

Fig. 4.8 Lymphedema can cause hyperkeratosis. (*Left*) 21-year-old male with primary lymphedema has had progressive overgrowth of his second toe that has impeded his ability to wear shoes, caused pain, and leaked fluid. (*Right*) 40-year-old female with a history of myelomeningocele and primary lymphedema has hyperkeratotic lesions on her left lower extremity

Massive Localized Lymphedema

Obesity can result in a large, localized area of overgrowth termed "massive localized lymphedema" (MLL) (Fig. 4.9) [21]. The condition is uncommon and affects extremely obese patients. The average age of individuals is 47 years and males and females are affected equally [22]. Mean patient body mass index is 61 [22]. MLL involves the thigh (49 %), lower abdomen (18 %), penis/scrotum (12 %), suprapubic area (7 %), vulva (4 %), distal leg (7 %), and arm (3 %) [22]. The average size and weight of MLL is 37.4 cm and 9.3 kg, respectively. Although MLL of the

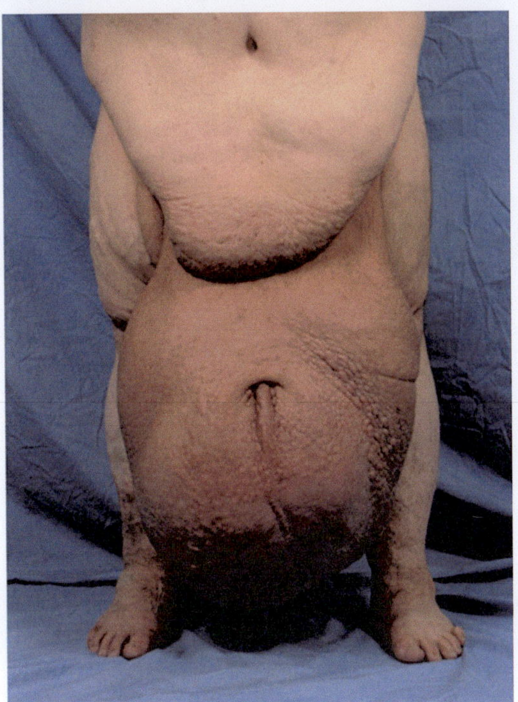

Fig. 4.9 Massive localized lymphedema. 48-year-old with obesity-induced lymphedema who developed massive localized lymphedema of his scrotum

extremities is typically unilateral, both lower extremities usually have underlying lymphatic dysfunction of the entire limb. Patients with MLL can have difficulty ambulating and fitting clothing. When the lesion involves the perineal area individuals may have problems sitting. Similar to other locations with lymphedema, angiosarcoma can develop in MLL [22].

MLL can be improved with weight loss, and patients are referred to a bariatric surgery center. Following massive weight loss, if the localized area remains symptomatic it can be removed. If an area of MLL is resected prior to weight loss the operative morbidity and recurrence rate are significantly higher than removing the area once the patient has lowered his/her body mass index.

Pain

Lymphedema generally is a painless; significant discomfort is not consistent with the disease. If a patient complains of significant pain, then he/she likely does not have lymphedema. However, as the circumferential overgrowth of the extremity worsens and the limb becomes heavier, underlying musculoskeletal discomfort can occur primarily because of stress on joints. The limb can feel heavy for the patient and cause fatigue, weakness, and or paresthesias [23].

Malignant Transformation

Chronic lymphedema can predispose an individual to lymphangiosarcoma in the affected extremity, although the risk is very low (~0.07–0.45 %) [24]. Stewart–Treves "syndrome" is not a syndrome and classically refers to a lymphangiosarcoma arising in a lymphedematous upper extremity following treatment for breast cancer (Fig. 4.10) [24]. The condition is better described as *Stewart–Treves Tumor*. The malignancy also can develop in chronic lower extremity lymphedema resulting from inguinal radiation and/or lymphadenectomy. Lymphangiosarcoma has been described in patients with primary lymphedema (in both the upper and lower extremity) as well as in areas of massive localized lymphedema [22, 24]. Prognosis is poor because of pulmonary metastasis and local recurrence. Mean survival is <2 years following diagnosis. If metastases are not present on imaging, early amputation may allow long-term survival. Chemotherapy and radiation have minimal efficacy [24].

Genitourinary

Generally, the primary morbidity of penile/scrotal lymphedema is psychosocial because patients do not like the appearance of their genitalia (Fig. 4.11). "Functional" problems with genital lymphedema are uncommon. Penile/scrotal lymphedema does not affect sexual function or sterility. Rarely, dysuria or phimosis can occur. Patients with severe penile/scrotal lymphedema may have difficulty fitting clothing, leaking lymphatic vesicles, and/or infections. Conservative management for symptomatic patients is to apply compression using tight fitting exercise shorts. Vesicles may be treated using sclerotherapy or

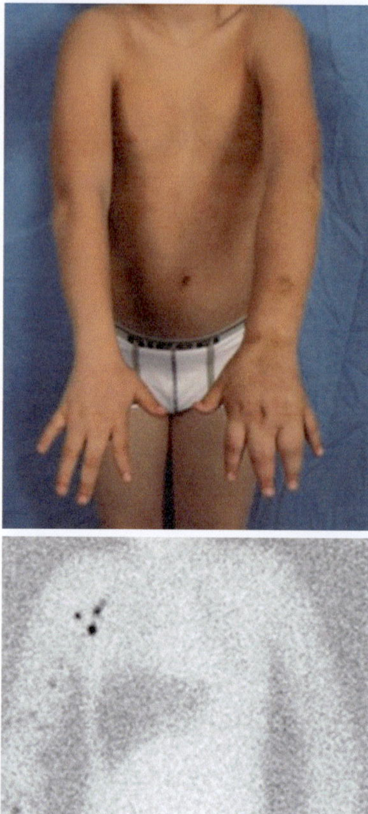

Fig. 4.10 Lymphangiosarcoma in a lymphedematous extremity. 12-year-old male with infant-onset primary lymphedema developed pain and hardening of this hand/forearm over the previous 3 months. Lymphoscintigraphy illustrated absence of tracer uptake in his left axilla. Biopsy showed lymphangiosarcoma

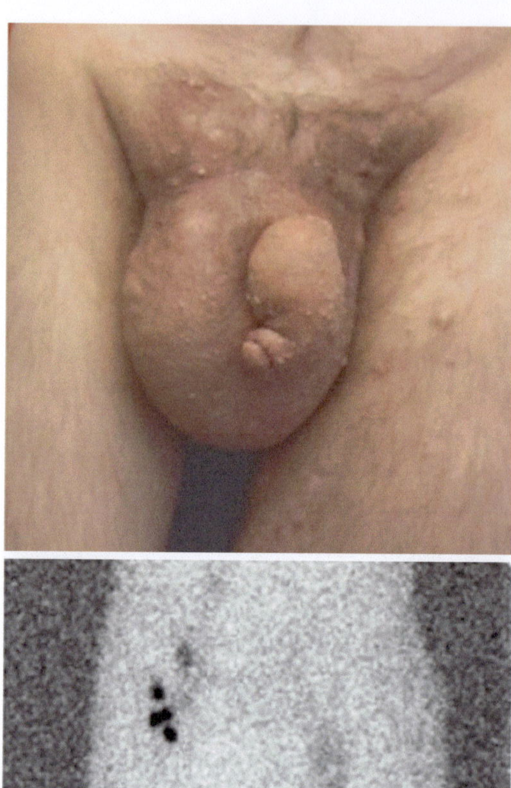

Fig. 4.11 Morbidity of genital lymphedema. 24-year-old with adolescent-onset primary lymphedema who was unhappy with the appearance of his genitalia; he also complained of leaking lymphatic vesicles. Lymphoscintigram shows absence of tracer in his left inguinal nodes 3.5 h following injection

carbon dioxide laser. The appearance of the genitalia and morbidity can be improved by resecting skin and subcutaneous tissue.

Congestive Heart Failure

The patient in our experience with the most severe manifestation of lymphedema developed congestive heart failure from his disease (Fig. 4.12). He had primary lymphedema of his right lower extremity that steadily worsened over the course of his life that caused him to be non-ambulatory. He developed high-output congestive heart failure because of the amount of blood flow that was being shunted to his massive extremity. Following staged subcutaneous excision of 45 lb of skin and subcutaneous tissue, his congestive heart failure resolved.

Conclusions

Lymphedema is a common condition. Most patients develop the disease following lymphadenectomy/radiation or from a parasitic condition. Patients may also develop idiopathic lymphedema from the anomalous development of the lymphatic system. Although many individuals

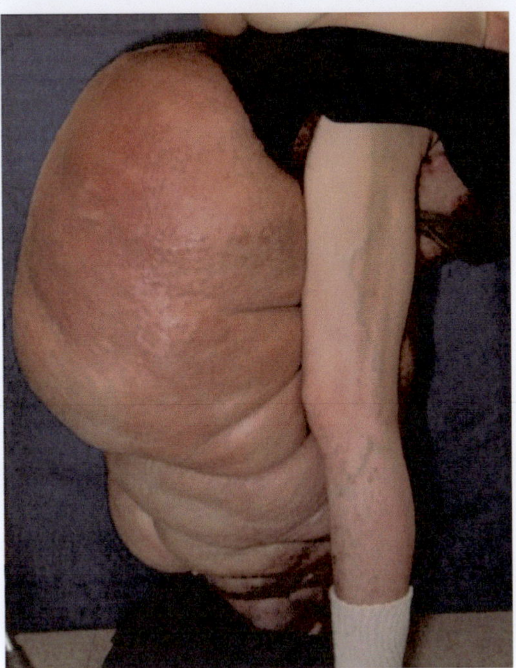

Fig. 4.12 32-year-old male with massive lower extremity lymphedema causing congestive heart failure because of excessive blood flow to the limb

with lymphedema have minimal morbidity, the disease can cause significant problems, e.g., psychosocial distress, infection, difficulty using the diseased area, malignant degeneration.

References

1. Schook CC, Mulliken JB, Fishman SJ, Grant F, Zurakowski D, Greene AK. Primary lymphedema: clinical features and management in 138 pediatric patients. Plast Reconstr Surg. 2011;127:2419–31.
2. Mendoza N, Li A, Gill A, Tyring S. Filariasis: diagnosis and treatment. Dermatol Ther. 2009;22:475–90.
3. Moffatt CJ. Lymphoedema: an underestimated health problem. QJM. 2003;96:731–8.
4. Rockson SG. Estimating the population burden of lymphedema. Ann N Y Acad Sci. 2008;1131:147–54.
5. Smeltzer DM, Stickler GB, Schirger A. Primary lymphedemas in children and adolescents: a follow-up study and review. Pediatrics. 1985;76:206–18.
6. Wolfe J, Kinmonth JB. The prognosis of primary lymphedema of the lower limbs. Arch Surg. 1981;116:1157–60.
7. Cormier JN, Askew RL, Mungovan KS, Xing Y, Ross MI, Armer JM. Lymphedema beyond breast cancer: a systematic review and meta-analysis of cancer related secondary lymphedema. Cancer. 2010;116:5138–49.
8. Gärtner R, Mejdahl MK, Andersen KG, Ewertz M, Kroman N. Development in self-reported arm-lymphedema in Danish women treated for early-stage breast cancer in 2005 and 2006 - a nationwide follow-up study. Breast. 2014;23:445. doi:10.1016/j.breast.2014.03.001. pii: S0960-9776(14)00042-3.
9. Johansson K, Branje E. Arm lymphoedema in a cohort of breast cancer survivors 10 years after diagnosis. Acta Oncol. 2010;49:166–73.
10. Petrek JA, Senie RT, Peters M, Rosen PP. Lymphedema in a cohort of breast carcinoma survivors 20 years after diagnosis. Cancer. 2001;92:1368–77.
11. Dayangac M, Makay O, Yeniay L, Aynaci M, Kapkac M, Yilmaz R. Precipitating factors for lymphedema following surgical treatment of breast cancer: implications for patients undergoing axillary lymph node dissection. Breast J. 2009;15:210–1.
12. Yen TW, Fan X, Sparapani R, Laud PW, Walker AP, Nattinger AB. A contemporary, population-based study of lymphedema risk factors in older women with breast cancer. Ann Surg Oncol. 2009;16:979–88.
13. McLaughlin SA, Wright MJ, Morris KT, Giron GL, Sampson MR, Brockway JP, Hurley KE, Riedel ER, Van Zee KJ. Prevalence of lymphedema in women with breast cancer 5 years after sentinel lymph node biopsy or axillary dissection: patient perceptions and precautionary behaviors. J Clin Oncol. 2008;26:5220–6.
14. Hayes SB. Does axillary boost increase lymphedema compared with supraclavicular radiation alone after breast conservation? Int J Radiat Oncol Biol Phys. 2008;72:1449–55.
15. Helyer LK, Varnic M, Le LW, Leong W, McCready D. Obesity is a risk factor for developing postoperative lymphedema in breast cancer patients. Breast J. 2010;16:48–54.
16. Van der Zee AG, Oonk MH, De Hullu JA, Ansink AC, Vergote I, Verheijen RH, Maggioni A, Gaarenstroom KN, Baldwin PJ, Van Dorst EB, Van der Velden J, Hermans RH, van der Putten H, Drouin P, Schneider A, Sluiter WJ. Sentinel node dissection is safe in the treatment of early-stage vulvar cancer. J Clin Oncol. 2008;26:884–9.
17. Flegal KM, Carroll MD, Ogden CL, Curtin LR. Prevalence and trends in obesity among US adults, 1999–2008. JAMA. 2010;303:235–41.
18. Greene AK, Grant FD, Slavin SA. Lower extremity lymphedema and elevated body mass in obese patients. N Engl J Med. 2012;366:2136–7.
19. Brorson H, Ohlin K, Olsson G, Karlsson MK. Breast cancer-related chronic arm lymphedema is associated with excess adipose and muscle tissue. Lymphat Res Biol. 2009;7:3–10.
20. Fu MR, Ridner SH, Hu SH, Stewart BR, Cormier JN, Armer JM. Psychosocial impact of lymphedema: a

systematic review of literature from 2004–2011. Psychooncology. 2013;22:1466–84.

21. Farshid G, Weiss SW. Massive localized lymphedema in the morbidly obese: a histologically distinct reactive lesion simulating liposarcoma. Am J Surg Pathol. 1998;10:1277–83.

22. Chopra K, Tadisina KK, Brewer M, Holton LH, Banda AK, Singh DP. Massive localized lymphedema revisited: a quickly rising complication of the obesity epidemic. Ann Plast Surg. 2015;74:126–32.

23. Brorson H, Ohlin K, Olsson G, Langstrom G, Wiklund I, Svensson H. Quality of life following liposuction and conservative treatment of arm lymphedema. Lymphology. 2006;39:8–25.

24. Sharma A, Schwartz RA. Stewart-Treves syndrome: pathogenesis and management. J Am Acad Dermatol. 2012;67:1342–8.

Myths Associated with Lymphedema

Arin K. Greene

5

Key Points
- Many myths about lymphedema exist.
- Limited randomized, prospective evidence about the clinical management of lymphedema is available.
- Any treatment recommendations must be made based on the best evidence available.
- Strong evidence has to support interventions that would negatively impact the patient's quality of life.
- Further study is necessary to definitively support or refute myths about lymphedema.

Introduction

Although lymphedema is a common condition, it is poorly understood and few physicians are focused on this disease. The lack of interest in lymphedema among health care providers is multifactorial. First, the disease typically is not covered during medical school or residency. Second, lymphedema does not fit easily into a specific medical discipline. Finally, because the disease is chronic and not curable, it may be less attractive to physicians.

A.K. Greene, M.D., M.M.Sc. (✉)
Department of Plastic and Oral Surgery,
Boston Children's Hospital, Harvard Medical School,
300 Longwood Avenue, Boston, MA 02115, USA
e-mail: arin.greene@childrens.harvard.edu

Lymphedema is not well-understood or popular among health care providers; thus, evidence-based management is minimal. Perhaps no disease has as many myths associated with it as does lymphedema. The less something is understood, the greater the risk that "superstitions" will be associated with it. Treatment of patients with lymphedema is primarily based on retrospective studies, extrapolation from other conditions (e.g., venous insufficiency), and physician expertise (i.e., Level 3–5 evidence) (Table 5.1) [1]. Consequently, when managing individuals with lymphedema the best available practices should be followed.

Many myths about lymphedema do not have evidence to support them. Some misconceptions can be harmful to patients because they might significantly inhibit their quality of life. For example, I met a patient in our Lymphedema Clinic in Boston who had lymphedema for 20 years. She drove to the appointment from San Diego because she was told that flying would worsen her lymphedema. She had not travelled on an airplane since the time of her diagnosis. Although I could not cure her lymphedema, I improved her quality of life by informing her that there was not convincing evidence that flying would worsen her lymphedema. In this chapter I address the most common potential myths about lymphedema that I have encountered in my practice (Table 5.2).

A.K. Greene et al. (eds.), *Lymphedema: Presentation, Diagnosis, and Treatment*,
DOI 10.1007/978-3-319-14493-1_5, © Springer International Publishing Switzerland 2015

Table 5.1 Levels of evidence for clinical research studies

Level	Definition
1	Randomized controlled prospective study
	Meta-analysis of randomized trials
2	Non-randomized controlled prospective study
	Prospective cohort study
3	Observational study (e.g., case–control study)
4	Retrospective study without controls (e.g., case-series)
5	Expert opinion

Table 5.2 Common lymphedema myths

Airplanes worsen lymphedema
Avoid injections into a lymphedematous extremity
Avoid blood pressure measurements in a lymphedematous extremity
Blunt trauma causes lymphedema
Certain foods can worsen lymphedema
Diuretics improve lymphedema
Do not exercise a limb with lymphedema
Extreme temperature may worsen lymphedema
Lymphedema occurs immediately following an insult to the lymphatic system
Operating on a lymphedematous extremity is contraindicated

Myths Associated with Lymphedema

Airplanes Worsen Lymphedema

It has been postulated that airplane flight might initiate lymphedema in patients at risk for the disease, or exacerbate the condition [2]. The proposed mechanism is low cabin pressures and/or reduced activity. However, both retrospective [3] and prospective [4, 5] studies have showed that air travel does not negatively affect lymphedema.

Avoid Injections into a Lymphedematous Extremity

Injections and venipuncture generally are avoided in an extremity with lymphedema because of the concern that these interventions will: (1) cause

cellulitis and/or (2) worsen the patient's lymphedema. Although incidental cuts are much more likely to cause cellulitis in a patient with lymphedema, *sterily* breaking the skin does not increase the risk of infection [1, 5, 6]. For example, cellulitis from venipuncture in a limb with lymphedema has never been reported [6]. Lymphangiography, which necessitates a sterile incision to access lymphatics for dye injection, did not cause an infection in 32,000 lymphangiograms [7]. Injections of radiolabelled colloid during lymphoscintigraphy do not cause cellulitis [8]. Sterile incisions during resection of lymphedematous tissue also are not associated with infection. Liposuction, which requires as many as twenty 1 cm incisions, is not complicated by infection and reduces the risk of cellulitis [9]. After staged skin and subcutaneous excision, which includes long incisions from the hand/foot to the axilla/groin, patients have a reduced incidence of cellulitis [10]. A prospective study did not find an association between needle sticks and lymphedema in breast cancer survivors [5]. Although no evidence exists that sterily penetrating lymphedematous skin worsens the disease or is harmful to the patient, it is reasonable to use the non-diseased limb when possible. Patients with bilateral disease can be reassured that injections or venipuncture in one of their affected limbs is not harmful to them.

Avoid Blood Pressure Measurements in a Lymphedematous Extremity

Many health care providers are hesitant to perform blood pressure measurements on patients with lymphedema or who are at risk for the disease because of the possibility that the pressure from the cuff will damage lymphatics. However, no evidence exists that using a blood pressure cuff increases the likelihood of lymphedema or worsens the disease. In fact, a blood pressure cuff might be beneficial to patients because pressure is the primary method used to treat a lymphedematous extremity (e.g., multilayer bandaging, massage, custom-made garments, pneumatic pumps).

Compression garments can exert pressures up to 80 mmHg, while pneumatic pumps emit a force up to 150 mmHg [6]. These compression modalities have been shown to be safe and significantly improve lymphedema [9, 11].

Additional evidence contradicting the possibility that blood pressure measurements are harmful to an extremity at risk for lymphedema is derived from data on extremity tourniquets. Tourniquets exert pressures of 250–350 mmHg to occlude all blood in an extremity (arterial, venous, lymphatic) for periods of up to 2 h without any evidence of lymphatic injury [12]. In addition, tourniquets are used during suction-assisted lipectomy to remove lymphedematous tissue [9] and have not caused lymphedema in patients at risk of developing lymphedema (i.e., have a history of lymph node dissection) [12]. If hours of using a pneumatic pump, months of continuous wearing of pressure garments, and tourniquet use are not harmful to the lymphedematous limb, then sporadic blood pressure readings will not cause injury either. A prospective study also has shown that blood pressure measurements do not increase the risk of lymphedema in women who have been treated for breast cancer [5]. Pressure from the blood pressure cuff may even improve lymph drainage proximal to the site of application.

Blunt Trauma Causes Lymphedema

Patients with lymphedema often associate an incidental blunt trauma with the onset of their disease. It may be possible that blunt trauma may expedite the onset of lymphedema in an individual who would have otherwise presented later with the condition. However, it is very unlikely that blunt trauma can result in lymphedema because secondary lymphedema is hard to cause. For example, even after removing axillary lymph nodes and radiating the area, only 1/3 of women with breast cancer develop upper extremity lymphedema [13]. Unlike blunt trauma, a penetrating injury to the axillary or inguinal

area could severe lymphatic vessels and nodes resulting in lymphedema; although the risk would be much lower than lymphadenectomy or radiation. Blunt traumas to extremities are very common and thus are likely to be temporarily related to the onset of lymphedema from another cause.

Certain Foods Can Worsen Lymphedema

No evidence exists that a certain diet is beneficial or harmful to patients with lymphedema [14]. Consequently, individuals are educated that they may eat any type of food as well as drink alcohol [5]. However, diet might indirectly affect lymphedema because obesity can increase the risk of developing the disease or cause the condition [15, 16]. Patients are advised to maintain a normal body mass index because obesity causes inflammation, which damages lymphatic vessels and worsens lymphedema [17]. Obese patients, or individuals at risk for obesity, are referred to a dietician or surgical weight loss center.

Diuretics Improve Lymphedema

Patients with lymphedema are often prescribed diuretics because of the misconception that patients have a "fluid" overload problem. Eight percent of patients referred to our center with lymphedema have been treated with a diuretic [18]. Unlike congestive heart failure, lymphedema is not caused by excess systemic fluid. Instead, high-protein fluid is located outside of the vasculature in the interstitial space. Consequently, diuretics (or fluid restriction by diet) will not improve lymphedema. Diuretics may worsen lymphedema by increasing the osmotic gradient between the vasculature and interstitial space; these drugs also can cause electrolyte abnormalities for patients. Diuretics or fluid restriction is not recommended for peripheral lymphedema by the International Society of Lymphology [14].

Do Not Exercise a Limb with Lymphedema

One of the most common misconceptions about lymphedema is that using the extremity will worsen the condition, possibly by increasing blood flow to the limb and thus lymph production [5]. Instead, the opposite is true. One of the primary forces propelling lymph fluid proximally is muscle contraction. Using the extremity facilitates lymph transport. Exercise has been shown to be beneficial for lymphedema in multiple randomized, prospective trials [5, 19–21]. In contrast, inactivity and muscle atrophy may predispose an individual to lymphedema and worsen the condition. For example, patients with myelomenigocele have an increased risk of idiopathic lymphedema compared to the rest of the population. In addition, obese individuals with minimal mobility and who have difficulty exercising also are at increased risk for developing lymphedema. Another benefit of exercise to patients with lymphedema is that it helps them maintain a normal body weight because elevated body mass index can worsen their condition [16]. Exercise also is beneficial to the patient's overall health, psychological well-being, and quality of life.

Extreme Temperature May Worsen Lymphedema

Some organizations advocate that patients who are at risk for lymphedema should avoid hot or cold temperature extremes. However, evidence suggests that heat does not increase the risk for lymphedema and may even improve the condition. For example, following severe burn injuries, less than 1 % of patients develop extremity lymphedema [22]. Application of heat to lymphedematous extremities has been shown to reduce extremity volume in patients with lymphedema [23]. It has been hypothesized that heating might create an immune response, change the extracellular matrix, and reduce edema [24]. Prospective evidence shows that exercise in warm weather, travel to a hot environment, submerging in a heated bath, and skin burns do not increase the risk of lymphedema

[5]. Sauna use has been associated with the development of lymphedema; although this finding is confounded, because patients who used a sauna also had more cuts on their arm [5] I currently recommend that patients avoid sauna use.

Lymphedema Occurs Immediately Following an Insult to the Lymphatic System

One misconception about secondary lymphedema is that its onset occurs shortly after the insult to the lymphatic system. In fact, edema presents at a median time of 11 months following injury to lymphatics [25]. Three-fourths of patients develop swelling within 3 years after the injury, and the risk of lymphedema is 1 % each year thereafter [26].

Operating on a Lymphedematous Extremity is Contraindicated

Opponents of operative intervention for lymphedema claim that a surgical procedure can damage functioning lymphatics and worsen the disease. However, both excisional (e.g., liposuction, staged skin/subcutaneous excision) and physiologic (e.g., lymphatic–venous anastomosis, lymph node transfer) procedures not only have been shown to not be harmful but may improve lymphatic flow. Lymphoscinitigraphy after staged skin and subcutaneous excision has shown improved lymphatic flow by lymphoscintigraphy [10]. Removal of excess subcutaneous adipose tissue likely reduces the amount of lymph fluid that is produced and improves drainage of lymph through the subfascial compartment. Lymphoscintigraphy following suction assisted lipectomy has shown that not only is lymphatic function not worsened [27], but cutaneous blood flow is increased and the risk of infection is reduced [9, 28]. Excisional procedures increase cutaneous blood flow to the skin by the delay phenomenon, thus likely improving the condition. Physiologic procedures also have not been shown to be harmful to a lymphedematous extremity; in some cases improvement in lymphatic flow by lymphoscintigraphy has been shown [29].

Conclusions

Despite its wide prevalence, lymphedema remains a poorly understood condition, and thus, many myths about the disease exist. Because Level 1 clinical evidence is limited, management strategies made to patients often are based on the provider's expert opinion (Level 5 evidence). Interventions for patients must be made based on the best evidence available. Before advising a patient of a strategy that might negatively impact their quality of life (e.g., do not fly on an airplane, do not exercise the limb), strong evidence must support the recommendation.

References

1. Cemal Y, Pusic A, Mehrara BJ. Preventative measures for lymphedema: separating fact from fiction. J Am Coll Surg. 2011;213:543–51.
2. Casley-Smith JR. Lymphedema initiated by aircraft flights. Aviat Space Environ Med. 1996;67:52–6.
3. Graham PH. Compression prophylaxis may increase the potential for flight-associated lymphedema after breast cancer treatment. Breast. 2002;11:66–71.
4. Kilbreath SL, Ward LC, Lane K, McNeely M, Dylke ES, Refshauge KM, McKenzie D, Lee MJ, Peddle C, Battersby KJ. Effect of air travel on lymphedema risk in women with history of breast cancer. Breast Cancer Res Treat. 2010;120:649–54.
5. Showalter SL, Brown JC, Cheville AL, Fisher CS, Sataloff D, Schmitz KH. Lifestyle risk factors associated with arm swelling among women with breast cancer. Ann Surg Oncol. 2013;20:842–9.
6. Greene AK, Borud L, Slavin SA. Blood pressure monitoring and venipuncture in the lymphedematous extremity. Plast Reconstr Surg. 2005;116:2058–9.
7. Koehler PR. Complications of lymphography. Lymphology. 1968;1:116–20.
8. Gloviczki P, Calcagno D, Schirger A, Pairolero PC, Cherry KJ, Hallett JW, Wahner HW. Noninvasive evaluation of the swollen extremity: experiences with 190 lymphoscintigraphic examinations. J Vasc Surg. 1989;9:683–9.
9. Brorson H, Svensson H. Liposuction combined with controlled compression therapy reduces arm lymphedema more effectively than controlled compression therapy alone. Plast Reconstr Surg. 1998;102:1058–67.
10. Miller TA, Wyatt LE, Rudkin GH. Staged skin and subcutaneous excision for lymphedema: a favorable report of long-term results. Plast Reconstr Surg. 1998;102:1486–98.
11. Johansson K, Lie E, Ekdahl C, Lindfeldt JA. Randomized study comparing manual lymph drainage with sequential pneumatic compression for treatment of postoperative arm lymphedema. Lymphology. 1998;31:56–64.
12. Dawson WJ, Elenz DR, Winchester DP, Feldman JL. Elective hand surgery in the breast cancer patient with prior ipsilateral axillary dissection. Ann Surg Oncol. 1995;2:132–7.
13. Gärtner R, Mejdahl MK, Andersen KG, Ewertz M, Kroman N. Development in self-reported arm-lymphedema in Danish women treated for early-stage breast cancer in 2005 and 2006 - a nationwide follow-up study. Breast. 2014;23:445. doi:10.1016/j.breast.2014.03.001. pii: S0960-9776(14)00042-3.
14. International Society of Lymphology. The diagnosis and treatment of peripheral lymphedema: 2013 consensus document of the International Society of Lymphology. Lymphology. 2013;46:1–11.
15. Ahmed RL, Schmitz KH, Prizment AE, Folsom AR. Risk factors for lymphedema in breast cancer survivors, the Iowa women's health study. Breast Cancer Res Treat. 2011;130:981–91.
16. Greene AK, Grant FD, Slavin SA. Lower-extremity lymphedema and elevated body-mass index. N Engl J Med. 2012;366:2136–7.
17. Savetsky IL, Torrisi JS, Cuzzone DA, Ghanta S, Albano NJ, Gardenier JC, Joseph WJ, Mehrara BJ. Obesity increases inflammation and impairs lymphatic function in a mouse model of lymphedema. Am J Physiol Heart Circ Physiol. 2014;307:H165.
18. Maclellan RA, Couto RA, Sullivan JE, Grant FD, Slavin SA, Greene AK. Management of primary and secondary lymphedema: analysis of 225 referrals to a center. Ann Plast Surg. 2014 (in press).
19. Schmitz KH, Ahmed RL, Troxel A, Cheville A, Smith R, Lewis-Grant L, Bryan CJ, Williams-Smith CT, Greene QP. Weight lifting in women with breast-cancer-related lymphedema. N Engl J Med. 2009;361:664–73.
20. Schmitz KH, Ahmed RL, Troxel AB, Cheville A, Lewis-Grant L, Smith R, Bryan CJ, Williams-Smith CT, Chittams J. Weight lifting for women at risk for breast cancer-related lymphedema: a randomized trial. JAMA. 2010;304:2699–705.
21. Brown JC, John GM, Segal S, Chu CS, Schmitz KH. Physical activity and lower limb lymphedema among uterine cancer survivors. Med Sci Sports Exerc. 2013;45:2091–7.
22. Hettrick H, Nof L, Ward S, Ecthernach J. Incidence and prevalence of lymphedema in patients following

burn injury: a five-year retrospective and three-month prospective study. Lymph Res Biol. 2004;2:11–24.

23. Gan JL, Li SL, Cai RX, Chang TS. Microwave heating in the management of postmastectomy upper limb lymphedema. Ann Plast Surg. 1996;36:576–80.

24. Liu NF, Olszewski W. The influence of local hyperthermia on lymphedema and lymphedematous skin of the human leg. Lymphology. 1993;26:28–37.

25. Togawa K, Ma H, Sullivan-Halley J, Neuhouser ML, Imayama I, Baumgartner KB, Wilder Smith A, Alfano CM, McTiernan A, Ballard-Barbash R, Bernstein L. Risk factors for self-reported arm lymphedema among female breast cancer survivors: a prospective cohort study. Breast Cancer Res. 2014;16(4):414.

26. Petrek JA, Senie RT, Peters M, Rosen PP. Lymphedema in a cohort of breast carcinoma survivors 20 years after diagnosis. Cancer. 2001;92:1368–77.

27. Brorson H, Svensson H, Norrgren K, Thorsson O. Liposuction reduces arm lymphedema without significantly altering the already impaired lymph transport. Lymphology. 1998;31:156–72.

28. Brorson H, Svensson H. Skin blood flow of the lymphedematous arm before and after liposuction. Lymphology. 1997;30:165–72.

29. Becker C, Vasile JV, Levine JL, Batista BN, Studinger RM, Chen CM, Riquet M. Microlymphatic surgery for the treatment of iatrogenic lymphedema. Clin Plast Surg. 2012;39:385–98.

The Lymphedema Center and Multidisciplinary Management

6

Arin K. Greene, Sumner A. Slavin, and Håkan Brorson

Key Points

- Lymphedema is a complex problem, and few physicians focus on the disease.
- Patients with lymphedema often feel isolated because they have difficulty finding a provider who understands their condition and can treat them.
- Plastic surgeons and compression experts are necessary components of a Lymphedema Center.
- More than one specialist is often needed to treat a patient with lymphedema.
- Individuals with lymphedema are best managed in a multidisciplinary Lymphedema Center.

A.K. Greene, M.D., M.MSc. (✉)
Department of Plastic and Oral Surgery, Boston Children's Hospital, Harvard Medical School, 300 Longwood Avenue, Boston, MA 02115, USA
e-mail: arin.greene@childrens.harvard.edu

S.A. Slavin, M.D.
Division of Plastic Surgery, Beth Israel Deaconess Medical Center, Harvard Medical School, Boston, MA, USA

H. Brorson, M.D., Ph.D.
Department of Clinical Sciences, Lund University, Malmö, Sweden

Plastic and Reconstructive Surgery, Skåne University Hospital, Malmö, Sweden

Introduction

Lymphedema is a complicated medical condition that is poorly understood. Few physicians care for patients with lymphedema and the condition is associated with many myths. Patients often are misdiagnosed, undergo unnecessary tests, and are managed incorrectly. For example, 25 % of individuals referred to our Lymphedema Center with "lymphedema" do not have the disease [1, 2]. One-third of patients sent to our Lymphedema Center previously had undergone tests that were non-diagnostic for lymphedema; 8 % had been treated erroneously with a diuretic [2].

"Lymphedema" often is used as a generic term to describe any condition that causes extremity overgrowth; incorrect diagnosis can lead to incorrect management [1, 3]. We believe patients with lymphedema are best managed in an interdisciplinary Lymphedema Center. Because the disease does not fit easily into one medical specialty, individuals usually require multiple providers. In this chapter we present our patient care model and current treatment algorithm.

Lymphedena Center

Patients with lymphedema typically are medical nomads, being referred from provider to provider until they find someone who can manage their

A.K. Greene et al. (eds.), *Lymphedema: Presentation, Diagnosis, and Treatment*, DOI 10.1007/978-3-319-14493-1_6, © Springer International Publishing Switzerland 2015

condition. One-third of patients treated in our Lymphedema Center reside outside of our referral area [2]. Our clinic meets monthly and is directed by plastic surgeons. New patient visits are scheduled for 1 h and they are initially seen by the plastic surgeon. Next, they undergo standardized photography as well as limb measurements by a physician's assistant or nurse. Individuals then are seen by a compression garment specialist and fitted for garments. In Boston patients also are measured for a pneumatic compression device. Individuals who are being considered for operative intervention undergo water displacement to most accurately determine the volume of their diseased extremity (Fig. 6.1).

All patients undergo lymphoscintigraphy to determine their lymphatic function. Patients who reside outside of our region have their lymphoscintigram performed at our institution the day before their scheduled appointment. We have a standard lymphoscintigraphy protocol (images at 45 min, 2 h, 4 h). The use of a consistent protocol enables us to compare patients as well as follow the same individual longitudinally. We have found that when patients undergo lymphoscintigraphy at outside institutions the test often is not performed properly or is difficult to interpret (e.g., only a 2 h image is taken). We prefer to obtain a lymphoscintigram for most patients because it definitively diagnoses the condition. In addition, the test gives a subjective measure of the severity of lymphedema in patients who likely have the condition. For example, an individual who has transit to the inguinal nodes by 2 h and no dermal backflow would be considered to have "mild" lymphatic dysfunction, whereas a patient with no tracer in the inguinal nodes by 4 h and dermal backflow would be labeled as "severe" dysfunction. Patients with worse lymphoscintigraphic findings are counseled that their prognosis may be less favorable and that they should be vigilant with conservative interventions.

All individuals evaluated in our Lymphedema Center are entered into a database to facilitate research. Using this strategy, we have been able to publish demographic data on patients referred to a Lymphedema Center as well as characterize the disease *obesity-induced lymphedema* [1–6]. Collecting patients in regional referral centers allows retrospective and prospective clinical

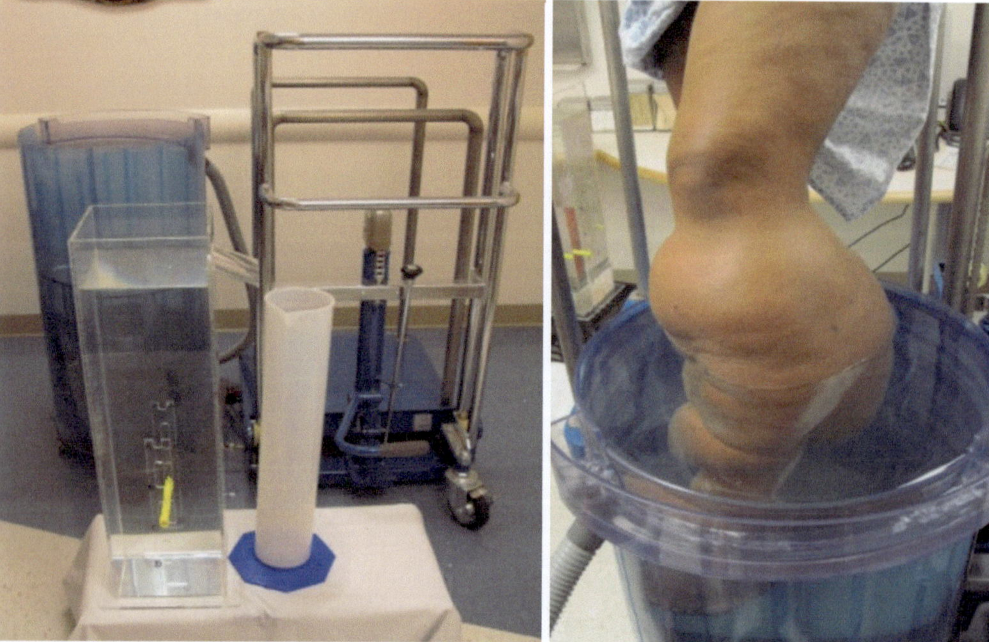

Fig. 6.1 Measurement of limb volumes using water displacement

research studies to be performed. In addition, insights into the condition are more easily formed when patients are concentrated among specific providers. Our database also has allowed us to help patients contact other individuals with lymphedema who reside in their area. Often individuals obtain psychological benefit from speaking or meeting with others who share their disease (particularly in the pediatric population).

Interdisciplinary Management

Although many types of specialists care for patients with lymphedema, plastic surgeons have been particularly involved in patient management because they are most capable of providing surgical intervention. Currently performed physiologic procedures (i.e., lymphatic–venous anastomosis, lymph vessel transplantation, lymph node transfer) require the microsurgical expertise of plastic surgeons. Excisional procedures that are carried out (i.e., liposuction, staged skin/subcutaneous excision, Charles procedure) also require plastic surgical training.

A Lymphedema Center should be staffed by a plastic surgeon capable of providing operative intervention if necessary (Table 6.1). Compression experts must participate as well (e.g., rehabilitation medicine physician, physical therapist, occupational therapist, physician assistant, and/or nurse). Our clinic in Boston is staffed by a compression garment specialist who measures, fits,

Table 6.1 Multidisciplinary lymphedema center specialists

Plastic surgeon
Compression garment expert (rehabilitation medicine, physical therapy, physician assistant, nurse)
Pneumatic compression expert
Nuclear medicine physician
Radiologist
Bariatric surgeon
Infectious disease physician
Specialists to rule out other causes of extremity edema (orthopedic surgeon, vascular surgeon, internist, pediatrician, rheumatologist)

and troubleshoots garments during the patient's appointment. In addition, we have a pneumatic compression expert who teaches pneumatic compression to patients during their visit.

Our multidisciplinary clinic in Boston also involves the following specialties who do not attend the clinic: nuclear medicine, radiology, bariatric surgery, and infectious disease. We have a close collaboration with our nuclear medicine department with whom we have developed our lymphoscintigraphy protocol. An interventional radiologist with expertise in the field of vascular anomalies is available to review imaging (e.g., MRI, CT, ultrasound) to diagnose patients who have normal lymphoscintigraphy. Patients with obesity-induced lymphedema, or at risk for the disease, are referred to our bariatric surgical collaborator. Individuals with >3 infections a year, or who are at risk for having filariasis, are referred to our infectious disease colleagues.

Current Treatment Algorithm

Almost all patients referred to our Lymphedema Center undergo lymphoscintigraphy to determine whether they have the disease and, if so, the severity of the condition (Fig. 6.2). Patients are prescribed compression garments as well as pneumatic compression. Management of patients diagnosed with lymphedema begins with patient education. Individuals are counseled about activities of daily living that may help or worsen their condition (e.g., exercise the affected extremity and avoid trauma). Often we answer questions regarding myths about lymphedema that can significantly improve the patient's quality of life (e.g., the individual can eat any type of food, take a warm bath, exercise (Nordic pole walking or running).

After counseling a patient with lymphedema about his/her condition, we initiate conservative compression strategies. We advocate that custom-fitted compression garments should be worn continuously. We also recommend pneumatic compression for 2 h each day if possible. The authors do not routinely use lymphatic

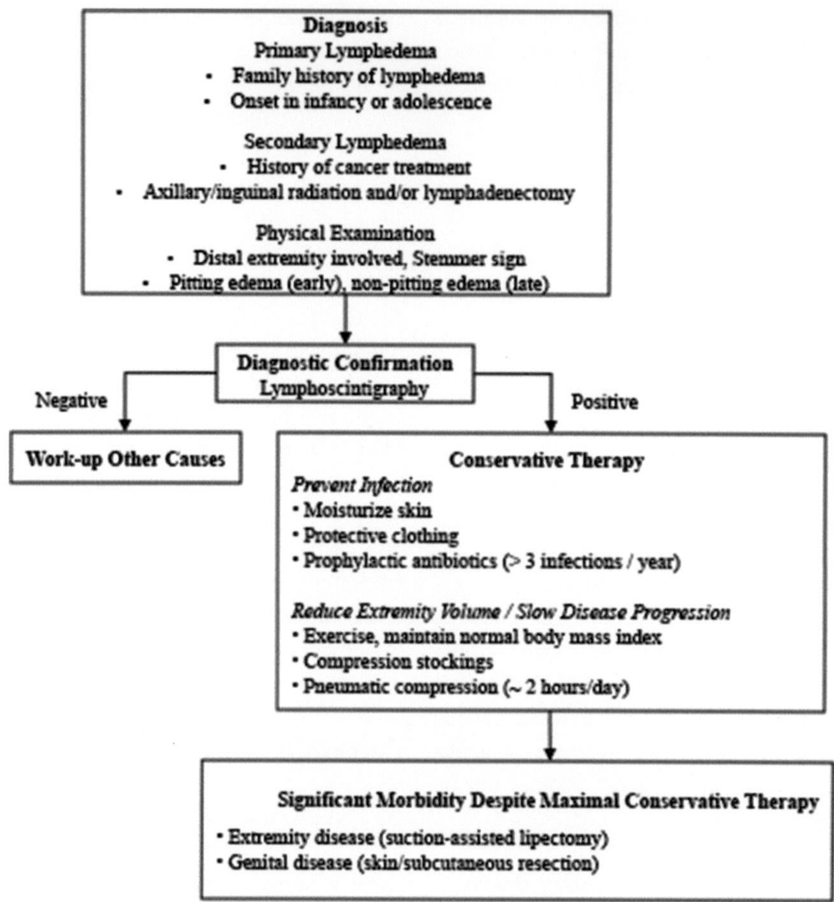

Fig. 6.2 Current lymphedema management algorithm used by the authors

massage or combination compressive regimens (e.g., complex decongestive therapy), although these modalities can be effective. Compared to complex decongestive regimens, compression garments and pneumatic compression are easier for the patient and can be done at their convenience in their home.

Approximately 95 % of our patients are able to be managed conservatively without operative intervention. Indications for surgical treatment include failure of conservative measures and repeated infection, difficulty using the extremity, and/or significant psychosocial morbidity. The authors favor excisional procedures over physiologic operations because we believe the results are most predictable and patients with severe disease are candidates. Our first-line operation for lymphedema is suction-assisted lipectomy (liposuction). Individuals with genital disease or very severe extremity lymphedema are managed by staged skin/subcutaneous excision.

Patients referred to our center that have a normal lymphoscintigram and are thought to have a condition other than lymphedema undergo further evaluation. Individuals with venous insufficiency are referred to a vascular surgeon. Typically, if we are unsure of the cause of the patient's swelling, we will obtain an MRI. MRI will illustrate whether or not the patient has a vascular malformation (e.g., Klippel–Trénaunay syndrome, venous malformation, lymphatic malformation) or an underlying orthopedic process (e.g., synovitis, ligament sprain, occult fracture). Individuals with suspected systemic fluid overload (e.g., cardiac, renal, hepatic pathology) are referred to their primary care physician. Occasionally, patients with a possible rheumatological process are sent to a rheumatologist.

Conclusions

Lymphedema is a poorly understood condition and patients often are misdiagnosed, managed incorrectly, and feel isolated. Individuals with this disease should be treated by providers focused on their condition. Because a single specialist can rarely manage a patient with lymphedema, individuals are treated in a multidisciplinary center where they can be diagnosed, educated, and managed both conservatively and operatively. Concentrating patients in regional centers also improves their condition by facilitating research.

References

1. Schook CC, Mulliken JB, Fishman SJ, Alomari AI, Greene AK. Differential diagnosis of lower extremity lymphedema in 170 pediatric patients. Plastic Reconstr Surg. 2011;127:1571–81.
2. Maclellan RA, Couto RA, Sullivan JE, Grant FD, Slavin SA, Greene AK. Management of primary and secondary lymphedema: analysis of 225 referrals to a center. Ann Plast Surg. Accessed 8 Apr 2014. [Epub ahead of print].
3. Hassanein A, Mulliken JB, Fishman SJ, Greene AK. Evaluation of terminology for vascular anomalies in current literature. Plastic Reconstr Surg. 2011;127: 347–51.
4. Schook CC, Mulliken JB, Fishman SJ, Grant F, Zurakowski D, Greene AK. Primary lymphedema: clinical features and management in 138 pediatric patients. Plast Reconstr Surg. 2011;127:2419–31.
5. Greene AK, Grant FD, Slavin SA. Lower-extremity lymphedema and elevated body-mass index. N Engl J Med. 2012;366:2136–7.
6. Greene AK, Grant F, Slavin SA, Maclellan RA. Obesity-induced lymphedema: clinical and lymphoscintigraphic features. Plastic Reconstr Surg (in press).

Part II

Classification of Lymphedema

Primary Lymphedema

7

Arin K. Greene

Key Points

- Primary lymphedema is a rare condition, affecting approximately 1/100,000 persons.
- Lymphoscintigraphy confirms the disease and illustrates the degree of lymphatic dysfunction.
- Patients are encouraged to maintain a normal body mass index, exercise, and engage in all activities.
- The mainstay of treatment is compression.
- Operative intervention is rarely necessary; our preferred method is suction-assisted lipectomy.

Introduction

Lymphedema is divided by etiology into *primary* and *secondary* disease [1]. Primary lymphedema is idiopathic and results from an error in lymphatic development. Secondary lymphedema is acquired and caused by injury to a normally developed lymphatic system. Primary lymphedema is rare, affecting approximately 1/100,000 children [2]. In the pediatric population idiopathic lymphedema is responsible for the disease in 97 % of patients who do not reside in areas endemic for filariasis [3]. Secondary lymphedema is rare in children (<3 % of cases), but is responsible for the disease in 99 % of adults with the condition [3]. The most common cause of secondary lymphedema worldwide is a parasitic infection (e.g., *Wuchereria bancrofti, Brungia malayi, Brugia timori*). In developed countries, secondary lymphedema usually results from treatment for malignancy (e.g., axillary/inguinal lymphadenectomy and/or radiation).

Regardless of whether a patient has primary or secondary lymphedema, the subsequent pathophysiology of the condition is equivalent. Over time, the diseased area increases in size because the interstitial lymphatic fluid causes adipose deposition [4, 5]. The term "lymphedema" is often used to describe an overgrown limb in a child, regardless of the underlying etiology [6, 7]. Consequently, it is important to accurately diagnose a patient with primary lymphedema so that the individual is managed correctly.

Etiopathogenesis

Genetic Causes

The majority of patients with primary lymphedema have a sporadic disease with an unknown somatic mutation However, several germ-line mutations can cause primary lymphedema: e.g., *VEGFR3* (Milroy), *FOXC2* (lymphedema–distichiasis), *SOX18* (hypotrichosis–telangiectasia–lymphedema), *CCBE1* (Hennekam) (Table 7.1). *VEFGR3* mutations typically are autosomal

A.K. Greene, M.D., M.MSc. (✉)
Department of Plastic and Oral Surgery,
Boston Children's Hospital, Harvard Medical School,
300 Longwood Avenue, Boston, MA 02115, USA
e-mail: arin.greene@childrens.harvard.edu

A.K. Greene et al. (eds.), *Lymphedema: Presentation, Diagnosis, and Treatment,*
DOI 10.1007/978-3-319-14493-1_7, © Springer International Publishing Switzerland 2015

Table 7.1 Lymphedema syndromes with known genetic mutations

Condition	Gene	Inheritance
Familial congenital primary lymphedema (Milroy)	*VEGFR3*	Dominant/recessive
Lymphedema–distichiasis	*FOXC2*	Dominant
Lymphedema–hypotrichosis–telangiectasia	*SOX18*	Dominant/recessive
Hennekam syndrome	*CCBE1*	Dominant/recessive
Noonan syndrome	*PTPN11/SOS1*	Dominant
Turner syndrome	*XO*	Sex-linked

dominant, but recessive transmission also can occur. *FOXC2* is autosomal dominant, *SOX18* can be dominant or recessive, and *CCBE1* can be dominant or recessive [8]. Also, patients with Noonan syndrome (*PTPN11/SOS1*) and Turner syndrome (*XO*) also can have lymphedema [8].

Table 7.2 Clinical progression of lymphedema

Stage	Definition
0	No edema clinically, but abnormal lymphatic function
1	Early edema that reverses with limb elevation
2	Pitting edema, not reversible with limb elevation
3	Fibroadipose deposition, skin changes

Morphology of Lymphatics

Primary lymphedema is a type of lymphatic malformation. Malformed lymphatic vessels in an extremity or genitalia cause accumulation of protein-rich fluid in the interstitial space. Kinmonth used lymphangiography to describe the lymphatic morphology of primary lymphedema as hypoplasia/aplasia (89 %) or hyperplasia (11 %) [9]. The maldeveloped lymphatics do not have the capacity to return interstitial fluid to the venous circulation, which causes lymphedema.

Progression of Lymphedema

Fifty-eight percent of patients with primary lymphedema exhibit progression of their disease (i.e., increased volume or symptoms) [3]. Patients with unilateral lower extremity lymphedema have a 9–25 % risk of ultimately developing the condition in their contralateral extremity [3, 9]. Lymphedema progresses through 4 stages (Table 7.2) [10]. *Stage 0* indicates a normal extremity clinically, but with abnormal lymph transport (i.e., illustrated by lymphoscintigraphy). *Stage 1* is early edema which improves with limb elevation. *Stage 2* represents pitting edema not resolved with elevation. *Stage 3* describes fibroadipose deposition and skin changes [10].

In the latent phase (*Stage 0*) the patient is unaware of his/her lymphatic dysfunction. Compensatory mechanisms, such as increased macrophage activity and spontaneous lymphaticovenous shunts, prevent swelling until lymphatic transport has been significantly reduced. Over time, pitting edema becomes non-pitting because the high-protein fluid in the interstitial space causes inflammation, fibrosis, and progressive adipose deposition [4, 5, 10]. The extremity continues to enlarge primarily because of adipogenesis. This cycle further damages functioning lymphatics. Fat in an extremity can increase by 73 % [5].

Clinical Features

Onset

Primary lymphedema can present during: (1) infancy, (2) childhood, (3) adolescence, or (4) adulthood. Although patients with primary lymphedema have malformed lymphatics at birth, individuals often develop swelling after infancy. Similar to adults with secondary lymphedema following lymph node removal and/or

Table 7.3 Onset of primary lymphedema

Historical classification		Current developmental classification	
Age of onset	Definition	Age of onset	Definition
Congenital	At birth	Infancy	Birth-1 Year
	Birth-3 months		
	Birth-1 year		
	Birth-2 years		
Praecox	Birth-35 years	Childhood	1–9 Years
	After birth-24 years	Adolescence	10–21 Years
	After birth-35 years		
	4 Months-20 years		
	1–35 Years		
Tarda	After 20 years	Adulthood	>21 Years
	After 35 years		

radiation, an interval exists between the onset of malfunctioning lymphatics and swelling. Fluid leaking out of the venous circulation is unable to be returned by the lymphatic vasculature. The high-protein interstitial fluid causes inflammation and further injures functioning lymphatics until edema is noticed clinically. Other factors, such as hormones, may influence the onset of lymphedema. For example, females most commonly present with the disease in adolescence.

Primary lymphedema traditionally has been divided according to the age of the patient when the swelling develops: "congenital," "praecox," or "tarda" [1]. This classification system is neither standardized nor precise, and the terms have been applied inconsistently (Table 7.3) [3, 11]. For example, "congenital" lymphedema is used if swelling was noted at birth, "shortly after birth," birth to 3 months, birth to 1 year, or birth to 2 years. Thus, some authors would consider a 6-month-old infant presenting with lymphedema to be "congenital," whereas others would label it "praecox." A "congenital" anomaly may not present at birth (a child or adolescent who develops primary lymphedema was born with malformed lymphatics). "Praecox" is synonymous with "early" and relative to another time point; it does not identify an age range. A 1-day-old child with "congenital" lymphedema is "praecox" to a 1 month-old infant with lymphedema (although both would be labeled "congenital"). Similarly, "tarda" is used to describe "late" onset lymphedema, but a 1-month-old child is "tarda" to a 1-day-old neonate with congenital swelling.

Developmental terminology should be used to define the onset of primary lymphedema: *infancy, childhood, adolescence, or adulthood* [3, 11]. These periods are defined and their use will facilitate communication and research.

In the pediatric population onset occurs in infancy (49.2 %), childhood (9.5 %), or adolescence (41.3 %) (Fig. 7.1) [3]. Primary lymphedema develops during adulthood in 19 % of patients (Fig. 7.2) [9]. Males are more likely to present in infancy (68 %), while females most commonly develop the disease during adolescence (55 %) [3]. The lower extremities are affected in 91.7 % of patients; 50 % have unilateral lymphedema and 50 % have bilateral disease [3]. Eighteen percent have genital lymphedema, which is usually associated with lower extremity lymphedema. Four percent of patients with primary lymphedema have isolated genital involvement. Sixteen percent of children with idiopathic lymphedema have upper extremity disease [3]. Rarely, a child can have lymphedema affecting the legs, genitalia, and/or arms (Fig. 7.3). Bilateral lower extremity lymphedema is more common in patients presenting in infancy (63 %), compared to adolescence (30 %) [3].

Syndromic Associations

Eleven percent of patients with primary lymphedema have a familial/syndromic association (e.g., Turner syndrome, Noonan syndrome, Milroy disease) (Fig. 7.4) [3]. Children with onset

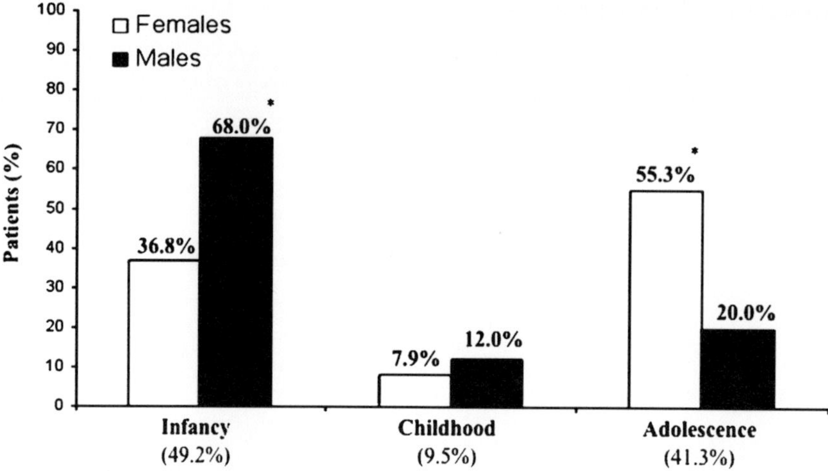

Fig. 7.1 Age-of-onset of primary pediatric lymphedema. With permission from Schook CC, Mulliken JB, Fishman SJ, Grant F, Zurakowski D, Greene AK. Primary lymph- edema: clinical features and management in 138 pediatric patients. Plast Reconstr Surg 2011; 127: 2419–2431 © Wolters Kluwer in 2011 [3]

in infancy and a familial history are referred to as having Milroy disease. This eponym often is erroneously applied to patients with any type of primary lymphedema. The term *Milroy disease* should be restricted to an infant with lower extremity lymphedema (unilateral/bilateral) present at birth with either: (1) a family history of the condition or (2) no family history of lymphedema, but a documented mutation in vascular endo- thelial growth factor receptor-3 (*VEGFR3*) [12]. Patients also should not be labeled as "Milroy dis- ease" if they have either: (1) lymphedema appearing after infancy; (2) lymphedema/lymphatic anoma- lies outside of the extremities; or (3) associated anomalies (e.g., dysmorphic face, epicanthal folds, cardiac anomalies, or biliary atresia) [12]. A mutation in *VEGFR3* is present in 75 % of chil- dren with familial lower extremity lymphedema, compared to 68 % of children without a family history of lymphedema [12]. Therefore, a positive family history of autosomal transmission is not essential for a diagnosis of Milroy disease. There can be *de novo* mutations in *VEGFR3* and reces- sive transmission also can occur. *Meige disease* refers to familial lymphedema of the lower extremity that manifests during adolescence. "Meige disease" should not be used for patients with adolescent onset of lymphedema without a family history of the disorder [13].

Patients with a *FOXC2* mutation causing lymphedema–distichiasis have an extra row of eyelashes and may exhibit eyelid ptosis and/or yellow nails. Hypotrichosis–lymphedema–telan- giectasia (*SOX18* mutation) causes sparse hair, and cutaneous telangiectasias. Hennekam syn- drome (*CCBE1* mutation) is characterized by generalized lymphedema with visceral involve- ment, developmental delay, flat faces, hyper- telorism, and a broad nasal bridge [8]. Patients with Turner syndrome have a 57 % percent risk of lymphedema; 76 % have onset in infancy and 19 % develop swelling during childhood or ado- lescence [14]. Noonan syndrome may manifest with generalized lymphedema, intestinal lym- phangiectasis and/or fetal hydrops. Patients with Noonan syndrome have a 3 % risk of lymph- edema [15]. Hennekam syndrome is character- ized by unusual facies, seizures, lymphedema of the lower limbs, genitalia and face, intestinal lymphangiectasis, and mental retardation. Overall, a genetic cause of primary lymphedema is present in 36 % of patients' familial disease, and in 8 % of individuals without a family his- tory of the condition [16]. Most of the known mutations for lymphedema involve proteins involved in the VEGFR3 pathway (e.g., *FLT4, GJC2, FOXC2, SOX 18, GATA2, CCBE1, PTPN14*) [16].

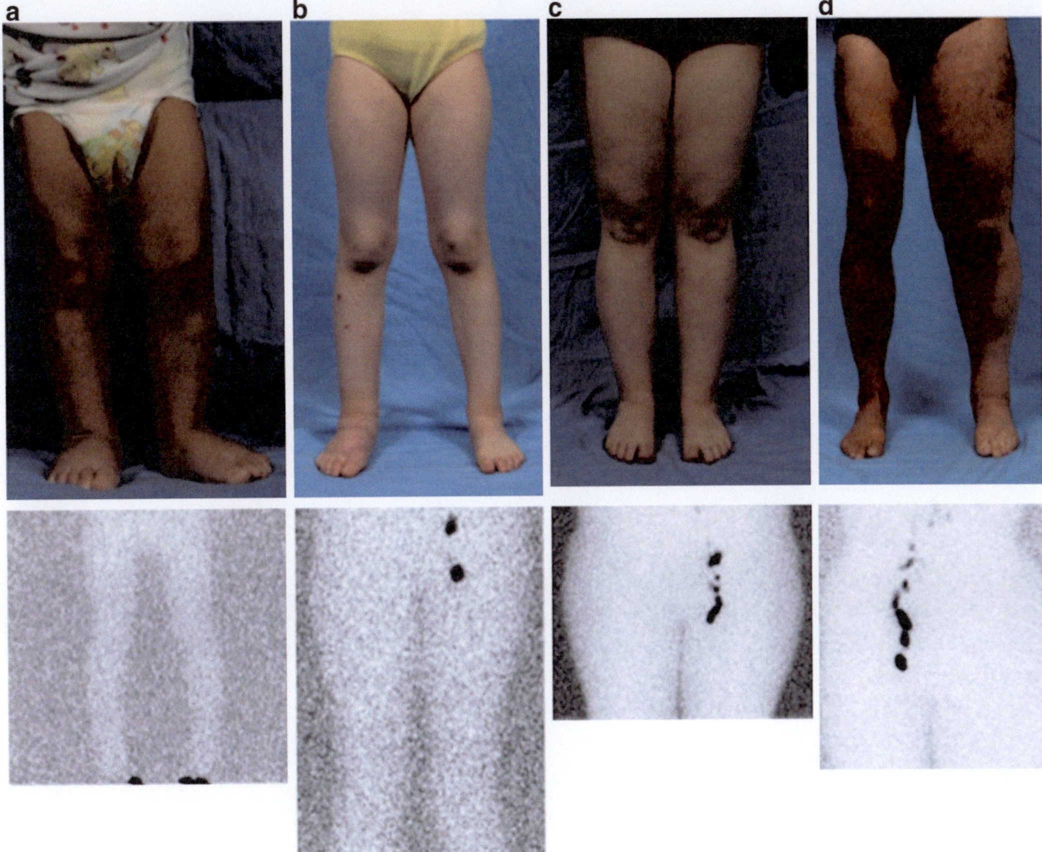

Fig. 7.2 Onset of primary lymphedema. (**a**) Presentation in infancy: 1-year-old female with bilateral lower extremity edema since birth. Lymphoscintigram demonstrates absence of lymph node tracer accumulation in the inguinal nodes 1.5 h following injection (normal transit time is 45 min). (**b**) Onset in childhood: 6-year-old female with 1-year history of progressive right lower extremity swelling. No proximal transit of tracer is noted by lymphoscin- tigraphy 1 h after injection. (**c**) Presentation in adolescence: 15-year-old female with a 1-year history of right lower extremity swelling. Lymphoscintigram shows absence of tracer accumulation in the right inguinal lymph node 2 h following injection. (**d**) Adult onset: 48-year-old male with a 3-year history of left lower extremity swelling. Lymphoscintigram illustrates no tracer in left inguinal nodes 4 h following injection

Morbidity

Primary lymphedema is a progressive condition and there is no cure. Generally, patients with primary lymphedema have less morbidity (e.g., enlarged limb size, infections, reduced function) compared to adults with secondary lymphedema (Table 7.4). One explanation may be that patients with primary lymphedema have compensated for the lack of lymphatic function because the defect occurred during embryogenesis. Lymphedema generally is not painful; significant discomfort is inconsistent with the disease. However, as the circumferential overgrowth of the extremity worsens and the limb becomes heavier, underlying musculoskeletal symptoms can occur.

Psychosocial

The most common problem caused by lymphedema is emotional distress (Fig. 7.5). Patients have lowered self-esteem because the involved area does not look normal. Unilateral limb involvement can be more distressing than bilateral disease because the asymmetry is more noticeable. Individuals may not feel comfortable wearing clothing that exposes their diseased limb.

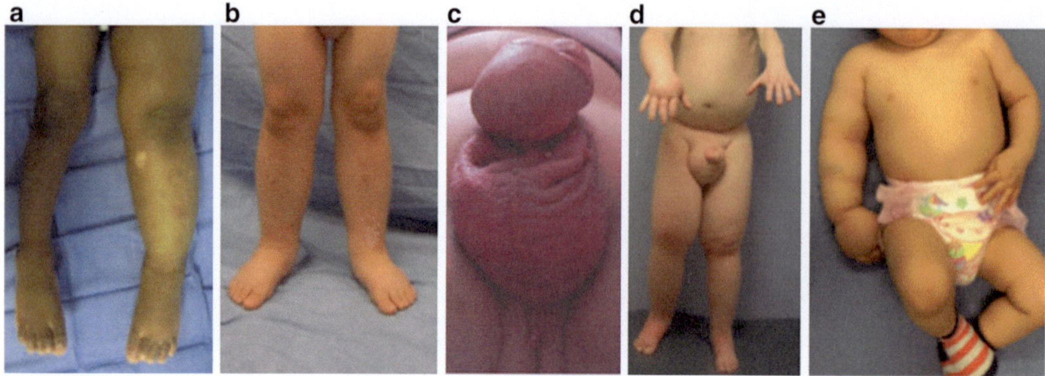

Fig. 7.3 Phenotypes of primary lymphedema. (**a**) Infant with unilateral lower extremity lymphedema. (**b**) Child with bilateral lower extremity disease. (**c**) 14-year-old male with isolated genital lymphedema. (**d**) Adolescent male with right upper extremity, bilateral lower extremity, and genital lymphedema. (**e**) 1-year-old male with right upper extremity lymphedema

Children may avoid changing clothes in front of their peers at school or refrain from swimming. Patients with moderate/severe disease can have significant psychosocial morbidity which negatively impacts their quality of life.

Infection

A lymphedematous extremity has a significantly increased risk of cellulitis compared to the non-affected limb. Lymph stagnation predisposes the area to infection after minor trauma because of: (1) impaired immunosurveillance (lymphatics function as an immunologic defense), (2) decreased oxygen delivery to the skin, and (3) a proteinaceous environment favorable for bacterial growth. Nineteen percent of patients with primary lymphedema have a history of cellulitis, 13 % have been hospitalized, and 7 % have >3 attacks each year [3]. Cutaneous infections in patients with lymphedema can spread more quickly compared to individuals without the disease. A superficial cellulitis can develop rapidly into a systemic infection and sepsis. Patients are counseled to seek medical attention quickly if they suspect an infection in a lymphedematous area. Often, individuals will carry oral antibiotics with them and administer the medication during the onset of the infection. Patients who have ≥3 episodes of cellulitis/year are placed on chronic suppressive antibiotic therapy following infectious disease consultation.

Skin Changes

Generally, patients with primary lymphedema have normal appearing skin. However, primary lymphedema can occur with other types of vascular malformations (usually capillary malformation). Because the disease is progressive, 15 % of patients will develop cutaneous problems such as bleeding from vesicles, fungal toenail lesions, hyperkeratosis, lymphorrhea, and verrucous changes [3]. Skin ulceration rarely affects patients with primary lymphedema because their arterial and venous circulations are intact. However, skin breakdown can occur in patients who also have venous insufficiency.

Orthopedic

Only 5 % of children with primary lymphedema have orthopedic problems, such as disturbance of gait or restriction of joint motion [3]. As adipose deposition increases the circumference of the affected area, patients can have difficulty using the extremity because of its weight. Individuals also may find it challenging to fit in clothes because of the soft-tissue overgrowth. The extra weight of the extremity causes the underlying muscle and bone to be hypertrophied from the added work of moving the extra subcutaneous tissue and skin [5]. Soft tissue overgrowth can be improved by removing hypertrophied tissue (e.g., suction-assisted lipectomy, staged skin/subcutaneous excision). Because lymphedema

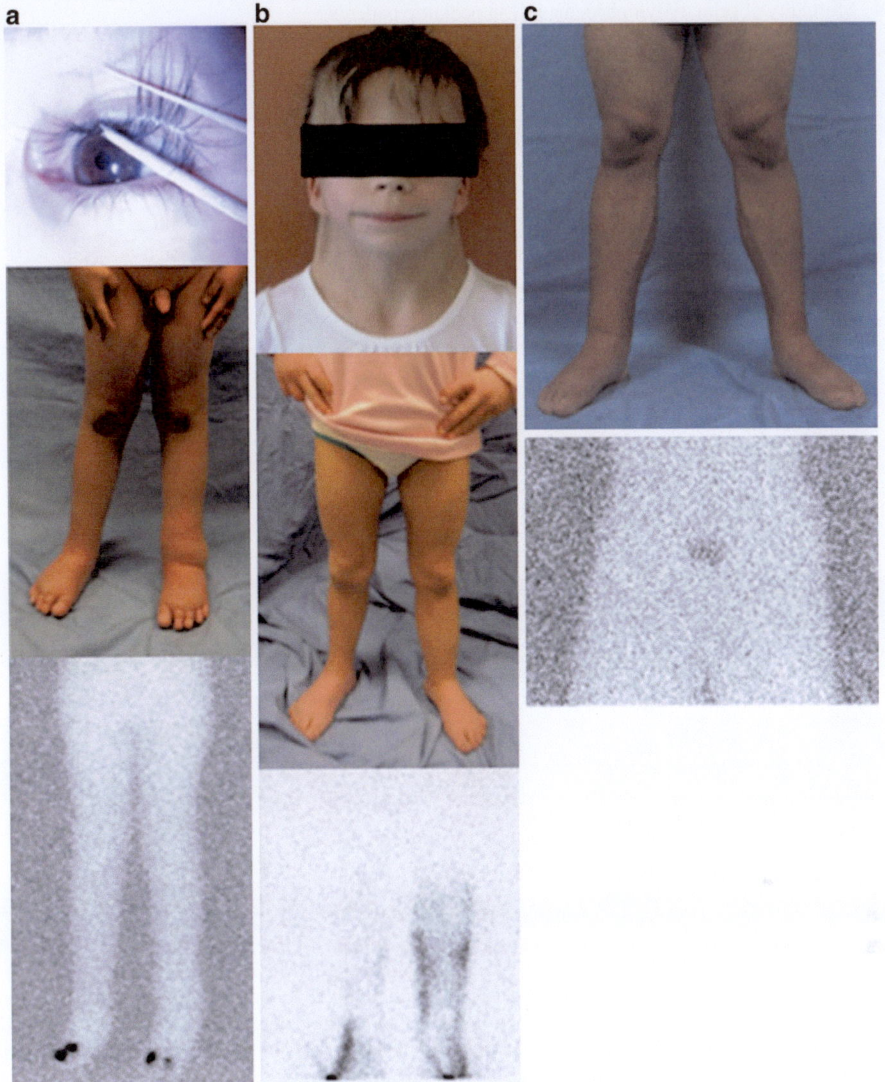

Fig. 7.4 Familial and syndromic lymphedema. (**a**) 6-year-old male with lymphedema–distichiasis syndrome causing bilateral lower-extremity swelling. No flow of tracer to his inguinal nodes 2 h following injection. His mother also has the condition (**b**) 9-year-old with Turner syndrome and lymphedema of all four extremities. Lymphoscintigraphy showed delayed transit to inguinal nodes and dermal backflow on 3 h image. (**c**) 23-year-old with Milroy disease. The patient has lymphedema of the lower extremities and scrotum since birth, as well as a family history of the disease. The tracer has not reached his inguinal nodes 3 h after the injection

only affects the skin and subcutis, the underlying muscle and bone are not primarily affected. Consequently, axial overgrowth of the extremity does not occur and patients do not need to be monitored for a leg-length discrepancy.

Malignant Transformation

Chronic lymphedema can predispose an individual to lymphangiosarcoma in the affected extremity, although the risk is very low (~0.07–0.45 %) [17]. Stewart–Treves "syndrome" classically refers to a

Table 7.4 Morbidity of primary lymphedema in 138 pediatric patients

Infection	Cellulitis	18.8 %	(26/138)
	Recurrent (>3/year)	7.2 %	(10/138)
	Hospitalization	13.0 %	(18/138)
	Chronic antibiotic prophylaxis	5.1 %	(7/138)
Cutaneous	Hyperkeratosis, lymphorrea, ulceration, verrucous changes	15.2 %	(21/138)
Orthopedic	Gait disturbance	5.0 %	(6/121)
Genitourinary	Dysuria, urethritis, phimosis, spraying of urine	16.0 %	(4/25)
Progression	Increased volume or worsening symptoms	57.9 %	(55/95)

With permission from Schook CC, Mulliken JB, Fishman SJ, Grant F, Zurakowski D, Greene AK. Primary lymphedema: clinical features and management in 138 pediatric patients. Plast Reconstr Surg 2011;127:2419–2431 © Wolters Kluwer in 2011 [3]

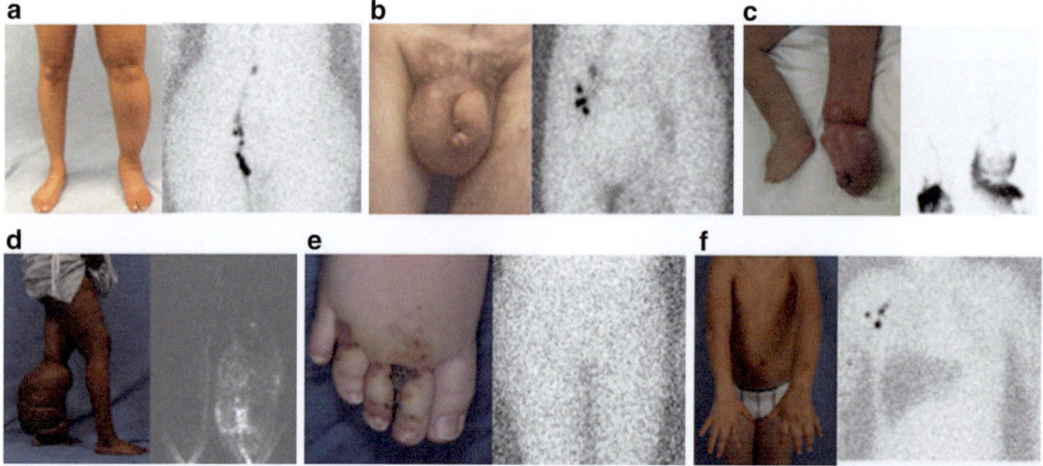

Fig. 7.5 Morbidity of primary lymphedema. (**a**) 37-year-old female with left lower extremity lymphedema causing low self-esteem because of the asymmetry between her legs. No flow of tracer to her left inguinal nodes 2 h following injection. (**b**) 24-year-old male with psychosocial distress because of genital lymphedema. Absent nodal uptake of tracer on left side 3.5 h after injection. (**c**) 26-year-old female with lower extremity lymphedema and dermal backflow on lymphoscintigram. She has cellulitis of her left leg that required intravenous antibiotics. (**d**) 37-year-old female with adolescent onset lymphedema. Her disease inhibited her ability to ambulate and fit clothing. Note dermal backflow on lymphoscintigram. (**e**) 11-year-old male with infant-onset lymphedema and cutaneous vesicles causing bleeding, lymphorrhea, and infection. Lymphoscintigram image illustrates no flow of tracer to inguinal nodes 2.5 h following injection. (**f**) 12-year-old male with infant-onset left upper extremity lymphedema. He had a 3-month history of arm pain and exacerbation of this disease. Histopathology showed lymphangiosarcoma. Note absence of tracer in left axillary lymph nodes on lymphoscintigram

lymphangiosarcoma arising in a lymphedematous upper extremity following treatment for breast cancer [17]. The tumor also can develop in chronic lower extremity lymphedema resulting from inguinal radiation and/or lymphadenectomy. Lymphangiosarcoma has been described in patients with primary lymphedema (in both the upper and lower extremity) [17]. Prognosis is poor because of pulmonary metastasis and local recurrence. Mean survival is <2 years following diagnosis. If metastases are not present on imaging, early amputation may allow long-term survival. Chemotherapy and radiation have minimal efficacy [17].

Diagnosis

History

Ninety percent of patients with primary lymphedema can be diagnosed by history and physical examination (Table 7.5). Onset of swelling is the first clue whether or not the patient has primary lymphedema. Males are more likely to present during infancy, while females usually have onset of edema in adolescence [3]. Males and females are affected equally, so the gender of the patient does not increase the risk of having the disease [3]. Patients are queried about a family history of extremity edema; if positive it raises the suspicion that the individual has lymphedema because many familial forms of the disease exist. If the patient has had infections in the affected area then the likelihood of lymphedema is increased. The swelling does not wax and wane, but almost always begins in the distal extremity and then moves proximally. Patients are asked about other medical problems that might be associated with lymphedema (e.g., double row of eyelashes, Turner syndrome, Noonan syndrome). Pain and skin ulceration are atypical for lymphedema.

Table 7.5 Presentation of primary lymphedema in 138 pediatric patients

Etiology	Nonfamilial/syndromic	88.4 %	(122/138)
	Familial/syndromic	11.6 %	(16/138)
Gender	Female	58.7 %	(81/138)
	Male	41.3 %	(57/138)
Location	Extremity	95.7 %	(132/138)
	Isolated	81.9 %	(113/138)
	Upper	16.7 %	(22/132)
	Unilateral	36.4 %	(8/22)
	Bilateral	63.6 %	(14/22)
	Lower	91.7 %	(121/132)
	Unilateral	47.1 %	(57/121)
	Bilateral	52.9 %	(64/121)
	Genitalia	18.1 %	(25/138)
	Isolated	4.3 %	(6/138)
	And lower extremity	13.8 %	(19/138)

With permission from Schook CC, Mulliken JB, Fishman SJ, Grant F, Zurakowski D, Greene AK. Primary lymphedema: clinical features and management in 138 pediatric patients. Plast Reconstr Surg 2011;127:2419–2431 © Wolters Kluwer in 2011 [3]

To ascertain whether the patient may have secondary lymphedema, he/she is asked about operations or radiation in the axilla or groin areas. A history of travel to areas endemic for filariasis also is ascertained. Although penetrating trauma to the axilla or groin can cause lymphedema, the risk is low because secondary lymphedema is very hard to cause. For example, only one-third of women who undergo axillary lymphadenectomy and radiation for breast cancer treatment develop lymphedema [18]. Patients frequently associate their onset of lymphedema with an episode of blunt trauma (e.g., twisting an ankle, a fall, injury playing sports). Blunt trauma, however, does not cause primary lymphedema although it theoretically might accelerate the onset of clinically noticeable edema sooner than the patient would have presented without the trauma.

Physical Examination

Initially, pitting edema is present over the hand, foot, or genitalia. Over time the edema is replaced by subcutaneous fibroadipose tissue and there can be less swelling. Lymphedema almost universally affects the distal extremity and then migrates proximally. If a patient does not have distal limb swelling, it is unlikely that he/she has lymphedema. A fairly sensitive and specific sign for lymphedema is the Stemmer sign [19]. If the examiner is unable to pinch the skin on the dorsum of the hand or foot (positive Stemmer sign), then it is likely the patient has lymphedema. Chronic swelling, inflammation, and adipose deposition cause the skin to thicken which reduces the ability to lift and pinch the integument of the distal extremity. Lymphedema is typically a painless condition and cutaneous ulceration is uncommon. Lymphedema does not affect the underlying bone, and thus patients do not have a leg-length discrepancy. Over time, individuals with lymphedema can develop lymphatic vesicles, usually involving the toes, which may bleed and leak lymph fluid (lymphorrhea). A double row of eyelashes is present in patients with lymphedema–distichiasis syndrome.

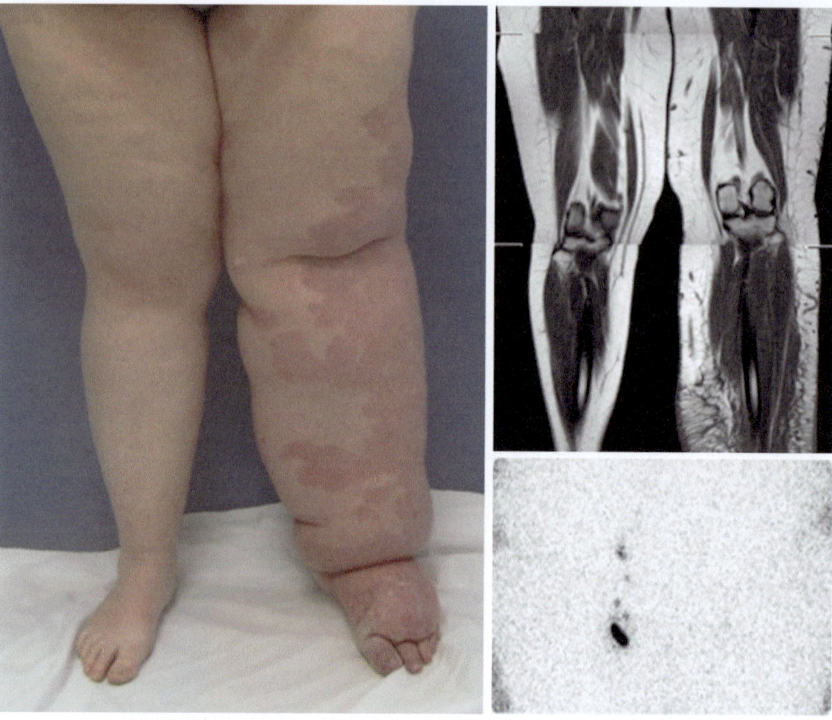

Fig. 7.6 Primary lymphedema and a combined vascular malformation. Adolescent female with a capillary malformation of the left extremity as well as primary lymphedema. MRI shows disease limited to skin and subcutaneous tissue with normal subfacial structures. Lymphoscintigram illustrates absence of tracer accumulation in left inguinal lymph nodes 2 h following injection

Yellow nails indicate cholestasis lymphedema syndrome. Overlying skin discoloration can occur, but is uncommon. Primary lymphedema can occur with other types of vascular malformations (Fig. 7.6).

Clinically, the severity of lymphedema can be categorized as minimal (<20 % increase in extremity volume), moderate (20–40 %), or severe (>40 %) [10]. Limb volume measurements can be made using a tape measure, perometer, or water displacement. Tape measurements are the least accurate method because extremity volume must be calculated and it is difficult to use the exact points again for future measurements. In addition, depending on how tight the examiner pulls the tape measure the circumference can change significantly. We do not routinely measure limb volumes because it does not affect the patient's management. In children, extremity measurements are particularly problematic because the extremities are still growing.

All patients who are being considered for operative intervention undergo water displacement to assess their limb volume before and after their procedure.

Imaging

Lymphoscintigraphy

Lymphoscintigraphy is the "gold-standard" test to determine whether a patient has lymphedema [10]. We use this imaging technique for almost all patients referred with "lymphedema" in order to: (1) obtain diagnostic confirmation and (2) quantitatively assess lymphatic dysfunction. Lymphoscintigraphy is 100 % specific and 92 % sensitive for lymphedema [20]. The test is safe and does not cause morbidity (e.g., infection, allergic reactions, worsening of lymphedema). A radiolabeled colloid (usually Tc-99 m filtered sulfur) is injected into the dorsum of the hand or foot.

Because of the large size of the protein, it is only taken up by lymphatic vessels. Delayed transit time to the regional lymph nodes (>45 min), dermal backflow, and collateral lymphatic channels represent abnormal proximal lymphatic transport and lymphedema. Even if a patient has a high clinical suspicion of having primary lymphedema, the study provides an objective measure of the severity of lymphatic dysfunction which affects clinical care. Patients are counseled whether they have "mild," "moderate," or "severe" lymphedema based on their lymphatic flow. For example, an individual who has tracer accumulation in the in inguinal nodes 2 h after the injection and no evidence of dermal backflow would be considered to have "mild" lymphedema. In contrast, a patient without evidence of nodal tracer accumulation after 24 h and dermal backflow would be labeled as having "severe" lymphedema. The individual with severe lymphatic dysfunction might be managed more aggressively than the patient with mild disease.

Lymphangiography

Lymphangiography has been replaced by lymphoscintigraphy as the first-line test to diagnose lymphedema. Lymphangiography involves the injection of dye into the lymphatic vasculature and is rarely used to evaluate lymphedema because: (1) it is technically difficult to perform, (2) an allergic reaction to the dye can occur, (3) lymphangitis is common, and (4) it may worsen the lymphedema. A lymphangiogram might be indicated to identify a localized anatomic obstruction in the thoracic duct if a bypass procedure is planned.

Other Diagnostic Modalities

MRI and CT are neither sensitive nor specific for lymphedema. These studies are only obtained to: (1) determine the amount of subcutaneous adipose tissue present if an excisional procedure is being considered and (2) assess for other causes of swelling if the lymphoscintigram is normal. Lymphedema appears as thickened skin and subcutaneous tissue with adipose hypertrophy, stranding, and edema. The tissues below the muscular fascia are normal (unlike Klippel–Trénaunay syndrome, Parkes Weber syndrome, hemihypertrophy, lymphatic malformation, venous malformation). Ultrasound is non-diagnostic for lymphedema, but can be used to rule out venous disease. Lymphedema cannot be diagnosed histopathologically because findings are nonspecific (i.e., adipose tissue with inflammation).

Differential Diagnosis

The term "lymphedema" is commonly misused to describe any condition that causes overgrowth of a limb. Approximately 25 % of patients referred to our center with a diagnosis of "lymphedema" do not have the disease (Table 7.6) [6, 7]. In the pediatric population, the most common lesions confused with primary lymphedema are other types of vascular anomalies: capillary malformation, lymphatic malformation, venous malformation, infantile hemangioma, kaposiform hemangioendothelioma, CLOVES syndrome, Klippel–Trénaunay syndrome, and Parkes Weber syndrome. Other conditions mistaken for primary lymphedema in children include hemihypertrophy, lipofibromatosis, lipedema, and

Table 7.6 Differential diagnosis of primary lymphedema

Capillary malformation
Hemihypertrophy
Infantile hemangioma
Kaposiform hemangioendothelioma
Klippel–Trénaunay syndrome
Lipedema
Lipofibromatosis
Lymphatic malformation
Noneponymous combined vascular malformation (e.g., lymphatic–venous malformation)
Obesity
Parkes Weber syndrome
Posttraumatic swelling (e.g., ligament sprain, occult fracture)
Rheumatologic disease (e.g., tenosynovitis, rheumatoid arthritis)
Systemic causes of edema (cardiac, renal, hepatic disease)
Venous malformation
Venous stasis disease

posttraumatic swelling. Adult-onset primary lymphedema is most frequently confused with obesity, lipedema, venous insufficiency, posttraumatic swelling, and systemic diseases (e.g., cardiac, renal, hepatic, rheumatologic). Usually, lymphedema can be differentiated from other causes of extremity overgrowth by history and physical examination. Lymphoscintigraphy provides diagnostic confirmation; only lymphedema shows delayed lymphatic function using this test. If lymphoscintigraphy is normal, then MRI is often used to determine the cause of the patient's enlarged limb. It is important to accurately diagnose a patient with lymphedema because the prognosis and treatment of this disease is very different than other causes of extremity overgrowth.

Nonoperative Management

Activities of Daily Living

Although there is no cure for lymphedema, most patients with primary disease are managed successfully with conservative therapy and do not require operative intervention [3]. Nonoperative management includes: (1) education/activities of daily living and (2) compression of the affected area. Patients are advised to moisturize the limb to prevent desiccation and subsequent skin breakdown that can cause cellulitis. Protective clothing is worn to prevent incidental trauma that can lead to cellulitis (e.g., patients with lower extremity disease should avoid walking barefoot). When reclining or sleeping, leg elevation is recommended.

Exercise is encouraged and patients are allowed to participate in all activities. Exercise improves lymphedema by stimulating muscle contraction and proximal lymph flow [21]. Patients should maintain a normal body mass index because obesity can worsen and cause lymphedema [22]. There are no dietary restrictions, although a low-salt, low-fat diet is likely beneficial because obesity can worsen lymphedema. Diuretics are ineffective and can exacerbate the disease by increasing the concentration

of interstitial protein. Coumarin, a benzopyrone immunomodulator, is not recommended because it has minimal efficacy and may cause hepatoxicity. Patients with >3 episodes of cellulitis each year may benefit from chronic suppressive antibiotic therapy against *Streptococcus*.

Compression

The mainstay of treatment for lymphedema is compression which: (1) decreases the size of the area by reducing edema and (2) slows progression of the disease by minimizing the high-protein fluid in the interstitial space that stimulates adipose deposition (Fig. 7.7). Pressure may reduce extremity volume by: (1) increasing lymph transport, (2) decreasing capillary filtration, (3) opening collapsed vessels, (4) minimizing interstitial pressure, and/or (5) widening the vessel wall by direct injury. We prescribe patients custom-fitted garments and pneumatic compression, rather than manual lymphatic drainage/combination compressive regimens, because we believe: (1) their efficacy is superior, (2) they are easier for the patient, and (3) treatment is not dependent on a therapist.

Static Garments

Static compression consisting of custom-fitted garments is the most effective compression method because the garments are worn continuously. When they are progressively tightened (controlled compression therapy), extremity volume may be reduced by 47 % over 1 year [4]. We prefer a single-layer garment for the upper extremity (30 mmHg) and two layers for the lower extremity (20 mmHg garment over a 30 mmHg sleeve). Patients with genital lymphedema are advised to wear a tight-fitting athletic undergarment. Custom-fitted garments are not popular for patients because: (1) they are uncomfortable, (2) the appearance of the garments is not appealing, and (3) they are a continuous reminder of their underlying disease. In children, these

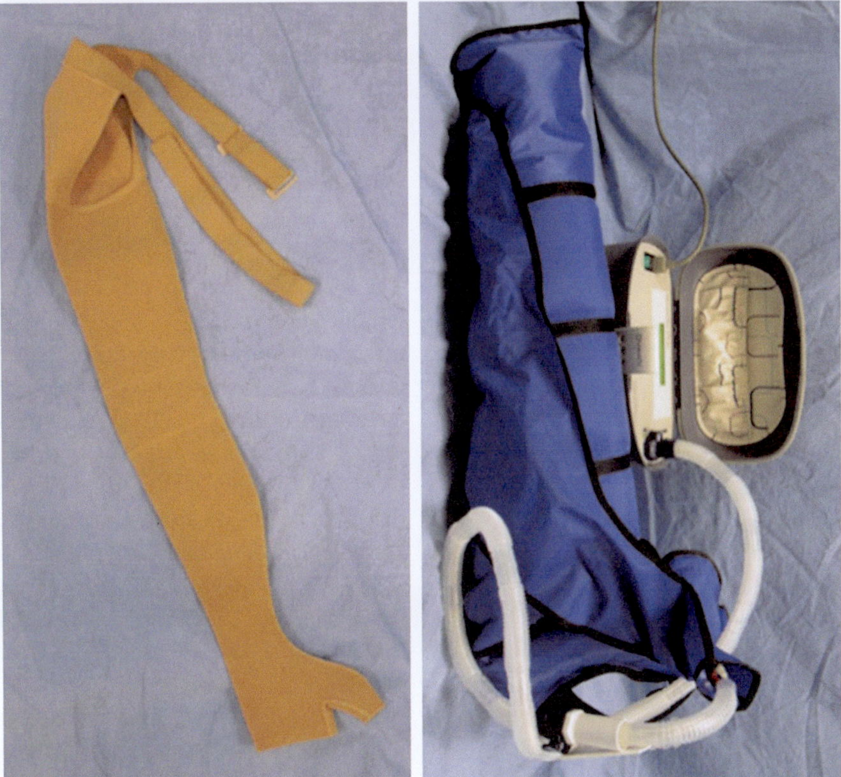

Fig. 7.7 Nonoperative management of primary lymphedema. (*Left*) Custom-fitted compression garment. (*Right*) Pneumatic compression machine

drawbacks are particularly problematic and compliance is more difficult. In addition, because children are rapidly growing they have to have frequent fittings and new garments which are expensive. Consequently, I often recommend commercially available stockings for pediatric patients instead of medical grade garments. Children are allowed to pick stockings that they like (e.g., "superhero" socks for boys, "princess" socks for girls), which increases compliance with compression and does not remind the patient of their disease. There is no evidence that wearing a tight, commercially available sock is inferior to using a medical grade compression garment. In fact, increasing compliance with a stocking that is most favorable to the child is likely more efficacious than using a custom medical grade garment that is worn less frequently.

Pneumatic Compression

Pneumatic compression devices deliver intermittent pressure through a power source and inflatable sleeve. Machines may be sequential/non-sequential, gradient/non-gradient and have single/multiple compartments. A sequential pump has multiple chambers that inflate distally followed by the expansion of more proximal chambers. A gradient pump delivers more force in the distal chambers. We prefer a sequential, gradient device with multiple compartments because it best recapitulates physiologic lymph flow. Extremity volume may be reduced 3–66 % using pneumatic compression, and we recommend pumping for at least 2 h/day [23]. Results depend on the type of device, outcome measures, and treatment regimen. In the pediatric population with primary lymphedema I only recommend pneumatic compression for: (1) adolescents or (2) younger children with severe disease. Generally, I have a high threshold to prescribe pneumatic compression for children because they are being "hooked up" to a machine which impedes their activities and quality of life. There is no evidence that children managed with pneumatic compression have a more favorable long-term course from their lymphedema. Consequently, I attempt to have children be as "normal" as possible and not use the compression unless they are older or have severe disease.

Manual Lymphatic Drainage and Combination Regimens

Manual lymphatic drainage uses massage to stimulate proximal lymphatic flow. Combination compressive regimens (e.g., complex decongestive therapy) are programs that combine skin care, manual lymphatic drainage, and compression bandaging [10]. A treatment phase of several weeks at an outpatient facility is initiated followed by maintenance, which is conducted at home by the patient/family. Manual lymphatic drainage alone has minimal efficacy [10]. Combination regimens may reduce limb volume 19–68 % for patients with secondary lymphedema, but studies have been small with unclear inclusion criteria. These techniques may be helpful in managing early/mild disease but are less likely to be effective with chronic lymphedema containing fibroadipose tissue. Disadvantages of these treatments include: (1) substantial time burden for patients, (2) reliance on a provider for treatment, and (3) cost. Massage and bandaging are particularly problematic in the pediatric population because they are burdensome to children and parents. Similar to pneumatic compression, there is no evidence that children managed with manual lymphatic drainage/combination regimens have better long-term outcomes compared to children who do not have these interventions. Consequently, I prefer static compression which is easiest for children and has the best efficacy of all nonoperative interventions for lymphedema [4].

Operative Management

Timing and Indications

Operative intervention is rarely indicated for patients with primary lymphedema. It is more common for individuals with genital disease (36 %), compared to patients with extremity lymphedema (6 %) [3]. Patients are considered for a surgical procedure if: (1) they have been compliant with conservative therapies and (2) have significant morbidity despite maximal conservative interventions. Indications for a surgical procedure include: (1) recurrent infections, (2) inhibition of daily activities, and/or (3) the patient is unhappy with the appearance of the affected area. Pubertal males often seek improvement for the appearance of their genitalia, while adolescent females are interested in improving the contour of their leg.

There are two categories of operative intervention: (1) physiologic and (2) excisional. Physiologic procedures attempt to produce new lymphatic connections to enhance lymph drainage. Excisional operations remove excessive subcutaneous fibroadipose tissue with or without overlying skin. I prefer excisional procedures because they have consistent and excellent long-term results. In addition, all patients (minor, moderate, or severe disease) are potential candidates. Suction-assisted lipectomy (liposuction) is my preferred technique. I reserve staged skin/subcutaneous resection for very severe disease. It is possible that excisional procedures also may have a physiologic benefit by: (1) reducing the amount of lymph load produced by the extremity, (2) increasing drainage from the superficial to deep system by removing tissue, and (3) increasing blood flow to the skin because the procedures delay the integument. Physiologic procedures have poor results for moderate/severe lymphedema. In early disease, results are inconsistent and long-term benefits are modest. Even if improved proximal lymph flow is achieved, the excess fibroadipose tissue cannot be reversed and may only be improved using an excisional procedure.

Physiologic Procedures

Physiologic operations attempt to reconnect, reconstruct, or stimulate lymphatic pathways. A superficial lymphatic system is separated from a deep system by muscle fascia. Lymphedema only affects the skin and subcutis; tissues beneath the muscle fascia are not affected. Handley (1908) unsuccessfully used subcutaneous silk threads to drain edematous areas into normal tissue. Kondoleon (1915) removed the muscle fascia in a failed attempt to allow the superficial lymphatics to drain into the deep lymphatic system. Flap transpositions to connect superficial lymphatics to the deep system have been abandoned because clear efficacy has not been proven and the procedures have greater morbidity compared to excisional or microsurgical operations [10]. Examples include: (1) transposition of a skin flap into muscle (Thompson procedure), (2) pedicled omental flap to drain the axillary/inguinal lymph nodes, (3) inferiorly based rectus myocutaneous flap transferred into the groin.

Microsurgical lymphatic–venous anastomosis is the most commonly performed physiological procedure. Results are variable, but reported improvement for minor/moderate disease is 55 % excess volume reduction [24, 25]. If lymphatic–venous anastomosis is performed, it should be carried out early in disease when there is still potentially functional drainage prior to progressive fibrosis and adipose deposition. More recently, microsurgical lymph node transfer to the axilla/inguinal region has been performed [26]. Although beneficial results have been reported, patients had early disease and the contribution of postoperative manual lymphatic drainage to the improvement is unclear. Lymphoscintigraphy has failed to show improved lymphatic function in most patients. This procedure also risks causing donor site lymphedema where the nodes were harvested.

The role of lymphatic–venous anastomosis or lymph node transfer is less clear in children than for adults. Patients with primary have lymphedema have hypoplastic/aplastic lymphatics, unlike individuals with secondary lymphedema who have normal lymphatic vessels. Consequently, the ability to find a lymphatic vessel to anastomose with a vein is unclear. It is unlikely that if a lymphatic vessel is found it will have a network of other lymphatics to drain into the venous system. Similarly, placing a vascularized lymph node into the axilla or inguinal region of a patient who has a paucity of lymphatics to drain is unlikely to work. In fact, operating in the axillary or inguinal region of a patient with primary lymphedema may injure functioning lymphatics/nodes, will create scar tissue, and may worsen the patient's lymphedema. Patients with primary lymphedema have either a germ-line or somatic mutation responsible for their disease and are at increased risk for developing lymphedema at other sites over the course of their life. Consequently, patients with primary lymphedema likely are at much higher risk of donor site lymphedema from the harvest of lymph nodes.

Excisional Procedures

Suction-Assisted Lipectomy

Excisional operations remove excess fat, fibrous tissue, and expanded skin that develops with lymphedema. Because the underlying disease is not cured, lifelong compression is required to minimize edema, inflammation, and recurrent fibroadipose deposition. Suction-assisted lipectomy (liposuction) is my first-line operative intervention for extremity lymphedema because of its efficacy, consistent results, and low-morbidity (Fig. 7.8). Excess volume reduction for upper extremity lymphedema can be as high as 106 % after 1 year, with no recurrence 15 years postoperatively [4]. Suction-assisted lipectomy for lower extremity lymphedema achieves 75 % volume reduction 18 months postoperatively [27, 28]. Liposuction increases cutaneous blood flow, reduces the annual risk of cellulitis by 30 %, and significantly improves quality of life [4]. Lymphatics are not injured by the procedure, and lymph flow is not affected.

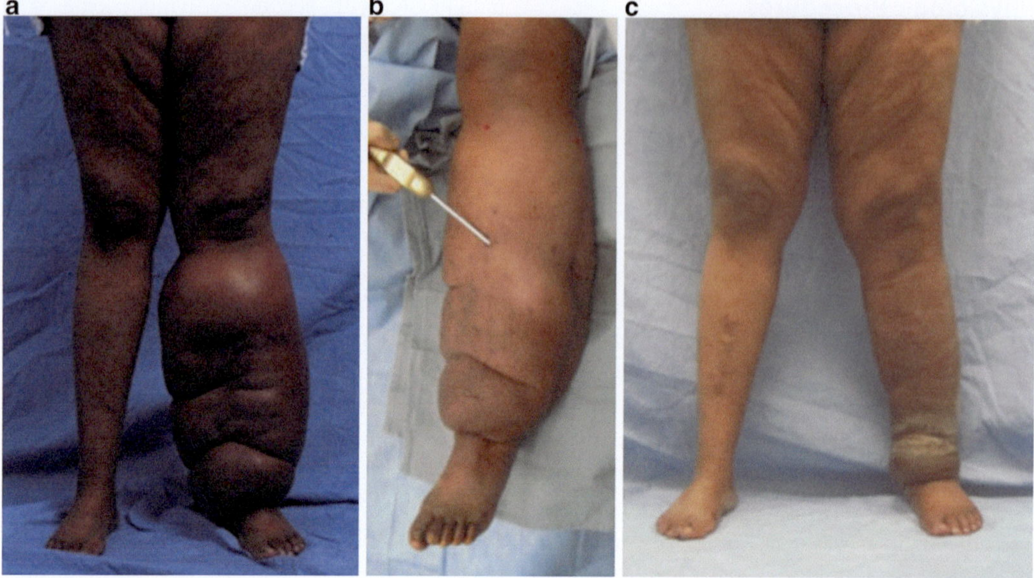

Fig. 7.8 Operative management of lymphedema. (**a**) 37-year-old female with adolescent-onset primary lymphedema of the left lower extremity. (**b**) Removal of excess subcutaneous adipose tissue using suction-assisted lipec- tomy. (**c**) Improved contour 5 months postoperatively. With permission from Greene AK. Vascular Anomalies: Classification, Diagnosis, and Management. CRC Press, Boca Raton, FL © 2013 [31]

Staged Cutaneous/Subcutaneous Excision

Staged cutaneous/subcutaneous excision is used for: (1) severe lymphedema with significant skin excess and (2) genital lymphedema. Disadvantages compared to suction-assisted lipectomy include: (1) two stages, (2) extended hospital stay, (3) long incisions/scars, and (4) greater operative morbidity. Sistrunk (1918) modified the Kondoleon procedure by removing tissue and fascia. Homans (1936) excised subcutaneous tissue, deep fascia and created thin skin flaps. Miller (1998) showed significant improvement in limb size in 79 % of patients and a reduction in the risk of infection [29, 30]. Postoperative lymphoscintigraphy illustrated increased lymphatic function, suggesting that this procedure might have physiologic benefit. Excision of skin and subcutaneous tissue is the first-line operative technique for genital lymphedema.

Charles Procedure

Charles (1912) described a method for treatment of tropical elephantiasis of the lower extremities that involved resection of all skin and subcutaneous

tissue and covering the muscle with split thickness skin grafts obtained from other areas of the body. Most surgeons do not advocate for this procedure, especially in children, because the appearance of the limb is usually significantly worse than its preoperative appearance. The skin grafts are susceptible to trauma, chronic ulceration, infections, and hyperkeratosis. The procedure is an option for severe lymphedema that has failed other operations.

Conclusions

One principle of management of patients with primary lymphedema is that the treatment should not hinder quality of life as much as possible, especially in children. Because the disease is incurable, children should grow up being as "normal" as possible. Consequently, commercially available tight fitting socks that the child likes is preferred over medical grade garments. Medical grade garments remind the child of their disease, and there is no evidence suggesting they are superior to tight fitting socks chosen by the patient.

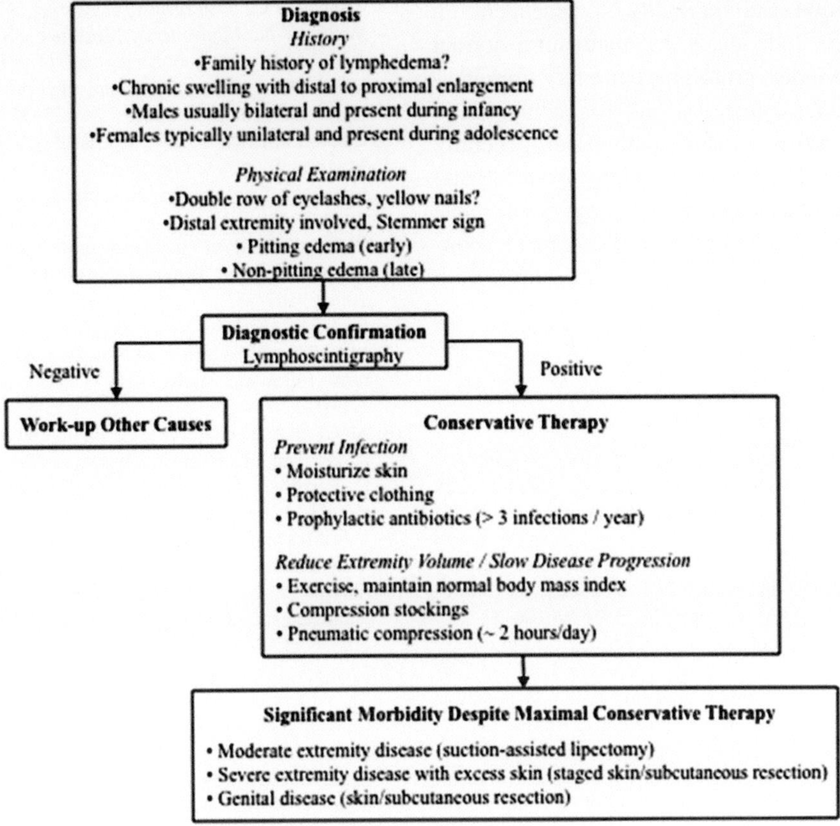

Fig. 7.9 Management algorithm for primary lymphedema

There is also no evidence that wearing compression for 24 h a day is superior to using a garment less frequently. Consequently, patients are advised to wear stockings as much as possible, but it is acceptable to abstain from the garment when needed (e.g., social events, warm weather, etc). Individuals are encouraged to engage in all activities.

Patients with primary lymphedema are best managed by an interdisciplinary team focused on the condition. A lymphedema clinic provides accurate diagnosis, education, static and pneumatic compression therapy, as well as the most effective operative techniques (Fig. 7.9). Most individuals can be managed conservatively with hygiene and compression strategies. Full activity should be encouraged. Nonoperative measures must be exhausted before a procedure is contemplated. We favor custom-fitted static compression garments for all patients. In young children we have them pick out commercially available stockings that they like and are tight to increase compliance. We also prescribe a pneumatic compression device and advocate its use for at least 2 h/day for patients with moderate or severe disease. We prefer pneumatic compression to massage therapy or combination compressive regiments because: (1) its efficacy is equivalent or superior; (2) it is easier for the patient (therapy is delivered at home when convenient); and (3) treatment is not dependent on a therapist. Excisional operations provide consistent, excellent results. We favor suction-assisted lipectomy for moderate disease and staged cutaneous/subcutaneous excision for severe extremity lymphedema.

Patients are advised that although lymphedema is an incurable disease, the progression of the condition and morbidity is dependent on compliance. Individuals that maintain a normal body mass index, protect the extremity from incidental trauma/infections, and use compression garments and pneumatic compression generally have minimal-moderate morbidity from the disease. In contrast, patients who are obese, have repeated infections which further damage lymphatics, and are noncompliant with compression can have significant morbidity.

References

1. Allen EV. Lymphedema of the extremities. Classification, etiology and differential diagnoses. A study of 300 cases. Arch Intern Med. 1934;56: 606–24.
2. Smeltzer DM, Stickler GB, Schirger A. Primary lymphedemas in children and adolescents: a follow-up study and review. Pediatrics. 1985;76:206–18.
3. Schook CC, Mulliken JB, Fishman SJ, Grant F, Zurakowski D, Greene AK. Primary lymphedema: clinical features and management in 138 pediatric patients. Plast Reconstr Surg. 2011;127:2419–31.
4. Brorson H, Svensson H. Liposuction combined with controlled compression therapy reduces arm lymphedema more effectively than controlled compression therapy alone. Plast Reconstr Surg. 1998;102: 1058–67.
5. Brorson H, Ohlin K, Olsson G, Karlsson MK. Breast cancer-related chronic arm lymphedema is associated with excess adipose and muscle tissue. Lymphat Res Biol. 2009;7:3–10.
6. Schook CC, Mulliken JB, Fishman SJ, Alomari AI, Greene AK. Differential diagnosis of lower extremity lymphedema in 170 pediatric patients. Plast Reconstr Surg. 2011;127:1571–81.
7. Maclellan RA, Couto RA, Sullivan JE, Grant FD, Slavin SA, Greene AK. Management of primary and secondary lymphedema: analysis of 225 referrals to a center. Ann Plast Surg. 8 Apr 2014. [Epub ahead of print].
8. Brouillard P, Boon L, Vikkula M. Genetics of lymphatic anomalies. J Clin Invest. 2014;124:898–904.
9. Wolfe J, Kinmonth JB. The prognosis of primary lymphedema of the lower limbs. Arch Surg. 1981; 116:1157–60.
10. International Society of Lymphology. The diagnosis and treatment of peripheral lymphedema: 2013 Consensus Document of the International Society of Lymphology. Lymphology. 2013;46:1–11.
11. Greene AK, Schook CC. Primary lymphedema: a standardized classification based on developmental age-of-onset. Plast Reconstr Surg. 2012;129:221e–2.
12. Connell FC, Ostergaard P, Carver C, Brice G, Williams N, Mansour S, Mortimer PS, Jeffery S. Analysis of the coding regions of VEGFR3 and VEGFRC in Milroy disease and other primary lymphoedemas. Hum Genet. 2009;124:625–31.
13. Connell F, Brice G, Jeffery S, Keeley V, Mortimer P, Mansour S. A new classification system for primary lymphatic dysplasias based on phenotype. Clin Genet. 2010;77:438–52.
14. Welsh J, Todd M. Incidence and characteristics of lymphedema in Turner's syndrome. Lymphology. 2006;39:152–3.
15. Shaw AC, Kalidas K, Crosby AH, Jeffery S, Patton MA. The natural history of Noonan syndrome: a long-term follow-up study. Arch Dis Child. 2007;92: 128–32.
16. Mendola A, Schlogel MJ, Ghalamkarpour A, Irrthum A, Nguyen HL, Fastre E, Bygum A, van der Vleuten C, Fagerberg C, Baselga E, Quere I, Mulliken JB, Boon LM, Brouillard P, Vikkula M. Mutations in the VEGFR3 signaling pathway explain 36 % of familial lymphedema. Mol Syndromol. 2013;4:257–66.
17. Sharma A, Schwartz RA. Stewart-Treves syndrome: pathogenesis and management. J Am Acad Dermatol. 2012;67:1342–8.
18. Dayangac M, Makay O, Yeniay L, Aynaci M, Kapkac M, Yilmaz R. Precipitating factors for lymphedema following surgical treatment of breast cancer: implications for patients undergoing axillary lymph node dissection. Breast J. 2009;15:210–1.
19. Stemmer R. A clinical symptom for the early and differential diagnosis of lymphedema. Vasa. 1976;5: 261–2.
20. Gloviczki P, Calcagno D, Schirger A, Pairolero PC, Cherry KJ, Hallett JW, Wahner HW. Noninvasive evaluation of the swollen extremity: experiences with 190 lymphoscintigraphic examinations. J Vasc Surg. 1989;9:683–9.
21. Schmitz KH, Ahmed RL, Troxel A, Cheville A, Smith R, Lewis-Grant L, Bryan CJ, Williams-Smith CT, Greene QP. Weight lifting in women with breast-cancer-related lymphedema. N Engl J Med. 2009; 361:664–73.
22. Greene AK, Grant FD, Slavin SA. Lower-extremity lymphedema and elevated body-mass index. N Engl J Med. 2012;366:2136–7.
23. Johansson K, Lie E, Edkahl C, Lindfeldt J. A randomized study comparing manual lymph drainage with sequential pneumatic compression for treatment of postoperative arm lymphedema. Lymphology. 1998;2: 56–64.
24. Koshima I, Nanba Y, Tsutsui T, Takahashi Y, Itoh S. Long-term follow-up after lymphaticovenular anastomosis for lymphedema in the legs. J Reconstr Microsurg. 2003;19:209–15.
25. Campisi C, Da Rin E, Bellini C, Bonioli E, Boccardo F. Pediatric lymphedema and correlated syndromes: role of microsurgery. Microsurgery. 2008;28:138–42.

26. Becker C, Arrive L, Saaristo A, Germain M, Fanzio P, Batista BN, Piquilloud G. Surgical treatment of congenital lymphedema. Clin Plast Surg. 2012;39:377–84.

27. Greene AK, Slavin SA, Borud L. Treatment of lower extremity lymphedema with suction-assisted lipectomy. Plast Reconstr Surg. 2006;118:118e–21.

28. Brorson H, Ohlin K, Olsson G, Svensson B, Svensson H. Controlled compression and liposuction treatment for lower extremity lymphedema. Lymphology. 2008;41:52–63.

29. Brorson H, Svensson H, Norrgren K, Thorsson O. Liposuction reduces arm lymphedema without significantly altering the already impaired lymph transport. Lymphology. 1998;31:156–72.

30. Miller TA, Wyatt LE, Rudkin GH. Staged skin and subcutaneous excision for lymphedema: a favorable report of long-term results. Plast Reconstr Surg. 1998;102:1486–98.

31. Greene AK. Vascular anomalies: classification, diagnosis, and management. CRC Press, Boca Raton, FL, 2013 © Francis and Taylor.

Secondary Lymphedema

Sumner A. Slavin

S.A. Slavin, M.D. (✉)
Division of Plastic Surgery, Beth Israel Deaconess
Medical Center, Harvard Medical School,
Boston, MA, USA

Lymphedema Program, Boston Children's Hospital,
Boston, MA, USA
e-mail: ssbsj@aol.com

Key Points

- Secondary lymphedema is the most common form of lymphedema in the USA, occurring most commonly after breast cancer treatment.
- Patients can be accurately diagnosed using lymphoscintigraphy. Indocyanine lymphography adds to our ability to perform physiologic imaging, especially in the operating room setting.
- Most cases of secondary lymphedema can be managed by combinations of compression therapy consisting of manual lymphatic drainage, compression garments, bandaging, and skin care. Sequential pumping devices can supplement these treatments.
- Microsurgical techniques that enhance lymphatic flow by creating lymphatico-venous anastomoses or by supplementing lymphatic function through the transfer of vascularized lymph nodes represent new surgical options showing promise. Older techniques of subcutaneous excision have a more limited role, reserved mostly for the severe end stage or near-end stage of lymphedema.
- The recognition that fat hypertrophies and accumulates in the subcutaneous compartment of a lymphedematous limb is an extremely important clinical observation that led to the application of liposuctioning as an effective technique for patients with moderate, non-fibrosed limbs. Only liposuctioning addresses this problem of adipose tissue buildup. Physiologic procedures improve lymphatic drainage but do not decrease accumulations of hypertrophied fat in a lymphedematous limb.

Introduction

Lymphedema is a chronic disease characterized by impairment of the lymphatic channels which normally transport lymph, resulting in a buildup of lymph and fluid within the extravascular interstitial spaces. Unlike primary lymphedema, in which developmental anomalies of the lymphatic system predominate, secondary lymphedema is usually caused by injury to the lymphatics by surgery, radiation, trauma, and other disease processes. Estimated to afflict 2–3 million people in the USA [1], it is a debilitating disease that causes chronic swelling, pain, inflammation, fibrosis, and infection. Additionally, patients with secondary lymphedema can suffer from severe interruption of activities of daily living, psychological dysfunction, and economic hardship from loss of function in both upper and lower extremities. Globally, the overwhelming majority of cases are filarial in origin caused by parasites such as the nematode *Wuchereria bancrofti*. In the USA,

A.K. Greene et al. (eds.), *Lymphedema: Presentation, Diagnosis, and Treatment*,
DOI 10.1007/978-3-319-14493-1_8, © Springer International Publishing Switzerland 2015

however, lymphatic filariasis is generally unknown, with the most common causes being surgical and radiation therapies, either combined or individually administered for malignant conditions. Secondary lymphedema results when the damage to the lymphatics in any specific anatomical area is sufficient to disrupt lymphatic transport on a prolonged or permanent basis, causing a level of obstruction that blocks normative physiologic processes. Apart from breast cancer, secondary lymphedema occurs following surgical treatment for urological cancers such as (prostatic and testicular), gynecological malignancies (uterine and ovarian) various head and neck tumors, lymphoma, melanoma and other cancerous conditions. The spread of cancer follows regional lymphatics to nodal basins as the principal path of progression. Current oncologic concepts call for local nodal sampling and excision in areas such as the axillary, inguinal, and pelvic nodal confluences, often leading to significant lymphatic disruption and subsequent failed function.

Clinical Findings and Diagnosis of Secondary Lymphedema

Most patients present with painless swelling of the extremity most closely related to the original surgical procedure, radiation course, or site of traumatic injury. Over time—sometimes weeks, but even months to multiple years, the swelling increases and can progress from the non-pitting edema of early stage disease to a more typically non-pitting edema of more advanced stages of lymphedema. Concomitant with these changes, the limb becomes more difficult to move, enlarging to a multiple of the volume of a normal, contralateral extremity. A positive Stemmer Sign [2, 3]—in which the examiner cannot pinch the skin on the dorsum of the second toe with his index finger and thumb—is strongly indicative of lymphedema [2]. Integumental thickening occurs in moderate to severe lymphedema with histological findings of parakeratosis and hyperkeratosis that are susceptible to fissure formation, and may predispose to bouts of cellulitis. As lymphedema progresses, there are increased

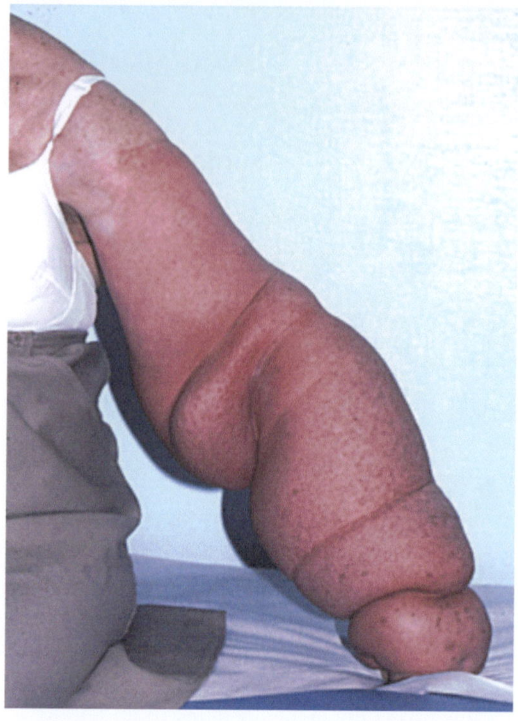

Fig. 8.1 Secondary lymphedema following mastectomy, axillary node dissection, and radiation therapy, complicated by cellulitis. Severe cellulitis, as depicted here, usually requires intravenous antibiotic therapy and possible hospitalization

fibrin deposits, diffuse fibrosis, and hyperplasia of fat in the subcutaneous compartment. Cracks in the thickened skin can lead to chronic drainage known as lymphorrea, delaying wound healing in all of the affected areas, or to outright infection (Fig. 8.1) [3]. Non-pitting edema, also, becomes more evident in the advanced stages. In order to provide a uniform international classification system for the stages of lymphedema, a Consensus Document was created by the International Society of Lymphology, which informs discussion of clinical cases; four stages are clearly defined in this system [4]. Stage 0 is a normal appearing extremity that has abnormal lymph transport on imaging (such as lymphoscintigraphy); Stage I is early edema responsive to elevation; Stage II has pitting edema unresponsive to elevation, and Stage III limbs have fibrosis, fat hypertrophy, and skin changes (Figs. 8.2 and 8.3).

Although advanced secondary lymphedema is obvious on clinical examination, the early stages can be less definitively determined, and are often confused with venous dysfunction, other vascular disorders, obesity, lipedema (Figs. 8.4 and 8.5) and various hematological-lymphatic congenital disorders. In a recent review [5] of referrals to a Lymphedema Center, patients were commonly misdiagnosed; only 75 % had a verifiable diagnosis of lymphedema. In 25 % of the group, a diagnosis other than lymphedema accounted for their

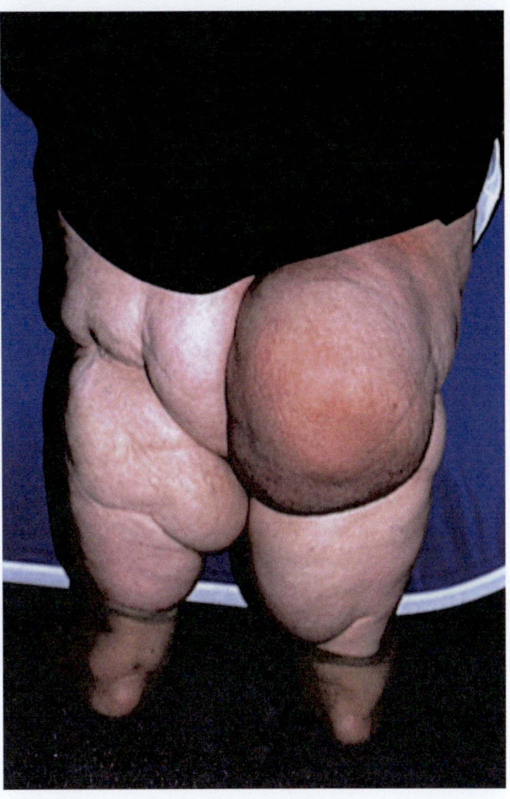

Fig. 8.4 A patient with extreme lipedema. The feet are spared, but extensive deposits of fat are present in both lower extremities above the ankle

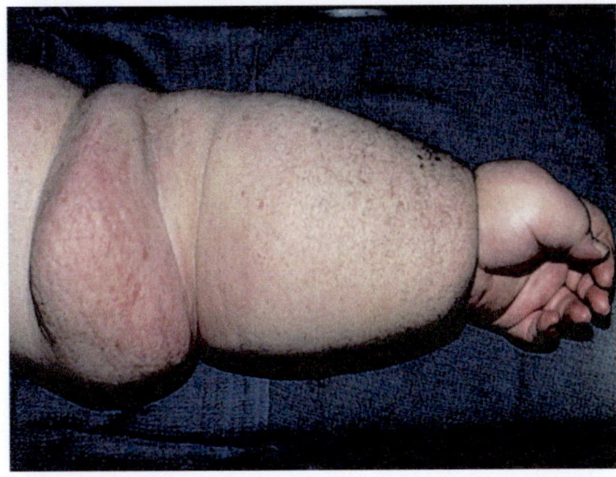

Fig. 8.2 Extreme swelling and skin thickening signifying advanced lymphedema

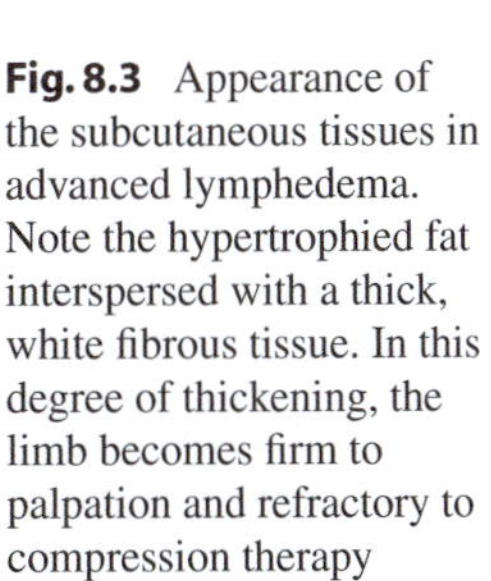

Fig. 8.3 Appearance of the subcutaneous tissues in advanced lymphedema. Note the hypertrophied fat interspersed with a thick, white fibrous tissue. In this degree of thickening, the limb becomes firm to palpation and refractory to compression therapy

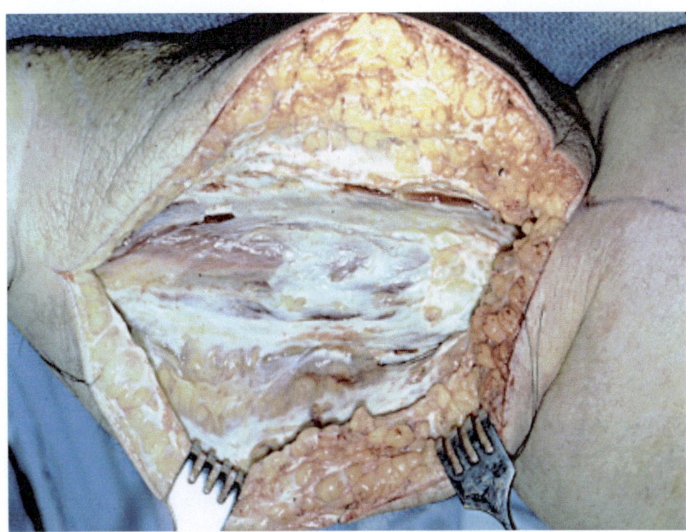

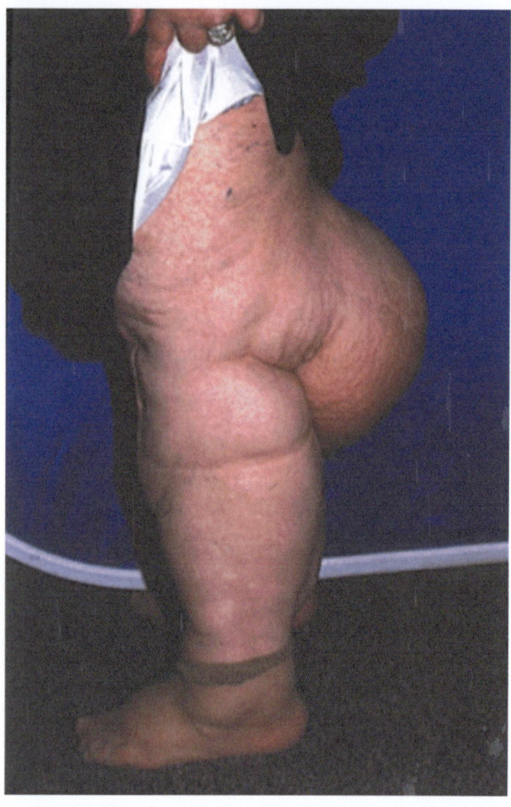

Fig. 8.5 In some patients with lipedema, fat deposition in the subcutaneous tissues leads to outpouchings of skin stretched by the accumulated adipose tissue. These extensions create folds of skin which can cause obstruction of the lymphatics localized within them. Areas of permanent lymphedema occur within such regions of a limb with lipedema. A basketball type of appearance usually indicates lymphedema that develops in the context of lipedema, and can be confirmed by lymphoscintigraphy

condition, leading to improper or delayed treatment. Limb volume circumferential measurement along with water displacement devices can assist in the assessment of a correct diagnosis and its severity, but they are not specific for lymphedema. Tape measurements, in particular, are notoriously unreliable because they are so easily influenced by the subjectivity of the strength of pull on the tape or the selection of anatomic landmarks, usually points on bones that are used as end points. Water displacement measurements performed preoperatively and postoperatively assist in an assessment of the efficacy of any surgical intervention. Other techniques under investigation use bioimpedance instruments and infrared laser perometry. Because all of these methods correlate, they can be used collectively in the diagnosis of lymphedema [6–8]. It is clearly difficult to assess edema in certain areas such as the head, neck, breast, and genitalia, especially if circumferential measurements are the mainstay. Patients tend to underreport extremity lymphedema, especially upper extremity edema following breast cancer treatment, either due to the inaccuracy of the method or other issues relating to self-reporting. For those who rely on a determination of upper extremity lymphedema prevalence following breast cancer based on the common instruments described, gross inaccuracies have led to a bewildering spectrum of range, and a confusing picture of how many are actually afflicted.

Diagnostic Imaging

Radiologic lymphography or lymphangiography was popularized by Kinmonth [6] who demonstrated with great clarity the anatomy of the lymphatic system using lipiodol contrast medium. However, toxicity by the contrast agent resulted in damage to lymphatic endothelium and subsequent occlusion of the vessel. Radiocolloid imaging with technetium-labelled antimony sulfide allows lymphoscintigraphic imaging of both lymphatics and nodal basins without toxicity and is virtually free of allergic reaction. Lymphoscintigraphy is not only 100 % specific for delineating lymphatic channels, but can also be used to evaluate lymphatic transport using transit times and demonstrations of lymphatic collateralization and dermal back flow. At our Lymphedema Center, a lymphoscintigram is required in all patients, confirming the correctness of the diagnosis and assisting in adjunctive classification of the degree of lymphatic dysfunction. Failed or markedly delayed nodal visualization documents the severity of the lymphedema; any improvement in the lymphoscintigraphic appearance is extremely useful in the selection of treatment management programs. Lymphoscintigraphy can be used to determine whether certain surgical approaches are indicated, such as a microsurgical or an excisional technique. The status of previously functioning lymphatic channels is an important postoperative finding, helping to validate the efficacy of the operation. Other diagnostic modalities include CT and MRI imaging, but unlike lymphoscintigraphy, are not specific for lymphedema. They do visualize pathologic components of lymphedema, such as hypertrophied fatty collections in the subcutaneous tissues, thickening in the skin, and fluid accumulations that occur in earlier stages with pitting edema, but their low specificity is a problem. Neither MRI nor CT examination is useful in the identification of areas of lymphatic obstruction, a useful observation for new microsurgical constructive techniques of lymph node transfer and lymphatico-venous anastomosis. The most commonly confused conditions—chronic venous insufficiency, lipedema, and obesity—can be differentiated by a combination of physical examination and radionuclide imaging, despite some overlap in these conditions. Lymphedema is not usually associated with chronic venous insufficiency, but such a combination is possible. A lymphoscintigram should be unremarkable in such a patient. Lipedema is distinguished by a number of factors, including bilaterality, female gender association, severity of fat accumulation (most commonly in the lower extremities), absence of iatrogenic causation such as oncological therapeutic intervention, and sparing of the dorsum of the foot when the lower extremity is involved.

Obesity is also distinguishable from secondary lymphedema, but less so with primary lymphedema (which is often bilateral). In extreme obesity [7]—BMI over 40—excess accumulation of adipose tissue causes obstruction of lymphatic by the formation of large skin folds and creases. Lymphoscintigraphy in such patients demonstrates obstruction, dilatation, and extravasation of radiotracer, consistent with a diagnosis of lymphedema. If the obesity persists—the exact timetable is unknown—lymphatic channels can fibrose on a permanent basis. It is also unknown whether effective treatment of obesity with attendant massive weight loss can reverse the lymphatic dysfunction. This risk of obesity to lymphatic function has not been previously appreciated. In addition, procedures associated with massive weight loss surgery such as medial

thigh lift can cause secondary lymphedema by injuring lymphatics during the removal of excess skin and fatty tissues.

Secondary Lymphedema and Risk Factors

Swelling of the arm following treatment of breast cancer constitutes the largest category of patients with secondary lymphedema most likely caused by various combinations of surgery and radiation therapy [8, 9]. Specifically, the extent of axillary lymph node dissection has been identified as a major factor, but large population based studies do not exist for confirmation. Lymphedema incidence assessment is complicated by widespread misunderstanding of the definition of lymphedema and its definitive diagnosis, and by major differences in the reporting of secondary lymphedema. Despite using important patient characteristics of extent of surgery, number of nodes, type and duration of postoperative radiotherapy, and the length of follow-up, a wide range of reported incidence, ranging approximately from 2 to 43 %, is known and accepted. When patients report upper extremity lymphedema following breast cancer treatment, an incidence of 14 % based on circumferential measurements is observed; when actual volume measurements are conducted with water displacement and perometry, the incidence of secondary lymphedema of the upper extremity rises to 25.5 %. Lymphedema occurs most often (38 % of patients) after combined axillary sampling and radiotherapy. Commonly accepted risk factors are patient age, body mass index, and length of follow-up. The latter factor adds confusion to the literature because of the wide variation in onset of lymphedema—from a few months to 10–20 years after surgery and radiotherapy. Also, despite the Consensus Document, different gradations of lymphedema severity are used internationally, and many physicians are ignorant of current grading systems.

Some controlled randomized trials have been reported comparing the incidence of lymphedema after sentinel node biopsy with axillary sampling.

Not surprising, sentinel node biopsy is associated with less arm swelling than axillary lymph node sampling, which is more extensive and therefore more likely to be by injurious to lymphatic function [10]. Patients reported that the incidence of moderate to severe lymphedema was less with sentinel node biopsy than with axillary sampling, 5 % versus 13 %. However, the reporting was conducted at 12 months after operation, a short follow-up given that most lymphedema occurs later than the first year [10–13]. Patients are usually aware of the risks of axillary sampling, but may not be expecting lymphedema following sentinel node biopsy because it is depicted as a much lesser operation. Unfortunately, secondary lymphedema has been observed in 6.9 % of patients at 6 months and in 5 % at a median of 5 years follow-up. In contrast, axillary lymph node sampling was found to be a cause of lymphedema in 16 % of patients for the same time interval.

Lymphedema remains incurable at this time, and prevention is controversial. Standard precautions include a program of elevation, elastic compression garments, compression pumps, exercise [14], and physiotherapy. Antibiotic therapy is needed as soon as the earliest symptoms and signs of cellulitis become evident: redness, swelling, pain, and fever. Some patients are urged to have antibiotics available immediately at the commencement of an attack, and to seek intravenous antibiotic therapy in a local emergency department. Cellulitis can be unpredictable in the earlier stage of secondary lymphedema. Patients with mild to moderate degrees may avoid attacks of cellulitis completely whereas others will suffer recurrent episodes. Multiple attacks of cellulitis can lead to increasing debility as an ever diminishing quantity of functioning lymphatic channels suffer inflammation, fibrosis, and obliteration of patency. These changes are demonstrable on serial lymphoscintigraphic images, which document the destruction. Patients are advised to avoid blood pressure monitoring and venipuncture in the affected extremity, but there is little if any proof that these precautions are either effective or necessary. The reported incidence of infection following venipuncture in an upper extremity afflicted with lymphedema essentially equals the clean wound infection rate in normal limbs.

Over time, the upper extremity in patients with secondary lymphedema increases in volume from a distal to proximal direction. Pitting edema—present in the early stages, becomes less evident as the high protein fluid in the interstitial space causes progressive inflammation, fibrosis, and fat deposition. Brorson [15–17] was among the first to note that the arm continues to enlarge in some patients, perhaps as part of the natural history of the disease. As a result of adipogenesis stimulated presumably by growth factors within lymphatic fluid—Veg F and others have been identified—a hypertrophy of fat in the subcutaneous compartment containing injured lymphatics and extravastated lymphatic fluid occurs and can continue indefinitely. An interval appears to exist clinically between the onset of lymphedema and the appearance of significant fat hypertrophy, but its duration is unknown. Similar to the mechanism in obese patients, the hypertrophied fat acts to obstruct adjacent lymphatics and abet inflammation and infection. Patients with secondary lymphedema have a 70 times increased risk of infection in the affected versus the unaffected limb.

Secondary upper extremity lymphedema has been associated with post-mastectomy and post-lumpectomy radiation therapy as a result of studies investigating sentinel node and axillary node sampling risks. Upper extremity [18] lymphedema appears to be at greatest risk for women who have both procedures, and the risk continues post-treatment for an indefinite period with this combination. Estimates of lymphedema risk range from 4 to 72 %. With the possible exception of lymphedema occurring in the early weeks or months after axillary dissection and post-lumpectomy radiation, arm lymphedema is not reversible. The chronicity of lymphedema raises the issue of possible malignant transformation over time. Fortunately this risk is extremely low, estimated at .07 to .45 %, but lymphangiosarcoma has been recorded arising in a lymphedematous upper extremity after treatment of breast cancer. When this tumor occurs in a lower extremity following inguinal lymphadenectomy and radiation therapy, prognosis is extremely poor because of the probability of pulmonary metastases. With the limited efficacy of either chemotherapy or radiation therapy, most patients live less than 2 years.

Psychosocial Problems in Secondary Lymphedema

The persistence of lymphedema in the upper extremity has been connected to a multitude of problems involving psychological, sexual, and physical aspects of daily activities. For those in whom the lymphedema develops in the dominant limb, there is greater negative impact and disruption of function. These patients should be supported with appropriate counseling, education, and medications as needed. Frustration, anxiety, and depression are some of the psychological needs to be addressed, along with increased attention directed to covariates of socioeconomic, social, and ethnic factors that determine quality of life (QOL). These factors may be ignored by physicians who, anecdotally, emphasize the sheer importance of "being alive' over all of the comorbidities associated with secondary lymphedema of the upper extremity.

Secondary Lymphedema of the Lower Extremity

This condition occurs in a manner that is similar to upper extremity lymphedema, but can be more severely debilitating because of the dependency of the lower limb and use in ambulation. Patients with malignancies of the urogenital tract, including prostate and testicular tumors in men and ovarian and uterine malignancies in women are at highest risk, but secondary lower extremity lymphedema has also been reported following trauma or any disease process that injures or destroys inguinal and pelvic nodes. Risk factors mimic those for the arm, including obesity, extent of nodal dissection, duration and intensity of radiotherapy, and characteristics of the tumor.

Scrotal lymphedema, while much less common, is a particularly disabling form of secondary lymphedema that can occur in the same context. Injury to inguinal nodes can obstruct scrotal lymphatics and lead to massive scrotal swelling. There is increased pain from the sheer heaviness

of the tissues and much greater risk of cellulitis. The enlargement can result in an appearance of a buried penis. Men can suffer from associated erectile dysfunction and social embarrassment.

Management of Secondary Lower Extremity Lymphedema

The overwhelming majority of cases of secondary leg lymphedema can be managed successfully with compression therapy, including custom-fitted, double layered garments, combined with daily pneumatic compression pumping. Surgical intervention has been reserved for those patients who fail conservative therapy as manifested by increasing bouts of cellulitis and worsening of swelling. Surgical intervention is indicated when conservative therapy fails, with suction assisted lipectomy (liposuctioning) considered to be the first choice technique. Popularized by Brorson (Figs. 8.6, 8.7, 8.8, 8.9,

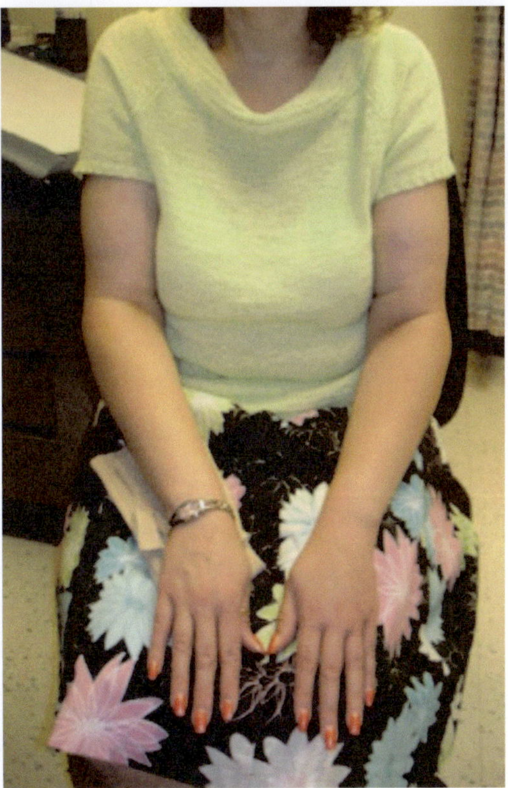

Fig. 8.6 Patient developed moderate lymphedema of both upper extremities following bilateral brachioplasties

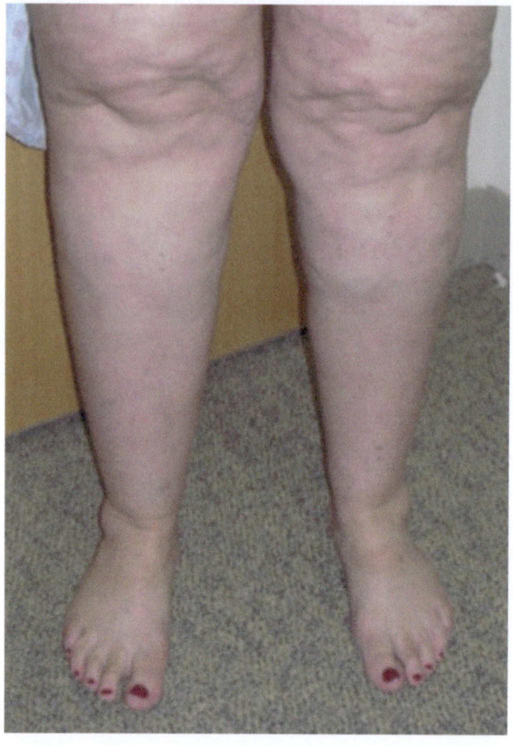

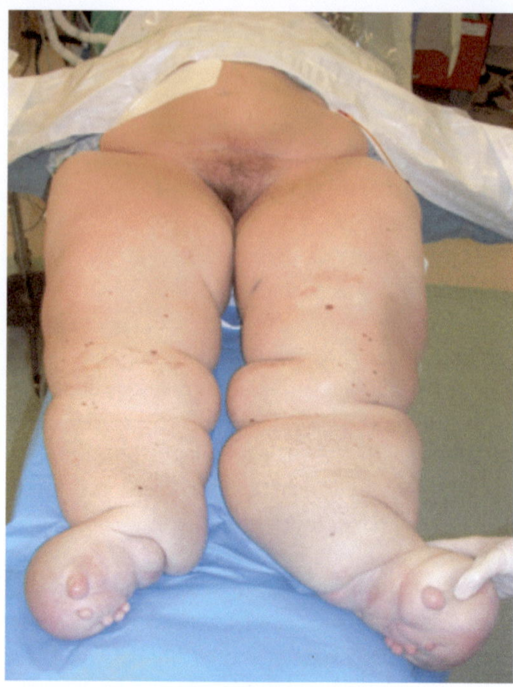

Fig. 8.8 Suction assisted lipectomy was offered to this patient with congenital limb disease who suffered recurrent bouts of cellulitis. Excess folds of skin create multiple areas of mechanical obstruction of lymphatics and secondary lymphedema

Fig. 8.7 Patient with bilateral lower extremity lymphedema after bilateral medial thighplasties

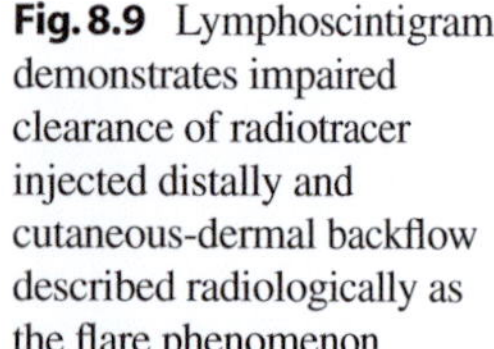

Fig. 8.9 Lymphoscintigram demonstrates impaired clearance of radiotracer injected distally and cutaneous-dermal backflow described radiologically as the flare phenomenon

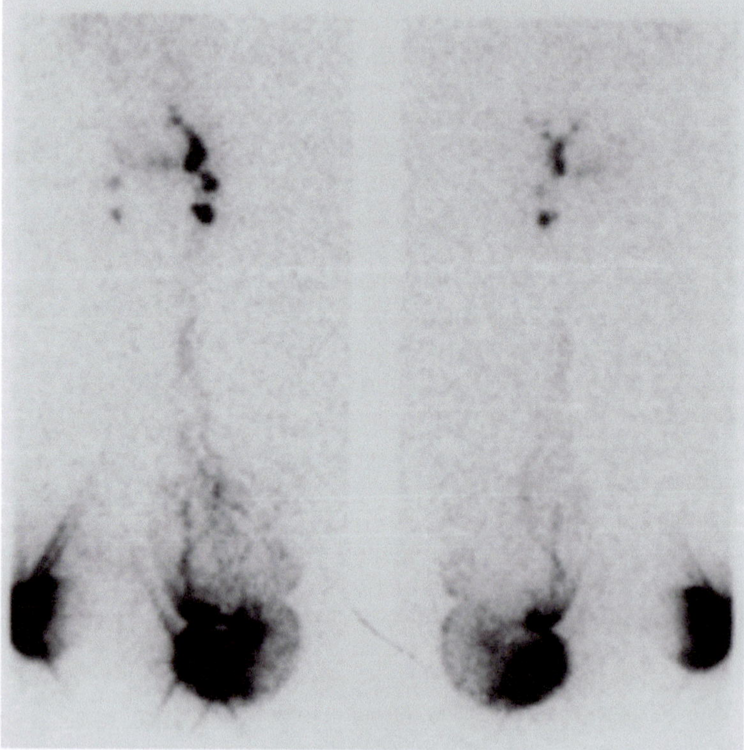

Fig. 8.10 Following debulking by liposuctioning, the patient has marked excess of skin which can be treated by direct excision

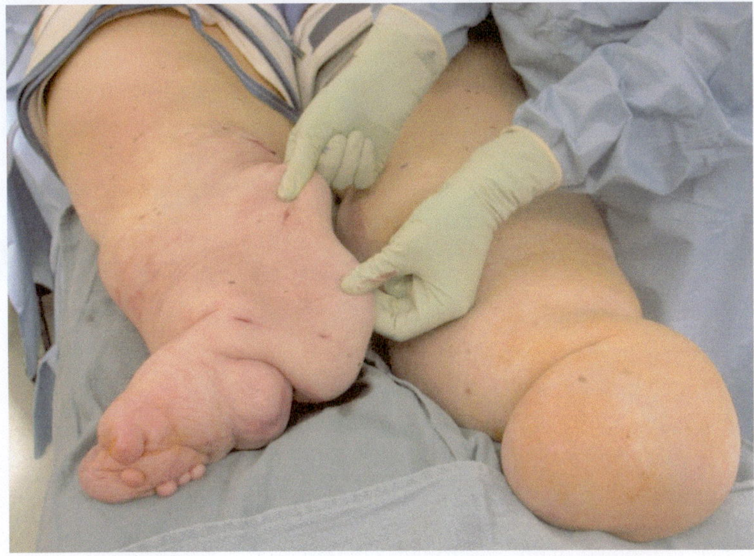

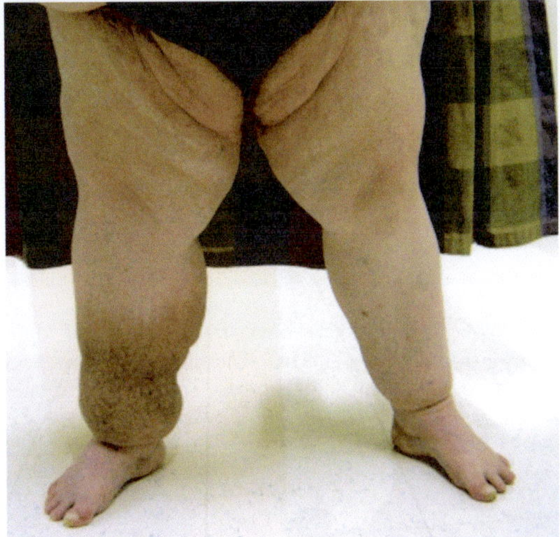

Fig. 8.11 Patient with lipedema and secondary lymphedema, preoperative appearance

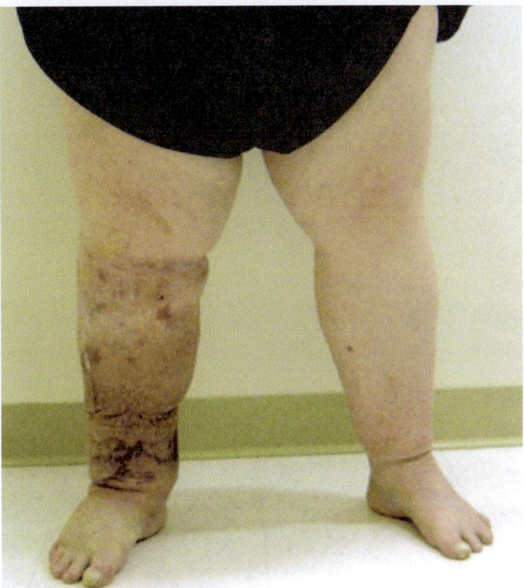

Fig. 8.12 Postoperative appearance after liposuctioning, the only technique which removes the hypertrophied fat present in the subcutaneous space

8.10, 8.11, and 8.12) and others [19, 21], the technique is based on the observation that excess fat in the subcutaneous space appears to be secondary to hyperplasia and adipogenesis. Suction lipectomy is not initiated until the pitting edema has been successfully eradicated by conservative treatment. Once that goal has been accomplished, complete reduction of the limb is achieved by liposuctioning. The patient is required to wear a compression garment custom-fitted for the limb continuously.

Follow-up of 11 years demonstrated a complete maintenance of normal leg volume in the involved leg. A significant reduction of morbidity was also seen following liposuctioning for secondary lower extremity lymphedema: frequency of episodes of cellulitis was reduced as were infection related hospitalizations. Patients continue after liposuctioning with exercises, elevation, compression garments, pumps, manual lymphatic drainage, and proper skin care practices.

Liposuctioning for Secondary Lymphedema of the Arm

Although controlled compression and elastic bandaging have been the best recognized treatment regimens for secondary arm lymphedema, these approaches can be disappointing in their ability to reduce existing lymphedema and control or prevent progression. Patients treated with liposuction [20] (Figs. 8.13, 8.14, 8.15, 8.16, and 8.17) combined with controlled compression therapy had a reduction of 106 % of arm volume at 1 year. In a follow-up study comparing liposuction and controlled compression therapy with controlled compression therapy alone, the combined therapy was significantly more effective with a mean difference of approximately 100 ml during the first year. When compression therapy was discontinued postoperatively, however, there was a severe recrudescence of swelling remedied by reinstitution of the garment. Despite the immediate and substantial improvement provided by liposuctioning, a lifetime commitment to

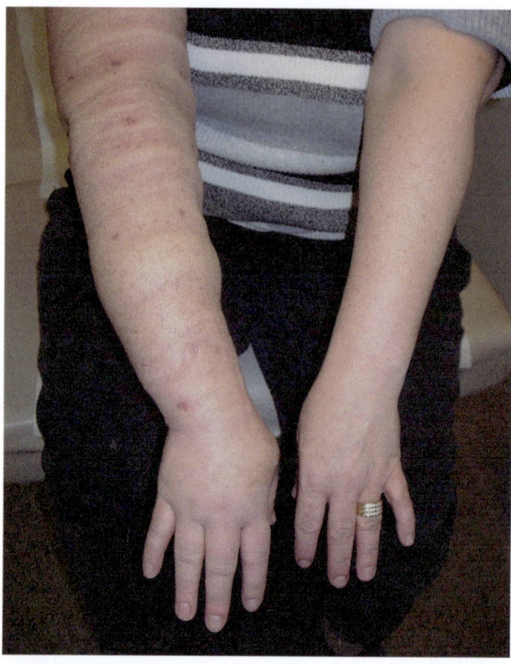

Fig. 8.14 Result 1 year after liposuctioning of right upper extremity lymphedema. The patient must wear a compression garment daily in order to preserve the reduction in arm volume

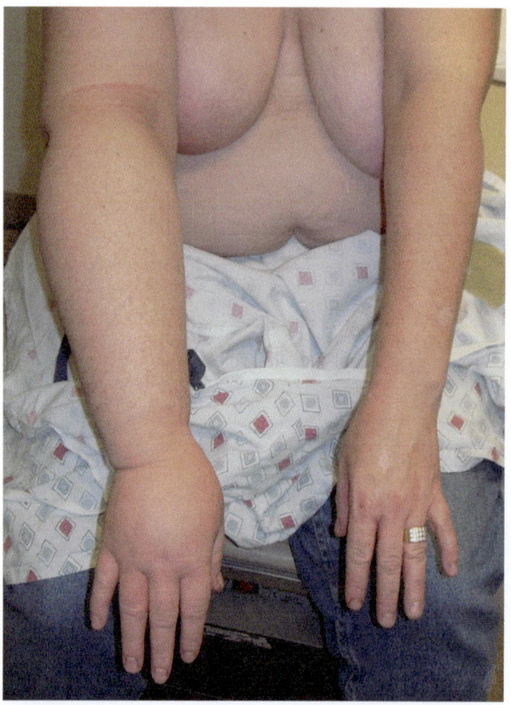

Fig. 8.13 Patient with right upper extremity lymphedema refractory to compression therapy and bandaging

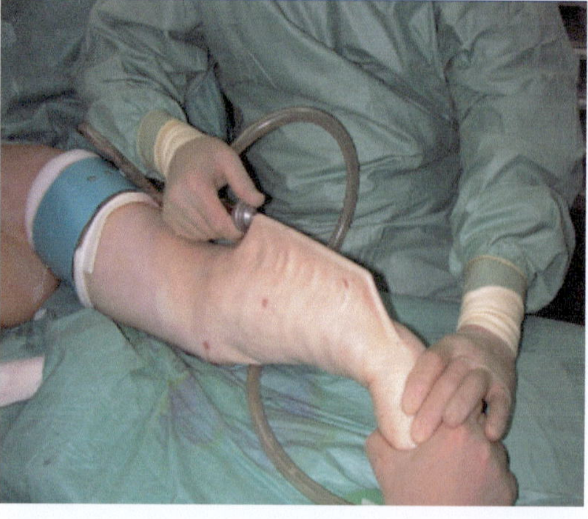

Fig. 8.15 Technique of liposuctioning for lymphedema popularized by Brorson. Corrections of up to 106 % of volume of the involved extremity have been recorded

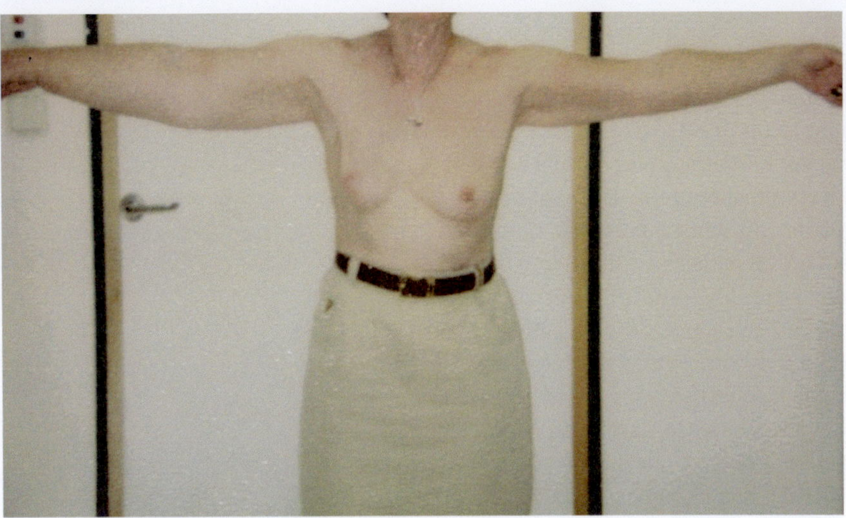

Fig. 8.16 Microlymphatic dissection. Preoperative appearance of a patient with right upper extremity lymphedema, prior to liposuctioning with Brorson's technique

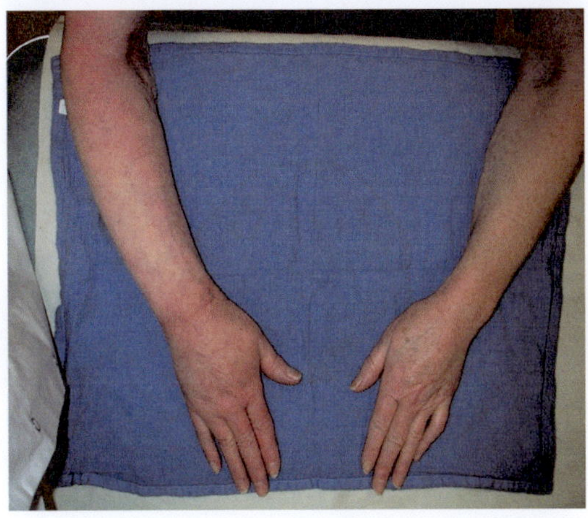

Fig. 8.17 Result 10 years after liposuctioning. The limb has been maintained with a favorable cosmetic outcome and essentially free of the stigmata of lymphedema

wearing a garment is mandated. The efficacy of this combined approach has been observed over a 20-year follow-up. Suction lipectomy is favored for patients with mild to moderate levels of lymphedema, but is not appropriate for advanced cases with severe fibrosis. The rigidity of the fibrotic tissues prevents passage of a liposuctioning cannula, and the fibrosed fatty layer resists removal by this means. Patients with extreme swelling, fibrosis of the subcutaneous tissues, and chronic skin changes of thickening require aggressive skin resection and subcutaneous debulking by direct excision down to fascia or muscle [22].

Liposuctioning is also less feasible in the setting of genital lymphedema. It represents one of the most important advances in the surgical management of both arm and leg edema through its augmentation of cutaneous blood flow, sparing of existing lymphatic structures in the area of treatment, and restoration of a normal quality of life.

Other Surgical Therapies: Staged Subcutaneous Excision

Because no surgical intervention is curative for lymphedema, initial management should always be conservative. Failure of conservative therapy is generally meant to include loss of function, increased morbidity, and a history of recurrent infections, often defined as three or more per year. Excisional procedures can provide long lasting reduction of limb volume, but do not achieve any physiologic improvements. Similar to suction lipectomy, staged subcutaneous excision preserves overlying flaps of skin, removing the underlying, hypertrophied fatty layer down to muscle fascia. Long flaps are mobilized for much of the full length of the extremity. Although it involves two stages (procedures), reductions in limb volume of up to 80 % are seen. When the skin is excessive or rigid, staged subcutaneous excision offers enhanced remodeling of the limb that is superior to suction lipectomy. In a long-term follow-up, 38 patients with lower extremity lymphedema were followed for an average of 14 years (range 3–27 years). Of the 38 patients, ten had developed lower extremity lymphedema after combined ablative surgery and radiation therapy for pelvic disease. Using photographic analysis as the principal means of assessment (though volume displacement, circumferential measurements, and lymphoscintigraphy were also utilized), 30 patients had prolonged improvement in function, aesthetic contour, and volume following this surgical method. There was an observed reduction in episodes of cellulitis and in some patients, these attacks subsided completely. Men did not have results as good as women, and minor complications of wound breakdown occurred in four patients. No differences in the result occurred regardless of cause, primary or acquired. These procedures can be associated with lengthy, unsightly scarring and numbness of the skin flaps. They can also be offered to patients with the most severe forms of elephantiasis often referred to as end-stage lymphedema, as a salvage effort prior to amputation.

Charles Procedure

Mostly discarded as a surgical alternative therapy, the Charles procedure (Fig. 8.18) involves the excision of skin, subcutaneous tissues, and fascia down to the underlying muscle surface, followed by extensive skin grafting for wound closure. Cutaneous tissues are prone to recurrent breakdown on multiple areas, usually secondary to fissuring in skin surfaces weakened by chronic keratotic processes. Most of these procedures are performed on the lower extremity from below the knee in a distal direction. In addition to skin breakdown because of increased susceptibility to trauma, the Charles Procedure can be complicated

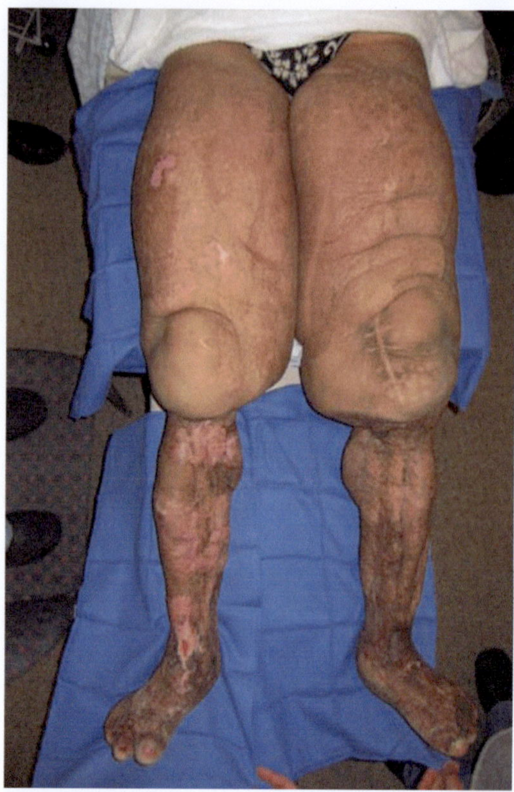

Fig. 8.18 Disfigured appearance after a Charles Procedure. The skin and soft tissues below the knee have been excised down to muscle fascia. Wound closure completed by split thickness skin grafting. Although this procedure reduces infections in the distal leg, it is painful to experience and most unsightly

by severe lymph leakage. It creates a permanent deformity of contour that is aesthetically unacceptable to many patients and surgeons. Its current use is largely relegated to the so-called tropical elephantiasis, the final stage of lymphedema.

Surgical Treatment of Secondary Lymphedema: Physiologic Procedures: Lymphatico-venous Anastomosis

Physiologic procedures [23–27] attempt to restore the normal lymphatic flow mechanism by creating new connections between the lymphatic and venous systems. They are comprised of many procedures that achieve this goal through microsurgically achieved lymphatico-venous anastomosis (LVA), or by transferring functioning lymphatics and associated nodes to areas of deficiency. Vascularized lymph node transfer is currently the most popular form of lymphatic supplementation, but a variety of procedures including lymphatic grafting, pedicled flap transposition, and free tissue transfer are being used to improve lymphatic drainage. These physiologic procedures work best in earlier stages of secondary lymphedema because they may be ineffective in a fibrosed field typically seen in later stages of lymphedema. They do not directly remove excessive areas of skin and fat, nor do they appear to diminish areas of established adipose tissue hypertrophy, thus limiting any opportunity for a diminution of limb volume. Although standard conservative therapy is considered first choice treatment for secondary lymphedema, microsurgical lymphatic reconstruction, and in particular lymphatic–venous anastomosis could be an alternate option.

Advances in the technology of microsurgery now permit microsurgically engineered connections between vessels in a size range of 0.3 to 0.5 mm, allowing small venules and lymphatics of similar size to be connected without creating the extreme pressure gradients that doomed earlier attempts of this type. By anastomosing microvessels to one another a better patency rate has been observed. When multiple such connections are performed, effective drainage has been achieved.

There are few prospective case series available for comparison with this technique (LVA). Ranges in the reduction of volume or circumference were as low as 2 % and as high as 30 % with follow-up times of 5–72 months. There were few if any complications in these studies because of the limited nature of the dissection, but most importantly, it was necessary to continue postoperative bandaging or compression in all case series.

The second largest category of physiologic procedures comprises vascularized lymphatic tissue transfer and lymphatic interposition grafts. These techniques, like lymphatico-venous anastomosis, restore lymphatic drainage pathways, either by directly supplying healthy, vascularized lymphatics, or by bypassing areas of obstruc-

tion. Afferent and efferent lymphatic pathways can be reconnected by interposing tissues as a bridge.

Evaluating whether these new microsurgical procedures have a role in the treatment of breast cancer related lymphedema is difficult when evidence-based medicine criteria are applied. In an area where there is an absence of randomized or comparative studies, the available data results in level IV evidence, but the methodology of these studies can be criticized for a number of inconsistencies. Patient selection criteria lack standardization regarding the status or extent of lymphedema that is present preoperatively. Hence, valid comparisons of outcomes in terms of symptom relief, reduction of limb volume, and improvements in lymphatic flow are difficult to determine when the lymphedema stage of the study population is not conclusively known. Another confounding fact was that different clinical criteria were used in the selection of patients for surgery. Given these heterogeneous populations of patients, the superiority of one physiologic technique over another cannot be stated. What is known is that all of these procedures are associated with reductions in limb volume; however, lymph fluid collections and collections of hypertrophied fat may not be responsive to these approaches. The extent of fatty accumulations in the limb should be assessed preoperatively and only patients with comparable findings preoperatively can be candidates for a valid postoperative comparison. Furthermore, the chronicity of the lymphedema should be assessed preoperatively because the lymphatic vessels may have suffered endothelial injury mediated by chronic hypertension within the lymphatic system.

Another method of postoperative assessment subjects the patient to a post-treatment lymphoscintigram. This safe radionuclide study provides an anatomic and quantitative evaluation of the involved lymphatics. Unfortunately, this critically important tool study was performed in less than half of the series reported. Another method that has gained popularity is indocyanine green fluorescence lymphangiography.

Tissue transfer techniques permit discontinuation of postoperative conservative therapies, liberating the patient from time consuming, immobilizing treatments which have been necessary following suction lipectomy. The best results using microsurgical techniques occur in patients with shorter duration of breast cancer related lymphedema. Despite the methodological drawbacks noted in the tissue transfer studies, vascularized lymph node transfer and in particular inguinal lymph node transfer holds special promise as an effective treatment for secondary lymphedema. The nodal transfer can be piggybacked onto an autologous breast reconstruction technique such as a perforator slap so that two objectives are met: breast reconstruction and placement of added, vascularized, functioning lymphatics intended to treat established lymphedema or prevent a future problem. Well-constructed prospective studies will be needed to give the answers to questions of what procedure works best and when is the optimal timing for the surgical intervention, but the early evidence is suggesting that these physiologic procedures reduce limb volume and circumference and have minimal complications.

New Microsurgical Techniques for Secondary Lymphedema Vascularized Lymph Node Transfer

Despite the success of vascularized lymph node transfer in the management of both upper and lower extremity secondary lymphedema, donor site lymphedema remains an important problem, based on the difficulty in knowing precisely which nodes drain the trunk on the extremity. To date, this problem has been a vexing one because it defies selection of nodal donors based on an anatomical landmarks alone. A new technique known as reverse lymphatic mapping uses alternate injections of technetium into the first and second web spaces and indocyanine green in the lower abdomen to differentiate nodes that are selectively draining each site. This physiologically based technique maps out appropriate nodes for harvest without harming those involved in the lymphatic drainage of the lymphedematous extremity. Thirteen consecutive patients with a mean age of 50 underwent vascularized groin lymph node

transfer for post-mastectomy upper extremity lymphedema. The superficial radial artery and the cephalic vein were used as recipient vessels. Outcomes were assessed by upper limb girth, incidence of cellulitis and lymphoscintigraphy.

Results: All flaps survived; no donor site morbidity. At a mean follow up of 56 months, the reduction in limb volume was 50.6%, a statistically significant measurement. Post-operative lymphoscintigraphy indicated improved lymphatic drainage of the upper arm, decreased lymph stasis, and rapid lymphatic clearance. To explain their results, the authors hypothesized that the vascularized lymph node transfer acts as an internal pump or suction pathway for lymphatic clearance.

Non-surgical Treatment of Secondary Lymphedema

Nonoperative management is considered the primary approach for the treatment of secondary lymphedema. Although not curative, when it is combined with patient education relating to the care of an affected limb, it can be successful. Most patients can be managed this way, but they must avoid any injury to the extremity, which could cause a break in skin integrity and lead to infectious complications such as cellulitis. Exercise is encouraged but is unlikely to reduce swelling by itself; swimming, in particular is helpful because it avoids dependency of both the upper and lower extremities. However, weight lifting and other upper body activities were discouraged out of fear that there was a risk of creating new lymphedema or worsening existing lymphedema. Despite an absence of factual support, this belief persists.

In order to determine if weight lifting affected lymphedema, researchers compared lymphedema risk in two groups of women [14]: women who lifted weights and those who did not. Of 134 patients studied, 11 % in the weight lifting group and 17 % in the no exercise group developed lymphedema. Among patients who had five or more nodes removed, 7 % of the weight lifting group and 22 % of the no weight lifting developed lymphedema. The authors concluded that

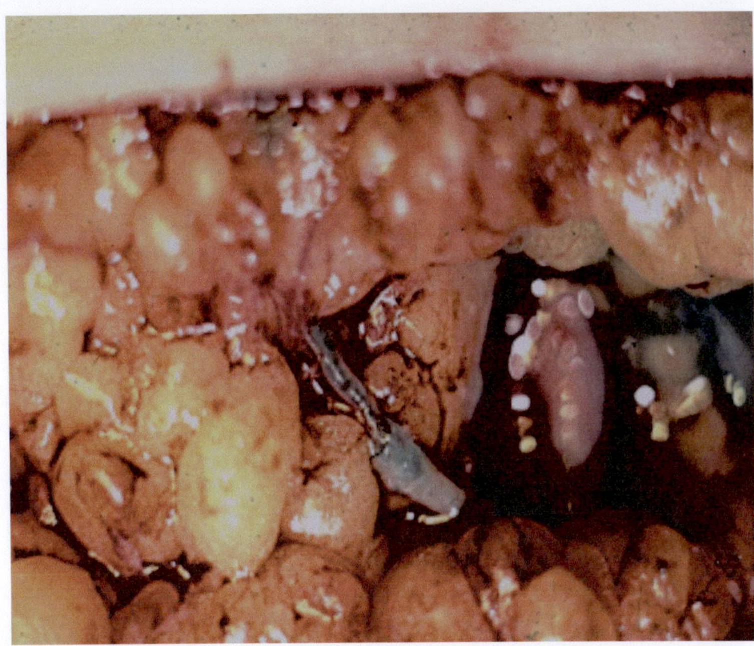

Fig. 8.19 Microlymphatico-venous anastomosis completed. The narrow lymphatic fills the larger, venous structure with lymph. A favorable gradient of flow from lymphatic to vein can be temporary, resulting in later occlusion of the lymphatic secondary to backflow of blood

weight lifting was not a risk factor for the development of lymphedema.

Compression therapy is successful because it achieves a real diminution of limb volume by expressing edema and reducing the quantity of high-protein levels in the interstitial space. It appears to increase the transport of lymph and may help to open lymphatics considered to be obstructed or fibrosed by decreasing the surrounding interstitial pressure. Pneumatic compression utilizes pumping devices that deliver intermittent pressures through a sleeve that is compartmentalized, allowing sequential inflations that fill distal and proximal chambers in a sequence that mimics physiologic mechanisms.

Complete decongestive therapy is a multi-component program for patients with established lymphedema that aims to control and reduce swelling and its attendant incidence of bacteria-induced infection. The program consists primarily of manual lymphatic drainage (MLD) accompanied by compression bandaging that follows immediately afterward. Other aspects of the program include exercise and skin and nail care. Manual Lymphatic Drainage is a specific technique performed by trained technicians who can expertly apply pressure to the superficial lymphatics beneath the skin and promote lymph transport to the venous system. By exercising light pressure in a distal to proximal direction, MLD works through lymphovenous anastomoses to promote evacuation of excess lymph fluid (Fig. 8.19). The compression bandaging that ensues creates a constant external compression between the fibrotic, non-elastic skin and the underlying fibrotic subcutaneous compartment. When successful, the limb softens and its circumference diminishes. Daily compression bandaging is necessary to prevent reaccumulation of lymphatic fluid in the tissues, most likely caused by decrease in tissue pressures related to loss of skin elasticity. Exercises supplement this effort by improving the natural pumping mechanism of skeletal muscle which surrounds lymphatic structures and stimulates lymphatic circulation.

Because data regarding the use of complete decongestive therapy are limited, prospective studies on the effect of CDT in lymphedema patients are needed. A study of 20 patients [28] reviewed those who were enrolled immediately after a diagnosis of lymphedema was made. Measurements were performed at 3 and 6 months, and after a year of treatment. There was a successful reduction in girth, with less pain, and Quality of Life and pain measurements continued to improve after the treatment was ended.

Conclusions

Secondary lymphedema, the most common form of lymphedema occurring in the USA, develops after injury to lymphatic channels following treatment of cancer. Although it can occur after disruption of any nodal group or basin, breast cancer treatment consisting of surgery of the axillary nodes, or even sentinel node harvest, combined with radiation therapy, is the single most important cause of secondary lymphedema. Other cancers treated by nodal and lymphatic interventions are similarly vulnerable, such as those associated with urological and gynecologic lesions. Reductions in the number of lymph nodes removed and increasing reliance on sentinel node biopsy have led to marked decreases in post-treatment lymphedema.

Although the disease is presently incurable, lymphedema treatments are showing promise. Established techniques of complex (complete) decongestive therapy have proven effective when combined with daily compressive bandaging. Microsurgical advances suggest that restoration of nodal and lymphatic physiological function may be realizable now or in the near future. Microsurgical lymphatico-venous anastomosis, abetted by significant technological improvement, can augment lymphatic function compromised by neoplasia. Vascularized lymph node transfer is perhaps the most exciting recent development because it offers the possibility of returning lymphatic drainage through functioning autologous transfers of tissues without incurring the feared complication of donor site induced lymphedema. These new surgical techniques have yet to be tested by prospective trials, but early evidence demonstrated by equally new techniques of imaging with indocyanine lymphography will be immensely useful in proving or disproving true functional improvement. Liposuctioning is extremely effective for early and moderate stages of lymphedema because it is the only technique that removes the hypertrophied fat in the subcutaneous compartment, yielding a 100 % reduction in limb circumferences. Long-term studies, at 15 years, show that volume is reduced and maintained if combined with daily bandaging.

References

1. Rockson SG, Rivera KK. Estimating the population burden of lymphedema. Ann NY Acad Sci. 2008;1131:147–54.
2. Stemmer R. A clinical symptom for the early and differential diagnosis of lymphedema. Vasa. 1976;5(3):261–2.
3. Schook CC, Mulliken JB, Fishman SJ, Almari AI, Green AK. Differential diagnosis of lower extremity lymphedema in 170 pediatric patients. Plast Recontr Surg. 2011;127:1571–81.
4. International Society of Lymphology. The diagnosis and treatment of peripheral lymphedema: 2013 Consensus Document of the International Society of Lymphology. Lymphology. 2013;46(1):2–11.
5. Maclellan RA, Couto R, Sullivan JE, Grant FD, Slavin SA, Greene AK. Management of primary and secondary lymphedema: analysis of 225 referrals to a center. Ann Plast Surg 2014 [Epub ahead of print].
6. Kinmonth JB. The lymphatics. London: Edward Arnold Ltd; 1982.
7. Greene AK, Grant FD, Slavin SA. Lower extremity lymphedema and elevated body-mass index. N Engl J Med. 2012;366(22):2136–7.
8. Ridner SH, Montgomery LD, Hepworth JT, Stewart BR, Armer JM. Comparison of upper limb volume measurement techniques and arm symptoms between healthy volunteers and individuals with known lymphedema. Lymphology. 2007;40(1):35–46.
9. Gloviczki P, Calcagno D, Schirger A, et al. Noninvasive evaluation of the swollen extremity: experiences with 190 lymphoscintigraphic examinations. J Vac Surg. 1989;9:683.
10. Erickson VS, Pearson M, Ganz PA, et al. Arm edema in breast cancer patients. J Natl Conc Inst. 2001;93:96–111.
11. Dayangac M, Makay O, Yeniay L, Aynaci M, Kapkac M, Yilmaz R. Precipitating factors for lymphedema following surgical treatment of breast cancer: implications for patients undergoing axillary lymph node dissection. Breast J. 2009;15(2):210–1.
12. Mansel RE, Fallowfield K, Kissin M. Randomized multicenter trial of sentinel node biopsy versus standard axillary treatment in operable breast cancer: the ALMANAC trial. J Natl Can Inst. 2006;98:599–609.
13. McLaughlin SA, Wright MJ, Morris KT, et al. Prevalence of lymphedema in women with breast cancer 5 years after sentinel lymph node biopsy or axillary dissection: patient perceptions and precautionary behaviors. J Clin Oncol. 2008;26:5220–8.

14. Schmitz KH, Ahmed RL, Troxel A, et al. Weight lifting in women with breast-cancer-related lymphedema. N Engl J Med. 2009;361:664.
15. Brorson H, Svensson H. Liposuction combined with controlled compression therapy reduces arm lymphedema more effectively than controlled compression therapy alone. Plast Reconstr Surg. 1998;102:1058.
16. Brorson H, Svensson H, Norrgren K, Thorsson O. Liposuction reduces arm lymphedema without significantly altering the already impaired lymph transport. Lymphology. 1998;31:156.
17. Brorson H, Ohlin K, Olsson G, Karlsson MK. Breast cancer-related chronic arm lymphedema is associated with excess adipose and muscle tissue. Lymphat Res Biol. 2009;7:3.
18. Passik SD, Newman SL, Brennan M, et al. Predictors of psychological distress, sexual dysfunctions and physical functioning among women with upper extremity lymphedema related to breast cancer. Psychooncology. 1995;4(4):255–63.
19. Greene AK, Slavin SA, Borud L. Treatment of lower extremity lymphedema with suction-assisted lipectomy. Plast Reconstr Surg. 2006;118:118e–21.
20. Brorson H, Ohlin K, Olsson G, Svensson B, Svensson H. Controlled compression and liposuction treatment for lower extremity lymphedema. Lymphology. 2008;41:52.
21. Johansson K, Lie E, Edkahl C, Lindfeldt J. A randomized study comparing manual lymph drainage with sequential pneumatic compression for treatment of postoperative and lymphedema. Lymphology. 1998;2:56.
22. Miller TA, Wyatt LE, Rudkin GH. Staged skin and subcutaneous excision for lymphedema: a favorable report of long-term results. Plast Recontr Surg. 1998;102:1486.
23. Lopez-Penha TR, Ijsbrandy C, Hendrix NAM, Heuts EM, Voogd AC, von Meyenfeldt MF, van der Hulst RRWJ. Microsurgical techniques for the treatment of breast cancer-related lymphedema: a systematic review. J Reconstr Microsurg. 2013;29(2):99–106.
24. Koshima I, Nanba Y, Tsutsui T, et al. Long-term follow-up after lymphaticovenular anastomosis for lymphedema in the legs. J Reconstr Microsurg. 2003;19:209.
25. Chang MH, Chen SC, Henry SL, Tan BK, Lin MC, Huang JJ. Vascularized groin lymph node transfer for post-mastectomy upper limb lymphedema: flap anatomy, recipient sites, and outcomes. Plast Reconstr Surg. 2013;131(6):1286–98.
26. Mihara M, Mihara M, Seki Y, et al. Comparison of indocyanine green lymphographic findings with the conditions of collecting lymphatic vessels of limbs in patients with lymphedema. Plast Reconstr Surg. 2013;132:1612–8.
27. Dayan JH, Dayan E, and Smith ML. Reverse lymphatic mapping: a new technique for maximizing safety in vascularized lymph node transfer. Plast Reconstr Surg 2014; [Epub ahead of print].
28. Mondry TE, Riffenburgh RH, Johnstone PA. Prospective trial of complete decongestive therapy for upper extremity lymphedema after breast cancer therapy. Cancer J. 2004;10(1):42–8. discussion 17–9.

Arin K. Greene

A.K. Greene, M.D., M.MSc. (✉)
Department of Plastic and Oral Surgery,
Boston Children's Hospital, Harvard Medical School,
300 Longwood Avenue, Boston, MA 02115, USA
e-mail: arin.greene@childrens.harvard.edu

Key Points

- Obesity-induced lymphedema affects both lower extremities.
- A BMI threshold of 50 exists at which point lymphatic dysfunction occurs.
- Definitive diagnosis of obesity-induced lymphedema is made using lymphoscintigraphy.
- Patients with obesity-induced lymphedema, or at risk for the disease, are referred to a bariatric weight loss center.
- Weight loss may improve lymphatic dysfunction, but might not reverse the condition.

Introduction

Obesity is a risk factor for developing secondary upper extremity lymphedema following radiation and/or lymphadenectomy. Obese individuals (i.e., body mass index (BMI) >30) have three times the risk of developing arm lymphedema, compared to patients with a BMI <25 [1]. BMI is the variable most closely associated with lymphedema after breast cancer treatment; the greater the BMI, the more likely the patient is to develop lymphedema [2]. BMI at the time of diagnosis appears to be a stronger risk factor for developing lymphedema than weight gain following treatment [3]. Although never studied, obese patients who undergo inguinal radiation and/or lymphadenectomy also are probably more likely to develop lower extremity lymphedema compared to normal-weighted individuals.

The mechanism by which an elevated BMI increases the risk of secondary lymphedema after lymphatic injury is unknown. Obese patients may have compromised extremity lymphatic function at baseline, and thus are more prone to develop lymphedema after suffering a "second hit" from nodal radiation or lymphadenectomy. Alternatively, obesity may impair lymphatic regeneration following lymph node trauma.

Recently, obesity has been shown to be a novel *cause* of lymphedema [4], a condition I termed "obesity-induced lymphedema." The relationship between obesity and lymphatic dysfunction has important consequences for public health. Obesity affects one-third of the US population, and 6 % has a BMI >40 [5]. The proportion of the population that is obese is increasing at a rate of 2–4 % every 10 years [5]. Lymphedema in obese individuals significantly affects their quality of life and further increases health care costs. It is important to recognize the relationship between obesity and lymphedema so that weight-loss interventions can be instituted before potentially irreversible lymphatic dysfunction occurs.

A.K. Greene et al. (eds.), *Lymphedema: Presentation, Diagnosis, and Treatment*,
DOI 10.1007/978-3-319-14493-1_9, © Springer International Publishing Switzerland 2015

Diagnosis

History

Prior to diagnosing a patient with obesity-induced lymphedema, all other potential causes of lymphatic dysfunction must be ruled out. Individuals are queried about a history of primary lymphedema and a family history of the disease. If an individual has developed swelling prior to becoming obese (usually during infancy, childhood, or adolescence), then he/she likely has primary lymphedema. Obese patients who have had lymph node radiation, lymphadenectomy, or penetrating trauma to the inguinal region have secondary lymphedema from the injury. Patients are asked if they have travelled to areas endemic for filariasis to rule out an infectious cause of lymphedema. Patients with obesity-induced lymphedema typically state that they were previously healthy and had either a normal (<25) or overweight (25–30) BMI as a teenager and young adult. As the individual gained weight they noted swelling of their extremities, followed by a worsening cycle of weight gain and lower extremity enlargement.

The most important risk factor for obesity-induced lymphedema is the patient's maximum BMI history. Individuals who currently or previously had a BMI >50 are at risk for the disease; the likelihood is much higher if a patient has had a BMI >60 [6]. An individual who has had massive weight loss following a bariatric surgical procedure and/or diet raises the suspicion of obesity-induced lymphedema. A history of cellulitis of the extremities suggests underlying lymphatic dysfunction and obesity-induced lymphedema. Because obesity affects both extremities, patients complain of bilateral symptoms. If an obese individual has unilateral findings, it is unlikely he/she has obesity-induced lymphedema.

Physical Examination

It is difficult to diagnosis obesity-induced lymphedema by physical examination; an obese leg with or without lymphedema appears the same. The amount of adipose tissue and pitting edema does not correlate well with lymphoscintigraphy findings. Patients with lymphedema typically have a positive Stemmer sign (i.e., the skin on the dorsum of the foot or hand can't be pinched with the examiner's fingers) [7]. However, because most obese patients without lymphedema have excess subcutaneous adipose deposition, a false-positive Stemmer sign is common. If a patient has a negative Stemmer sign, then it is unlikely he/she has had lymphedema.

Imaging

Definitive diagnosis of obesity-induced lymphedema is made using lymphoscintigraphy. All patients with possible obesity-induced lymphedema undergo this imaging study to determine whether or not they have lymphatic dysfunction. Lymphoscintigraphy is the "gold-standard" test for lymphedema and is 92 % sensitive and 100 % specific for the disease [8]. An abnormal lymphoscintigram is defined as delayed transit of radio-labelled colloid, dermal backflow, and/or tortuous collateral lymphatic channels [7–10].

Clinical Findings

Lower Extremity

Obesity-induced lymphedema always affects the lower extremities. In our series of 51 obese patients (BMI >30) referred for possible lymphedema, the mean age was 54 years (range, 14–86 years) [6]. Thirty-eight females and 13 males were in the cohort (Table 9.1). Twenty subjects had lower extremity lymphatic dysfunction by lymphoscintigraphy (12 female, 8 male); 75 % had abnormal findings bilaterally and 25 % had unilateral lymphatic dysfunction. The only variable that predicted lymphoscintigram result was the patient's BMI. Subjects with an abnormal lymphoscintigram had a greater BMI [64.9 (range 43.9–83.3)] compared to individuals with a normal study [BMI 38.8 (range, 30.0–55.8)] ($p < 0.0001$) [6]. Gender, comorbidities, and duration of obesity were not different between patients with normal and abnormal lymphoscinitigrams.

Table 9.1 Obese patients (BMI ≥30) referred to a lymphedema program with possible lower extremity lymphedema (*n*=51)

	Normal lymphoscintigram	Abnormal lymphoscintigram	*p*
n	31	20	
Female	26	12	
Male	5	8	
Age	54	54	
Body mass index (mean)	39	65	<0.0001
Diabetes	2	5	0.1
Heart failure	1	0	1
Hypercholesterolemia	4	0	0.15
Hypertension	12	12	0.16
Venous insufficiency	2	0	0.51

With permission from Greene AK, Grant F, Slavin SA, Maclellan RA. Obesity-induced lymphedema: clinical and lymphoscintigraphic features. Plast Reconstr Surg (in press)

Table 9.2 Cohort of obese patients at their maximum BMI at time of lymphoscintigraphy (*n*=33)

	Normal lymphoscintigram	Abnormal lymphoscintigram	*p*
n	22	11	
Female	19	6	
Male	3	5	
Age	53.3 years (range, 14–86)	55.0 years (range, 30–73)	
Body mass index	37.7 (range, 30.0–55.8)	72.0 (range, 54.1–83.3)	<0.0001

With permission from Greene AK, Grant F, Slavin SA, Maclellan RA. Obesity-induced lymphedema: clinical and lymphoscintigraphic features. Plast Reconstr Surg (in press)

Table 9.3 Cohort of obese patients with a history of weight loss and not at their maximum BMI at time of lymphoscintigraphy (*n*=18)

	Normal lymphoscintigram	Abnormal lymphoscintigram	*p*
n	9	9	
Female	7	6	
Male	2	3	
Age	54.0 years (range, 34–63)	54.0 years (range, 35–71)	
Maximum body mass index	63.1 (range, 44.3–85.4)	78.6 (range, 60.4–105.6)	0.03
Current body mass index	41.6 (range, 30.0–53.1)	56.1 (range, 43.9–73.3)	0.005
Body mass index change	20.1 (range, 5.3–36.2)	22.5 (range, 4.4–45.2)	0.7

With permission from Greene AK, Grant F, Slavin SA, Maclellan RA. Obesity-induced lymphedema: clinical and lymphoscintigraphic features. Plast Reconstr Surg (in press)

Two cohorts of patients with obesity-induced lymphedema exist: (1) individuals who do not have a history of significant weight loss and are at their maximum BMI at the time of the lymphoscintigram (Table 9.2) and (2) subjects with a history of massive weight loss following a bariatric surgical procedure or dieting and are not at their maximum BMI at the time of lymphoscintigram (Table 9.3). Patients without a history of weight loss who have lymphedema have a greater BMI [72.9 (range, 54.1–83.3)] compared to individuals without lymphedema [37.7 (range, 30.3–55.8)] ($p < 0.0001$) [6]. In these patients a BMI threshold between 50 and 60 exists at which point lymphatic dysfunction occurs. All subjects with a BMI <50 had normal lymphatic function and

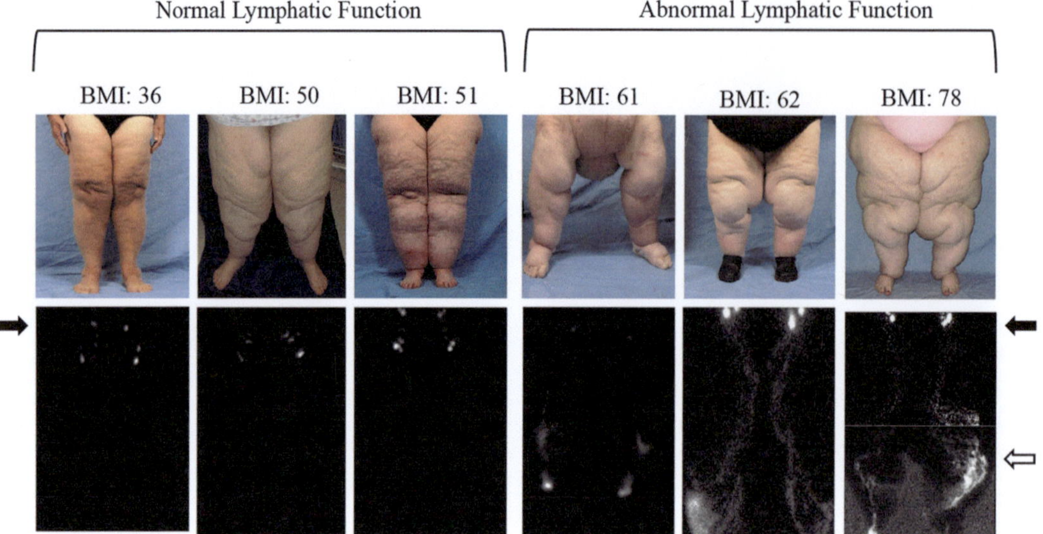

Fig. 9.1 Increasing BMI causes lower extremity lymphatic dysfunction. Patients without a history of massive weight loss and a BMI <50 have normal lower extremity lymphatic function. Individuals with a BMI >60 have abnormal findings on lymphoscintigraphy consistent with lymphedema. A BMI threshold exists between 50 and 60 at which point lymphatic dysfunction occurs. Patients on the left with a normal lymphoscintigram exhibit inguinal lymph node uptake of technetium Tc-99m sulfur colloid 45 min after injection into the feet. Subjects on the right with an abnormal lymphoscintigram illustrate delayed transport of tracer and/or dermal backflow on 3 h images. *Black arrows* identify inguinal lymph nodes, and the *white arrow* marks dermal backflow. With permission from Greene AK, Grant F, Slavin SA, Maclellan RA. Obesity-induced lymphedema: clinical and lymphoscintigraphic features. Plast Reconstr Surg (in press)

every person with a BMI >60 had lymphatic dysfunction. Individuals with a BMI between 50 and 60 had either normal or abnormal lymphatic function (Fig. 9.1) [6].

Patients who have lost significant weight prior to their lymphoscintigram have more variable findings compared to the homogenous group without a history of weight loss. Individuals who have lost weight and have abnormal lymphoscintigraphy findings have a greater historical BMI (78.6; $p = 0.03$) and BMI at the time of the lymphoscintigram (56.1; $p = 0.005$) compared to patients with normal lymphatic function (BMI 63.1 and 41.6, respectively) [6]. The amount of weight loss, duration of obesity, and time since the patient has been at his/her maximum weight does not affect lymphoscintigram result. Approximately 50 % of patients with a history of having a BMI >60 (and thus are assumed to have lower extremity lymphatic dysfunction at that time) who lowered their BMI to <50 (and thus would be predicted to have normal lymphatic function) had normal lymphatic function (Fig. 9.2). Consequently, obesity-induced lymphedema might be reversible in some patients following weight loss.

Upper Extremity

Similar to the lower extremity, a BMI threshold may exist at which point upper extremity lymphatic dysfunction occurs. We have had two obese patients, without any risk factors for arm lymphedema, complain of upper extremity swelling in addition to their lower extremity edema. Both individuals had abnormal lymphatic function of the lower extremities by lymphoscintigraphy. The patient with the highest BMI history in our cohort (105.6) had bilateral upper extremity lymphatic dysfunction by lymphoscintigraphy (his BMI at the time of the study was 60.3) (Fig. 9.3) [11]. The second patient was at his

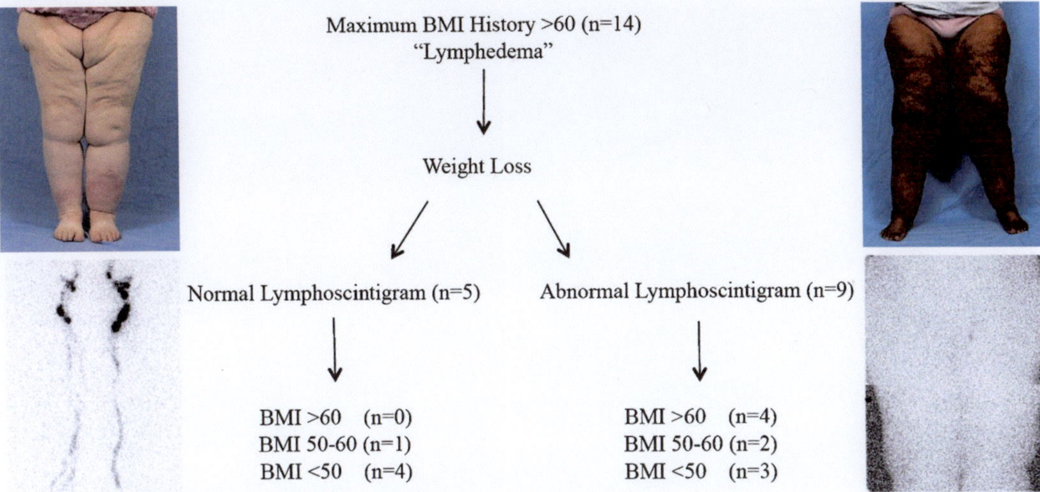

Fig. 9.2 Cohort of patients with a maximum BMI history >60 who subsequently lost weight. Although these patients did not have a lymphoscintigram while they were at their peak BMI, if we *assume* that they would have had abnormal findings (similar to all other individuals in the cohort with a BMI >60), then information about the effects of weight loss on lymphatic function might be ascertained. Of the ten patients who reduced their BMI to <60 and then had a lymphoscintigram, five had normal lymphatic function and five had abnormal findings. Weight loss may improve lymphatic function in some individuals but not others. (*Left*) 55-year-old female with a maximum BMI history of 75.3 and a BMI of 53.1 at the time of lymphoscintigraphy exhibits normal transit of radiolabelled tracer to the inguinal nodes 45 min following injection into the feet. (*Right*) 52-year-old female with a maximum BMI of 60.5 and a BMI of 45.0 during lymphoscintigraphy with no significant tracer uptake in the inguinal nodes at 45 min. With permission from Greene AK, Grant F, Slavin SA, Maclellan RA. Obesity-induced lymphedema: clinical and lymphoscintigraphic features. Plast Reconstr Surg (in press)

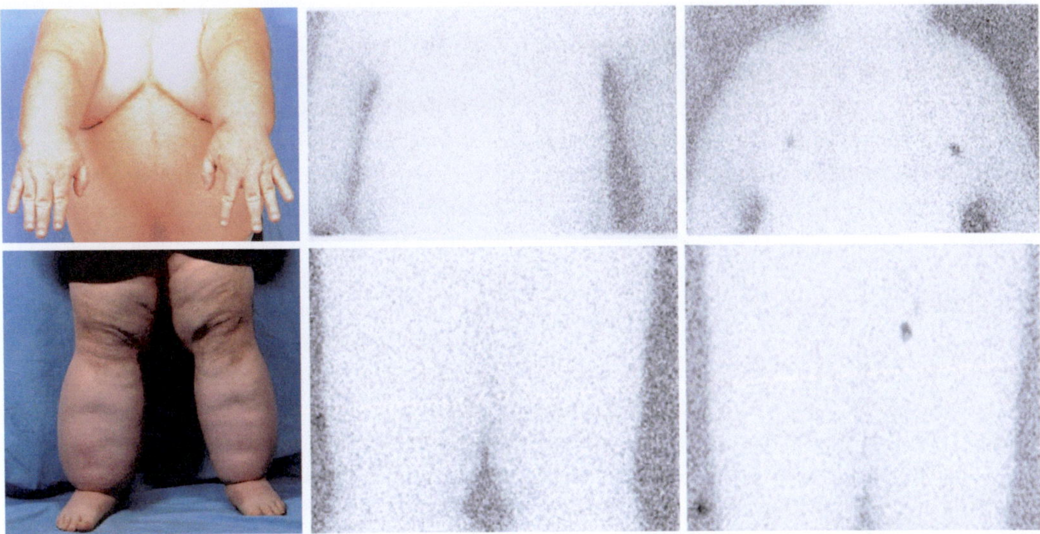

Fig. 9.3 Obesity-induced upper extremity lymphedema. 62-year-old male with a maximum BMI history of 105.6, presented with a BMI of 60.3 after dieting. He complained of swelling of all four limbs (*left*). Lymphoscintigraphy showed absence of tracer in the axillary and inguinal nodes 45 min following radiolabelled colloid injection into the hands and feet (*middle*). Minimal, delayed tracer accumulation into the axillary and inguinal nodes occurred 2 h after injection (*right*). These findings indicated lymphatic dysfunction of all four extremities consistent with lymphedema. With permission from Greene AK, Maclellan RA. Obesity-induced upper extremity lymphedema. Plast Reconstr Surg Glob Open. 2013;1:e59

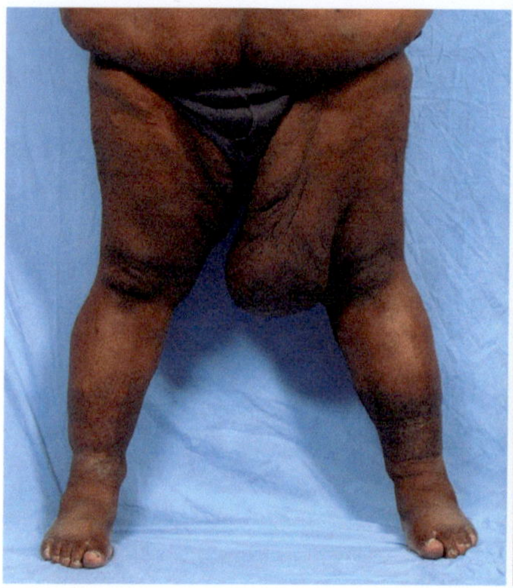
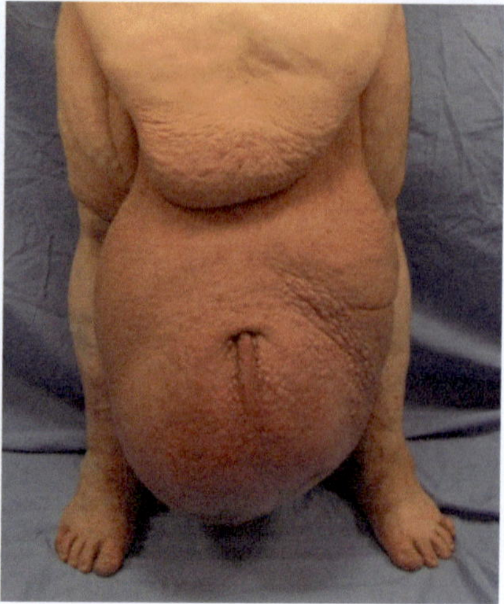

Fig. 9.4 Massive localized lymphedema (MLL). (*Left*) Male with bilateral obesity-induced lower extremity lymphedema and MLL of the thigh (BMI 78). (*Right*) Individual with obesity-induced lymphedema of the legs and MLL of the scrotum (BMI 62)

maximum BMI (81.2) at the time of lymphoscintigraphy and had a normal upper extremity lymphoscintigram. Consequently, a maximum BMI history above 81 might exist at which point arm lymphedema occurs. The upper limbs should be more resistant to developing obesity-induced lymphedema, compared to the lower extremities, because: (1) adipose deposition in obese patients preferentially affects the legs rather than the arms and (2) lymph drainage from the upper limbs is closer to the central venous circulation and is less affected by dependent positioning and proximal transport against gravity.

Localized

Obesity can result in a large, localized area of overgrowth termed "massive localized lymphedema" (MLL) [12]. The average age of patients is 47.4 years; males and females are affected equally [13]. Mean patient BMI is 61 (range, 26–91) [13]. MLL affects the thigh (49 %), lower abdomen (18 %), penis/scrotum (12 %), suprapubic area (7 %), vulva (4 %), distal leg (7 %), and arm (3 %) (Fig. 9.4) [13]. Average size is 37.4 cm (range, 4–98) and weight 9.3 kg (range 638 g–34 kg). Angiosarcoma ("Stewart–Treves tumor") can develop in areas of MLL [14]. Although MLL of the extremities is typically unilateral, both lower extremities usually have underlying lymphatic dysfunction of the entire limb.

Pathophysiology

Several factors are probably responsible for lymphatic dysfunction in obese individuals because secondary lymphedema is hard to cause. For example, despite axillary lymphadenectomy and radiation for breast cancer treatment, only 1/3 of women develop upper extremity lymphedema [15]. Lymph transport is dependent on the function of the lymphatic vasculature (clearance) and the volume of lymph produced by the tissues (load). One hypothesis to explain obesity-induced lymphedema is that the lymphatics in the extremity are normal, but are unable to transport the volume of lymph that is being produced. As the patient's BMI rises the amount of lymph produced by the leg increases, while ambulation/muscle contraction to transport the fluid decreases. In addition, excessive pressure from the weight of the tissue and/or progressive skin folds might collapse lymphatic vessels.

Another hypothesis for the mechanism of obesity-induced lymphedema is that lymphatic vasculature is damaged as the size of the extremity increases. Because approximately one-half of patients with an initial BMI >60 continued to have lymphatic dysfunction after reducing their BMI below 50, extreme obesity likely causes lymphatic injury. Inflammation from elevated subcutaneous adipose may destroy lymphatic vasculature [16]. Obese mice have decreased lymphatic transport as well as abnormal lymph node architecture and function [17].

Based on our cohort of patients with a BMI history >60 that had normal lower extremity lymphatic function following massive weight loss, obesity-induced lymphedema may be the first example of reversible lymphedema. Although lymphatic damage may occur, lymphatics might recover following weight loss and/or sufficient non-damaged vessels remain to adequately drain the limb.

Management

Patients with obesity-induced lymphedema are initially managed like other individuals with primary or secondary lymphedema. They are prescribed compression garments as well as pneumatic compression. Individuals are advised to avoid incidental trauma that might lead to cellulitis. Exercise is encouraged because it helps the patient lower his/her BMI and muscle activity aids the transport of lymph fluid [18]. Although conservative intervention may slow the progression of the disease, patients will not have significant improvement.

Definitive management of obesity-induced lymphedema is to treat the underlying cause of the disease which is the patient's weight. Individuals are referred to a bariatric weight loss center, and a minority are able to lose significant weight by diet and exercise; most patients benefit from a surgical weight-loss procedure. Our experience suggests that if a patient can reduce his/her BMI to <50, there is an approximately 50 % chance that lower extremity lymphatic function will reverse. Even if lymphatic dysfunction remains it may be improve; the patient's quality of life also will be better because his/her legs will be smaller.

Obese patients who do not have lower extremity lymphedema by lymphoscintigraphy also are referred to a bariatric surgical center prior to their BMI reaching 50, at which point permanent lymphedema may occur. Unlike other comorbidities that are reversible with weight loss (e.g., diabetes, hypertension, hyperlipidemia), lymphedema may not resolve following a bariatric procedure. We counsel individuals who are at risk for lymphedema (e.g., family history of lymphedema, axillary/inguinal operations) to maintain a normal BMI.

Resection of excess lower extremity tissue is best reserved after the patient has had a bariatric surgical procedure. Following weight loss, a patient may no longer need a procedure to reduce the size of his/her legs. If a debulking procedure is indicated, the intervention is facilitated and associated with much less morbidity, compared to attempting resection when the patient is at his/her maximum BMI. After weight loss, removal of redundant skin and a smaller area of MLL will facilitate the procedure and reduce the risk of complications. In addition, because the patient's BMI and lymphatic function is likely improved, the risk of recurrence is much lower. For example, resection of MLL prior to weight loss has a recurrence rate of at least 50 % [13]. Surgical options to improve overgrown tissues following weight loss include suction-assisted lipectomy, or staged-subcutaneous excisions.

Obesity-induced lymphedema has implications for body contouring procedures after massive weight loss. Post-bariatric surgery of an extremity may be a "second-hit" to a limb at high risk for lymphedema. Patients could have residual or resolving lymphatic dysfunction at the time of their thigh-lift. An inguinal incision in an area of potentially compromised lymphatic function may place the patient at higher risk for lymphedema. A thigh lift might also cause a patient who would have had normalization of lymphatic function to have permanent lymphedema. Patients with a maximum BMI history >50 may benefit from lymphoscintigraphy prior to lower extremity body contouring procedures to assess their lymphatic function. A post-bariatric surgical patient who attributes leg edema to a thigh-lift procedure may have had unrecognized obesity-induced lymphedema before the operation.

Conclusions

Severe obesity causes lymphedema of the lower extremities and may result in upper extremity disease as well as MLL. A BMI threshold of 50 appears to exist at which point lymphatic dysfunction can occur. Patients with obesity-induced lymphedema (or at risk for the disease) are referred to a bariatric center because weight loss will improve the condition.

References

1. Helyer LK, Varnic M, Le LW, Leong W, McCready D. Obesity is a risk factor for developing postoperative lymphedema in breast cancer patients. Breast J. 2010;16:48–54.
2. Werner RS, McCormick B, Petrek J, Cox L, Cirrincione C, Gray JR, Yahalom J. Arm edema in conservatively managed breast cancer: obesity is a major predictive factor. Radiology. 1991;180:177–84.
3. Ridner SH, Dietrich MS, Stewart BR, Armer JM. Body mass index and breast cancer treatment-related lymphedema. Support Care Cancer. 2011;19:853–7.
4. Greene AK, Grant FD, Slavin SA. Lower extremity lymphedema and elevated body mass in obese patients. N Engl J Med. 2012;366:2136–7.
5. Flegal KM, Carroll MD, Ogden CL, Curtin LR. Prevalence and trends in obesity among US adults, 1999–2008. JAMA. 2010;303:235–41.
6. Greene AK, Grant F, Slavin SA, Maclellan RA. Obesity-induced lymphedema: clinical and lymphoscintigraphic features. Plast Reconstr Surg (in press).
7. Stemmer R. A clinical symptom for the early and differential diagnosis of lymphedema. Vasa. 1976;5:261–2.
8. Gloviczki P, Calcagno D, Schirger A, Pairolero PC, Cherry KJ, Hallett JW, Wahner HW. Noninvasive evaluation of the swollen extremity: experiences with 190 lymphoscintigraphic examinations. J Vasc Surg. 1989;9:683–9.
9. Szuba A, Shin WS, Strauss HW, Rockson S. The third circulation: radionuclide lymphoscintigraphy in the evaluation of lymphedema. J Nucl Med. 2003;44:43–57.
10. Scarsbrook AF, Ganeshan A, Bradley KM. Pearls and pitfalls of radionuclide imaging of the lymphatic system. Part 2: evaluation of extremity lymphoedema. Br J Radiol. 2007;80:219–26.
11. Greene AK, Maclellan RA. Obesity-induced upper extremity lymphedema. Plast Reconstr Surg Glob Open. 2013;1:e59.
12. Farshid G, Weiss SW. Massive localized lymphedema in the morbidly obese: a histologically distinct reactive lesion simulating liposarcoma. Am J Surg Pathol. 1998;10:1277–83.
13. Chopra K, Tadisina KK, Brewer M, Holton LH, Banda AK, Singh DP. Massive localized lymphedema revisited: a quickly rising complication of the obesity epidemic. Ann Plast Surg. Accessed 30 May 2013. [Epub ahead of print].
14. Shon W, Ida CM, Boland-Froemming JM, Rose PS, Folpe A. Cutaneous angiosarcoma arising in massive localized lymphedema of the morbidly obese: a report of five cases and review of the literature. J Cutan Pathol. 2011;38:560–4.
15. Gärtner R, Mejdahl MK, Andersen KG, Ewertz M, Kroman N. Development in self-reported arm-lymphedema in Danish women treated for early-stage breast cancer in 2005 and 2006 – a nationwide follow-up study. Breast. Accessed 7 Apr 2014. [Epub ahead of print].
16. Savetsky IL, Torrisi JS, Cuzzone DA, Ghanta S, Albano NJ, Gardenier JC, Joseph WJ, Mehrara BJ. Obesity increases inflammation and impairs lymphatic function in a mouse model of lymphedema. Am J Physiol Heart Circ Physiol. Accessed 23 May 2014. [Epub ahead of print].
17. Weitman ES, Aschen SZ, Farias-Eisner G, Albano N, Cuzzone DA, Ghanta S, Zampell JC, Thorek D, Mehrara BJ. Obesity impairs lymphatic fluid transport and dendritic cell migration to lymph nodes. PLoS One. 2013;8:e70703.
18. Schmitz KH, Ahmed RL, Troxel A, et al. Weight lifting in women with breast-cancer-related lymphedema. N Engl J Med. 2009;361:664–73.

Arin K. Greene

A.K. Greene, M.D., M.M.Sc. (✉)
Department of Plastic and Oral Surgery,
Boston Children's Hospital, Harvard Medical School,
300 Longwood Avenue, Boston, MA 02115, USA
e-mail: arin.greene@childrens.harvard.edu

Key Points

- 25 % of patients referred to a lymphedema center with "lymphedema" do not have the condition.
- Approximately 90 % of patients with lymphedema can be accurately diagnosed by history and physical examination.
- A history of injury to axillary or inguinal lymph nodes is the most significant risk factor for lymphedema.
- Lymphedema almost always affects the distal extremity.
- The Stemmer sign is a moderately specific, but sensitive physical examination finding for lymphedema.

Introduction

Lymphedema is divided into *primary* and *secondary* disease [1]. Primary lymphedema is idiopathic and results from an error in lymphatic development. Secondary lymphedema is acquired and caused by injury to a normally developed lymphatic system. Primary lymphedema is rare, affecting approximately 1/100,000 children [2]. In the pediatric population idiopathic lymphedema is responsible for the disease in 97 % of patients who do not reside in areas endemic for filariasis [3]. Secondary lymphedema is rare in children (~3 % of cases), but is responsible for the disease in 99 % of adults [3]. The most common cause of secondary lymphedema world-wide is a parasitic infection (e.g., *Wuchereria bancrofti*, *Brugia malayi*, *Brugia timori*). In developed countries, secondary lymphedema usually results from treatment for malignancy (e.g., axillary/inguinal lymphadenectomy, radiation). Regardless of whether a patient has primary or secondary lymphedema, the subsequent pathophysiology of the condition is equivalent. Over time, the diseased area increases in size because the interstitial lymphatic fluid causes subcutaneous adipose production [4, 5].

The term "lymphedema" is often used to describe an overgrown limb regardless of the underlying etiology; 25 % of patients referred to our center with "lymphedema" do not have the disease [6, 7]. Many conditions are confused with lymphedema: capillary malformation, lymphatic malformation, venous malformation, infantile hemangioma, kaposiform hemangioendothelioma, CLOVES syndrome, Klippel–Trénaunay syndrome, Parkes Weber syndrome, hemihypertrophy, lipedema, lipofibromatois, obesity, posttraumatic swelling, systemic diseases (e.g., cardiac, renal, hepatic, rheumatologic), and venous insufficiency [6, 7]. It is important to accurately determine if a patient has lymphedema so that the individual is managed correctly. Although ~90 %

A.K. Greene et al. (eds.), *Lymphedema: Presentation, Diagnosis, and Treatment*,
DOI 10.1007/978-3-319-14493-1_10, © Springer International Publishing Switzerland 2015

of patients with lymphedema can be diagnosed by history and physical examination, confirmation requires lymphoscintigraphy.

History

Onset

Primary Lymphedema

Primary lymphedema is much less common than secondary disease, and usually presents prior to adulthood. In the pediatric population onset occurs in infancy (49.2 %), childhood (9.5 %), or adolescence (41.3 %) [3]. Males and females are equally at risk for developing primary lymphedema; boys are more likely to present in infancy (68 %), while girls commonly develop the disease during adolescence (55 %) [3]. Primary lymphedema presents during adulthood in 19 % of patients [8].

Secondary Lymphedema

Injury to the lymphatic system is responsible for approximately 3 % of pediatric cases and >99 % of adult disease [3]. In developed countries, most people have lymphedema because of treatment for malignancy (i.e., lymphadenectomy, axillary/inguinal radiation). Upper extremity lymphedema from breast cancer treatment is the most common etiology of the disease in the USA. Pelvic or abdominal malignancy is the most frequent reason for lower extremity lymphedema. A misconception exists that edema begins immediately after lymphatics are injured. Edema following lymphadenectomy and/or radiation typically begins several months following the injury to lymph vessels. Three-fourths of patients develop swelling within 3 years after the injury and the risk of lymphedema is 1 % each year thereafter [9]. Compensatory mechanisms (e.g., spontaneous lymphatic–venous anastomoses, increased macrophage activity) delay the onset of clinical swelling. Consequently, patients with a possible history of secondary lymphedema are queried about the interval between the insult to their lymph nodes and the onset of swelling. Edema that forms immediately following the injury is not consistent with lymphedema.

Axillary or Inguinal Injury

Axillary or inguinal injury is the most significant risk factor for developing lymphedema. An individual with upper extremity edema and a history of breast cancer treatment is likely to have lymphedema. Similarly, a patient who has had inguinal lymphadenectomy/radiation and complains of swelling probably has lymphedema.

Trauma to the lymphatic vasculature must be severe to cause lymphedema. For example, only 1/3 of women who have axillary lymphadenopathy and radiation develop the condition [10]. Although penetrating trauma to lymph nodes can cause lymphedema, the risk is much lower compared to removal of lymph nodes or radiation. While patients may present with a history of incidental trauma to an extremity with subsequent edema, blunt injury should not be severe enough to cause lymphedema. Usually the trauma is coincidental to another source of the individual's edema. Alternatively, blunt trauma may precipitate the clinical appearance of primary lymphedema sooner than it would have presented without the insult.

Travel

All patients with suspected lymphedema are asked if they have a travelled to areas where filariasis is prevalent. Eighty-three countries are endemic to the disease; 70 % of cases are in Bangladesh, India, Indonesia, and Nigeria [11]. Other affected areas include Africa (central), Brazil, Burma, China (southern), Dominican Republic, Guiana, Guyana, Haiti, Malaysia, Nile delta, Pacific Islands, Pakistan, Sri Lanka, Surinam, and Thailand [11]. If filariasis is suspected, the patient is referred to an infectious disease specialist.

Family History

Individuals with possible primary lymphedema are asked whether either of their parents have extremity swelling. If a patient's mother or father has primary lymphedema, then it is likely that he/she has the condition. Familial lymphedema typically presents during infancy. If neither parent has lower extremity swelling, the patient still may have lymphedema because 89 % of individuals with primary lymphedema have non-familial disease [3]. A known mutation is present in only 36 % of patients with familial lymphedema, and in 8 % of individuals without a family history of the condition [12]. *VEFGR3* mutations (Milroy disease) typically are autosomal dominant, but recessive transmission also can occur. *FOXC2* (hypotrichosis–lymphedema–telangiectasia syndrome) is autosomal dominant, *SOX18* (hypotrichosis–lymphedema–telangiectasia syndrome) can be dominant or recessive, and *CCBE1* (Hennekam syndrome) may be dominant or recessive [13].

Comorbidities

Patients suspected of having lymphedema are queried about comorbidities that are associated with the condition. Individuals with suspected primary lymphedema are asked whether they have Noonan or Turner syndrome. Patients with Turner syndrome have a 57 % risk of lymphedema; 76 % develop the disease in infancy, and 19 % present with swelling later [14]. Noonan syndrome has a 3 % risk of lymphedema which may manifest with generalized swelling, intestinal lymphangiectasis, and/or fetal hydrops [15]. Other risk factors for lymphedema include myelomeningocele and obesity. Patients with a body mass index (BMI) >30 are more likely to develop lymphedema after lymphadenectomy and nodal radiation compared to non-obese individuals [16]. Severely obese patients with a BMI >60 can develop lymphedema without a prior history of lymphatic injury, termed "obesity-induced lymphedema" [17, 18].

Infection

Individuals with lymphedema have an increased risk of infection in the affected area. Because the lymphatic system contributes to immunological defense, when it is not functioning correctly

Table 10.1 Patient medical history consistent with lymphedema

A parent has lymphedema
Turner syndrome, Noonan syndrome
Cancer treatment with inguinal/axillary lymphadenectomy or radiation
Travel to areas endemic for filariasis
Extreme obesity
Onset several months after injury to the lymphatic system
Progressive enlargement of the area
Cellulitis
Minimal discomfort

patients are more likely to develop cellulitis. Nineteen percent of patients with primary lymphedema have a history of cellulitis, 13 % have been hospitalized, and 7 % have >3 attacks each year [3]. If a patient has a history of infections in the diseased extremity or genitalia then he/she is more likely to have lymphedema. Other causes of extremity edema (e.g., venous insufficiency, cardiac failure) do not increase the risk of cellulitis.

Progression

Lymphedema is a chronic condition that does not improve and slowly worsens. If an individual has intermittent or resolving swelling, it is unlikely that he/she has lymphedema. Patients who provide a history of worsening edema are more likely to have the disease. Lymphedema progresses through four stages (Table 10.1) [19]. *Stage 0* indicates a normal extremity clinically, but with abnormal lymph transport (i.e., illustrated by lymphoscintigraphy). *Stage 1* is early edema which improves with limb elevation. *Stage 2* represents pitting edema that does not resolve with elevation. *Stage 3* describes fibroadipose deposition and skin changes [19]. A lymphedematous extremity continues to gradually enlarge over time because of subcutaneous adipose production.

Symptoms

The most common problem caused by lymphedema is lowered self-esteem because the disease creates a deformity. Consequently, patients often cover their extremities and avoid activities that would expose their abnormal limb to others (e.g., swimming, wearing shorts). The condition also continually reminds cancer survivors of their malignancy. Genital lymphedema can negatively affect a patient's sexual activity. The second most common morbidity of lymphedema is infection. Patients often state that they have had cellulitis of the involved area, and many have required inpatient intravenous antibiotics.

Lymphedema typically is painless; if a patient complains of significant pain it is unlikely he/she has the condition. As the size of the extremity enlarges, however, secondary musculoskeletal discomfort can occur. Patients often state that the extremity feels heavy, and some individuals have decreased cutaneous sensation. Lymphedema only affects the skin and subcutaneous tissue leading to circumferential overgrowth. The disease does not involve the muscles or bone, and thus, patients do not have axial overgrowth and a leg-length discrepancy. Individuals with severe overgrowth can have difficulty fitting clothing and using the enlarged limb. It can be hard to lift a lymphedematous upper extremity when getting dressed. A markedly enlarged lower extremity can inhibit ambulation. Lymphatic vesicles may bleed or leak lymph fluid (lymphorrhea). Cutaneous ulceration is not typical for lymphedema and should suggest an alternate diagnosis (e.g., venous insufficiency).

Physical Examination

Location

The anatomical distribution of lymphedema includes: an extremity (99 %), isolated genitalia (1 %), or localized to another area of the body (<1 %). Lymphedema almost always affects the distal extremity; if the hand or foot is not involved, then the diagnosis of lymphedema should be questioned. If a patient complains of swelling outside of the limbs or genitalia, then lymphedema likely is not the cause. However, primary generalized lymphedema (including the face and trunk) can occur rarely. Children or adults with secondary lymphedema have lymphedema of the extremity ipsilateral to the site of axillary/inguinal lymph node injury.

Primary lymphedema affects the lower extremities in 92 % of cases; 50 % have unilateral lymphedema and 50 % have bilateral disease [3]. Eighteen percent of patients with primary lymphedema have genital involvement, which usually is associated with lower extremity lymphedema (4 % have isolated genital disease). Sixteen percent of children with idiopathic lymphedema have upper extremity disease [3]. Rarely, a child can have lymphedema affecting the legs, genitalia, and/or arms. Approximately 2/3 of patents with lymphedema in infancy have bilateral lower extremity disease, while 2/3 of patients who present in adolescence have unilateral lower extremity lymphedema [3].

Severity

Clinically, the severity of lymphedema can be categorized as mild (<20 % increase in extremity volume), moderate (20–40 %), or severe (>40 %) (Fig. 10.1) [19]. Limb volume measurements can be made using a tape measure, perometer or by water displacement. Tape measurements are the least accurate method to determine extremity volume because it must be calculated; it is also difficult to use the exact reference points for future assessments. In addition, depending on how tight the examiner pulls the tape measure the circumference can change significantly. In children, extremity measurements are particularly problematic because the limbs are still growing. We do not routinely record limb volumes because it does not affect the patient's management. However, an individual who is being considered for operative intervention undergoes water displacement to assess extremity volume before and after the procedure.

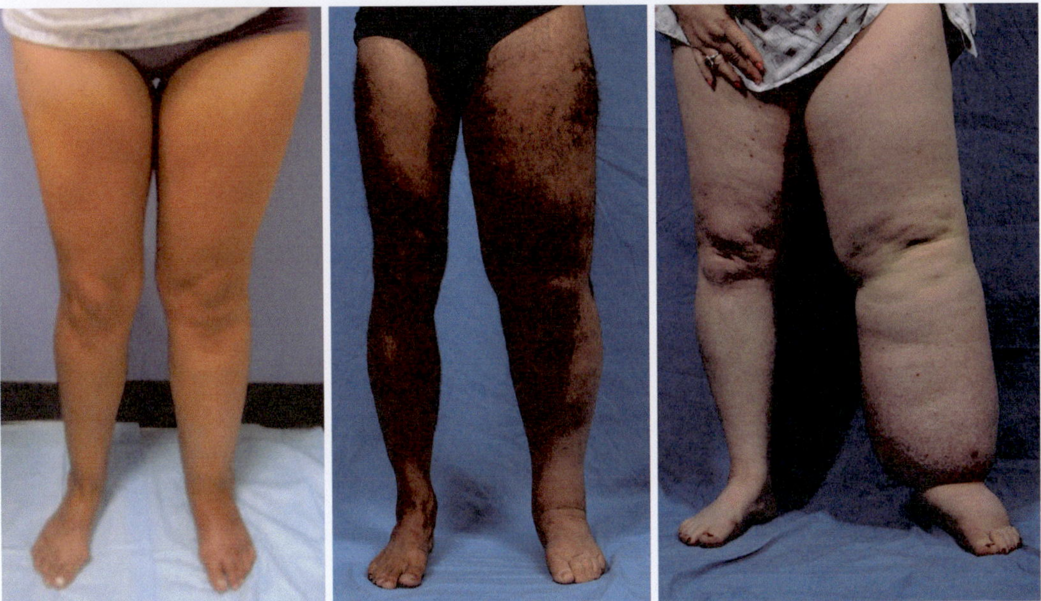

Fig. 10.1 Severity of lymphedema. (*Left*) mild. (*Center*) moderate. (*Right*) severe

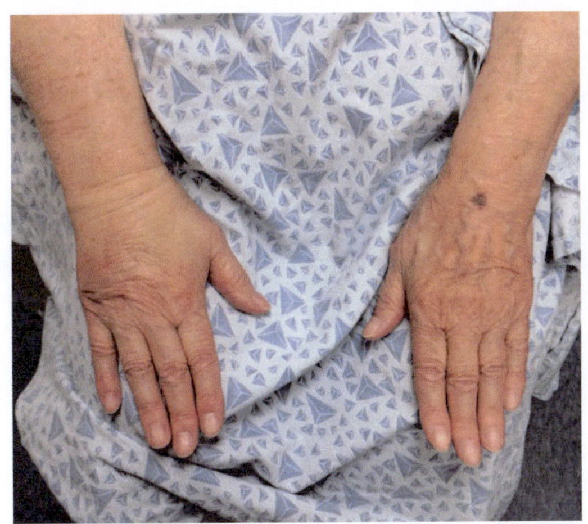

Fig. 10.2 Lymphedema of the right arm causes superficial veins to be less visible

Pitting Edema

Patients with lymphedema exhibit pitting edema early in their disease. Even minor swelling can be appreciated because superficial veins are less visible (Fig. 10.2). Pressing the thumb into the dorsum of the hand or foot for 60 s will illustrate the degree of pitting edema (Fig. 10.3) [20]. Significant pitting (measured in millimeters) indicates that fluid is primarily responsible for limb enlargement and the patient can be managed using compression (Grade 1 edema) [20]. Over time, the body reacts to the lymphedematous fluid in the extremity by producing subcutaneous fibro-adipose tissue. Consequently, on physical examination the amount of pitting edema is reduced. Individuals with long-standing lymphedema may not exhibit pitting edema on physical examination (Grade 2 edema); these patients will have minimal benefit from conservative interventions and are candidates for surgical excisional procedures [20].

Stemmer Sign

A fairly sensitive and specific sign for lymphedema is the Stemmer sign [21]. If the examiner is unable to pinch the skin on the dorsum of the hand or foot (positive Stemmer sign), then it is likely the patient has lymphedema (Figs. 10.4 and 10.5). Swelling, inflammation, and adipose

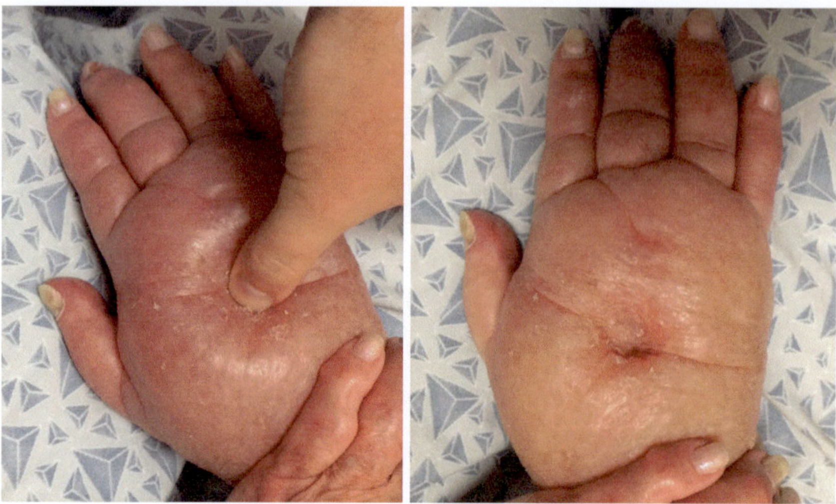

Fig. 10.3 Pitting edema in early lymphedema

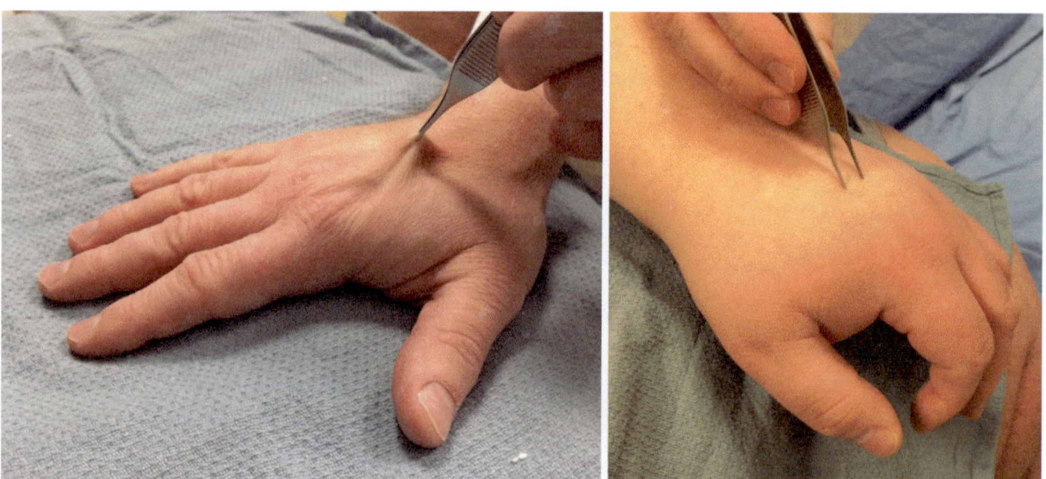

Fig. 10.4 Stemmer sign. (*Left*) negative Stemmer sign in an individual without lymphedema. The skin is able to be pinched. (*Right*) positive Stemmer sign in a patient with left upper extremity lymphedema following breast cancer treatment. Note that the skin cannot be pinched

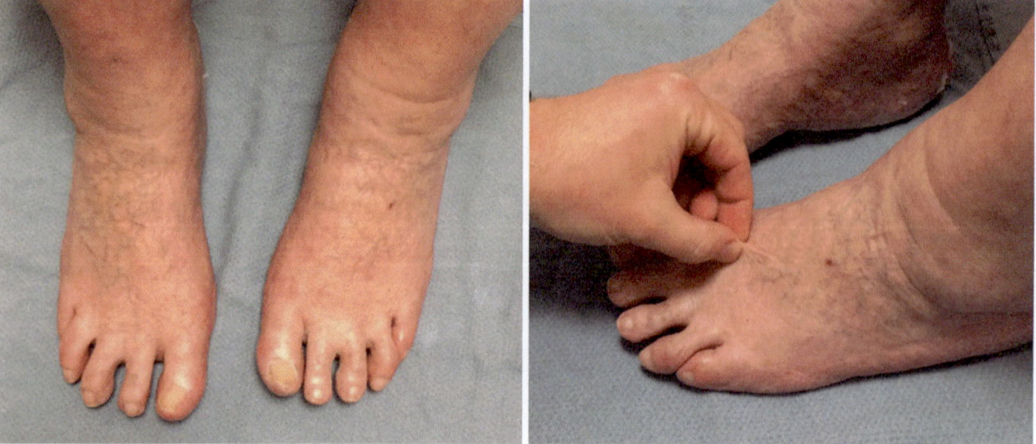

Fig. 10.5 A patient referred with bilateral lower extremity swelling and possible "lymphedema." The individual was diagnosed with venous insufficiency and had a negative Stemmer (the examiner was able to pinch the skin of her foot)

deposition cause the skin to thicken which reduces the ability to lift and pinch the integument of the distal extremity. The Stemmer sign is more sensitive than specific. If the test is positive, it is likely the patient has lymphedema. However, if the exam is negative, the patient may still have lymphedema depending on the severity of their condition and the length of time they have had the disease.

Scars

Patients with possible lymphedema are examined for scars in the axillary and inguinal regions. Injury to these locations can damage lymphatics and cause lymphedema. The presence of radiation skin fibrosis also is ascertained.

Body Mass Index

Individuals referred with possible lymphedema have their height and weight recorded at the time of their consultation. Patients with a body mass index (BMI) >50 are at risk for obesity-induced lymphedema, and individuals with a BMI >60 likely have the disease [17, 18]. Obese patients are also examined for areas of massive localized lymphedema (MLL) which can develop in the background of extremity lymphedema [22]. These large areas of pannus most commonly affect the thigh, abdomen, or pubic area.

Skin Appearance

Patients with primary lymphedema typically have normal appearing skin. However, primary lymphedema can occur with other types of vascular malformations (usually capillary malformation). Because lymphedema is progressive, 15 % of patients will develop cutaneous problems such as bleeding from vesicles, hyperkeratosis, and lymphorrhea [3]. Skin ulceration rarely affects patients with primary lymphedema because their arterial and venous circulations are intact.

However, skin breakdown can occur in older patients who also have venous insufficiency.

Syndromic Features

Children with suspected primary lymphedema are examined for syndromic characteristics that are associated with the disease: (1) an extra row of eyelashes, eyelid ptosis, yellow nails (lymphedema–distichiasis syndrome); (2) sparse hair, cutaneous telangiectasias (hypotrichosis–lymphedema–telangiectasia syndrome); (3) generalized edema, visceral involvement, developmental delay, flat faces, hypertelorism, and a broad nasal bridge (Hennekam syndrome) [13]. Patients with Noonan syndrome may have short stature, pectus excavatum, webbed neck, hypertelorism, low set ears, and/or a flat nasal bridge [15]. Individuals with Turner syndrome might exhibit short stature, webbed neck, broad chest, and/or low set ears [14].

Conclusions

Lymphedema often is confused with other causes of extremity edema and enlargement. Understanding the risk factors (Table 10.1) and physical examination signs (Table 10.2) of lymphedema should allow the health care practitioner to accurately diagnose patients approximately 90 % of the time. Confirmatory diagnosis of the disease is made using lymphoscintigraphy. It is important to correctly diagnose patients with lymphedema so that they can be managed appropriately.

Table 10.2 Physical examination findings consistent with lymphedema

Swelling involves arms, legs, and/or genitalia
Distal extremity is involved
Pitting edema
Positive Stemmer sign
Circumferential (not axial) overgrowth
Scars in axillary or inguinal regions
No skin ulceration
Body mass index >60
Lymphatic vesicles, lymphorrhea

References

1. Allen EV. Lymphedema of the extremities. Classification, etiology and differential diagnoses. A study of 300 cases. Arch Intern Med. 1934;56:606–24.
2. Smeltzer DM, Stickler GB, Schirger A. Primary lymphedemas in children and adolescents: a follow-up study and review. Pediatrics. 1985;76:206–18.
3. Schook CC, Mulliken JB, Fishman SJ, Grant F, Zurakowski D, Greene AK. Primary lymphedema: clinical features and management in 138 pediatric patients. Plast Reconstr Surg. 2011;127:2419–31.
4. Brorson H, Svensson H. Liposuction combined with controlled compression therapy reduces arm lymphedema more effectively than controlled compression therapy alone. Plast Reconstr Surg. 1998;102: 1058–67.
5. Brorson H, Ohlin K, Olsson G, Karlsson MK. Breast cancer-related chronic arm lymphedema is associated with excess adipose and muscle tissue. Lymphat Res Biol. 2009;7:3–10.
6. Schook CC, Mulliken JB, Fishman SJ, Alomari AI, Greene AK. Differential diagnosis of lower extremity lymphedema in 170 pediatric patients. Plast Reconstr Surg. 2011;127:1571–81.
7. Maclellan RA, Couto RA, Sullivan JE, Grant FD, Slavin SA, Greene AK. Management of primary and secondary lymphedema: analysis of 225 referrals to a center. Ann Plast Surg. 2014 (in press).
8. Wolfe J, Kinmonth JB. The prognosis of primary lymphedema of the lower limbs. Arch Surg. 1981;116:1157–60.
9. Petrek JA, Senie RT, Peters M, Rosen PP. Lymphedema in a cohort of breast carcinoma survivors 20 years after diagnosis. Cancer. 2001;92:1368–77.
10. Gärtner R, Mejdahl MK, Andersen KG, Ewertz M, Kroman N. Development in self-reported arm-lymphedema in Danish women treated for early-stage breast cancer in 2005 and 2006—a nationwide follow-up study. Breast. 2014;23:445–52.
11. Mendoza N, Li A, Gill A, Tyring S. Filariasis: diagnosis and treatment. Dermatol Ther. 2009;22:475–90.
12. Mendola A, Schlogel MJ, Ghalamkarpour A, Irrthum A, Nguyen HL, Fastre E, Bygum A, van der Vleuten C, Fagerberg C, Baselga E, Quere I, Mulliken JB, Boon LM, Brouillard P, Vikkula M. Mutations in the VEGFR3 signaling pathway explain 36 % of familial lymphedema. Mol Syndromol. 2013;4:257–66.
13. Brouillard P, Boon L, Vikkula M. Genetics of lymphatic anomalies. J Clin Invest. 2014;124:898–904.
14. Welsh J, Todd M. Incidence and characteristics of lymphedema in Turner's syndrome. Lymphology. 2006;39:152–3.
15. Shaw AC, Kalidas K, Crosby AH, Jeffery S, Patton MA. The natural history of Noonan syndrome: a long-term follow-up study. Arch Dis Child. 2007;92: 128–32.
16. Helyer LK, Varnic M, Le LW, Leong W, McCready D. Obesity is a risk factor for developing postoperative lymphedema in breast cancer patients. Breast J. 2010;16:48–54.
17. Greene AK, Grant FD, Slavin SA. Lower-extremity lymphedema and elevated body-mass index. N Engl J Med. 2012;366:2136–7.
18. Greene AK, Grant F, Slavin SA, Maclellan RA. Obesity-induced lymphedema: clinical and lymphoscintigraphic features. Plast Reconstr Surg. (in press).
19. International Society of Lymphology. The diagnosis and treatment of peripheral lymphedema: 2013 Consensus Document of the International Society of Lymphology. Lymphology. 2013;46:1–11.
20. Bagheri S, Ohlin K, Olsson G, Brorson H. Tissue tonometry before and after liposuction of arm lymphedema following breast cancer. Lymphat Res Biol. 2005;3:66–80.
21. Stemmer R. A clinical symptom for the early and differential diagnosis of lymphedema. Vasa. 1976; 5:261–2.
22. Chopra K, Tadisina KK, Brewer M, Holton LH, Banda AK, Singh DP. Massive localized lymphedema revisited: a quickly rising complication of the obesity epidemic. Ann Plast Surg. 2015;74:126–32.

Volume Measurements and Follow-Up

Håkan Brorson, Barbro Svensson, and Karin Ohlin

Key Points

- Outcomes of surgical treatment of lymphedema very seldom present results as excess volume or excess volume reduction. Instead circumference measurements, taken at random sites along the extremity, are used making it very difficult to estimate the true outcome as well as to compare various studies.
- Volume measurement, either using plethysmography or based on circumference measurements, is an easy and quick method to objectively assess treatment outcome and to increase the scientific impact when presenting results.

Introduction

Measurement of extremity volumes with plethysmography or indirect via circumference measurement is essential for assessing the size of the lymphedema and for treatment monitoring. It is important that both the normal and diseased limb is measured in exactly the same way at all time points to eliminate natural volume variations. The normal arm volume variations are between 2 and 13 % in healthy individuals. The dominant arm is usually about 1.5 % larger [1]. Lymphedema is usually defined as a relative extremity volume difference > 10 percent (the edematous extremity is 10 % larger than the normal) [2, 3]. Both plethysmography and circumference measurements are useful and show satisfactory validity and reliability [4–9], plethysmography is recommended if only one method is used [10].

Volume Measurements Using Plethysmography

The most reliable way to measure the volume of an extremity is plethysmography according to Archimedes' principle, i.e., the limb is immersed in a water bath and the drained water is weighed [1–11]. The weight in grams equals the volume in milliliter and also includes the hand and foot volume. For description of the volume meter see Figs. 11.1 and 11.2.

For both the arm and leg volume meter it is important that the draining pipe is be placed high enough so that the entire limb can be measured. The diameter of the draining hose should be large so that the water can flow quickly. It is important that the limb is immersed into the volume meter at exactly the same depth each time.

H. Brorson, M.D., Ph.D. (✉)
• B. Svensson, B.S., P.T. • K. Ohlin, B.S., O.T.
The Lymphedema Unit, Department of Clinical Sciences, Lund University, Plastic and Reconstructive Surgery, Jan Waldenströms gata 18, 2nd floor, Skåne University Hospital, Malmö SE-205 02, Sweden
e-mail: hakan.brorson@med.lu.se
http://www.plasticsurg.nu

A.K. Greene et al. (eds.), *Lymphedema: Presentation, Diagnosis, and Treatment*,
DOI 10.1007/978-3-319-14493-1_11, © Springer International Publishing Switzerland 2015

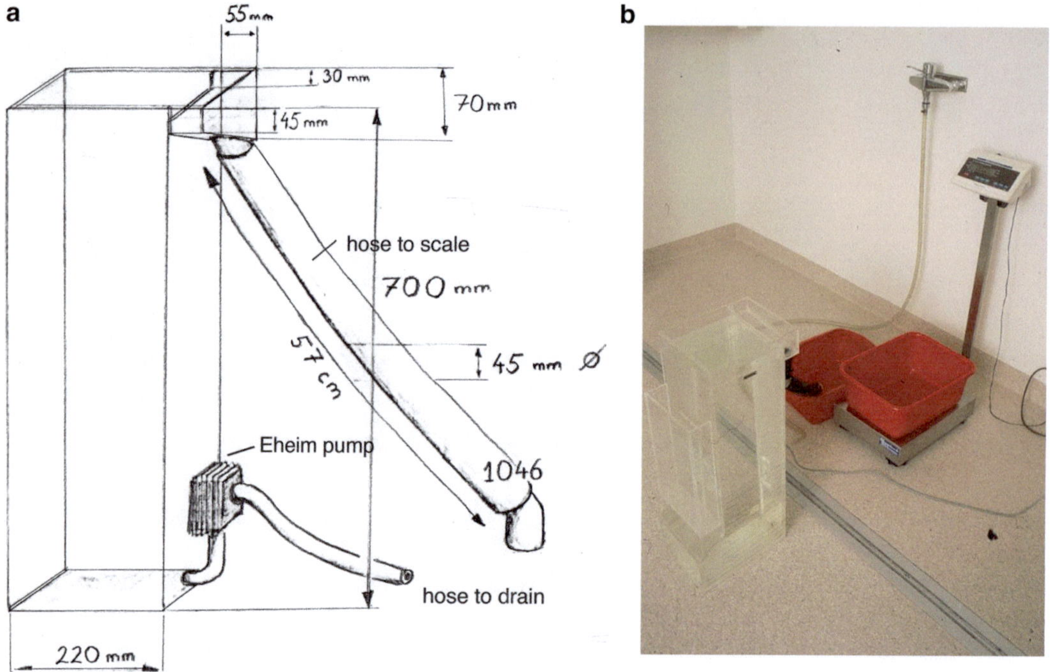

Fig. 11.1 (a) Arm volume meter. Figures in millimeter. (b) The clinical setup

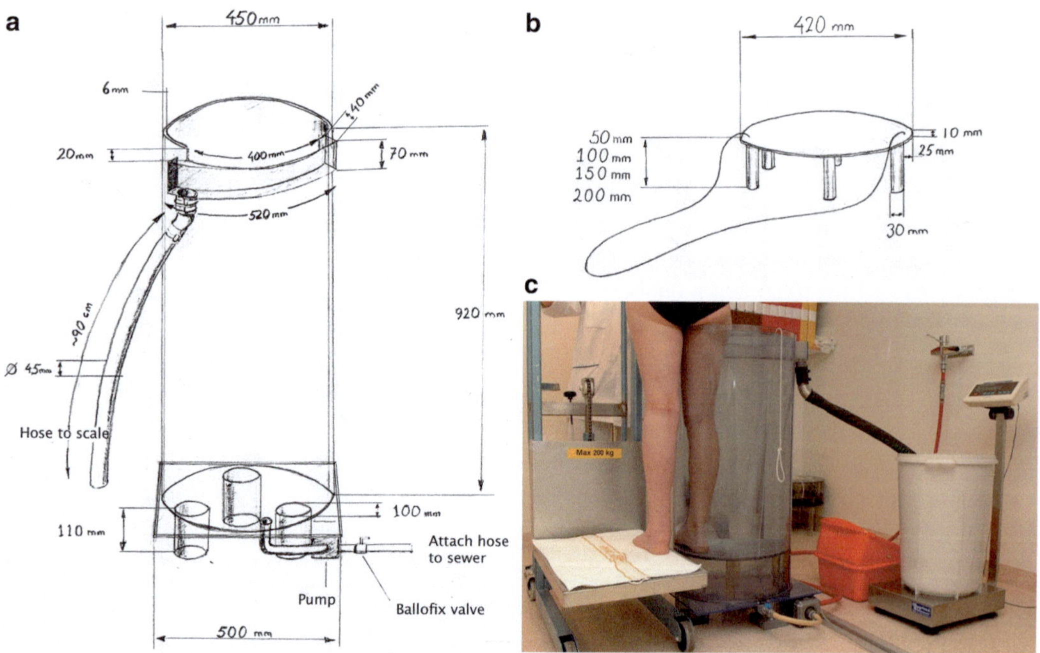

Fig. 11.2 (a) Leg volume meter. Figures in millimeter. (b) Leg volume meter. Spacers to compensate for various leg lengths. Figures in millimeter. (c) The clinical setup

Arm Volume Meter (Fig. 11.1)

The hose is connected to a standard faucet with a threaded bayonet mount and the volume meter is filled with water through a hose at the bottom of tank. The arm is brought down into the volume meter with the palm against the wall to avoid surge. The fingers are held outstretched and brought down until the tip of the middle finger reaches the bottom. Wait a few seconds to allow the water to flow out. There are gradation lines with 1-cm intervals for patients who do not reach down to the bottom of the volume meter. Measurements can be reproduced from time to time by noting the distance between the volume meter's bottom and the tip of the middle finger. The drained water is collected in a plastic tray (Orth Plast, for example, model 101-8: 40 cm× 34 cm×16 cm), which holds about 17 L. To empty the volume meter the hose is led down a drain in the floor or to a sink so the water can drain. An electric pump accelerates the runoff (Eheim 1046, Eheim, http://www.eheimparts.com). A drawing of a volume meter is shown in Fig. 11.1. The scale should have an accuracy of 5 g (digital max 30 kg/5 g). The volume meter has an average measurement error (CV%) of 0.24.

Leg Volume Meter (Fig. 11.2)

To compensate for different leg lengths, different spacers are put into the volume meter so that the entire leg volume can be measured up to the crotch. The measuring cylinder's height minus the leg length=the height of the spacer. An electric pump accelerates the runoff when emptying (Eheim 1060, Eheim, http://www.eheimparts.com). To hoist the patient a commercially available "lift" (Santo Lift SC 200, PMH International AB, http://www.pmh.se) is used. The water is collected in a large plastic laundry basket (Idealplast; model 0519; 33 cm×55 cm), which holds about 40 L (Fig. 11.2).

Volume Measurements Based on Circumference Measurements

Another method is circumference measurements on well-defined distances along the limb. Circumference measurements also provide information of the localization of the swelling. Hand and foot volumes cannot be calculated. To only make single circumference measurements (for example the middle of the upper arm, elbow, middle of the forearm) is not adequate either for clinical use or scientific study.

Volume measurements based on plethysmography or circumference measurements are useful and show satisfactory validity and reliability [4–9], plethysmography is recommended if only one method is used [10].

How Volumes Are Calculated Using Circumference Measurements

The circumferences of the limb measured every 4 cm along the limb. The volume of each segment is calculated according to the formula of the truncated and added together to get the limb volume (Fig. 11.3):

$$V = \frac{1}{3} \times \pi \times h \times \left(r_1^2 + r_2^2 + r_1 \times r_2 \right)$$

You need:
- A long ruler to mark every the 4 cm
- Marker pen (eyeliner pen)
- Narrow tape measure for circumference measurements
- Protocol.

How to measure:
- Arm lymphedema: The patient sits on a chair with the arm straight and abducted 90 ° on a table
- Highlight the 0 point in the wrist level
- The tape is placed around the extremity distal to each mark
- Read the circumferences measured and record

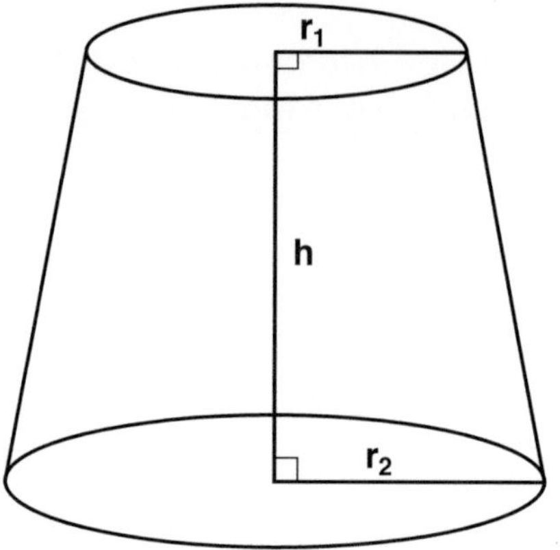

Fig. 11.3 Truncated cone segment. *H* height of the cone. r_1 radius at upper end of the segment. r_2 radius at lower end of the segment

- Leg lymphedema: The patient sits with the hip flexed at 90° with extended knee and foot in 0-position.

The measurement programs for arms and legs can be downloaded from: https://lu.box.com/s/9abvigfbx2rw7afgk9kz or by contacting the first author.

Other Methods

The following methods are not used routinely, but mainly for research purposes.

Perometry

This is an *optoelectronic measuring* method using a square frame with multiple perpendicular light beams. The frame is moved along the limb and the cross-sectional area is calculated continuously and thereby the volume. The equipment is expensive, but the method is accurate and fast [12]. Foot and hand volume are not measured [13, 14].

Bioelectric Impedance (BIS)

Extracellular fluid can be measured by bioelectrical impedance, which is recorded with a low current with different frequencies, transmitted through the tissue [15]. The method is particularly useful for diagnosing early lymphedema of the arm after breast cancer treatment [16].

Local Tissue Fluid, Tissue Dielectric Constant (TDC)

Tissue fluid may be measured by means of electromagnetic waves transmitted via a measuring head, which is set against the skin. The instrument measures a few millimeters into the skin and a constant (tissue dielectric constant), directly proportional to the tissue fluid content, is calculated. The method is useful for measuring tissue water anywhere in the body where the skin is not too close to the skeleton. The method has been used to measure edema in the extremities [17], legs [18, 19].

Other methods include *computed tomography* (CT) [20] and *magnetic resonance imaging* (MRI) [21].

Volume Calculations

A large number of computational methods have been presented for reporting treatment results [5, 7, 8]. The *excess volume* of a unilateral lymphedema is calculated as the difference between the edematous and the contralateral healthy extremity.

The *absolute excess volume* (volume of the affected limb − volume of the unaffected limb) of a lymphedema [22, 23] together with the *relative value* in percent (affected limb/unaffected limb × 100) gives optimal information before and after treatment. The relative value provides information about the extent of the edema [1, 10]. The same absolute excess volume provides greater relative value (swollen extremity/healthy extremity) in a skinny person as compared to a corpulent [1, 10].

Absolute Excess Volume and Percentage Reduction

Edematous arm (EA), Normal arm (NA), Before treatment (bt), After treatment (at).

	EA	NA	Excess volume	Excess volume reduction (%)
bt	5,000 ml	2,000 ml	Δ3,000 ml	
				67 %
at	3,000 ml	2,000 ml	Δ1,000 ml	

By measuring the normal arm at the same time as the edematous arm one takes into account the daily variations in arm volumes as well as weight gain or loss. It is very important that this is done at every time when volumes are measured.

$$\frac{\left(EA_{bt}-NA_{bt}\right)-\left(EA_{at}-NA_{at}\right)}{\left(EA_{bt}-NA_{bt}\right)}\times100 = \frac{\left(5,000\text{ ml}-2,000\text{ ml}\right)-\left(3,000\text{ ml}-2,000\text{ ml}\right)}{5,000\text{ ml}-2,000\text{ ml}}\times100$$

$$=\frac{3,000\text{ ml}-1,000\text{ ml}}{3,000\text{ ml}}\times100 = \mathbf{67\,\%}$$

Follow-up controls

	EA	NA	Excess volume	% Excess volume reduction
bt	5,000 ml	2,000 ml	Δ3,000 ml	
at1	4,000 ml	2,200 ml	Δ1,800 ml	$\dfrac{3,000\text{ ml}-1,800\text{ ml}}{3,000\text{ ml}}\times100$ $= \mathbf{40\,\%}$
at2	3,000 ml	1,800 ml	Δ1,200 ml	$\dfrac{3,000\text{ ml}-1,200\text{ ml}}{3,000\text{ ml}}\times100$ $= \mathbf{60\,\%}$
at3	2,000 ml	2,000 ml	Δ0 ml	$\dfrac{3,000\text{ ml}-0\text{ ml}}{3,000\text{ ml}}\times100$ $= \mathbf{100\,\%}$

The same calculation applies also for a leg.

In bilateral lymphedema the excess volume cannot be determined. Instead the change in volume, also in percent, for each limb is calculated, i.e.,

$$\left(\frac{EA_{bt}-EA_{at}}{EA_{bt}}\right)\times100 = \left(1-\frac{EA_{at}}{EA_{bt}}\right)\times100.$$

When scientific material is presented, the mean excess volume for all patients at baseline is calculated, as well as at follow-up. The percentage reduction for each patient is calculated and the mean percent edema reduction for all patients is calculated at follow-up.

The Relative Value of the Excess Volume

The excess volume can also be calculated in relation to the normal arm as a ratio, i.e., edematous arm/normal arm.

	EA	NA	Ratio
bt	5,000 ml	2,000 ml	2.5
$\dfrac{EA_{bt}}{NA_{bt}} = \dfrac{5,000\text{ ml}}{2,000\text{ ml}}\times100 = 2.5$			
at	3,000 ml	2,000 ml	1.5
$\dfrac{EA_{at}}{NA_{at}} = \dfrac{3,000\text{ ml}}{2,000\text{ ml}}\times100 = 1.5$			

The absolute excess volume is not always sufficient to describe a lymphedema. The same absolute excess volume of 200 ml (difference between the edematous arm and the normal arm) in a lean and in a corpulent person results in 10 % relative excess volume in a lean subject as opposed to 5 % in a corpulent subject.

Lean subject			Corpulent subject		
EA	NA	Excess volume	EA	NA	Excess volume
2, 200 ml--2, 000 ml			4, 200 ml--4, 000 ml		
= 200 ml			= 200 ml		

Excess volume in percent:

$$\frac{200\ \text{ml}}{2,000\ \text{ml}} \times 100 = 10\ \% \qquad \frac{200\ \text{ml}}{4,000\ \text{ml}} \times 100 = 5\ \%$$

Potential Sources of Errors

Potential Sources of Error

A common source of error is when the normal limb volume is measured only at baseline or not at all. This leads to incorrectly calculated values when the normal limb increases or decreases in volume [11].

Diurnal variation and weight loss or gain are sources of error, especially in patients with a small lymphedema.

Examples

Example of calculations of percent excess volume reduction when even the *normal* limb volume *decreases* (see Table 11.1).

The percentage reduction is calculated correctly when the normal limb volume is measured both before treatment and at follow-up (*). The left side of the table shows data from one arm while the right shows data from a leg. Note that if the initial normal limb volume is used at all subsequent measurements incorrect values are achieved. In the example of the arm an incorrect reduction of 53.9 % is calculated instead of 32.5 %, which is the correct excess percentage reduction. In the example of the leg an erroneous reduction of 91.2 % is calculated instead of the correct value of 7.3 % (see Table 11.1).

Example of calculations of percent excess volume reduction when even the normal limb volume *increases* (see Table 11.2):

The percentage reduction will be calculated correctly by the normal limb volume measured

Table 11.1 Example of calculations of percent excess volume reduction when even the *normal* limb volume *decreases* [11]

	Arm			Leg		
	Extremity volume			Extremity volume		
	Before	Follow-up	Follow-up*	Before	Follow-up	Follow-up*
Edematous extremity	4,798	4,297	4,297	9,441	8,366	8,366
Normal extremity	**3,869**	3,670	**3,869**	**8,262**	7,273	**8,262**
Excess volume	929	627	428	1,179	1,093	104
% Reduction		32.5 %	53.9 %		7.3 %	91.2 %
		Correct	Incorrect		Correct	Incorrect

The percentage reduction is calculated correctly when the normal limb volume is measured both before treatment and at follow-up (*). Bold numbers represent the use of the same volume of the normal extremity both at initial and final measurement, which is incorrect

Table 11.2 Example of calculations of percent edema reduction when even the *normal* limb volume *increases* [11]

	Arm			Leg		
	Extremity volume			Extremity volume		
	Before	Follow-up	Follow-up*	Before	Follow-up	Follow-up*
Edematous extremity	3,784	3,212	3,212	12,268	9,681	9,681
Normal extremity	**2,500**	2,599	**2,500**	**7,168**	7,877	**7,168**
Excess volume	1,284	613	712	5,100	1,804	2,513
% Reduction	52.3 %	44.5 %		64.6 %		50.7 %
		Correct	Incorrect		Correct	Incorrect

The percentage reduction is calculated correctly whem the normal limb volume is measured both is measured both before treatment and at follow-up (*). Bold numbers represent the use of the same volume of the edematous extremity both at initial and final measurement, which is incorrect

both at initial measurement and the final measurement (*). The left side of the table shows data from one arm while the right shows data from a bone. Note that if the normal limb initial measured value is used all the time to get the wrong values. In the example on an arm improperly obtained an edema reduction of 44.5 % instead of 52.3 %, which is the correct edema reduction. In the example on one leg got an error reduction of 50.7 % instead of the correct 64.6 % (see Table 11.2).

Conclusion

Volume measurement should be used when presenting outcomes of lymphedema treatment.

References

1. Godal R, Swedborg I. A correction for the natural asymmetry of the arms in the determination of the volume of oedema. Scand J Rehabil Med. 1982;14(4): 193–5.
2. Swedborg I. Effects of treatment with an elastic sleeve and intermittent pneumatic compression in postmastectomy patients with lymphoedema of the arm. Scand J Rehabil Med. 1984;16(1):35–41.
3. Borup Christensen S, Lundgren E. Sequelae of axillary dissection vs. axillary sampling with or without irradiation for breast cancer. A randomized trial. Acta Chir Scand. 1989;155(10):515–9.
4. Kuhnke E. Volumenbestimmung aus Umfangsmessungen. Folia Angiologica. 1976;24:228–32.
5. Kuhnke E. Die Volumenbestimmung entrundeter Extremitäten aus Umfangsmessungen. Lymphologie. 1978;2:35–44.
6. Stranden E. A comparison between surface measurements and water displacement volumetry for the quantification of leg edema. J Oslo City Hosp. 1981; 31(12):153–5.
7. Casley-Smith JR. Measuring and representing peripheral oedema and its alterations. Lymphology. 1994; 27(2):56–70.
8. Sitzia J. Volume measurement in lymphoedema treatment: examination of formulae. Eur J Cancer Care (Engl). 1995;4(1):11–6.
9. Brorson H, Höijer P. Standardised measurements used to order compression garments can be used to calculate arm volumes to evaluate lymphoedema treatment. J Plast Surg Hand Surg. 2012;46(6):410–5.
10. Swedborg I. Voluminometric estimation of the degree of lymphedema and its therapy by pneumatic compression. Scand J Rehabil Med. 1977;9(3):131–5.
11. Bernas MWM, Witte C, Belch D, Summers P. Limb volume measurements in lymphedema: issues and standards. Lymphology. 1996;29(Suppl):199–202.
12. Stanton AW, Northfield JW, Holroyd B, Mortimer PS, Levick JR. Validation of an optoelectronic limb volumeter (Perometer). Lymphology. 1997;30(2): 77–97.
13. Goltner E, Fischbach JU, Monter B, Kraus A, Vorherr H. Objective measurement of lymphedema after mastectomy. Dtsch Med Wochenschr. 1985;110(24): 949–52.
14. Bednarczyk JH, Hershler C, Cooper DG. Development and clinical evaluation of a computerized limb volume measurement system (CLEMS). Arch Phys Med Rehabil. 1992;73(1):60–3.
15. Cornish BH, Thomas BJ, Ward LC, Hirst C, Bunce IH. A new technique for the quantification of peripheral edema with application in both unilateral and bilateral cases. Angiology. 2002;53(1):41–7.
16. Cornish BH, Chapman M, Thomas BJ, Ward LC, Bunce IH, Hirst C. Early diagnosis of lymphedema in postsurgery breast cancer patients. Ann N Y Acad Sci. 2000;904:571–5.
17. Mayrovitz HN, Weingrad DN, Davey S. Local tissue water in at-risk and contralateral forearms of women

with and without breast cancer treatment-related lymphedema. Lymphat Res Biol. 2009;7(3):153–8.

18. Jensen MR, Birkballe S, Norregaard S, Karlsmark T. Validity and interobserver agreement of lower extremity local tissue water measurements in healthy women using tissue dielectric constant. Clin Physiol Funct Imaging. 2012;32(4):317–22.

19. Mayrovitz HN, Davey S, Shapiro E. Localized tissue water changes accompanying one manual lymphatic drainage (MLD) therapy session assessed by changes in tissue dielectric constant inpatients with lower extremity lymphedema. Lymphology. 2008;41(2):87–92.

20. Uhl JF. 3D multislice CT to demonstrate the effects of compression therapy. Int Angiol. 2010;29(5):411–5.

21. Sagen A, Karesen R, Skaane P, Risberg MA. Validity for the simplified water displacement instrument to measure arm lymphedema as a result of breast cancer surgery. Arch Phys Med Rehabil. 2009;90(5):803–9.

22. Tracy GD, Reeve TS, Fitzsimons E, Rundle FF. Observations on the swollen arm after radical mastectomy. Aust N Z J Surg. 1961;30:204–8.

23. Treves N. An evaluation of the etiological factors of lymphedema following radical mastectomy; an analysis of 1,007 cases. Cancer. 1957;10(3):444–59.

Bioelectrical Impedance Spectrometry for the Assessment of Lymphoedema: Principles and Practice

Leigh C. Ward

Key Points

- Bioimpedance spectroscopy is a causally related direct measure of lymph accumulation.
- Bioimpedance spectroscopy is the method of choice for early detection of lymphoedema. It is a rapid non-invasive and relatively inexpensive method.
- Originally limited to the assessment of unilateral lymphoedema of the arms, assessment can now be extended to bilateral lymphoedema of both the arms and legs.
- The method is suitable for home care monitoring of those at risk of developing lymphoedema.

Introduction

Secondary lymphoedema occurs as a consequence of lymphatic dysfunction, frequently as a result of surgical and/or radiological intervention for the treatment of cancer. In its earliest stages it presents as swelling of the affected body region as a consequence of accumulation of lymphatic fluid. Measurement of the volume increase of tissue is frequently used as a criterion of detection for early stage lymphoedema and for later staging [1]. Since there is general consensus that early detection of lymphoedema presents the optimal opportunity for instituting therapy, much effort has been expended in developing methods to detect lymphoedema as early as possible with high sensitivity and specificity. Bioelectrical impedance spectroscopy is at the forefront of these efforts [2].

Bioelectrical Impedance Background and Lymphoedema

What Is Bioelectrical Impedance Spectroscopy?

Bioelectrical impedance spectroscopy (BIS) is one of a number of technologies that are generically known as bioelectrical impedance analysis (BIA) techniques; all of which have the same theoretical basis [3].

Bioelectrical impedance techniques measure the opposition of the body's tissues to the flow of an electrical current. This opposition is known as impedance where the applied electrical current is an alternating current and is, by convention, denoted by the symbol, Z (Fig. 12.1). Impedance comprises two components, reactance (X_c) and resistance (R). Reactance is the opposition of current flow due to the cell membranes and tissue interfaces whereas resistance is the opposition to

L.C. Ward, B.Sc. (Hons), Ph.D. (✉)
School of Chemistry and Molecular Biosciences,
The University of Queensland, St Lucia, Brisbane,
QLD 4072, Australia
e-mail: l.ward@uq.edu.au

A.K. Greene et al. (eds.), *Lymphedema: Presentation, Diagnosis, and Treatment*,
DOI 10.1007/978-3-319-14493-1_12, © Springer International Publishing Switzerland 2015

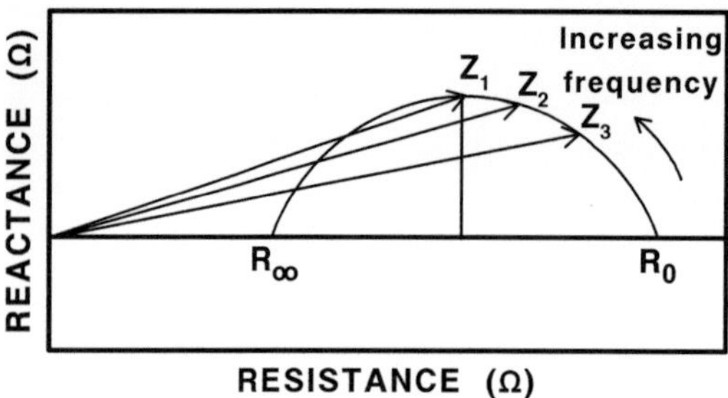

Fig. 12.1 Relationship between impedance (Z), reactance (X_c), resistance (R) and frequency of an applied electrical current. Biological tissue presents specific Z, R and X_c for each applied frequency (e.g. Z_1, Z_2, Z_3). The loci of R and X_c for a range of frequencies plot a semicircle, eponymously known as a Cole plot. Experimentally measured data are fitted to this theoretical semicircle to allow estimation of resistance at the otherwise immeasurable frequencies of zero (R_0) and infinite (R_∞) Hz. R_0 is the measure of extracellular fluid, including lymph, volume

the flow of electric current through tissue fluids. The magnitude of resistance is inversely proportional to the volume of the conductor and is determined by the inherent electrical properties of the conductor, the specific resistance or resistivity (ρ). The magnitude of resistance is also proportional to conductor length. These relationships are described by

$$V = \rho \frac{l^2}{R} \qquad (12.1)$$

where V is volume (mL), ρ is resistivity (Ω cm), l is conductor length (cm) and R is resistance (Ω).

In BIA, the applied current is an alternating current, i.e. with a sine wave of a given frequency, typically 50 kHz. In BIS, alternating currents are applied over a range of frequencies, typically between 5 and 1000 kHz. At low frequencies, the capacitive nature of cell membranes is such that they present a barrier to current flow and current flows only through the extracellular fluids while at high frequencies current can pass across the cell membranes and current flows through both intra- and extracellular water, i.e. total tissue water (Fig. 12.2). Thus in Eq. (12.1) if R is the measured resistance at a low frequency, ideally zero (R_0), then the volume of the extracellular fluid may be calculated if the resistivity of extracellular fluid and the conductive length is known.

Application of Bioimpedance Spectroscopy in Lymphoedema

The concept underlying the use of BIS to assess lymphoedema is that lymph is an extracellular fluid. Consequently, if the lymph content of a tissue or body region changes, this should be reflected in a change in the electrical resistance measured at a low (zero) frequency. One of the earliest publications to suggest the use of BIS for lymphoedema quantification was the work of Watanabe et al. in 1989 [4], but the approach was not systematically developed until some years later with the publication of Ward et al. [5]. The reasons for this delay were both practical and analytical. At this time there were no suitable impedance analysers commercially available; instruments were developed by research groups for their sole use. In the early 1990s two companies, Xitron and SEAC, both now incorporated in the one company ImpediMed, simultaneously developed BIS analysers. The analytical problems were twofold. Extracellular fluid including lymph is optimally quantified from the resistance measured at zero frequency (R_0). Unfortunately, a number of technological and safety issues preclude being able to measure R_0 directly. Instead R_0 is estimated by modelling the impedance data obtained from measurements made within the practical measurement region of 5–1000 kHz. The development of theoretical models and availability of computer programs at this time allowed for the first time the ready estimation of R_0 [6]. An additional problem is readily seen from consideration of Eq. (12.1). In order to quantify volume, resistivity and true conductor length are required. In biological systems both are unknown. The linear distance between the measurement points on the body is used as a surrogate for l while an apparent value for resistivity can be approximated from empirical studies. However, since both are approximations to the true values, their use can introduce error into the prediction of volume. Consequently, an index approach was adopted to "quantify" lymphoedema. In a manner analogous to use of inter-limb volume differences to assess unilateral limb lymphoedema, the ratio of R_0 values

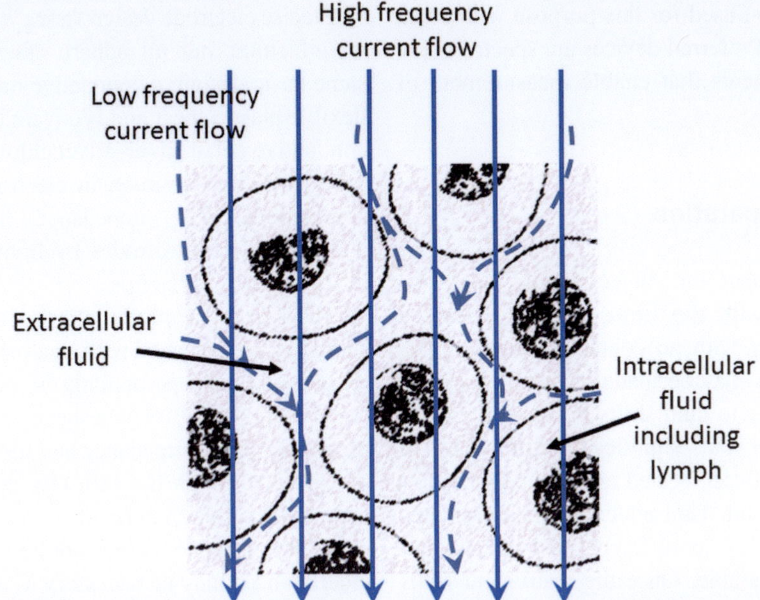

Fig. 12.2 Representation of the frequency-dependent flow of an applied electric current through biological tissue. At high frequencies, ideally infinite frequency but generally considered to be any frequency greater than 50 kHz, current can cross the cell membrane and hence flows through total tissue water. At low frequency, ideally zero frequency or below approximately 10 kHz, current cannot pass across the cell membrane owing to the capacitive nature of the bi-lipid structure of the membrane. Consequently current flows only through the extracellular fluid. Resistance measured at a low frequency is therefore a measure of extracellular fluid volume. With permission from Impedimed

between an at-risk or affected tissue region and a comparable unaffected region was used as a measure of the excess intracellular (lymph) volume [5]. This approach continues to be used to this day [7, 8].

Assessment of bilateral lymphoedema requires a different approach that makes use of BIS' ability to distinguish between intra- and extracellular water. Lymphoedema is considered to be purely accumulation of extracellular water; the intracellular water compartment volume remains unchanged. Consequently in lymphoedema, the ratio of extra- to intracellular water increases; this ratio in an affected body region can be indexed or standardised against the equivalent ratio in an unaffected body region, for example, the ratio observed in affected legs in bilateral lymphoedema is compared to the "normal" ratio found in the unaffected arms of the same individual [9].

Bioimpedance Spectroscopy for Assessment of Lymphoedema in Practice

Choice of Instrument

Many different impedance analysers are commercially available. They fall into two main groups according to the type of electrical connection to the body: stand-on and lead devices. Stand-on devices are rarely used for lymphoedema assessment and will not be discussed further. Lead type devices can be further categorised according to the number of frequencies of measurement. Single frequency devices are designed primarily for body composition analysis and are generally not recommended for lymphoedema assessment since they operate at 50 kHz, a frequency too high to quantify specifically extracellular fluid although they have been used for this purpose with some success [10]. Preferred devices are spectroscopic (BIS) instruments that enable measurement of R_0 [11].

Subject Preparation

For measurement, the subject should ideally be lying down with the limbs slightly abducted from the body with no contact between limbs. Measurements may be made in the seated position but, owing to fluid shifts in the body due to gravity, small but significant differences in impedance between seated and supine measurements are found. Consequently, measurements made in patients in different postures are not directly comparable. Once the instrument leads are connected to the appropriate electrodes, measurement of impedance takes only a few seconds and during this time the subject should refrain from making any movement. Measurements should always be made in replicate and outlying values discarded.

Electrodes

Universally, commercially available BIS instruments are designed as tetra-polar instruments. In theory, the impedance of a conductor can be measured with the use of a pair of electrodes that span the conductor of interest; each electrode acts to apply the electric current and, using, separate circuitry, also to measure the opposition to the flow of current. This approach is not suitable in most biological applications since it measures the total impedance between the electrodes. This includes not only the deep tissue impedances, i.e. of tissue fluids, but also the much larger contact impedance at the interface between the electrode and the skin surface. This contact impedance can be mitigated by separating the measurement or sensing circuitry and the current application circuitry. In this arrangement, the region of interest is spanned by a pair of sense or measurement electrodes with the current being applied by a pair of distally located current electrodes.

Precise electrode design varies with instrument manufacturer but all adhere essentially to the same basic design; a conductive material coats a flexible plastic sheet and is covered with a sticky conductive gel of silver–silver chloride. This type of electrode is common in electrocardiography applications. The impedance instrument is attached to the electrodes by light-weight wire leads and crocodile clips.

The site of electrode attachment to the skin should be well cleaned with an alcohol wipe prior to measurement particularly if oil-based skin creams are likely to have been used. Both the measurement of impedance and the transmission of current through the skin rely upon the naturally conductive nature of normally hydrated skin. Dry or papery skin is not uncommon in the elderly and it may be necessary to use extra conductivity (ultrasound) gel to obtain good electrical contact in such individuals. The electrode sites should be free of jewellery such as watches and bracelets particularly if made of conductive materials.

Electrode Locations

The precise body sites for electrode application are generally determined by what is desired to be measured, but the guiding principles are that the sense electrodes span the region of interest, that the sites are easily anatomically identifiable and reproducible and that the body extends distally to provide sites for application of the current drive electrodes. The most common applications of BIS are for assessment of limb, either arm or leg, lymphoedema. Consequently, sense electrodes are typically located at the wrist and ankle with current drive electrodes placed at the base of the toes and fingers. It is recommended that manufacturers' instructions specific to their impedance instruments and electrodes are consulted. In order to measure the arm or leg, in addition to the sense electrode at the wrist and ankle respectively, the second electrode sense electrode needs to be placed proximally along the limb. In early studies, these were located using either the acromion or anterior superior

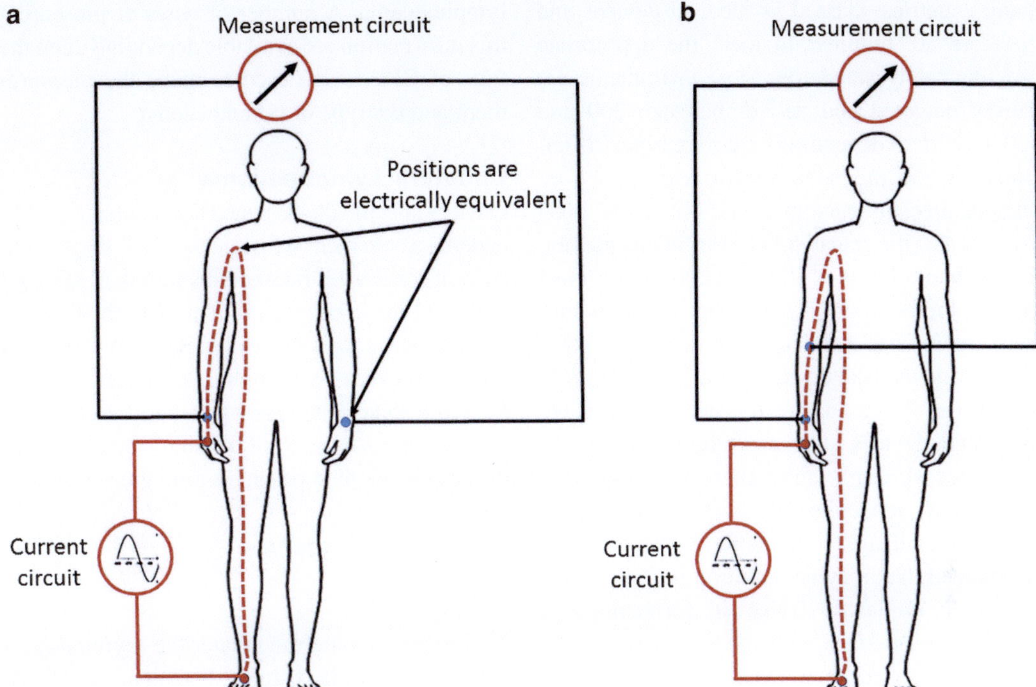

Fig. 12.3 Electrode locations for the measurement of whole arm impedance utilising the principle of equipotentials (**a**) and for the measurement of sub-limb segment, e.g. the forearm (**b**). Distally located electrodes (*red circle*) on the foot at the base of the toes and hand at the base of the fingers provide the current drive circuit. In *figure a* electrodes (*blue circle*) precisely located on the wrist on the mid-line between the bony prominences provide the impedance measuring sites. In the example shown, the impedance of the right arm is being measured with the electrode at the left wrist being electrically equivalent to a point at the junction of the arm and torso. Although the precise point is not known, it will be identical for each arm. For measurement of the left arm, these electrode positions are a mirror image. The same principle for locating electrodes can be applied to the legs. In *figure b*, the location of electrodes is shown for measurement of a segment of the arm. In this case the equipotential approach is not used and the location of the two measurement electrodes (*blue circle*) defines the measured volume

iliac spine as easily identified and reproducible sites. However, subsequent research found that, based on the principle of equipotentials, better precision of measurement could be obtained by using electrodes located on the contralateral wrist or ankle (Fig. 12.3a). If an intermediate segment of a limb, for example the forearm only, is to be measured, sense electrodes are located at a defined distance apart along the limb (Fig. 12.3b). Current drive electrodes can remain on the hand and foot as the only requirement is that current flows past the site of the sense electrodes. Measurement of non-cylindrical regions of the body such as the breast or hand requires arrangements of electrodes particularly suited to the anatomically irregular shape of these regions [12, 13].

Irrespective of measurement region, it is imperative that electrodes are placed with the greatest care and attention to reproducibility of location particularly where data are to be expressed as ratios between limbs; electrodes must be identically located on both limbs.

Contraindications for Use

There are few contraindications for the use of BIS. Since the widespread adoption of impedance technology for body composition analysis, there have been no reported adverse consequences due to the use of the equipment. Impedance devices when used in a clinical setting are, in many countries, classed as medical devices and therefore are required to meet the appropriate exacting safety standards. Most instruments are battery powered and deliver between 200 and 800 μA current depending on device type. In general its use in pregnant women is precluded on prudent precautionary grounds, but it has been used for specific research purposes in this population without reports of ill effects. Similarly most manufacturers do not recommend its use in subjects fitted with cardiac pacemakers or other implantable medical devices. Bioimpedance techniques can be used in subjects with passive implanted devices such as orthopaedic screws and plates although, since these can provide a preferential conductive track owing to their lower resistance compared to tissue fluid, interpretation of obtained data may be compromised. Presence of metallic implanted devices in, for example, a leg will not interfere with measurements in the arms. Rarely some individuals show an allergic reaction to the conductive gel coating electrodes. Propensity to such allergic reactions to, for example, adhesive wound dressings should be established prior to measurement.

It should also be appreciated that BIS is measuring tissue fluid. Consequently, the greatest value of BIS lies in the early stages (0 and 1) of lymphoedema development when it is primarily accumulation of excess fluid lymph. In later stage lymphoedema, when tissue fibrosis and fat infiltration is occurring, BIS will be less sensitive and of more limited value.

Measurements Obtained and Data Presentation

The format of data output will depend upon the particular instrument and manufacturer. Typically, the measured impedance, resistance and reactance at each frequency of measurement will be available and the derived value of interest, R_0. While these data are of primary interest to researchers, manufacturers have recognised that the output of primary interest to clinicians is a value or index that can be directly interpreted as indicative of the presence of lymphoedema or a change in the magnitude of pre-established

lymphoedema. A number of ways of presenting this information are available depending upon the type of BIS device used to make the measurement and the type of lymphoedema.

Unilateral Lymphoedema

Devices specifically designed for unilateral lymphoedema assessment will calculate and display the ratio of resistances between the at-risk or affected limb and the contralateral control limb. By convention, since R_0 is inversely related to volume, a limb with excess lymph fluid will have a smaller R_0 value than a control limb; consequently the ratio is expressed as R_0 of the unaffected to that of the affected limb to provide a ratio greater than 1:

$$\text{Lymphoedema index} = \frac{R_0 \text{unaffected}}{R_0 \text{affected}} \quad (12.2)$$

The larger the ratio the greater the asymmetry in extracellular fluid volume between the limbs. Since the body is naturally asymmetric due to dominance, typically the dominant arm for example is 1–2 % larger than the non-dominant arm, ratios are compared either to pre-lymphoedema ratios for the patient, if known, or to normative standards that account for limb dominance [14–16]. An important question is what magnitude of difference between a measured ratio and the normative standard is indicative of lymphoedema, i.e. the diagnostic cut-off or threshold value? This was originally set as being the mean value for a control population plus 3 standard deviations [14]. For women at risk of unilateral breast cancer-related lymphoedema, this equates to ratios ≥ 1.139 if their dominant side is at risk and a ratio ≥ 1.066 for those in whom breast cancer and treatment was on the non-dominant side [14]. More recently the specificity and sensitivity of these cut-offs for detection of lymphoedema has been questioned and cut-offs of the mean plus 2 standard deviations proposed as being more sensitive [17].

The use of simple ratios necessitates the need for separate standards for each limb dependent upon dominance. In addition, the use of ratios to compare affected and unaffected regions is not familiar to many clinicians and practitioners who are more accustomed to interpreting absolute differences. Indeed the International Society of Lymphology (ISL) Consensus Document [1] suggests that staging of lymphoedema be based on % difference between limbs while absolute volume differences in millilitres are also used [18]. Consequently, the L-Dex® score was introduced [17, 19, 20]. The L-Dex score linearizes and scales the ratios such that a change of +10 L-Dex units from baseline may indicate early lymphoedema. The L-Dex scale is based on the mean plus 3 SD detection cut-off. An example of the L-Dex report for an impedance measurement is presented in Fig. 12.4.

Bilateral Lymphoedema

For bilateral lymphoedema data are expressed as the ratio of impedances representing the extracellular fluid to intracellular ratio:

$$\frac{ECF}{ICF} = \frac{\rho_{ECF} R_i}{\rho_{ICF} R_0} \tag{12.3}$$

If it is assumed that the resistivities of the intra- and extracellular fluids are relatively constant [13], then Eq. (12.3) simplifies to:

$$\frac{ECF}{ICF} = \frac{R_i}{R_0} \tag{12.4}$$

The $R_i{:}R_0$ ratio is calculated for the body region affected by lymphoedema and this ratio compared to the same ratio measured in a body region of similar tissue composition but unaffected by lymphoedema. A larger ratio for the affected body region is taken as indicative of lymphoedema [9]. A graphical presentation of data is used to facilitate the comparison of ratios [9] where normative data are presented as tolerance ellipses (for a specified confidence interval) for the bivariate distribution of the ratio of the at-risk or affected body region and the ratio of the control body region. Patient data are then plotted as points on this graph; if the patient data fall outside the ellipse, this is interpreted as presumptive of lymphoedema (Fig. 12.5).

Absolute Volumes

According to Eq. (12.1), it should be possible to transform the measured resistance to an absolute quantity of extracellular fluid if the resistivity of extracellular fluid (ρ_{ECF}) and the inter-electrode length (l) is known. The latter is readily determined where the measured region is an arm or leg. This can be measured directly with a tape or estimated as a proportion of stature using readily available anthropometric ratios [21]. Determination of ρ_{ECF} is more difficult and can only be estimated empirically from whole body bioimpedance measurements and independent measurements of ECF volume by tracer dilution [22]. Although validation of this approach has been encouraging [22], the accuracy of determination of resistivity coefficients is of concern and suggests that until these can be determined, caution should be exercised when adopting this approach.

Clinical Value of Bioimpedance Spectroscopy for Assessment of Lymphoedema

A number of validation studies of the use of BIS for early detection of lymphoedema and its monitoring have been undertaken (e.g. [5, 7, 14, 17, 23–27]). It is an extremely reliable and reproducible measurement tool, intra-class correlation coefficients are 0.95 or greater, [26] that inherently has high specificity since the parameter being measured (R_0) is directly related to accumulation of lymph (Eq. 12.1). This has been supported in formal specificity and sensitivity analyses [28] although it has been suggested that adoption of a 2 SD threshold improves sensitivity to 80 % and specificity to 90 % for detection of those with breast cancer-related lymphoedema [17]. Consequently, its use as the method of choice for early detection of lymphoedema has been strongly advocated [2] and this is its primary indication for use. Studies have demonstrated that, under the appropriate measurement conditions, BIS has a resolution of approximately 35 mL of ECF in the whole arm. The minimal detectable change ($1.96 \times \sqrt{2} \times$ standard error of the mean) is approximately 0.04 unit change in inter-arm impedance ratio [2]. Bioimpedance spectroscopy has proven useful in the monitoring of various treatment interventions including water-based exercise programmes [29] and pneumatic compression for arm lymphoedema in post-breast cancer treatment patients [30].

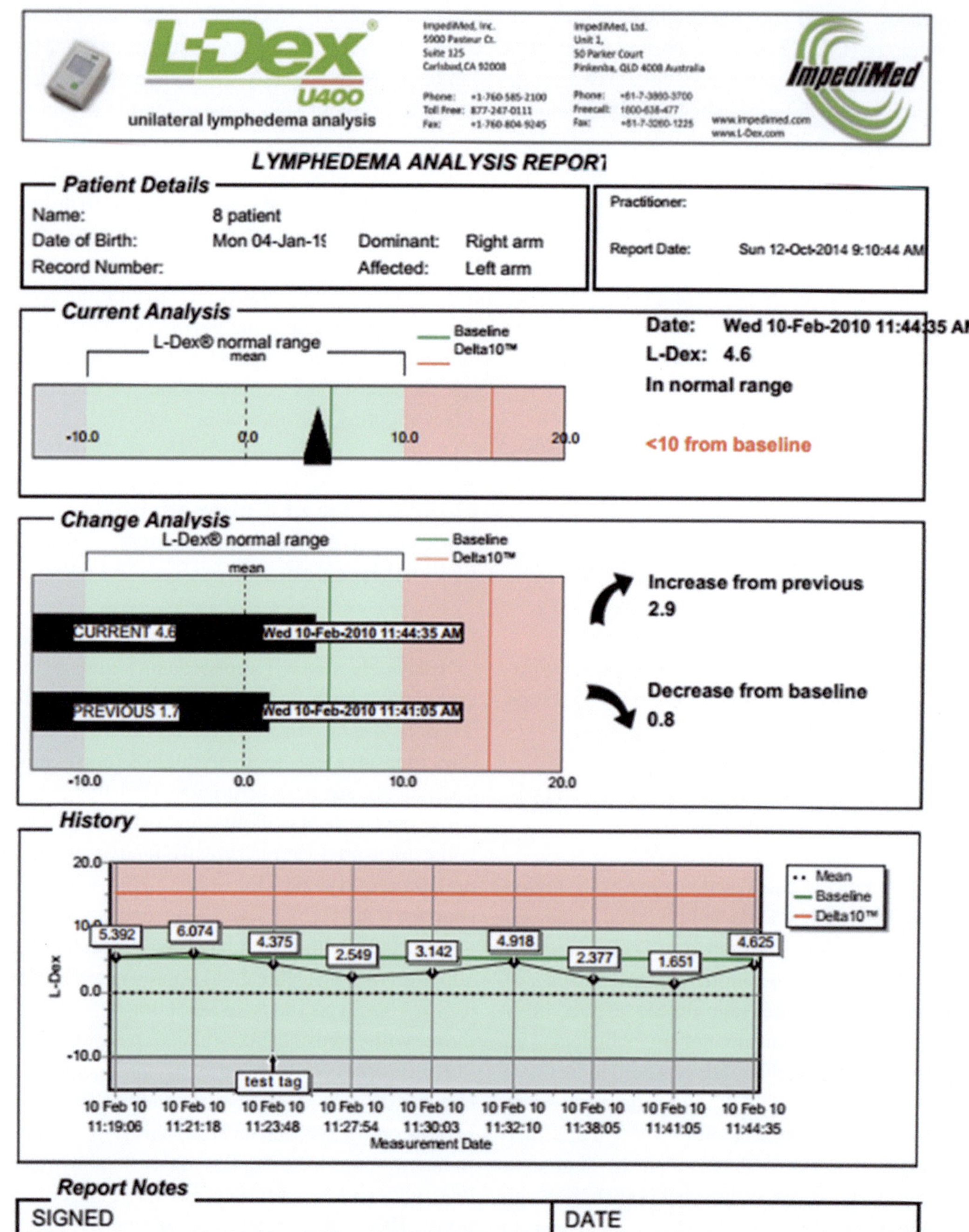

Fig. 12.4 An example of a bioimpedance spectroscopy assessment of unilateral arm lymphoedema using an L-Dex score as the index of lymphoedema. Image courtesy of ImpediMed

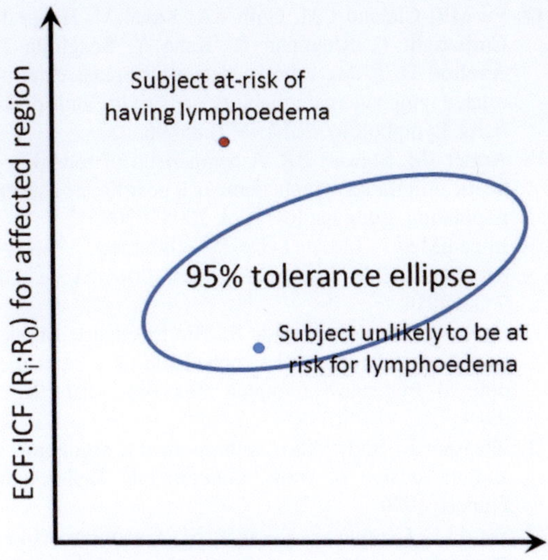

Fig. 12.5 Presentation of impedance measurements for bilateral lymphoedema. The ratio of impedances representing the ratio of extra- to intracellular fluid in non-lymphoedema tissues is plotted against the same ratio for the affected body region. Normative data for healthy individuals is plotted as a tolerance ellipse for a given confidence interval; in this example 95 %. The loci for individual subjects are plotted on this ellipse. Loci that fall within the ellipse are statistically, with the given level of confidence, unlikely to have lymphoedema; loci that fall outside the ellipse are considered, on a statistical basis, at risk of having lymphoedema

Conclusion

The past two decades have seen bioimpedance spectroscopy mature to play an important role in the early detection and management of lymphoedema. Technological advances have been made in both the necessary instrumentation and methods of data analysis. Originally impedance analysers designed for whole body composition analysis were adapted for the assessment of regional lymphoedema. While proving the principle of the method, they were not suitable for routine clinical practice. Instruments are now commercially available specifically designed for lymphoedema assessment, which are relatively inexpensive and easy to use. The data are presented to the clinician in a readily understandable form that can be used to aid diagnosis or assess the efficacy of therapeutic interventions (Fig. 12.4).

In addition to improving the general utility and accessibility of the technology, moving it from a predominantly research tool into clinical practice, research has continued to extend the applicability of the technology. Originally used for the assessment of unilateral lymphoedema principally in the arms of those with breast cancer-related lymphoedema, bioimpedance spectroscopy can now be used for the assessment of both unilateral and bilateral lymphoedema in both arms, legs and hands. The measurement of breast or truncal oedema remains challenging. Bioimpedance spectroscopy, and impedance measurements in general, are most suited to measurements of cylindrical body parts. This is dictated by the need for a linear array of electrodes spanning the region of interest. The breast is not cylindrical and being orthogonal to the body axis provides few suitable locations for electrodes. Although the trunk is cylindrical, its larger cross-sectional area in relation to its length means that measured resistances are small and errors in measurement are therefore proportionally larger. Undoubtedly, these obstacles can be overcome and the future holds the promise that bioimpedance spectroscopy can become the universal measurement modality for early detection of lymphoedema irrespective of where it is located in the body.

Funding No funding was used in the preparation of this document.

Conflict of interest: The author declares that he provides consultancy services to ImpediMed Ltd. ImpediMed Ltd had no involvement in the preparation of this chapter.

References

1. International Society of Lymphology. The diagnosis and treatment of peripheral lymphedema: 2013 Consensus Document of the International Society of Lymphology. Lymphology. 2013;46(1):1–11.
2. Ward LC. Early diagnosis in the latent phase. In: Lee BB, Bergan J, Rockson S, editors. Lymphedema: a concise compendium of theory and practice. 1st ed. Vienna: Springer-Verlag GmbH; 2010.
3. Cornish B. Bioimpedance analysis: scientific background. Lymphat Res Biol. 2006;4(1):47–50.

4. Watanabe R, Miura A, Inoue K, Haeno M, Sakamoto K, Kanai H. Evaluation of leg edema using a multi-frequency impedance meter in patients with lymphatic obstruction. Lymphology. 1989;22:85–92.

5. Ward LC, Bunce IH, Cornish BH, Mirolo BR, Thomas BJ, Jones LC. Multi-frequency bioelectrical impedance augments the diagnosis and management of lymphoedema in post-mastectomy patients. Eur J Clin Invest. 1992;22(11):751–4.

6. Cornish BH, Thomas BJ, Ward LC. Improved prediction of extracellular and total body water using impedance loci generated by multiple frequency bioelectrical impedance analysis. Phys Med Biol. 1999;38(3):337–46.

7. Ridner SH, Bonner CM, Doersam JK, Rhoten BA, Schultze B, Dietrich MS. Bioelectrical impedance self-measurement protocol development and daily variation between healthy volunteers and breast cancer survivors with lymphedema. Lymphat Res Biol. 2014;12(1):2–9.

8. Dylke ES, Alsobayel H, Ward LC, Liu M, Webb E, Kilbreath SL. Use of impedance ratios to assess hand swelling in lymphoedema. Phlebology. 2014;29(2):83–9.

9. Ward L, Winall A, Isenring E, Hills A, Czerniec S, Dylke E, Kilbreath S. Assessment of bilateral limb lymphedema by bioelectrical impedance spectroscopy. Int J Gynecol Cancer. 2011;21(2):409–18.

10. de Godoy JM, Valente FM, Azoubel LM, Godoy MF. Evaluation of lymph drainage using bioelectrical impedance of the body. Phlebology. 2011;26(7):298–300.

11. Shah C, Vicini F, Beitsch P, Laidley A, Anglin B, Ridner SH, Lyden M. The use of bioimpedance spectroscopy to monitor therapeutic intervention in patients treated for breast cancer related lymphedema. Lymphology. 2013;46(4):184–92.

12. Ward LC, Dylke ES, Kilbreath SL. Measurement of hand volume by bioelectrical impedance spectroscopy. Lymphat Res Biol. 2012;10(2):81–6.

13. Cornish BH, Thomas BJ, Ward LC, Hirst C, Bunce IH. A new technique for the quantification of peripheral edema with application in both unilateral and bilateral cases. Angiology. 2002;53(1):41–7.

14. Cornish BH, Chapman M, Hirst C, Mirolo B, Bunce IH, Ward LC, Thomas BJ. Early diagnosis of lymphedema using multiple frequency bioimpedance. Lymphology. 2001;34(1):2–11.

15. Ward LC, Dylke E, Czerniec S, Isenring E, Kilbreath SL. Confirmation of the reference impedance ratios used for assessment of breast cancer-related lymphedema by bioelectrical impedance spectroscopy. Lymphat Res Biol. 2011;9(1):47–51.

16. Svensson BJ, Dylke ES, Ward LC, Kilbreath SL. Segmental impedance thresholds for early detection of unilateral upper limb swelling. Lymphat Res Biol. 2014. doi:10.1089/lrb.2013.0050.

17. Fu MR, Cleland CM, Guth AA, Kayal M, Haber J, Cartwright F, Kleinman R, Kang Y, Scagliola J, Axelrod D. L-dex ratio in detecting breast cancer-related lymphedema: reliability, sensitivity, and specificity. Lymphology. 2013;46(2):85–96.

18. Armer JM, Stewart BR. A comparison of four diagnostic criteria for lymphedema in a post-breast cancer population. Lymphat Res Biol. 2005;3:208–17.

19. ImpediMed Ltd. L-Dex® (internet). http://international.l-dex.com/what-is-l-dex/ (2014). Accessed 9 Oct 2014.

20. Gaw R, Box R, Cornish B. Bioimpedance in the assessment of unilateral lymphedema of a limb: the optimal frequency. Lymphat Res Biol. 2011;9(2):93–9.

21. Pheasant S. Body space anthropometry, ergonomics and the design of work. London: UK Taylor and Francis; 1990.

22. Ward LC, Czerniec S, Kilbreath SL. Quantitative bioimpedance spectroscopy for the assessment of lymphoedema. Breast Cancer Res Treat. 2009;117(3):541–7.

23. Vicini F, Shah C, Lyden M, Whitworth P. Bioelectrical impedance for detecting and monitoring patients for the development of upper limb lymphedema in the clinic. Clin Breast Cancer. 2012;12(2):133–7.

24. Czerniec SA, Ward LC, Lee MJ, Refshauge KM, Beith J, Kilbreath SL. Segmental measurement of breast cancer-related arm lymphoedema using perometry and bioimpedance spectroscopy. Support Care Cancer. 2011;19(5):703–10.

25. Smoot BJ, Wong JF, Dodd MJ. Comparison of diagnostic accuracy of clinical measures of breast cancer-related lymphedema: area under the curve. Arch Phys Med Rehabil. 2011;92(4):603–10.

26. Moseley A, Piller N. Reliability of bioimpedance spectroscopy and tonometry after breast conserving cancer treatment. Lymphat Res Biol. 2008;6(2):85–7.

27. Warren AG, Janz BA, Slavin SA, Borud LJ. The use of bioimpedance analysis to evaluate lymphedema. Ann Plast Surg. 2007;58(5):541–3.

28. Hayes S, Cornish B, Newman B. Comparison of methods to diagnose lymphoedema among breast cancer survivors: 6-month follow-up. Breast Cancer Res Treat. 2005;89(3):221–6.

29. Johansson K, Hayes S, Speck RM, Schmitz KH. Water-based exercise for patients with chronic arm lymphedema: a randomized controlled pilot trial. Am J Phys Med Rehabil. 2013;92(4):312–9.

30. Ridner SH, Murphy B, Deng J, Kidd N, Galford E, Bonner C, Bond SM, Dietrich MS. A randomized clinical trial comparing advanced pneumatic truncal, chest, and arm treatment to arm treatment only in self-care of arm lymphedema. Breast Cancer Res Treat. 2012;131(1):147–58.

Harvey N. Mayrovitz

Key Points

1. Tissue dielectric constant (TDC) measurements using the MoistureMeterD provide a way to assess an individual's local skin-to-fat water rapidly and noninvasively.
2. Assessments can be done in virtually any anatomical site of clinical interest.
3. TDC and thereby relative water can be assessed at different depths, which is a feature that could aid in better characterizing edematous and lymphedematous characteristics.
4. Tracking of changes in lymphedematous status over time is easily and rapidly done.
5. In cases of potential unilateral lymphedema, inter-side TDC ratios may serve as markers of subclinical lymphedema.

Introduction

The MoistureMeterD (MMD) is a multiprobe device (Fig. 13.1) manufactured by Delfin Technologies (Kuopio Finland) that is used to measure skin and upper subcutis tissue dielectric constant (TDC) at a frequency of 300 MHz by touching the skin's surface with a handheld probe

for about 10 s (Fig. 13.2). Probe outer diameters range from 10 mm for a 0.5 mm effective measurement depth (Fig. 13.3) to 55 mm for a 5 mm measurement depth. Effective measurement depth is defined as the depth at which the electric field decreases to $1/e$ of its surface field as illustrated in Fig. 13.4 for a 2.5 mm depth measurement probe.

Dielectric constant, also known as relative permittivity, is a dimensionless number equal to the ratio of the permittivity of tissue to the permittivity of vacuum. Because TDC values in part depend on tissue water content, TDC values and their change provide indices of water content and quantitative estimates of water content changes. For reference the dielectric constant of distilled water at 32 °C is about 76. Because the measuring devices operate at a frequency of 300 MHz the measured skin TDC values are sensitive to both free and bound water within the measurement volumes. The vertical dimension for the measurement volume ranges between 0.5 mm and 5.0 mm below the epidermis with the total volume depending on the probe diameter.

Currently available devices come in two flavors. One is the original MMD, the multi-probe version with four separate probes as shown in Fig. 13.1 for effective measurement depths of 0.5, 1.5, 2.5, and 5.0 mm with the largest size probe measuring the deepest. The other device (Fig. 13.5) is a compact version (MMDC) in which the sensor and processing electronics are built into the handheld unit. The MMDC has a bar

H.N. Mayrovitz, Ph.D. (✉)
Department of Physiology, College
of Medical Science, Nova Southeastern University,
3200 S. University Drive, Fort Lauderdale,
FL 33322, USA
e-mail: mayrovit@nova.edu

A.K. Greene et al. (eds.), *Lymphedema: Presentation, Diagnosis, and Treatment,*
DOI 10.1007/978-3-319-14493-1_13, © Springer International Publishing Switzerland 2015

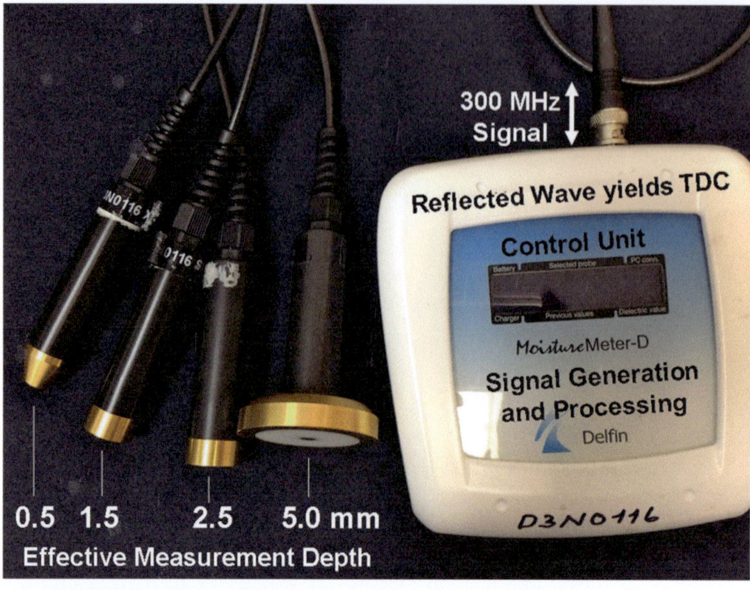

Fig. 13.1 Multiprobe Tissue Dielectric Constant (TDC) device. Effective measurement depth depends on probe construction and dimensions with larger diameter probes penetrating deeper. Operating principle is that a 300 MHz signal is transmitted to the tissue and the reflected wave is processed to obtain the dielectric constant of the tissue volume measured. The TDC is strongly dependent on the free and bound water contained within the measurement volume

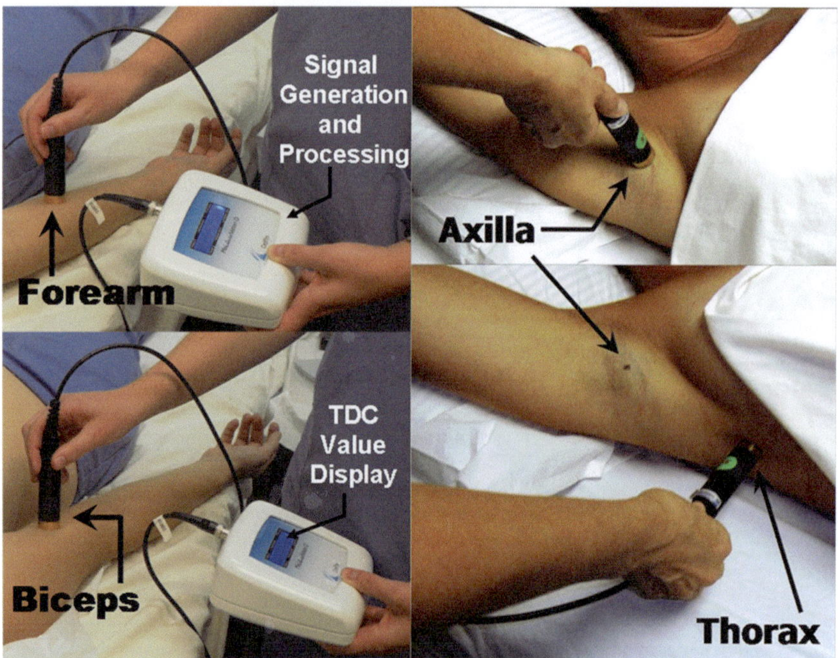

Fig. 13.2 Measuring TDC at multiple sites. Probes can be used to measure TDC at virtually any anatomical site of interest. Here is shown measurements using a probe measuring to an effective depth of 1.5 mm at forearm, biceps, axilla, and lateral thorax. Measurement activates when skin is touched and takes about 10 s

indicator showing the relative amount of contact pressure being exerted on the skin. The MMD and to a lesser extent the MMDC have been used in basic and clinical research studies in which skin tissue water and its change were of interest. Because either probe system can be used in virtually any anatomical location, data and findings are available for multiple anatomical sites on

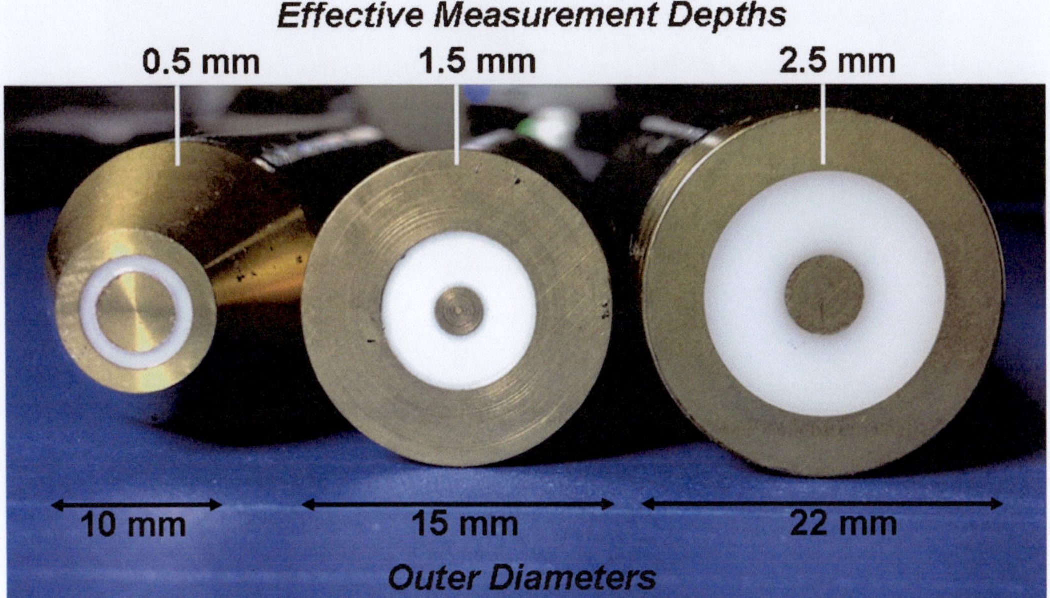

Fig. 13.3 Variation in probe design determines effective measurement depth. TDC measurements are used to assess localized tissue water and its change with the wider probe penetrating more deeply. Choice of probe to use depends on application and available space for placing the probe. The largest effective measurement depth is 5 mm achievable with a probe that has a diameter of 55 mm

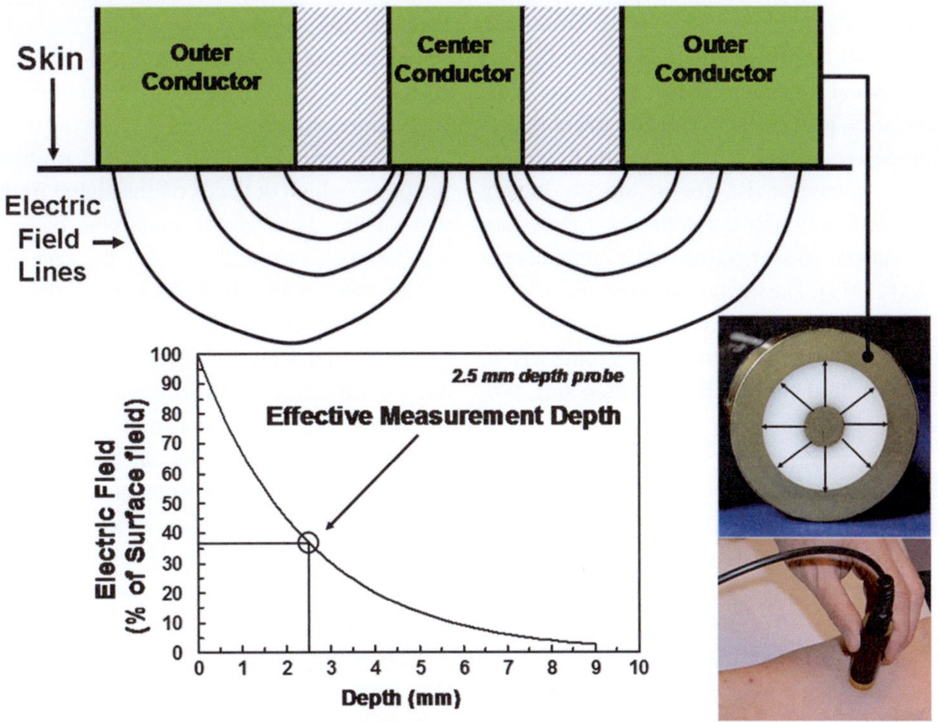

Fig. 13.4 Effective measurement depth concept. Effective measurement depth is defined as that depth at which the electric field produced by the probe on the skin surface is reduced to $1/e$ (36.7 %) of its value. The *electric field lines* are schematically illustrated emanating from and then terminating on the concentric electrodes of the probe

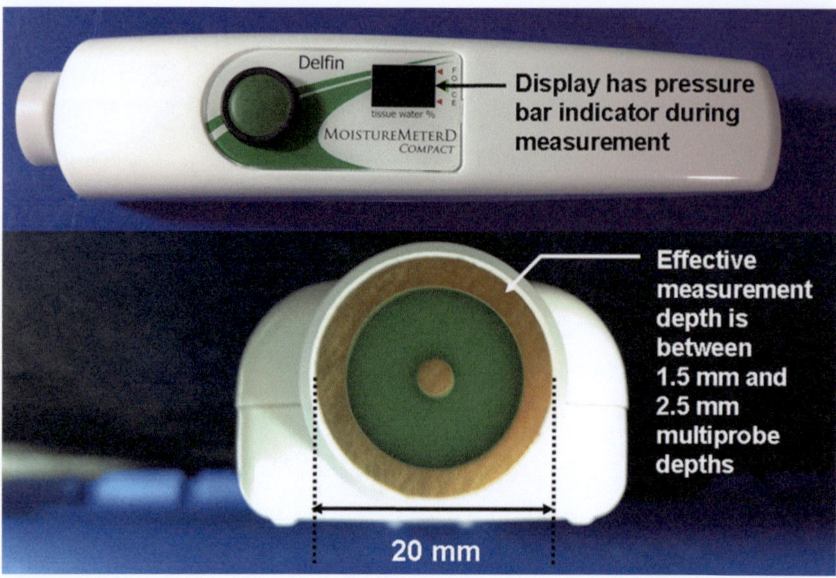

Fig. 13.5 Compact Tissue Dielectric Constant (TDC) measurement device. All functions are built into the single handheld device. Its effective measurement depth is between that of the 1.5 mm and 2.5 mm depth multiprobes and TDC readings would be about 6 % greater than those of the 2.5 mm probe. The display contains a series of *horizontal bars* that when aligned indicate the proper applied pressure. The display reads out in percent water rather than TDC values directly

the upper body including face [1, 2], breast [3], forearm [4–7], biceps, axilla, and thorax [8] and on the leg and foot [1, 9, 10]. One of the most frequent uses to date has been for tracking and possible early detection of subclinical lymphedema in women at-risk for or already having lower extremity lymphedema or upper extremity breast cancer treatment-related lymphedema (BCRL) [11–17]. The method also may have value in differentiating lower extremity lymphedema from lipedema [18], characterizing changes in postsurgical fluid status [19], and assessing skin irradiation effects [3].

Measurement Principles

The control unit (Fig. 13.1) generates and transmits a very low power 300 MHz signal into the probe that is in contact with the skin (Fig. 13.2). The signal is transmitted into the tissue via the probe that acts as an open-ended coaxial transmission line [20]. Part of the signal is absorbed by the tissue, mainly by water, and part is reflected back to the control unit where the complex reflection coefficient is determined [21, 22] from which the dielectric constant is determined [23, 24]. Reflections from the end of this coaxial transmission line depend on the complex permittivity of the tissue which depends on the signal frequency and on the dielectric constant (the real part of the complex permittivity) and the conductivity of the tissue with which the probe is in contact. At 300 MHz the contribution of the conductivity to the overall value of the permittivity is small and the dielectric constant is mainly determined by water molecules (free and bound). Consequently, the device includes and analyzes only the dielectric constant (TDC) that is directly proportional to tissue water content in a manner close to that predicted by Maxwell mixture theory for low water content but a slightly less good prediction for high water content tissues [25]. In all cases TDC is strongly dependent on relative water content with TDC values that decrease with water reductions during hemodialysis [26] and that correlate with whole body water percentages as illustrated in Fig. 13.6 in which forearm TDC

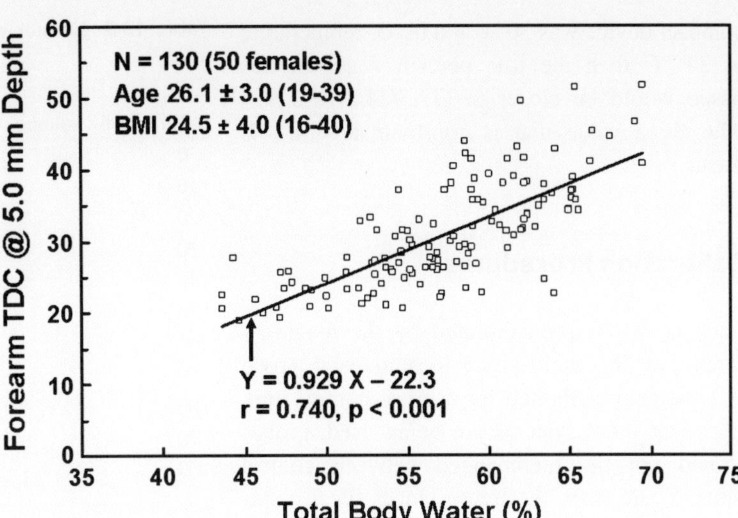

Fig. 13.6 Tissue Dielectric Constant (TDC) values in relation to total body water. TDC values are directly related to percentage of total body water (TBW). TBW was measured via bioimpedance. Relationship between TDC and TBW is illustrated for a 5 mm TDC forearm measurement depth in 130 young adults. The *solid line* is the linear regression equation with parameters as indicated in the figure

values are seen to highly correlate with total body water percentage as determined using bioimpedance measures.

The induced electric field within the tissue falls off exponentially and the effective measurement depth, defined as that depth at which the field is $1/e$ its surface value, depends on the dimensions of the probe [27] with larger dimensions being associated with deeper penetration. If the tissue measurement volume is viewed as being comprised of two layers, one being the skin including stratum corneum, epidermis and dermis with combined skin depth δ, and the other part being the subcutaneous tissue including fat, then it can be shown that measured TDC values depend on dielectric constants of skin (ε_{skin}) and fat (ε_{fat}) and on δ [3, 27]. This relationship can be expressed [2] as $TDC = (\varepsilon_{skin} - \varepsilon_{fat})(1 - e^{-q\delta}) + \varepsilon_{fat}$ in which q is a device constant that depends on probe dimensions and is about 0.82 for the 1.5 mm depth probe. Changes in TDC values largely reflect changes in skin water content because of the normally large fraction of skin water. However, because TDC values also depend on skin thickness (δ) comparisons of absolute water content between individuals or groups should be done with caution. An equation linking percentage of tissue water content (PWC%) to TDC values has been proposed [26] for high water content tissues and is given by PWC% = 100

Table 13.1 Dielectric constant of water versus temperature

Temperature (°C)	Dielectric constant
20	80.1
23	79.0
25	78.5
26	78.0
28	77.3
30	76.6
32	75.9
34	75.2
35	74.9
37	74.2
40	73.2

The most appropriate value for use in converting percentage water to Tissue Dielectric Constant (TDC) when using the compact probe would be to use the skin temperature at which the measurement is being made

(TDC − 1)/77.5. The denominator of this equation (77.5) is based on a TDC value for water of about 78.5 at 25 °C. However, since water's dielectric constant depends on temperature, the tissue temperature being measured should be taken into account. For example, at a skin temperature of 34 °C, water's dielectric constant is about 75.2. Table 13.1 lists water dielectric constants for various temperatures. Temperature corrections may result in small TDC changes but under certain circumstances such corrections are useful and easily done. For example if a PWC% reading on the compact device was 36 % at a tissue temperature of 34 °C then the true percent water in this tissue would be closer to $(77.5/74.2) \times 36\ \% = 37.6\ \%$, a value that is approximately 4.4 % greater.

Calibration Procedures

Each device is pre-calibrated by the manufacturer. For the multi-probe system each probe is separately calibrated for a given control unit. If two or more systems are being used, probes should not be interchanged between control units. There may be circumstances when independent calibrations or calibration checks are useful. This can be done by exposing the probe tips to various ethanol–water concentrations and comparing values obtained with known solution dielectric constants. The static dielectric constant for ethanol at 25 °C, averaged from multiple sources, is 24.8. The approximate dielectric constant values for various ethanol–water mixtures that are listed in Table 13.2 may be used to compare values obtained with any probe and if needed take appropriate calibration adjustments into account. An example of a full calibration curve is shown in Fig. 13.7, but only a few ethanol–water mixture concentrations would be sufficient.

Measurement Procedure

Touching skin with one of the probes of the multiprobe device or touching it with the compact device activates the measurement that is heralded by short distinctive sound. A single measurement takes about 10 s or less to complete with completion signaled by another distinct audible sound. The TDC value is displayed on the control unit of the multiprobe readout. For the compact device the readout is not directly that of the TDC value, but instead it is a calculated percentage water PCW% determined via the equation previously given. If one is using both multiprobe and compact devices, it is useful to convert compact readings to TDC to achieve uniformity of measures for comparison purposes between results obtained

Table 13.2 Ethanol–water mixture dielectric constant at 25 °C

% Ethanol by volume	Dielectric constant of ethanol–water mixture
0	78.3
10	73.0
20	67.6
30	62.3
40	56.9
50	51.6
60	46.2
70	40.9
80	35.5
90	30.2
100	24.8

For calibration or calibration checks the Tissue Dielectric Constant (TDC) probe can be exposed to ethanol–water mixtures to determine either calibration factors or to determine how well measured values agree with the values listed in the table

from the two systems. The conversion equation that can be used is $TDC = 1 + [(PWC\%)(\varepsilon_{water} - 1)]/100$ in which PWC% is the number displayed on the compact probe (calculated percentage water) and ε_{water} is the dielectric constant of water used by the device for its calculation which is 78.5. For example, a reading of 36 % would correspond to a TDC value of $1 + (36 \times 77.5)/100 = 28.9$.

Short- and Long-Term Measurement Repeatability

One or Multiple Measurements Averaged

TDC measurements taken in triplicate and averaged are the method most frequently employed. However, it has been shown that for TDC measurements on forearms of healthy women and women with BCRL the average difference in TDC value between the first measurement and the average of three sequential measurements to a depth of 2.5 mm is less than ± 1 TDC unit [6]. This suggests that for many purposes a single measurement may be sufficient; however, similar data on other anatomic sites is not yet available.

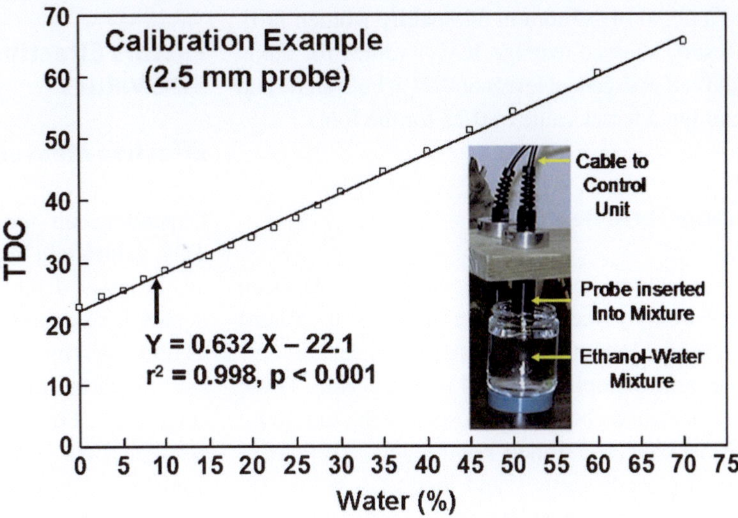

Fig. 13.7 Tissue Dielectric Constant (TDC) probe calibration check using various alcohol-water concentrations. Each probe is calibrated by exposing the probe measuring head to varying ethanol–water concentrations. This figure is for a 2.5 mm effective measurement depth probe and illustrates the essentially linear dependence of the TDC value with water concentration (%Water)

Short-Term Intrarater and Interrater Repeatability

Because some applications use pre- and post-TDC measurements to assess single treatment therapeutic modalities [11, 15] the measurement repeatability over intervals of the order of 60 min are of interest. Intrarater reliability has been assessed based on bilateral forearm TDC measurements to 2.5 mm depth on five subjects at 0, 30, and 60 min by a person with familiarity with TDC measurements. Intrarater repeatability has been assessed using intraclass correlation coefficients (ICC) that broadly express the percentage of variability attributable to true subject variance as opposed to measurement related variability (between-subject variation/total variation). Results revealed a single measure ICC value ($ICC_{2,1}$) of 0.996 with a 95 % confidence interval of 0.96–1.000. Additional tests based on measurements of a minimally trained rater under the same circumstances yielded $ICC_{2,1}$ values 0.999 with 95 % confidence intervals of 0.994–1.000. Interrater reliability ($ICC_{2,2}$) has also been assessed via triplicate measurements made on four subjects at 30 min intervals by two medical students who were minimally trained in TDC measurements. $ICC_{2,2}$ values obtained were quite good at 0.997 with a 95 % confidence interval of 0.988–0.999.

Table 13.3 Intraclass correlation coefficients (ICC) for Tissue Dielectric Constant (TDC) measurements

Measurement site	ICC	95 % Confidence interval
Forearm		
2.5 mm depth	0.962	(0.852–0.994)
1.5 mm depth	0.793	(0.394–0.994)
Leg		
2.5 mm depth	0.945	(0.792–0.991)
1.5 mm depth	0.941	(0.778–0.991)
Foot		
2.5 mm depth	0.887	(0.615–0.982)
1.5 mm depth	0.923	(0.720–0.988)

Measurements were made by two measurers on five subjects with TDC measurements made 1 week apart. Subjects were young healthy adults. Forearm site is on the dominant arm 5 cm distal to the antecubital space. Leg site is on the lateral calf 10 cm proximal to the malleolus. Foot site is mid dorsum of the foot. All measurements were made with subjects supine

Assessments of interrater reliability of TDC measurements made 1 week apart by two other minimally trained medical students yielded reasonable ICC values for both the 2.5 mm and the 1.5 mm depth probes as summarized in Table 13.3 for forearm, leg, and foot. Interobsever agreement of absolute TDC measurements in lower extremities has also been assessed based on measurements of three minimally trained measurers who each measured TDC at calf, ankle, and foot to a depth of 2.5 mm in 34 healthy women [10]. Results showed average $ICC_{2,3}$ values for ankle and calf at excellent levels of 0.94 at both ankle and calf but a lesser value of 0.77 for the foot.

Long-Term Reliability

Longer term intrarater repeatability has been assessed by measurements of normal control arms in 32 women on six separate occasions by the same therapist over a 24 month period. These women had been diagnosed with unilateral breast cancer and their contralateral arms measured prior to surgery and then at 3, 6, 12, 18, and 24 months post-surgery. Intraclass correlation coefficients ($ICC_{2,1}$) determined for forearm TDC measurements to a depth of 2.5 mm was 0.900 with a 95 % confidence interval of 0.835–0.946.

Factors Effecting Measured TDC Values

Effective Measurement Depth

Depending on the anatomical site, measured TDC values will vary with generally higher values at lesser depths and lesser values at greater depths. This dependence is not necessarily linear as illustrated by measurements made on the anterior forearm of a large group of women (Fig. 13.8). For this data set the TDC averaged between both arms decreased according to a nonlinear power regression equation given by $TDC = 32.44\,\delta^{-0.185}$ in which δ is measurement depth. This observed pattern is at least in part due to the inclusion of increasing amounts of low water content fat in the measurement volume with increasing depth [8]. Although this pattern is

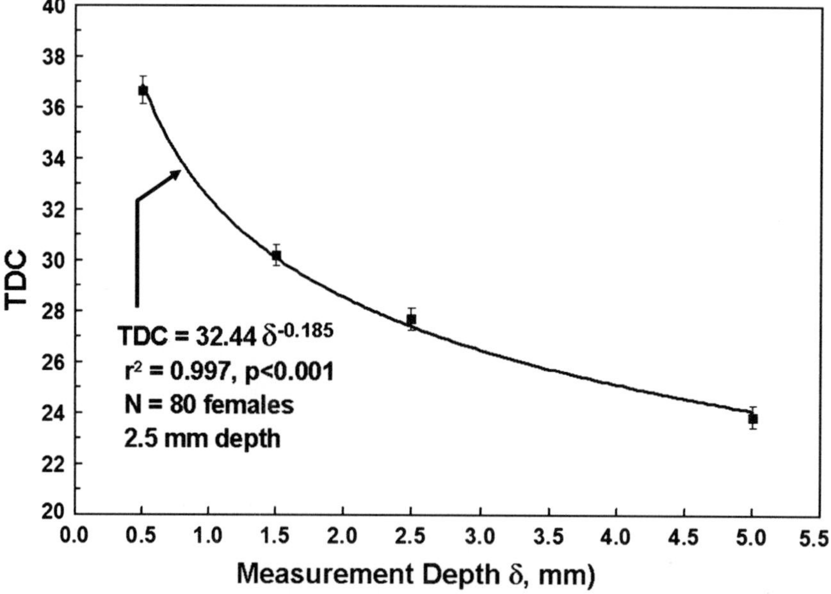

Fig. 13.8 Tissue Dielectric Constant (TDC) measurement depth-dependence: pre-surgery. Data points are pre-surgery mean TDC values for 80 patients with individual patient TDC values calculated as the average of both forearms. Error bars are ± 1 sem. *Solid line* is nonlinear (power-law) regression with the equation $TDC = 32.44\,\delta^{-0.185}$ determined based on 80 TDC measurements at each depth. *Inset* shows at-risk/control arm ratio with associated SD

Table 13.4 Site variations of Tissue Dielectric Constant (TDC) values

Measurement site	TDC at indicated effective measurement depths		
	0.5 mm	1.5 mm	2.5 mm
Forehead[a]	40.7±3.4	36.8±2.7	35.0±3.6
Cheek	33.4±6.4	32.5±3.6	32.2±4.1
Forearm[a] (Anterior)	29.5±4.0	28.2±2.4	24.9±3.4
Thenar Eminence[a]	34.0±5.6	35.1±4.5	39.3±5.1
Hand (Dorsum)	36.4±3.4	34.5±5.4	35.3±4.1
Calf[a] (Medial)	32.4±5.3	31.4±5.8	28.2±4.6
Peri-malleolar (Medial)	27.1±4.6	26.7±3.6	26.6±3.5
Foot (Dorsum)	27.9±4.1	28.2±3.2	28.2±3.5
Great Toe (Dorsum)	33.0±5.5	33.6±4.0	34.0±4.3
Great Toe[a] (Plantar)	31.6±5.0	33.9±3.9	38.1±3.9

Data (mean±SD) is for 32 females (33.0±13.9 years) with BMI of 24.8±5.4 kg/m². All measurements are with subjects supine. Forearm and hand values are for the dominant arm
[a]TDC values were significantly different among depths ($p<0.001$)

Table 13.5 Tissue Dielectric Constant (TDC) variations along nondominant forearm

Distance distal to the antecubital crease	TDC measurement depth	
	2.5 mm	1.5 mm
4 cm	26.3±2.8	28.5±2.5
8 cm	27.4±3.4	29.4±2.7
12 cm	28.4±3.7	30.1±2.5

Values are mean±SD for 30 young adult females with average age of 27.4±6.5 years and body mass index (BMI) of 22.9±3.4 kg/m². TDC values at 1.5 mm depth were all greater than corresponding values at 2.5 mm depth ($p<0.001$). The small TDC increase with increasing distance from the antecubital crease is statistically significant ($p<0.001$)

commonly observed in tissues such as forearm and biceps it may be different in other anatomical sites. For example no significant difference in TDC values was detected among depths of 0.5, 1.5, and 2.5 mm on the cheek or the dorsum of hand or foot [1]. Contrastingly, significant differences in TDC values as a function effective measurement depth were observed for forehead; forearm; and medial, lateral, and anterior gaiter areas of the leg [1].

Anatomical Site Variations

Not unexpectedly TDC values depend on the anatomical site being measured. There appears to be no specific guiding principle that will predict which anatomical site for a given effective measurement site will have a particular value range. Table 13.4 summarizes some absolute TDC values previously measured [1] at various sites and effective depths for a group of 32 healthy women. Local TDC values may also vary slightly depending on the exact location of the measurement. The range of such potential variations has been assessed on the forearm of 30 healthy females [5]

with triplicate measurements along and on either side of the forearm midline at various distances (Z, cm) from the antecubital crease for a total of nine separate sites. Mean TDC differences between adjacent longitudinal sites along the midline separated by 4 cm ranged from 0.7 to 4.2 % for 2.5 mm depth and 0.4 to 3.1 % for 1.5 mm depth. Variations among adjacent sites 1.2 cm distant from the midline in the medial direction ranged from 0.0 to 1.8 % for 2.5 mm depth and from 0.8 to 2.4 % for 1.5 mm depth. Table 13.5 summarizes absolute TDC values measured along the forearm midline [5]. For the 2.5 depth probe the regression equation was $TDC = 0.26Z + 25.2$ ($r^2 = 0.999$) and for 1.5 mm depth $TDC = 0.20Z + 27.7$ ($r^2 = 0.994$).

Gender and Age as Factors

Comparisons of TDC values measured to a depth of 1.5 mm in young adult males and females [2, 28] indicates that TDC values measured at the forehead, cheek, and forearm are all significantly greater in males than in females ($p<0.001$). On average male TDC values were found to be about 13 % greater than females on the forearm [28] and about 5.6 % and 9.5 % greater on the forehead and cheek respectively [2]. These TDC differences may be related to male–female differences in skin thickness or to actual differences in water content. In either case male–female differences should be considered in any protocol that includes both genders.

The role of age has been investigated by comparing forearm TDC values at multiple depths in two groups of women divided by age above and below 55 years [12]. The results showed that to depths of 0.5 mm and 1.5 mm the older group TDC values were significantly greater than for the younger group but for the deeper depths of 2.5 mm and 5.0 mm there was no detectible difference. Table 13.6 summarizes the comparative TDC values.

Body Fat Percentage as a Factor

TDC values tend to decrease with increasing body fat percentage and also to decrease with the percentage of arm fat. This feature is illustrated in Fig. 13.9 that is based on whole body and segmental body composition measurements via bioimpedance in 130 subjects. The fat dependence is greater when the effective measurement depth is greatest since for this condition the contribution of the low water content fat to the overall measurement is also greatest.

Table 13.6 Age as a factor in Tissue Dielectric Constant (TDC) values

| | Forearm TDC values | |
Measurement depth (mm)	Younger ($N=34$)	Older ($N=35$)
0.5	31.5 ± 4.7	$35.6\pm5.9^{**}$
1.5	30.0 ± 4.9	$33.2\pm4.9^{*}$
2.5	24.8 ± 3.4	25.9 ± 3.8
5.0	21.7 ± 3.7	21.9 ± 3.5

Entries are forearm TDC mean±SD determined as the average TDC values of the dominant and nondominant arm in 69 females with ages below 55 years (younger) and equal to or greater than 55 years of age (older). $^{**}p<0.001$ vs. younger, $^{*}p<0.01$ vs. younger

Vascular Factors

The potential impact of skin blood flow and vascular volume on TDC values has been investigated by measuring arm TDC values under various test conditions [4]. Arm vascular volume and skin blood flow was changed using an upper arm cuff inflated to 50 mmHg as illustrated in Fig. 13.10 with TDC measurements before and after inflation. Changes in skin blood flow were

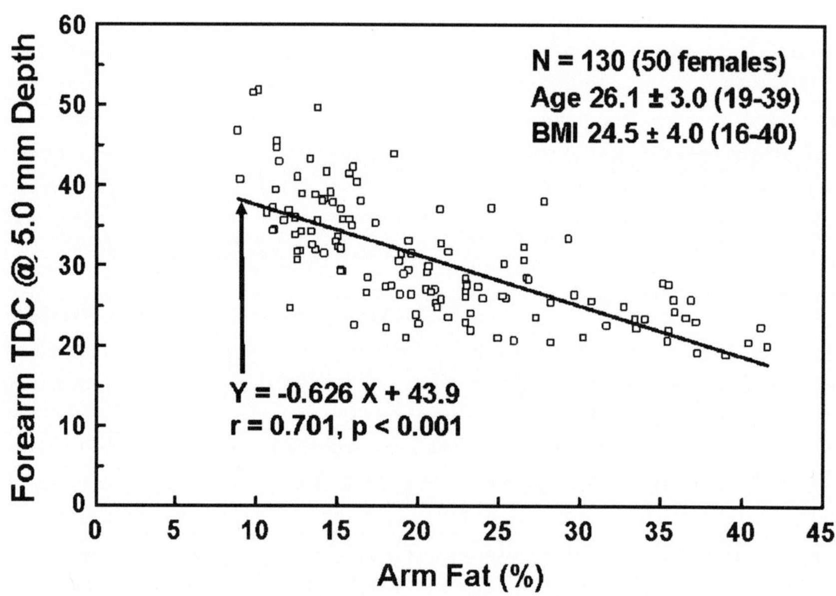

Fig. 13.9 Tissue Dielectric Constant (TDC) values in relation to percentage of fat in the arm. In contrast to a direct dependence on total body water, there is an inverse relationship between TDC values and total body fat percentage. TDC values to a depth of 5 mm are shown in relation to arm fat percentage determined via segmental bioimpedance. *Solid line* is linear regression equation with parameters shown in the figure

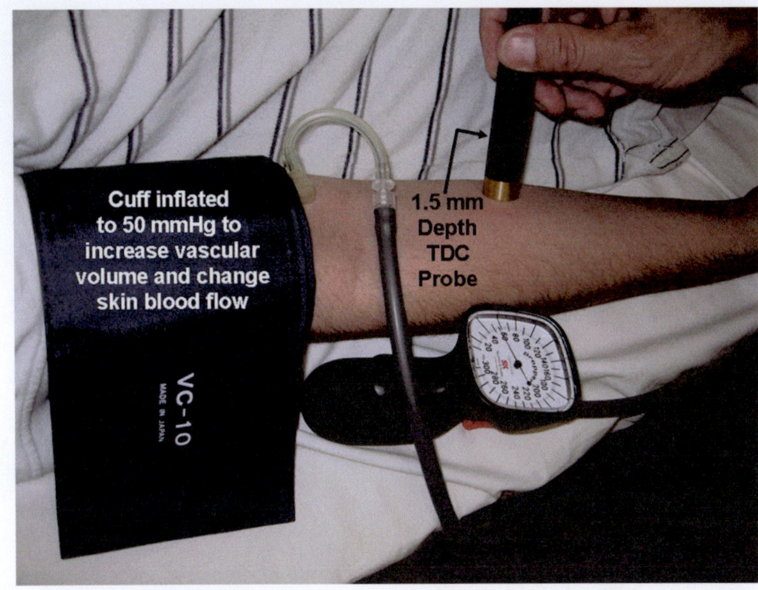

Fig. 13.10 Setup to assess vascular volume effects on Tissue Dielectric Constant (TDC). Forearm TDC measurement with a probe having an effective measurement depth of 1.5 mm is illustrated. Cuff around the upper arm is used to increase vascular volume and reduce blood flow. TDC measurements made before and during cuff inflation

also produced via changes in arm position ranging from horizontal positioning to arm elevated above the head. Illustrative results of such perturbations on skin blood flow measured via laser Doppler methods are shown in Fig. 13.11. As anticipated the various maneuvers caused significant vascular volume and blood flow changes but only minor effects on measured TDC values in the range of ±3 %. This suggests that vascular changes in most conditions are of minor importance vis-à-vis measured TDC values. However, from a technical viewpoint one should avoid placing the measuring probes directly over visible blood vessels.

Hormonal Factors

Because at least one anticipated application of the TDC method is the evaluation of edema and lymphedema in female patients the potential impact of hormonal influences associated with the menstrual cycle are of interest. This issue has been addressed via TDC measurements in pre-menopausal and postmenopausal women with premenstrual measurements made at three time points in the monthly cycle [7]. Results as summarized in Table 13.7 showed that forearm TDC values were not significantly different over the menstrual cycle at any measurement depth.

Diabetes Mellitus (DM)

Given the incidence of diabetes and its possible impact on skin physiology, awareness of possible impacts on skin tissue water is useful. This aspect has been investigated by comparing TDC values at multiple depths in forearm and foot dorsum in persons with and without diabetes mellitus [9]. Forearm TDC values tended to be slightly greater at all depths for the DM group but did not reach statistical significance. Contrastingly TDC values measured on foot dorsum were on average about 15 % greater in persons with DM. Absolute TDC values for persons with and without DM are summarized in Table 13.8. Although average foot TDC values were significantly ($p<0.05$) greater for the DM group, inter-foot TDC ratios were similar at all depths with no significant differences between groups.

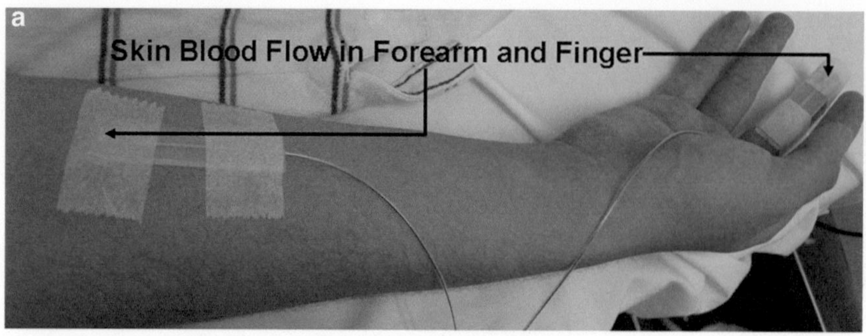

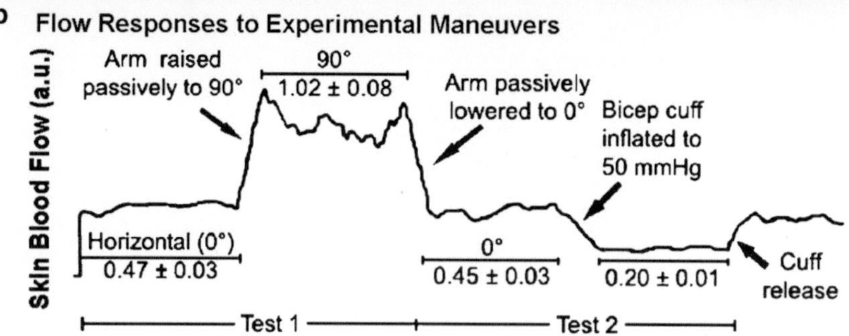

Fig. 13.11 Skin blood flow changes during experimental maneuvers. (**a**) Location of laser Doppler probes on forearm and finger to measure skin blood flow. (**b**) Typical example of blood flow changes associated with the various maneuvers. Forearm TDC is measured in triplicate near the end of each maneuver

Table 13.7 Menstrual cycle as a factor in Tissue Dielectric Constant (TDC) values

	Day of menstrual cycle		
TDC measurement depth (mm)	4	12	22
0.5	27.7±3.6	27.8±2.7	26.8±3.4
1.5	26.6±2.5	26.8±2.8	25.7±2.9
2.5	25.6±3.3	25.6±3.0	25.2±2.8
5.0	20.8±3.8	21.4±3.2	21.3±4.1
Hormones (pmol/L)			
Estradiol	5.7±1.5	11.8±6.8	3.4±1.0
Progesterone	105.7±35.9	138.3±64.4	266.8±220.4

Entries are mean±SD with each depth measured in triplicate and averaged. TDC values are measured on the dominant arm forearm. TDC values did not significantly differ among cycle day for any depth. Estradiol concentration at day 12 was significantly greater than for either day 4 or day 22 ($p<0.05$). Progesterone concentrations at day 22 were significantly greater than for either day 4 or day 12

Breast Cancer

Earlier published work evaluated TDC values at four strategic anatomical sites in women diagnosed with unilateral breast cancer [8]. These sites, forearm, biceps, axilla, and lateral thorax, were measured, and values obtained were compared to those obtained from a control group of women. Subsequently forearm TDC values were compared among three groups of women with groups classed as (1) healthy controls, (2) with breast cancer but prior to surgery, and (3) those patients who had developed BCRL [13]. The most current data available for these comparisons is for TDC measurements made in 80 women who were diagnosed with unilateral breast cancer and who were evaluated prior to their surgery. A summary of TDC values for the at-risk (cancer) side and for the contralateral (healthy) side as well as at-risk/contralateral side ratios are shown in Fig. 13.12.

Table 13.8 Diabetes Mellitus (DM) as a factor in Tissue Dielectric Constant (TDC) values

TDC site and depth	TDC values	
	NODM	DM
Forearm		
0.5 mm	32.4±3.7	34.3±4.6
1.5 mm	30.2±2.7	32.0±3.6
2.5 mm	27.5±3.3	29.1±3.9
Foot		
0.5 mm	28.4±4.8	31.9±3.7*
1.5 mm	28.9±32.5	32.5±5.9*
2.5 mm	29.1±4.1	33.3±6.4*

Entries are mean±SD for 18 persons with and 18 persons without DM. * indicates significantly different from NODM ($p<0.05$). Forearm TDC values decrease with increasing depth ($p<0.001$), but foot dorsum values are not different among depths

Side-to-side TDC values did not significantly differ for any site, but differences among sites were significant ($p<0.001$) with each site being significantly different from any other site. Contrastingly, side-to-side TDC ratios did not differ among measured sites.

Lymphedema

The presence of clinical lymphedema is associated with a significant increase in TDC values [13, 17] with affected arm values having average TDC values between 44 % to 65 % greater than contralateral arm values depending on the effective measurement depth [17]. Further, TDC values have been observed to decrease with various forms of therapy in lymphedematous legs [14, 15] and in arms and legs [11] by amounts ranging between 10 % and 16.8 % for legs and 8.2 % for arms. Table 13.9 summarizes the most recent data for TDC values measured at 2.5 mm depth in arms of 80 women with BCRL, in 80 women with breast cancer (BC) but no lymphedema and in 80 women without breast cancer (NOBC). TDC values of the lymphedematous arm greatly exceed TDC values obtained from contralateral arms. In patients with BCRL, contralateral arm TDC values are not significantly different from those measured in patients with breast cancer without lymphedema or in healthy women free of breast cancer.

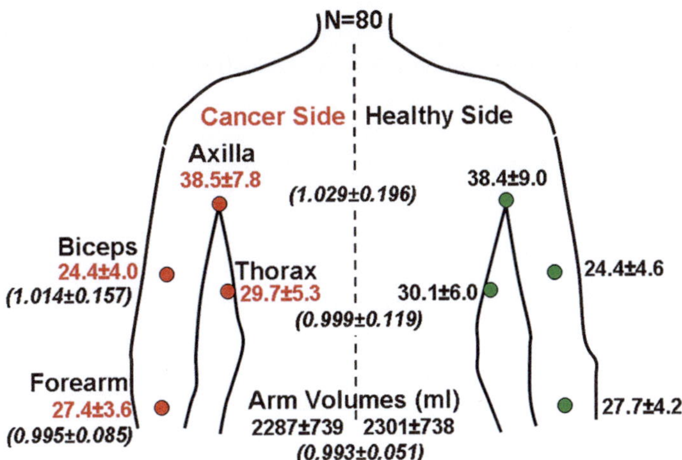

Fig. 13.12 Tissue Dielectric Constant (TDC) reference values from patients with breast cancer prior to surgery. TDC values, measured to a 2.5 mm depth, are given as mean±SD and in parenthesis is the ratio of at-risk side (cancer side) TDC values to the contralateral side (healthy side) values. Volumes are the arm volumes. Side-to-side values did not differ for any site but TDC values among sites were significantly different one from another ($p<0.001$)

Table 13.9 Tissue Dielectric Constant (TDC) values for women with and without breast cancer related lymphedema

| Group[a] | Tissue Dielectric Constant (TDC) | | |
	Affected (A) side	Control (C) side[b]	TDC ratio (A/C)
NOBC (N=80)	26.8±4.9	26.4±4.7	1.001±0.050
BC (N=80)	24.8±3.3	24.9±3.8	0.998±0.082
BCRL (N=80)	42.9±8.2**	26.0±4.0	1.663±0.319§

Data entries are TDC mean±SD measured on forearms to an effective depth of 2.5

[a]For breast cancer (BC) and lymphedema (BCRL) groups affected (A) sides refers to at-risk arms and lymphedema arms respectively; control sides are contralateral arms. For the group without breast cancer (NOBC) side A corresponds to the dominant arm and side C corresponds to the nondominant arm

[b]Control side TDC values are not significantly different among groups

** TDC values of BCRL affected arms were significantly greater than for BC or NOBC groups ($p<0.001$). For BC and NOBC groups, TDC values were insignificantly different between paired-arms and between groups yielding similar A/C ratios

§A/C ratios for the LE group were significantly greater than for either the BC or NOBC groups ($p<0.001$)

Multiprobe Versus Compact Probe as a Factor in TDC Values

All reported TDC measurements so far are based on use of the multiprobe system (Fig. 13.1). Because of construction and design feature differences of the compact TDC probe (Fig. 13.5) an assessment of comparative TDC values produced by the different devices is useful. For that purpose TDC values obtained with the compact probe were compared with the multiprobe system for probes to depths of 1.5 mm and 2.5 mm in forearms and biceps of 32 males and 32 females. Results of this comparison are summarized in Table 13.10. The compact device measurements were found to be between the 1.5 mm and 2.5 mm measurements. Including both male and female values, compact device values are 5.6 % to 5.8 % higher than the 2.5 mm probe.

Table 13.10 Compact versus multiprobe Tissue Dielectric Constant (TDC) values

| Probe | Forearm | | Biceps | |
	Female	Male	Female	Male
1.5 mm	30.9±2.7	35.7±3.4**	31.3±2.5	36.6±3.3**
Compact	28.2±2.0	33.9±3.2**	28.3±2.0	34.4±3.3**
2.5 mm	26.7±2.3	32.0±3.2**	26.5±2.4	32.9±3.7**

Data entries are TDC values (mean±SD) determined as the average of both arms for 32 males and 32 females. **=Male TDC values were greater than corresponding female values ($p<0.001$) for each probe at each site. The compact probe TDC values lie between the 1.5 and 2.5 mm depth probes and exceed the 2.5 mm depth probe by 5.6 % to 5.8 %

Potential Use of TDC for Early Lymphedema Detection

Based on the normal variance in TDC values among persons it is possible to develop criteria potentially useful to aid in the detection of early incipient lymphedema in persons at risk of developing unilateral arm lymphedema. To this end TDC bilateral forearm and biceps measurements were made to a depth of 2.5 mm in 103 women (60.6±13.2 years) who had been diagnosed with breast cancer. Measurements were made prior to their scheduled surgery to eliminate surgery as a variable. Because of the relative site independence of inter-arm TDC ratios, inter-arm TDC ratios were chosen as the potential detection parameter and determined as the ratio of TDC values measured on the at-risk arm to the TDC value measured on the contralateral arm. This ratio is designated by the symbol γ and is for the forearm $\gamma_{forearm}$ and for the biceps as γ_{biceps}. A summary of these measurements is shown in Table 13.11. Theoretical lymphedema detection thresholds might be based on $\gamma+2.5$ SD (includes 99.4 % of cases) or on $\gamma+3.0$ SD (includes 99.9 % of cases). A determination of the number of patients that exceed the $\gamma+3.0$ SD threshold was investigated in the course of tracking 104 different patients evaluated on average 26.3± 17.5 months post-surgery. Ten patients (9.6 %) exceeded the forearm threshold and six (5.8 %)

Table 13.11 Arm Tissue Dielectric Constant (TDC) values and ratios for breast cancer patients prior to treatment

Site	At-risk arm	Control arm	γ	$\gamma+2.5$ SD	$\gamma+3.0$ SD
Forearm TDC	25.7 ± 3.8	25.8 ± 4.1	1.003 ± 0.097	1.243	1.291
Biceps TDC	23.3 ± 4.5	23.3 ± 4.7	1.012 ± 0.143	1.369	1.441

Entries are mean $\pm$ SD for TDC values and at-risk/control arm ratios (γ) for 103 patients with age of 60.6 ± 13.2 years. Forearm site is 6 cm distal to the antecubital crease and the bicep site is 8 cm proximal. Theoretical lymphedema detection thresholds might be based on $\gamma+2.5$ SD (includes 99.4 % of cases) or $\gamma+3.0$ SD (includes 99.9 % of cases)

exceeded the biceps threshold. Further, patients reporting at least one lymphedema-related symptom ($N=34$, 32.7 %) also had a significantly greater value for γ_{biceps} than patients with no symptoms (1.113 ± 0.335 vs. 1.001 ± 0.119, $p=0.014$) and also had a greater value for $\gamma_{forearm}$ (1.100 ± 0.231 vs. 1.026 ± 0.129, $p=0.038$). Although these findings are encouraging vis-à-vis threshold detection, the concept remains theoretical at this time while awaiting outcomes of ongoing prospective sequential studies.

Conclusion

Measurements of the tissue dielectric constant (TDC) of the skin are a noninvasive, rapid, and reliable way to assess skin-to-fat relative water content and its change at almost any anatomical site. As described, the method has a well-documented physical basis and has a fairly extensive background of use in a variety skin sites and has been investigated for use in several conditions including lymphedema evaluation. The ability to measure water rapidly and locally provides the advantage of tracking changes in anatomical sites of particular interest either for pretreatment and posttreatment reasons or for longer-term follow-up assessments. In addition, the method allows for easy tracking of those anatomical sites deemed to be particularly at risk of developing lymphedema or those sites that on clinical examination already appear slightly edematous. Investigations into the use of TDC measures for early detection of incipient lymphedema have indicated significant potential, but studies are as yet incomplete and thresholds not yet validated.

References

1. Mayrovitz HN, Bernal M, Brlit F, Desfor R. Biophysical measures of skin tissue water: variations within and among anatomical sites and correlations between measures. Skin Res Technol. 2013;19(1): 47–54.
2. Mayrovitz HN, Bernal M, Carson S. Gender differences in facial skin dielectric constant measured at 300 MHz. Skin Res Technol. 2012;18:504–10.
3. Nuutinen J, Lahtinen T, Turunen M, Alanen E, Tenhunen M, Usenius T, et al. A dielectric method for measuring early and late reactions in irradiated human skin. Radiother Oncol. 1998;47(3):249–54.
4. Mayrovitz HN, Guo X, Salmon M, Uhde M. Forearm skin tissue dielectric constant measured at 300 MHz: effect of changes in skin vascular volume and blood flow. Clin Physiol Funct Imaging. 2013;33(1):55–61.
5. Mayrovitz HN, Luis M. Spatial variations in forearm skin tissue dielectric constant. Skin Res Technol. 2010;16(4):438–43.
6. Mayrovitz HN, Davey S, Shapiro E. Local tissue water changes assessed by tissue dielectric constant: single measurements versus averaging of multiple measurements. Lymphology. 2008;41(4):186–8.
7. Mayrovitz HN, Brown-Cross D, Washington Z. Skin tissue water and laser Doppler blood flow during a menstrual cycle. Clin Physiol Funct Imaging. 2007; 27(1):54–9.
8. Mayrovitz HN, Davey S, Shapiro E. Local tissue water assessed by tissue dielectric constant: anatomical site and depth dependence in women prior to breast cancer treatment-related surgery. Clin Physiol Funct Imaging. 2008;28(5):337–42.
9. Mayrovitz HN, McClymont A, Pandya N. Skin tissue water assessed via tissue dielectric constant measurements in persons with and without diabetes mellitus. Diabetes Technol Ther. 2013;15(1):60–5.
10. Jensen MR, Birkballe S, Nørregaard S, Karlsmark T. Validity and interobserver agreement of lower extremity local tissue water measurements in healthy women using tissue dielectric constant. Clin Physiol Funct Imaging. 2012;32(4):317–22.
11. Mayrovitz HN, Davey S. Changes in tissue water and indentation resistance of lymphedematous limbs accompanying low level laser therapy (LLLT) of fibrotic skin. Lymphology. 2011;44(4):168–77.

12. Mayrovitz HN. Local tissue water assessed by measuring forearm skin dielectric constant: dependence on measurement depth, age and body mass index. Skin Res Technol. 2010;16(1):16–22.

13. Mayrovitz HN, Weingrad DN, Davey S. Local tissue water in at-risk and contralateral forearms of women with and without breast cancer treatment-related lymphedema. Lymphat Res Biol. 2009;7(3):153–8.

14. Mayrovitz HN. Assessing lymphedema by tissue indentation force and local tissue water. Lymphology. 2009;42(2):88–98.

15. Mayrovitz HN, Davey S, Shapiro E. Localized tissue water changes accompanying one manual lymphatic drainage (MLD) therapy session assessed by changes in tissue dielectric constant inpatients with lower extremity lymphedema. Lymphology. 2008;41(2):87–92.

16. Mayrovitz HN, Macdonald J, Davey S, Olson K, Washington E. Measurement decisions for clinical assessment of limb volume changes in patients with bilateral and unilateral limb edema. Phys Ther. 2007; 87(10):1362–8.

17. Mayrovitz HN. Assessing local tissue edema in postmastectomy lymphedema. Lymphology. 2007;40(2): 87–94.

18. Birkballe S, Jensen MR, Noerregaard S, Gottrup F, Karlsmark T. Can tissue dielectric constant measurement aid in differentiating lymphoedema from lipoedema in women with swollen legs? Br J Dermatol. 2014;170(1):96–102.

19. Petaja L, Nuutinen J, Uusaro A, Lahtinen T, Ruokonen E. Dielectric constant of skin and subcutaneous fat to assess fluid changes after cardiac surgery. Physiol Meas. 2003;24(2):383–90.

20. Stuchly MA, Athey TW, Stuchly SS, Samaras GM, Taylor G. Dielectric properties of animal tissues in vivo at frequencies 10 MHz–1 GHz. Bioelectromagnetics. 1981;2(2):93–103.

21. Aimoto A, Matsumoto T. Noninvasive method for measuring the electrical properties of deep tissues using an open-ended coaxial probe. Med Eng Phys. 1996;18(8):641–6.

22. Grant JP, Clarke RN, Symm GT, Spyrou NM. In vivo dielectric properties of human skin from 50 MHz to 2.0 GHz. Phys Med Biol. 1988;33(5):607–12.

23. Alanen E, Lahtinen T, Nuutinen J. Measurement of dielectric properties of subcutaneous fat with open-ended coaxial sensors. Phys Med Biol. 1998;43(3): 475–85.

24. Alanen E, Lahtinen T, Nuutinen J. Variational formulation of open-ended coaxial line in contact with layered biological medium. IEEE Trans Biomed Eng. 1998;45(10):1241–8.

25. Smith SR, Foster KR. Dielectric properties of low-water-content tissues. Phys Med Biol. 1985;30(9): 965–73.

26. Nuutinen J, Ikaheimo R, Lahtinen T. Validation of a new dielectric device to assess changes of tissue water in skin and subcutaneous fat. Physiol Meas. 2004; 25(2):447–54.

27. Lahtinen T, Nuutinen J, Alanen E. Dielectric properties of the skin. Phys Med Biol. 1997;42(7): 1471–2.

28. Mayrovitz HN, Carson S, Luis M. Male-female differences in forearm skin tissue dielectric constant. Clin Physiol Funct Imaging. 2010;30(5): 328–32.

Conventional Imaging Modalities for the Diagnosis of Lymphedema

Pradeep Goyal, Gulraiz Chaudry, and Ahmad I. Alomari

Key Points

- Although the diagnosis of lymphedema is largely clinical, it is crucial to choose the appropriate imaging modalities and have awareness of the common imaging features of lymphedema.
- Conventional modalities (MRI, CT scan, and Ultrasound) not only show indirect evidence of impaired function of lymphatic channels but also provide anatomical details that may complement the functional assessment provided by lymphoscintigraphy and can be occasionally necessary to establish the diagnosis.
- These complementary imaging studies may be necessary to rule out the causes of secondary lymphedema and assess the response to therapy.

Introduction

Although the diagnosis of lymphedema is largely clinical, it is crucial to choose the appropriate imaging modalities and have awareness of the common imaging features of lymphedema.

P. Goyal, M.D. • G. Chaudry, M.B.Ch.B.
A.I. Alomari, M.D., M.Sc., F.S.I.R. (✉)
Division of Vascular and Interventional Radiology, Boston Children's Hospital and Harvard Medical School, 300 Longwood Avenue, Boston, MA 02115, USA
e-mail: ahmad.alomari@childrens.harvard.edu

Lymphedema has been divided into primary and secondary (acquired) [1]. Primary lymphedema results mainly from impaired drainage of lymph due to congenital defect in the peripheral lymph transporting system, including collecting lymphatic channels and nodes (i.e., aplasia, hypoplasia, and hyperplasia) [1, 2]. Primary lymphedema is occasionally associated with central conducting lymphatic anomaly. Secondary lymphedema results from obstruction or disruption of the normal collecting lymphatic system due to different pathologic processes such as metastatic disease, radiation, surgical injury, or infection [2–4].

Limb swelling and edema of the extremity, which may simulate lymphedema, can be caused by other local disorders (such as venous hypertension) or systemic disease (such as congestive heart failure, liver disease, renal disease, and hypoalbuminemia) [5]. Conventional imaging modalities are not only helpful in confirming the diagnosis of lymphedema but also in excluding other etiologies of limb swelling.

History and clinical examination can usually establish the diagnosis of lymphedema and differentiate the type (primary or secondary). Nevertheless, additional tests are sometimes necessary, particularly in the early stages of the disease and in edemas of combined etiology.

The imaging studies primarily confirm the presence of impaired lymphatic flow and/or the typical pattern of abnormal fluid distribution within the tissues [4].

A.K. Greene et al. (eds.), *Lymphedema: Presentation, Diagnosis, and Treatment*,
DOI 10.1007/978-3-319-14493-1_14, © Springer International Publishing Switzerland 2015

The diagnosis of primary lymphedema can be confirmed by functional assessment of the lymphatic channels by modalities like bipedal lymphangiography, lymphoscintigraphy, lymphatic capillaroscopy, and near-infrared (NIR) fluorescence imaging. These modalities are discussed in different chapters.

In this chapter, we discuss the role of conventional imaging modalities (including magnetic resonance imaging (MRI), magnetic resonance lymphangiography, computer tomography (CT) scan, ultrasonography, and plain radiography) in confirming the diagnosis of lymphedema, identifying any underlying causes and gauging response to therapy. These modalities not only show indirect evidence of impaired function of lymphatic channels but also provide anatomical details that complement the data provided by the aforementioned functional tests.

Magnetic Resonance Imaging

MRI relies on the fact that when a radiofrequency pulse is briefly applied to tissues in a magnetic field, the proton relaxation time is dependent on the type of tissue. As the magnetic vector returns to its resting state, this causes a radio wave to be emitted, which is then used to create an image. Usually MRI is performed with a 1.5–3.0 Tesla scanner equipped with high-performance gradients. Imaging of the lower extremity may require more than one station: the calf and the foot region; around the knee region; and proximal thigh and the pelvic region. A dedicated peripheral surface coil is used to examine the upper and lower leg while a phased-array body coil is used to image the pelvic region. MR pulse sequences that are most useful in the imaging of lymphedema include fat-sensitive T1-weighted sequence and fluid-sensitive sequences such as inversion recovery (STIR) or fat-suppressed T2-weighted sequences.

Gadolinium-enhanced, fat-suppressed T1-weighted sequences are required if diagnosis of secondary lymphedema is considered or in follow up cases of already diagnosed primary lymphedema in context of lymphangitis or cellulitis. Flow-sensitive gradient echo sequences to assess vascularity (magnetic resonance angiography) are not generally necessary.

In primary lymphedema, the images reveal a characteristic distribution of edema within the epifascial compartment with a classic reticular (honeycomb) pattern and thickening of the subcutaneous layer (see Fig. 14.1 a, b). These changes are typically circumferential. In chronic primary lymphedema, stasis of lymph stimulates progressive fat deposition and tissue fibrosis [6, 7]. The enlarged lymph channels and fat thickening can be identified on MRI (Fig. 14.1 c, d).

MRI can also be useful in the differential diagnosis of lymphedema [8–10]. In edema due to venous disease both the epifascial and subfascial compartments may be affected; the characteristic reticular pattern may or may not present. While in lipidemia, the fat accumulation occurs without signs of lymphatic congestion or reticular appearance [10]. The anatomic details provided by MRI may complement the functional assessment provided by lymphoscintigraphy and can be occasionally necessary to establish the diagnosis [11].

MRI may be helpful in differentiating the various causes of lymphatic obstruction in secondary lymphedema by demonstrating dilated lymphatic trunks and identification of abnormal lymph nodes. Malignant nodal involvement can be assessed further by lymphotropic nanoparticle-enhanced magnetic resonance imaging (LNMRI). These nanoparticles produce a significant susceptibility effect which can be detected as a drop in signal intensity on T2-weighted images [12]. Within a normal lymph node, nanoparticles accumulate within the reticuloendothelial system (phagocytized by macrophages) and show homogeneous uptake resulting in dark signal on T2-weighted images. In a node which is either partially or completely infiltrated by malignant cells, there is absence of functioning macrophages, leading to a lack of nanoparticle uptake resulting in focal or complete area of bright signal intensity on T2-weighted images. This technique is highly

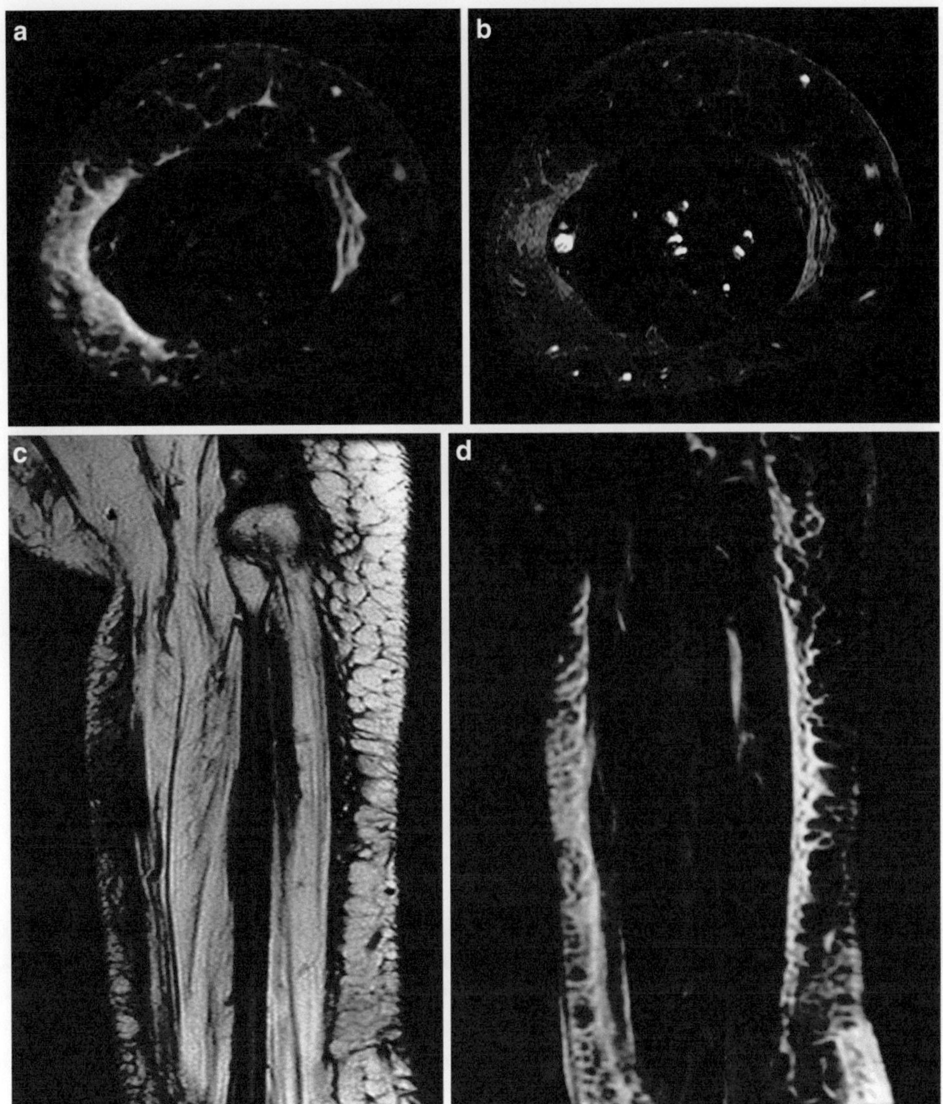

Fig. 14.1 MRI of the right leg in primary lymphedema. Axial T2-W fat-saturated (**a**) and T1-W fat-saturated, contrast-enhanced (**b**) MR images of the calf demonstrate extensive circumferential subcutaneous soft tissue thickening and reticular (honeycomb) pattern above the fascia with thickening of the subcutis and dermis. Note reticular post-contrast enhancement suggestive of lymphangitis/cellulitis. Coronal T1-W (**c**) and T2-W fat-saturated (**d**) MR images of right calf demonstrate predominantly subcutaneous extrafascial distribution of fluid and fat accumulation; a classic feature of chronic primary lymphedema

effective in identifying metastases in non-enlarged and partially replaced nodes; however, due to the negative-contrast nature of the detection, small lesions can be missed [13]. In one study, sensitivity and specificity of LNMRI was 76.5 % and 98.4 % in diagnosing nodal metastasis [14]. Lymphatic flow velocities can be assessed in lymphedema by visualization of lymphatic flow using principles of spin labeling MR imaging, and thus, lymphedema etiogenesis and therapies may be interrogated without exogenous contrast agents [15].

Magnetic Resonance Lymphography (MRL)

Magnetic resonance lymphangiography (MRL) is a recently added technique in which gadolinium-based, MRI contrast agent is injected for the visualization of lymphatic vessels in patients with primary and secondary lymphedema [16, 17]. A mixture of MRI contrast agent (gadobenate dimeglumine 0.1 mmol per kilogram or gadopentetate dimeglumine 0.2 mmol per kilogram of body weight) and 2 mL of Bupivacaine hydrochloride 0.25 % or Mepivacaine hydrochloride 1 % is injected intracutaneously into the interdigital webs of the dorsal aspect of both feet. Before MR lymphangiography, the extent and distribution of the lymphedema is evaluated using a heavily T2-weighted 3D turbo spin-echo sequence. For MR lymphangiography a 3D spoiled gradient-echo sequence [volumetric interpolated breath hold examination (VIBE)] is used. The three stations are first imaged without contrast material and subsequently repeated at 5, 15, 25, 35, 45, and 55 min after intracutaneous application of contrast. To emphasize the gadolinium-containing structures, baseline images are subtracted before 3D maximum intensity projection (MIP) reconstructions are calculated.

In one study, contrast MRL was capable of evaluating the anatomical and functional status of lymphatic vessels and lymph nodes in primary and secondary lymphedema by real-time visualization of enhanced lymph flow in lymphatic channels and within lymph nodes. In primary lymphedema, there were three major types of lymphatic system malformation: (a) only lymph nodes affected, (b) only lymph vessels affected, and (c) both lymph vessels and lymph nodes affected. In secondary lymphedema, MRL demonstrated tortuous and dilated collecting lymphatics in lymphedematous limbs [18].

In other study, diagnostic accuracy of magnetic resonance imaging (MR-lymphangiography) was calculated relative to the lymphoscintigraphy gold standard for assessment of focal lesions of the peripheral lymphatic system. MR-lymphangiography had sensitivity of 68 %, specificity of 91 %, positive predictive value of 82 %, and negative predictive value of 83 %. There was substantial correlation of results between the two modalities [19].

MR lymphangiography using interstitial injection of gadofosveset trisodium (Ablavar®, Lantheus Medical, North Billerica, MA) alone or premixed with 10 % human serum albumin (HSA) was used to visualize thoracic duct (TD) in a pig model [20]. Intradermal injection of nano-sized gadolinium-labeled dendrimer was also shown to rapidly opacify the deep lymphatic system, including the thoracic duct, in mice and pigs [21].

MRL is relatively noninvasive and can be used to identify anatomic and physiological abnormalities associated with lymphatic dysfunction in order to determine further treatment strategies [16, 17].

Computed Tomography

Although MRI is the preferred modality for assessing lymphedema, computed tomography (CT) can also be used, particularly when MRI cannot be technically or safely performed (e.g., uncooperative patients, unstable cardiovascular or respiratory status, contraindications to MRI). Acquiring CT scan studies is faster and can be performed without sedation or general anesthesia in infants and young children.

In lymphedema (see Fig. 14.2), CT scan demonstrates the characteristic reticular pattern and thickening of the subcutaneous tissue [22, 23]. It also provides anatomic localization of the edema which helps differentiate epifascial versus epifascial and subfascial edema. CT venography can also assess increased interstitial fluid formation due to venous hypertension (incompetent valves, venous obstruction). CT may be used to monitor responses to compression therapy in lymphedema through serial measurements of the cross-sectional area and tissue density in the tissue compartments of interest [24].

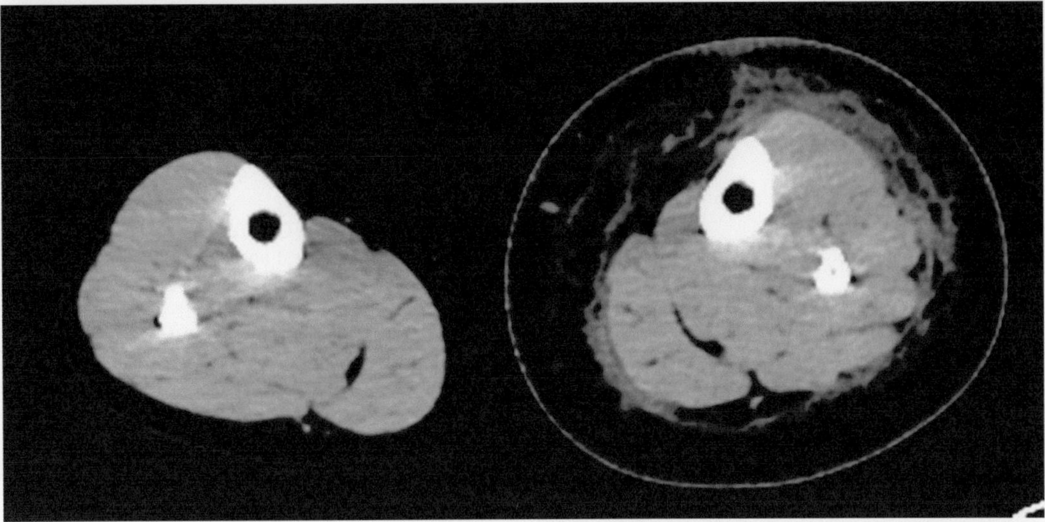

Fig. 14.2 Axial CT scan of the lower extremities in primary lymphedema. Circumferential reticular density is noted within the subcutaneous layer of the calf coalescing in the immediate epifascial plane. There is thickening of skin and subcutaneous fat

Ultrasonography

Ultrasonography (US) is utilized as a noninvasive diagnostic tool for the evaluation of lymphedema. US can be used to rule out the cause of increased interstitial fluid formation due to systemic disease (congestive heart failure, liver disease, renal disease). High-frequency linear-array probes are best for evaluation of superficial tissue. Gray-scale images are routinely obtained in transverse and longitudinal planes. In patients with lymphedema, it shows the thickening of the cutaneous, epifascial tissue compartments, interstitial fluid accumulation and occasionally may allow evaluation of the degree of fibrosis (Fig. 14.3). High frequency sonographic images reveal the characteristic patterns of cutaneous fluid localization in various types of edema [25]. In one study of patients with secondary lymphedema, the relative proportion of fluid and fibrosis identified on sonography correlated well with the clinical findings of soft, medium, hard, or pitting type of edema [26].

Low-flow color Doppler settings permits optimal visualization of small vessels and detection of low-flow vessels and thus help in the evaluation of deep and superficial venous systems, epifascial structure, confirming venous anomalies (i.e., valvular incompetence, obstruction, ectasia,) or excluding venous obstruction [27].

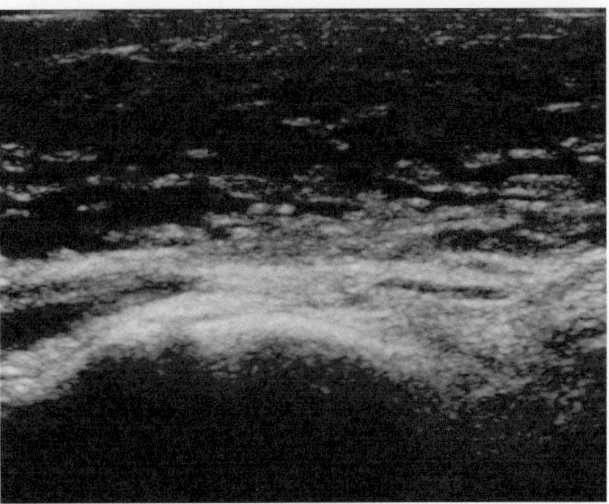

Fig. 14.3 Sonographic image of the dorsal aspect of the foot in lymphedema revealing thickening of skin and subcutaneous fat. The echogenic subcutaneous fat is interlaced with hypoechoic fluid-filled layers

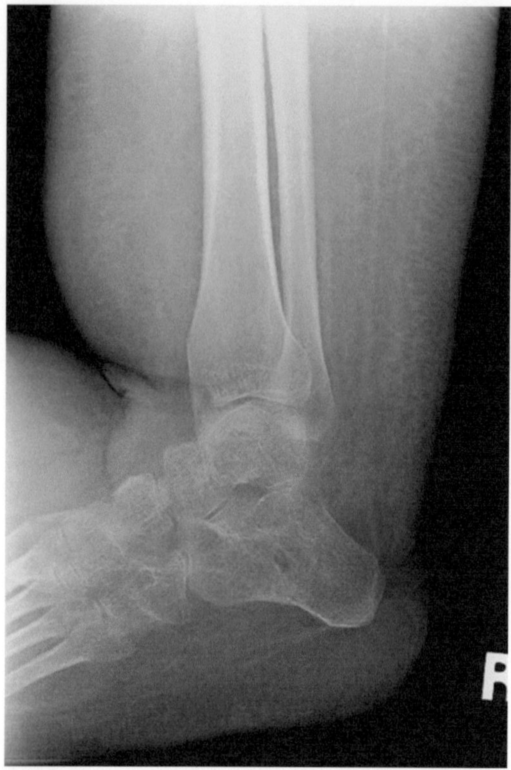

Fig. 14.4 Lateral radiograph of the right ankle and calf in lymphedema demonstrates circumferential soft tissue thickening with dense reticular markings. Note diffuse osteopenia

Plain Radiographs

The role of plain radiographs of extremities in the diagnosis of lymphedema is limited. Plain radiographs may show the epifascial soft tissue thickening of affected limb, secondary bone changes due to edema (Fig. 14.4) and limb-length discrepancies.

Conclusion

Conventional imaging modalities like MRI, CT scan, and US can be used to diagnose lymphedema. These studies also may provide information regarding the anatomical distribution of lymphedema, and assess response to therapy. MRI, CT scan, and US also are used to diagnose causes of extremity swelling other than lymphedema.

Statement of Financial Interest No financial support or benefits were given to the authors from any source that is related to the scientific work reported in the paper.

References

1. Kinmonth JB, Taylor GW, Tracy GD, Marsh JD. Primary lymphœdema. Clinical and lymphangiographic studies of a series of 107 patients in which the lower limbs were affected. Br J Surg. 1957;45(189):1–10.
2. Browse NL, Stewart G. Lymphoedema: pathophysiology and classification. J Cardiovasc Surg. 1985;26(2):91–106.
3. Rockson SG. Lymphedema. Am J Med. 2001;110(4):288–95.
4. Szuba A, Rockson SG. Lymphedema: classification, diagnosis and therapy. Vasc Med (Lond, Engl). 1998;3(2):145–56.
5. Szuba A, Razavi M, Rockson SG. Diagnosis and treatment of concomitant venous obstruction in patients with secondary lymphedema. J Vasc Interv Radiol. 2002;13(8):799–803.
6. Zampell JC, Aschen S, Weitman ES, Yan A, Elhadad S, De Brot M, et al. Regulation of adipogenesis by lymphatic fluid stasis: part I. Adipogenesis, fibrosis, and inflammation. Plast Reconstr Surg. 2012;129(4):825–34.
7. Aschen S, Zampell JC, Elhadad S, Weitman E, De Brot M, Mehrara BJ. Regulation of adipogenesis by lymphatic fluid stasis: part II. Expression of adipose differentiation genes. Plast Reconstr Surg. 2012;129(4):838–47.
8. Duewell S, Hagspiel KD, Zuber J, von Schulthess GK, Bollinger A, Fuchs WA. Swollen lower extremity: role of MR imaging. Radiology. 1992;184(1):227–31.
9. Haaverstad R, Nilsen G, Myhre HO, Saether OD, Rinck PA. The use of MRI in the investigation of leg oedema. Eur J Vasc Surg. 1992;6(2):124–9.
10. Haaverstad R, Nilsen G, Rinck PA, Myhre HO. The use of MRI in the diagnosis of chronic lymphedema of the lower extremity. Int Angiol. 1994;13(2):115–8.
11. Case TC, Witte CL, Witte MH, Unger EC, Williams WH. Magnetic resonance imaging in human lymphedema: comparison with lymphangioscintigraphy. Magn Reson Imaging. 1992;10(4):549–58.
12. Guimaraes R, Clement O, Bittoun J, Carnot F, Frija G. MR lymphography with superparamagnetic iron nanoparticles in rats: pathologic basis for contrast enhancement. AJR Am J Roentgenol. 1994;162(1):201–7.
13. Saksena MA, Saokar A, Harisinghani MG. Lymphotropic nanoparticle enhanced MR imaging (LNMRI) technique for lymph node imaging. Eur J Radiol. 2006;58(3):367–74.
14. McDermott S, Thayer SP, Fernandez-Del Castillo C, Mino-Kenudson M, Weissleder R, Harisinghani MG. Accurate prediction of nodal status in preoperative

patients with pancreatic ductal adenocarcinoma using next-gen nanoparticle. Transl Oncol. 2013;6(6): 670–5.

15. Rane S, Donahue PM, Towse T, Ridner S, Chappell M, Jordi J, et al. Clinical feasibility of noninvasive visualization of lymphatic flow with principles of spin labeling MR imaging: implications for lymphedema assessment. Radiology. 2013;269(3):893–902.

16. Lohrmann C, Foeldi E, Bartholoma JP, Langer M. Interstitial MR lymphangiography—a diagnostic imaging method for the evaluation of patients with clinically advanced stages of lymphedema. Acta Trop. 2007;104(1):8–15.

17. Liu NF, Lu Q, Jiang ZH, Wang CG, Zhou JG. Anatomic and functional evaluation of the lymphatics and lymph nodes in diagnosis of lymphatic circulation disorders with contrast magnetic resonance lymphangiography. J Vasc Surg. 2009;49(4):980–7.

18. Liu N, Zhang Y (2014) Magnetic Resonance Lymphangiography for the Study of Lymphatic System in Lymphedema. J Reconstr Microsurg (in press).

19. Weiss M, Burgard C, Baumeister R, Strobl F, Rominger A, Bartenstein P, et al. Magnetic resonance imaging versus lymphoscintigraphy for the assessment of focal lymphatic transport disorders of the lower limb: first experiences. Nuklearmedizin. 2014;53(5):190–6.

20. Turkbey B, Kobayashi H, Hoyt Jr RF, Choyke PL, Nakajima T, Griffiths GL, et al. Magnetic resonance lymphography of the thoracic duct after interstitial injection of gadofosveset trisodium: a pilot dosing study in a porcine model. Lymphat Res Biol. 2014;12(1):32–6.

21. Sena LM, Fishman SJ, Jenkins KJ, Xu H, Brechbiel MW, Regino CA, et al. Magnetic resonance lymphangiography with a nano-sized gadolinium-labeled dendrimer in small and large animal models. Nanomedicine (Lond). 2010;5(8):1183–91.

22. Hadjis NS, Carr DH, Banks L, Pflug JJ. The role of CT in the diagnosis of primary lymphedema of the lower limb. AJR Am J Roentgenol. 1985;144(2):361–4.

23. Marotel M, Cluzan R, Pascot M, Ghabboun S, Alliot F, Lasry JL. Computerized tomography of 150 cases of lymphedema of the leg. J Radiol. 1998;79(11):1373–8.

24. Collins CD, Mortimer PS, D'Ettorre H, A'Hern RP, Moskovic EC. Computed tomography in the assessment of response to limb compression in unilateral lymphoedema. Clin Radiol. 1995;50(8):541–4.

25. Gniadecka M. Localization of dermal edema in lipodermatosclerosis, lymphedema, and cardiac insufficiency. High-frequency ultrasound examination of intradermal echogenicity. J Am Acad Dermatol. 1996;35(1):37–41.

26. Balzarini A, Milella M, Civelli E, Sigari C, De Conno F. Ultrasonography of arm edema after axillary dissection for breast cancer: a preliminary study. Lymphology. 2001;34(4):152–5.

27. Lee B, Andrade M, Bergan J, Boccardo F, Campisi C, Damstra R, et al. Diagnosis and treatment of primary lymphedema. Consensus document of the International Union of Phlebology (IUP)-2009. Int Angiol. 2010;29(5):454–70.

Lymphoscintigraphy and Other Imaging Methods

15

Pierre Bourgeois

Key Points

- Edema is one clinical symptom. The symptom becomes a lymphedema when morphologic and/or functional abnormalities affecting the lymphatic system can be demonstrated. *But* the lymphedematous problem must always be placed in its overall context and presented with the (eventually) associated symptoms and with the specific patient's history. The clinician has to then formulate the question(s) to be answered. These questions will determine not only the technique to be proposed to the patient but also the methodology that will be applied by the specialist who will perform the investigation.

- Materials that allow whole-body and/or three-dimensional imaging(s) of the lymphatic system in relation to their surrounding anatomical structures, acquisition techniques, and the ability to quantify and dynamically analyze lymphatic system functions, and the applications of clinically based protocol(s) for investigation place, the specialists in Nuclear Medicine at the center of the diagnosis and management of edematous presentations.

- The physiological basis and limitations of current examinations should be well known and understood. Especially with lymphoscintigraphically based functional and morphological analysis of the lymphatic system, results must be interpreted by taking into account the patient's clinical symptoms and history as well also the results of other examinations. These investigations may seem time-consuming in terms of equipment needs and human investment (they are certainly not "fast-food" medicine), but no more so than many other currently available investigations. These investigations must also be planned and adapted to answer clinician's questions and meet patient's expectations. If these considerations are explained to both the patient and the referring clinicians, they will be more acceptable and tolerated.

- Lymphoscintigraphies have, until now, occupied a central place in the management of edema of suspected lymphatic origin. These imaging approaches must be well understood by clinicians requesting these exams, the specialists who perform them, and patients for in whom they are proposed. Lymphoscintigraphies must be performed with care and thought, using available materials in the most appropriate ways, with the best applied methodological approaches, and always analyzed and interpreted taking into account the specific patient's situation and expectations and the clinician's demands. The specialist in Nuclear Medicine who performs lymphoscintigraphy also must integrate lymphoscintigraphic

P. Bourgeois, M.D., Ph.D. (✉)
Service of Nuclear Medicine and Clinic of
Lymphology, Institute Jules Bordet, Université Libre
de Bruxelles, 121, Bd de Waterloo,
1000 Brussels, Belgium
e-mail: pierre.bourgeois@bordet.be

A.K. Greene et al. (eds.), *Lymphedema: Presentation, Diagnosis, and Treatment*,
DOI 10.1007/978-3-319-14493-1_15, © Springer International Publishing Switzerland 2015

investigations into the growing field of other imaging techniques now proposed for investigating patients with edema while never forgetting that the primary duty of a doctor of medicine is service to the patient.

Introduction

Physicians currently face three main problems when imaging lymphedema. The first issue is related to the clinical symptom—the edema, which can be observed anywhere on the body. The term "lymphedema" can be used only if the edema has been demonstrated as caused (either partly or totally) by an abnormality involving the lymphatic system. This causality can be obvious in the case of secondary edema related to prior events, such as surgery with removal of lymph nodes, radiotherapy on diseased lymph nodes, trauma or surgery that damages the lymphatic vessels, and infections that damage the lymphatic vessels or lymph nodes; however, the causality can frequently be less clear with other types of edema. Some clinical presentations may directly suggest a diagnosis of primary lymphedema, as is the case in the familial setting (i.e., with other members of the family presenting with an edematous limb, the true familial hereditary lymphedemas); in association with other symptoms (i.e., part of a syndrome that includes lymphedema); and when they are either present at birth (congenital lymphedemas) or arise typically within the first decades of life (lymphedema praecox). However, most of these primary lymphedemas frequently affect a single individual in one family and may be clinically apparent only later in the patient's life (i.e., lymphedema tarda). Additionally, clinicians more frequently face edematous situations that are associated with other symptoms and for which lymphatic system involvement represents only one of the pathogenic factors (e.g., phlebo-lymphedema, lipo-lymphedema, cyclic edemas).

The second problem for the clinician is which questions to ask and which answers to seek for the purposes of establishing a diagnosis, ruling out differential diagnoses, and selecting the appropriate treatment for the patient (Table 15.1). Along with symptoms, these questions and the answers being sought will guide the imaging technique to be used and the methodological approach to take.

The third problem clinicians will encounter is related to the imaging technique itself [1–3]. Many imaging approaches of the lymphatic system are available (Table 15.2). Scintigraphic investigations of the lymphatic system using the injection of a radiolabeled pharmaceutical, known as lymphoscintigraphies, are now the best established techniques to investigate edema in which the lymphatic system is either involved or its involvement is suspected [4–7]; however, lymphoscintigraphies, like other imaging techniques of the lymphatic system, carry both advantages and limitations (Table 15.3).

Table 15.1 Reasons to perform a lymphoscintigraphy in patients with lymphedema

To establish:
- In edemas clinically staged 0, 1 or 2: to establish the diagnosis of lymphedema
- In edemas clinically staged 1, 2, 3, or 4: as a pre-therapeutic "inventory" of the lymphatic system

An investigation useful for the physical therapist:
- To be reimbursed by the Health Insurance System for the physical treatment (in Belgium) [30]
- To show where manual lymphatic drainage maneuvers have to be applied
- To show the lymphatic collateralization pathways present in the patient

One way to select the surgical procedure(s)?
- "If no lymph node present, one indication for lymph node grafting?"
- "If no lymphatic vessels present, one indication for liposuction?"
- "If good lymphatic vessels are present, one indication for lymphatic to vein anastomosis?"
- "If lymph nodes are present, one indication for lymph node to vein anastomosis?"

For prevention:
- In case of unilateral lower limb lymphedema, to confirm that the other limb is not affected
- To investigate other family members (if clinical questions raise the possibility of familial hereditary lymphedema)
- Before any operation with damage to the lymphatic system, especially in patients with a familial history and/or mild symptoms of edema.

Table 15.2 The imaging techniques of the lymphatic system in 2014: can lymph nodes and/or lymph vessels be directly viewed and can lymph node and/or lymph vessel morphology and/or function be evaluated?

Imaging technique	Direct?	Indirect?	Lymph nodes		Lymph vessels		Comments
			Morphology	Function	Morphology	Function	
Vital dyes	**Yes**		Yes	No	**Yes**	**Yes**	Sentinel Node
Fatty meal!	**Yes**		No	No	**Yes**	"No"	Chyliferous!
Radio-colloids							
Lymphoscintigraphy		**Yes**	Yes	No[a]	**Yes**	**Yes**[a]	Dedicated protocols[a]!
PLUS Vital dyes	**Yes**	**Yes**					
Lympho-SPECT-CT		yes	**Yes**	Yes[a]	yes	Yes[a]	See text[a]
Positron Emitting Molecules		**Yes**	Yes	No	No	No	See footnote[a]
Ultrasound (see Chap. 14)		**Yes**	**Yes**	No	**Yes**[a]	**Yes**[a]	**High frequency and /or injection of micro-bubbles
X-rays (see Chap. 14)							
Lymphangiography		**Yes**	**Yes**	Yes	**Yes**	**Yes**	No longer performed?
CT		**Yes**	**Yes**	No	**Yes**[a]	No	Only if enlarged[a]!
MRI (see Chap. 14)							
Hydrography		**Yes**	No	No	**Yes**	No	
Lymphangiography		**Yes**	**Yes**	No	**Yes**	**Yes?**	
Lymphadenography		**Yes**	**Yes**	No	No	No	
Fluorescent molecules		**Yes**	Yes	No	**Yes**	**Yes**	See text

SPECT, single photon emission computed tomographic; *CT*, Computed tomography; *MRI*, magnetic resonance imaging
[a]Only for the demonstration of primary and/or secondary tumoral process involving the lymphatic system

Table 15.3 Respective contribution of the various imaging techniques in the management of the lymphedematous diseases

		Lymphoscintigraphies		Lympho-SPECT-CT		CT		Lympho-fluoroscopies		MRI	
		Diagnosis	Treatments	Diagnosis	Treatments	Diagnosis	Treatments	Diagnosis	Treatments	Diagnosis	Treatments
Upper Limb Edemas (ULE)											
Primary		++++	++++[a]	++++	++++[a]					++[b]	<
Secondary	Oncologic	++	++++[a]	+++	++++[a]	+/++	+	GP +++	GP +++	++[b]	++++[b]
	Others	++++	++	++++	<	+++	<	?	?		
Lower Limb Edemas (LLE)											
Primary	Congenital	++	++++[a]	+	++++[a]	+		? (see text)	? (see text)	+[b]	++++[b]
	Praecox	+++	++++[a]	++	++++[a]	++	+	P +++ ?	P +++ ?	++[b]	++++[b]
	Tarda	++++	++++[a]	+++	++++[a]	+++	++	GP ++	GP +++	+++[b]	++++[b]
Secondary	Oncologic	++	++++[a]	++	++++[a]	+/++	+	GP ++	GP ++	?	++++[b]
	Others	+++	++	++++	<	+++	<	?	?		
Lipo(-lymph-)edema		++	+/++	+++	+	++		?	?	?	?
Phlebo-lymphedemas		+++	+/++	++	+?	++		P ++?	?	?	?
Lymphangioma		+		++		++++	<	?	?	++++[b]	+++[b]
Lymphangiomatosis		+		+		++++	<	?	?	++++[b]	+++[b]
Chylous reflux disorders		++	+/++	'++++	+++	++		?	?	++++[b]	++++[b]
Genital LE	Males	++	+/++	'++++	'++	+		?	?	++[b]	++++[b]
	Females	++	+/++	'++++	'++	+		?	?	++[b]	++++[b]

In some indications ("lymphedematous diseases"), data are lacking for the "Lympho-fluoroscopies" and the technique (its contribution) has been classified as "?" (undetermined). In other indications, the contributions of the "lympho-fluoroscopies" have been classified—on the basis of the existing literature—as "GP" ("of great potential") and/or "P" ("of potential" to be established)

SPECT, single photon emission computed tomographic; *CT*, Computed tomography; *MRI*, magnetic resonance imaging; *LE*, lymphedema

[a]With additional injections at the root of the limbs

[b]With injection of contrast

The first key message of this chapter is as follows:

Key Point
Edema is one clinical symptom. The symptom becomes a lymphedema when morphologic and/or functional abnormalities affecting the lymphatic system can be demonstrated. But the lymphedematous problem must always be placed in its overall context and presented with the (eventually) associated symptoms and with the specific patient's history. The clinician has then to formulate well the question(s) to be answered. These questions will determine not only the technique to be proposed to the patient but also the methodology that will be applied by the specialist who will perform the investigation.

The following paragraphs primarily present and discuss two imaging approaches of the lymphatic system: **the lymphoscintigraphies** and the **lympho-fluoroscopies** (other "radiological" imaging approaches of the lymphatic system—Magnetic Resonance Imaging, classical Computed Tomography, Ultrasound, and Echo-Doppler—are presented and discussed in other chapters).

The Lymphoscintigraphies

Principle of the Lymphoscintigraphies

The principle of lymphoscintigraphies has to be kept in mind by the non-specialists in imaging. This principle in its application can be formulated as follows: if of adequate size (usually under 100 nM) and if labeled with a gamma-emitting radioisotope (usually Technetium (Tc)-99 m), these radiolabeled particles (also called the "tracer" in this chapter; in Europe, the most frequently used radiopharmaceutical is obtained by heating human serum albumin (HSA) that is filtered so that the particles are under 100 nM in size) and using scintigraphic techniques will allow, (1) study and quantification of their removal by the initial lymphatics from the tissue where they are injected; (2) study and visualization of the lymphatic vessels efferent from the injected site and where they will be transported and will transit; (3) demonstration of the lymph nodes that are part of these lymphatic pathways and where these particles, if colloidal, will be partly trapped by the reticuloendothelial cells during their intra-nodal transit; and (4) when they reach the systemic circulation (after their transit in the thoracic duct when the tracer is injected in the lower limbs), study of their accumulation in the liver (and sometimes the spleen and bone marrow), where their uptake is finally representative of the lymphatic load extracted from the limb or organ studied.

Scintigraphic Material and Qualitative Imaging of the Lymphatic System

The evolution and the current state of the art of scintigraphic techniques when applied to the evaluation of the lymphatic system must be emphasized. These images can be centered on one part of the lymphatic system (i.e., "spot" pictures) but can also cover the entire body [from the injected sites; for instance, at the level of the feet, up to the level of the head, including the transit of the tracer in the thorax, i.e., whole-body scanning (WBS)]. Most gamma camera systems are now dual-headed, which allows simultaneous acquisition of anterior and posterior views of the lymphatic system, and which also, by acquiring images when rotating around the patient [as with the single photon emission computed tomographic (or SPECT) devices], allow three-dimensional images of the lymphatic structures. Using adequate software, it is now possible to merge the acquired transverse, sagittal, and coronal lymphoscintigraphic slices with the corresponding pure anatomic slices showing the structures surrounding the lymph vessels and/or nodes and obtained using classical X-ray computed tomographic (CT) systems or, less widely available, magnetic resonance imaging (MRI) systems. Finally, many nuclear medicine services are now equipped with hybrid devices combining SPECT and CT (SPECT-CT) in a single system, which yields direct images of the lymphatic structures within their anatomical surroundings.

Table 15.4 What can be seen on lymphoscintigraphic imaging? [8]

- From one injected site, the "normal" lymphatic (superficial and/or deep) vessels—pathways expected on the basis of the historical anatomical data (Rouvière remains the "must")—including sometimes (and in the case of lower limb lymphoscintigraphies) the Ductus Thoracicus (and sometimes abnormalities of/on this great intra-thoracic lymphatic vessel: see Fig. 15.9)
- The radio-colloidal activities transiting ("in transit") in these lymphatic vessels
- The lymph nodes that are "normal" part of these lymphatic pathways, where these radio-colloids remained trapped and as expected on the basis of the historical anatomical data (Rouvière also remains the "must")
- The liver (and sometimes the spleen and bone marrow) where the radio-colloids (when they reach the systemic circulation) are taken up
- Sometimes (varying with the characteristics of the injected radio-colloids), activities in the "great" systemic circulation, in the kidneys, in the bladder
- From the injected site, one (abnormal) progression of the radio-colloidal tracer (not in well-delineated lymphatic vessels but diffuse), in and through the superficial lymphatic collateralization network without visualization of lymph nodes and/or lymphatic vessels
- From the injected site, one (abnormal) progression of the radio-colloidal tracer (not in well delineated lymphatic vessels but diffuse), in and through the superficial lymphatic collateralization network (sometimes limited to one small area and sometimes extended to the whole limb) with visualization of (superficial and/or deep) lymphatic vessels draining the corresponding area
- On any part of these lymphatic pathways, (abnormal) "blockade" of the lymph flows with lymphatic vascular reflux (see Figs. 15.1, 15.4, 15.7, and 15.10) into the (surrounding) superficial lymphatic collateralization network (the "dermal backflows," sometimes limited to one small area (see Figs. 15.1, 15.7, and 15.10) and sometimes extensive (see Fig. 15.4) and/or into, with visualization of (superficial and/or deep) lymphatic vessels draining the corresponding area (see Fig. 15.9) and/or of the lymph nodes that are "normal" and/or abnormal part of these lymphatic pathways and where these radio-colloids remained trapped (see Fig. 15.7, arrow 4)
- (Usually in secondary lower limb lymphedemas), lymph nodes "absent" in one limited and/or extended anatomical area, sometimes with:
  - From "normal" lymph nodes, reflux of the lymph (coming in the nodes from "large" collecting lymphatic vessels) in the "smaller" lymphatic vessels connected to these nodes (see Fig. 15.2, arrow 2 and Fig. 15.9, arrow 1) with lymphatic "vascular" reflux that may reach the (surrounding) superficial lymphatic collateralization network (the "dermal backflows," sometimes limited to one small area (see Fig. 15.9: arrows 2 and 3) and sometimes extensive (see Fig. 15.2: arrow 7) and/or into, with visualization of (superficial and/or deep) lymphatic vessels draining the corresponding area and/or of the lymph nodes that are "normal" and/or abnormal part of these lymphatic pathways and where these radio-colloids remained trapped
  - Collection of lymphatic activities [that does not correspond on single photon emission computed tomographic –computed tomography (SPECT-CT)] to a lymph node but to a "true" lymphocela and, in case of lower limb investigations, sometimes to reflux of lymph into the digestive tract (see Figs. 15.2, 15.6, and 15.9)
  - In cases of secondary upper limb edema, one "effusion" of lymphatic activities in one axilla and/or at the level of the thoracic wall, one "lymphorrea," and the lymphatic drainages of this area (see Figs. 15.10, 15.11, and 15.12)
  - Direct and/or indirect signs of (spontaneously opened) lymph to vein anastomosis
  - In cases of ascitis and/or or chylo-thorax and/or chylo-peritoneum, it is possible using dedicated protocols to show and to precise the level of one lymphatic leakage

Thus, lymphoscintigraphies can yield morphologic images of the lymphatic system (normal or abnormal at each of its parts: Table 15.4), with a definition that might be considered "limited" when compared to other imaging techniques but, when applied with the most advanced approaches (lymphoscintigraphic SPECT-CT), are still are very informative [8].

Scintigraphic Acquisitions and Quantitative Functional Imagings of the Lymphatic System

It must be reminded that these images, even if static, always contain useful quantitative information. Additionally, the acquisitions can be dynamic and thus allow the study and quantifica-

Table 15.5 The quantitative and functional parameters that can be obtained in the framework of lymphoscintigraphic investigations

- Extraction of the tracer by the lymphatic system at the level of the injected site(s)
- The speed of the lymphatic flows in the lymphatic vessels (a)
- The activities remaining in the lymphatic vascular structures (a)
- The time of the tracer to reach the first lymph nodes (for instance, from the foot to the first inguinal lymph nodes)
- The activities in the lymph nodes (a)
- The time to reach the half of the maximal activity in these lymph nodes
- The activity in the liver (a)

tion of, for instance, transit of the tracer in the lymphatic vessels (the lymphatic flows) and/or the accumulation of the tracer in the lymph nodes (and/or in the liver) under various conditions and during various periods. Lymphoscintigraphies allow not only acquisition of morphologic–qualitative information about the lymphatic system, but also provide information about the functional parameters describing the lymphatic system of the studied edematous structures. The functional parameters that can be obtained using this method (with radio-colloids) are listed in Table 15.5. Each of the parameters followed by (a) listed in Table 15.5 are usually expressed in percentages of the activities injected. They provide quantitative information about the ability of the lymphatic system to transport the radiolabeled colloids; in addition, they can be compared to a normal population, and in case of lateralized edema, between the edematous and healthy areas. The most refined quantitative approaches for studying the lymphatic system have been developed by Mortimer's team [9–13].

The Scintigraphic Methodological Approaches

As already noted, static or dynamic lymphoscintigraphic images can be obtained under various conditions. When facing a case of edema with a diagnostic goal, these acquisitions seem to be obtained in at least three conditions [14–16]:

(a) During and after a resting period (because the edema can appear and be present only in this condition); for instance, with the patient lying on the examination table for 30 min. This phase ("Phase 1") allows identification of the insufficiency of the lymphatic system in resting conditions and/or functional asymmetry in lymphatic function between the edematous limb site and its normal contralateral part. However, this approach requires a well-standardized protocol (See Fig. 15.1).

(b) During and after a period of exercise; for instance, performed with the patient lying on the examination table for 15 min and then after performing one standardized exercise (tiptoeing, handgripping). This "Phase 2" is frequently essential because it allows dynamic study of the lymphatic vessels (for instance, to identify localized lymphatic reflux, which can be masked by dermal backflows on delayed imaging; see next point and Fig. 15.2) and shows functional asymmetry in the lymphatic function between the edematous limb site and its normal contralateral part. This phase allows identification of lymphatic insufficiency under exercise conditions.

(c) After a period of for instance 1 h after the patient's normal activities (in case of lower limb edema, after walking, for example, but be aware that the patient should not remain sitting in the waiting room during this period; in case of upper limb edema, after having performed movements with the fingers, hands, and limbs in ways that would be part of normal daily activity) ("Phase 3"). The images and their information then will be representative of the response of the lymphatic system to lifestyle activities that patients typically report precede the appearance of edema.

These images are thus morphological–qualitative and also morpho-functional.

The specialist in Nuclear Medicine, however, will have to keep in mind that the dynamic and/or static acquisitions (and their consecutive results)

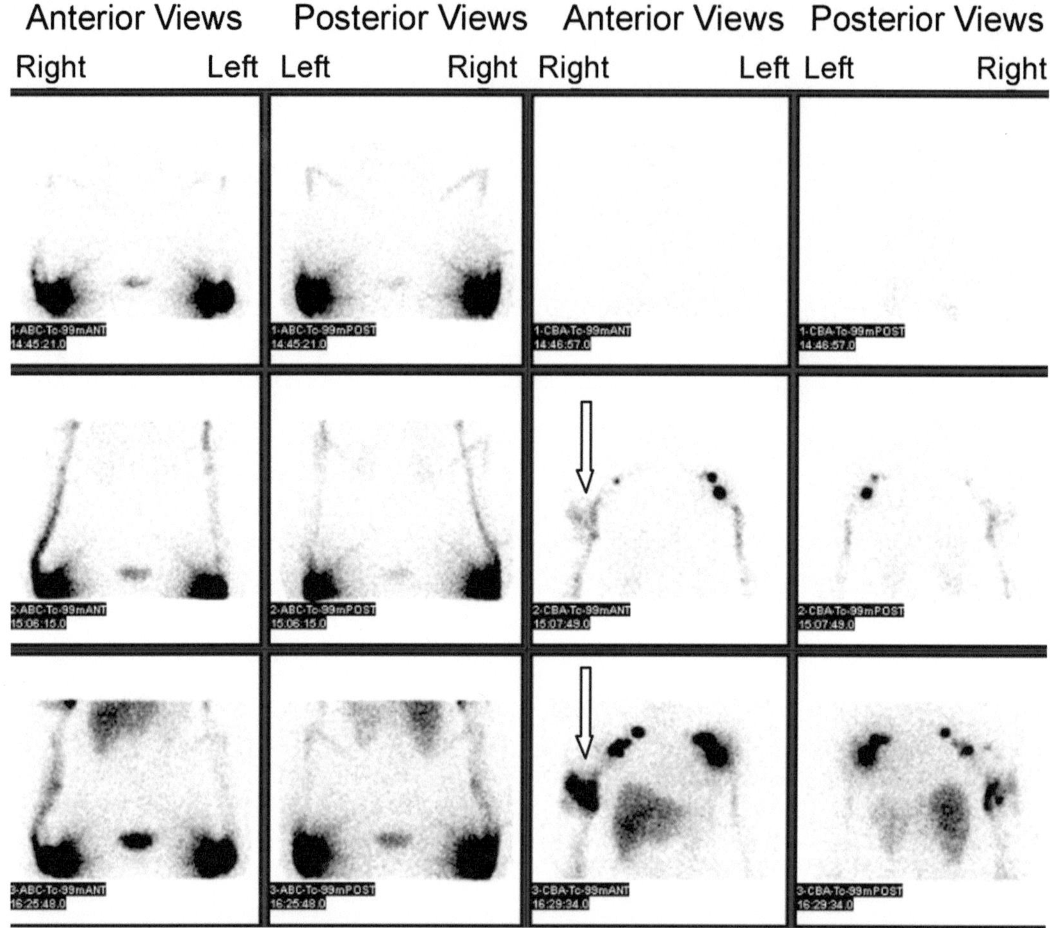

Fig. 15.1 Pictures (anterior and posterior views) centered on the hands, wrists, forearms, and elbows (on the *left* sided part of the figure) and on the elbows, arms, and axillas (on the *right* sided part of the figure) obtained (from up to down after 30 min without movements, after 15 min of handgripping and after 1 h of normal activities) in one woman with edema limited at the level of her right arm 2 years after one radical mastectomy with complete axillary node dissection. The *vertical arrows* show one lymphatic reflux limited after the 15 min of exercise but extended to the superficial network after 1 h of normal activities.

Key point for Figure 15.1:
The tracer has not reached the left axillary lymph nodes after 30 min without movements. This is observed in more than 90 % of the women referred for the investigation of one secondary upper limb lymphedema and supports the hypothesis that these women who are developing such lymphedema had one preexisting latent lymphatic functional insufficiency

will have sometimes to be considered and adapted to answer specific questions as listed, but not limited to, the examples in Table 15.6.

The Type of Injection

How the tracer is injected is of great importance [17]. In case of edema at the level of the skin, two kinds of injections can be performed: either subcutaneous or intradermal. The latter will usually allow rapid entry of the tracer into the initial lymphatics, fast transport into the lymphatic vessels, and rapid arrival in the lymph nodes. The former is, however, more physiological and sensitive to the pathophysiological parameters underlying the observed edema. Removal of the injected tracer will indeed depend on the characteristics

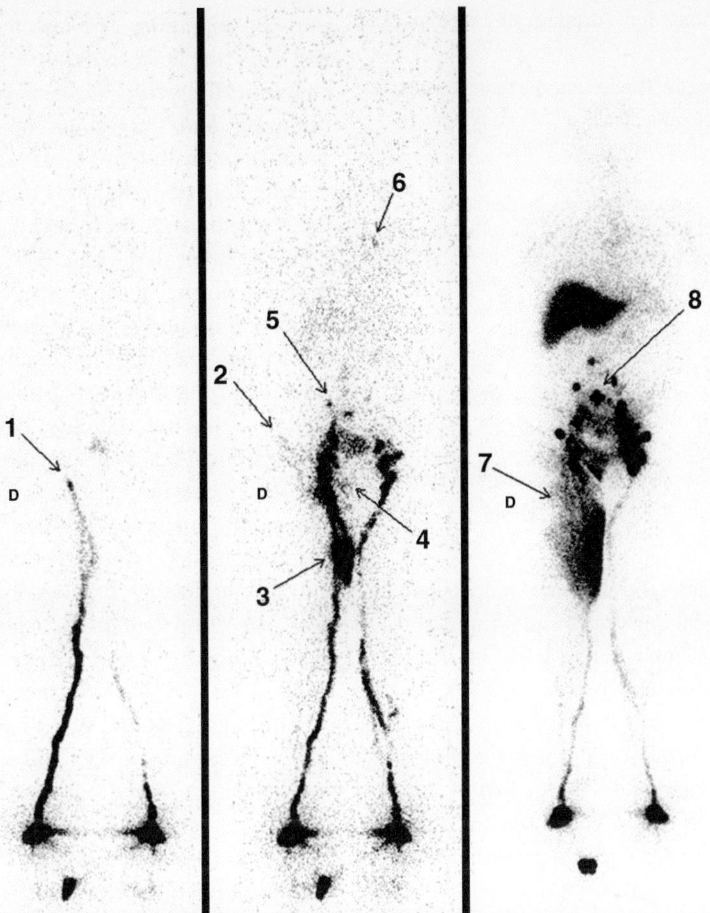

Fig. 15.2 Anterior whole-body scanning (WBS) obtained (after one subcutaneous injection of 99mTc-labeled HSA nanosized colloid in the first interdigital space of each foot, the patient lying on the examination table), from right to left, after 30 min without movement, after 5 min of tiptoeing, and after 1 h of walking. This man was sent for evaluation of right lower limb lymphedema (he also had pre-pubic edema on clinical examination) secondary to surgery and radiotherapy for prostatic carcinoma. After 30 min without movement, the tracer has reached the first inferior inguinal node on the right side (*arrow 1*), but progressed only to the level of the knee on the left side. After 5 min of tiptoeing, lymphatic reflux is seen in collaterals toward the external part of the right buttock (*arrow 2*), up to and in the mid internal part of the thigh (*arrow 3*), and in the right prepubic area (*arrow 4*). One right common iliac node is observed (*arrow 5*), as well as—faintly—two left retro-clavicular lymph nodes (*arrow 6*) proving that the thoracic duct is pervious. After 1 h of walking, the reflux of lymph in the superficial collaterization lymphat-ics extends to the upper and inner half of the right thigh (*arrow 7*), but one abnormal zone of activity is also demonstrated in the mid supra-pubic part of the abdomen (*arrow 8*). With permission from Bourgeois P. Combined Role of Lymphoscintigraphy, X-ray Computed Tomography, Magnetic Resonance Imaging, and Positron Emission Tomography in the Management of Lymphedematous Disease. In: Lee BB, Bergan J, Rockson SG, eds. Lymphedema: A concise compendium of theory and practice © Springer 2011.

Key points for Figure 15.2:
Lymph can normally flow from the right foot up and into the first inguinal lymph node (*arrow 1*) in resting conditions (→ "good indication for one lymph node to vein anastomosis?")
True lymphatic vascular reflux can (sometimes) be seen (only) with exercise (see *arrow 2*)
"Dermal backflows may mask the normally functioning lymphatic vessels (*arrow 1* versus *arrow 7*)

Table 15.6 Reasons for adapting the methological approach

- To study the Ductus Thoracicus, the thoracic duct
- To precisely determine the level of one lymphatic leakage (in the abdomen, in the thorax …)
- To demonstrate the patency-functionality of the lymphatico-venous anastomoses, of the node to vein anastomoses, of grafted lymphatic vessels (or veins: used to "bridge" the lymphatic "gap," to reconstruct the lymphatic pathway, to switch the lymph flow from one side to the other), so that grafted lymph nodes remain functional and/or viable
- To study the effects of specific manual lymphatic drainage maneuvers, pressotherapy systems, and wearing specific bandaging and/or elastic stockings, of drugs
- To investigate edema at the level of the face (see Fig. 15.13) and breast, limited to (part of) the genitals

of the injected interstitial tissue and, more precisely, on the local density of the lymphatic vessels network, but more importantly on the local hydrostatic and oncotic pressures. Once in the lymphatic vessels, transport of the tracer will depend on the normal or abnormal contractility of these vessels and on the forces that eventually oppose the lymph flows. The choice of injection will depend on the type of information desired.

The Importance of Standardization of Subcutaneous Injections

When performing subcutaneous injection of radio-colloids, it is important to work with standardized products, especially in the framework of a protocol with quantitative parameters. The amount of the labeled particles and the volume of injection in which they are diluted clearly influence the quantitative results obtained in terms of both what is removed by the lymphatic system and what will be found in the lymph nodes [18].

Where Is the Tracer Injected? The Superficial and the Deep Lymphatic System

In case of limb edemas, the anatomical site where the tracer is injected should also be taken into consideration. The injected site will define and show the corresponding a priori normal and anatomically well described lymphatic vascular drainage, and the lymph nodes that will be finally demonstrated. For instance, one subcutaneous injection in the *first interdigital* space of the feet and hands will show the superficial lymphatic system; in the case of lower limb edema, it is not normal to see popliteal lymph nodes, which are related to the deep lymphatic system. Such visualization of the popliteal lymph nodes is a sign of functional insufficiency and/or overload of the superficial lymphatic system. Conversely, it has to be considered that a subcutaneous injection in a more external interdigital space, i.e., in the *fourth interdigital* space may normally lead to lymphatic drainage toward and into the popliteal lymph nodes. At the level of the upper limbs, it is also not normal to see interosseous antebrachial and/or humeral lymph nodes after a single injection in the first interdigital space. Two (or more) injections in different interdigital spaces are certainly more representative of the whole edematous studied area than a single injection in the first interdigital space; in more practical terms, however, multiple injections can lead to misdiagnosis of some pathological conditions that affect the superficial lymphatic system.

To date, the deep lymphatic system has been the subject of relatively few studies [19]. However, mounting evidence indicates that some edemas are not related to a morphological and/or functional attempt of the superficial lymphatic system but of the deep lymphatic system. Typically, we are more and more frequently investigating women who complain of edema located at the level of the ankle, with associated pain and tension in the calves ("heavy limbs"), and sometimes with edema extending to the dorsum of the foot but usually not involving the toes. Investigation of the superficial lymphatic system after subcutaneous injection of the tracer in the first interdigital space of such patients is frequently normal but, in case of unilateral edema, may also show a paradoxical functional asymmetry with one superficial lymphatic system of the affected limb that seems to work better than the non-edematous side. Investigations of the deep lymphatic system of the two limbs in these women in fact show that the deep lymphatic system of the edematous side is either absent or functionally insufficient, when compared to the normal side. As a consequence, the lymph normally transiting through the deep lymphatic system is redirected toward the superficial which, when investigated, is overloaded when compared to the normal opposite side. Various sites of injection for studying the deep lymphatic system of the limbs have been proposed and/or are used, each with advantages and disadvantages: for example, at the level of the lower limbs, in the calf muscles, the medial part of the tissular space between the Achilles' tendon and the distal part of the tibia, the periosteum of the calcaneum, deep in the sole of the foot.

Apart from their interest in the diagnosis and evaluation of some edemas, these injections to visualize the deep lymphatic vessels are also used by some surgeons who seek other less superficial lymphatic vessels to use for lymphatico-venous anastomoses.

Additional Injections

In our clinical experience, one third of the patients (with upper and/or lower limb lymphedema) show none of the lymph nodes expected to be seen at the root of the limb, either in the axillary area or in the inguinal and/or iliac area. This outcome raised two possibilities: either the tracer injected peripherally was not transported up and into these lymph nodes, which are in fact present, or these lymph nodes are absent as either a normal variant, or a symptom of a lymphatic disease. This question can be addressed by the use of an additional injection.

In three fourths of upper limb lymphedemas, intradermal injection of 99mTc-labeled Human Serum Albumin (HSA) nanocolloids (twice what is injected into the hands) in the lateral part of the arm under the shoulder led either spontaneously or after massage to the lymphatic drainage of the tracer towards the homolateral axillary lymph nodes. In some cases, collateralization lymphatic pathways reaching lymph nodes in the ipsilateral supra and/or retro-clavicular area were also demonstrated (the Caplan's and Mascagni's pathways), as were the ipsilateral posterior scapular and/or cervical lymph nodes, the ipsilateral internal mammary, and the contralateral parasternal and/or axillary lymph nodes (see Fig. 15.3).

In cases of lower limb lymphedemas, an intradermal injection at the level of the lateral part of the thigh in front of the great trochanter led (spontaneously or after massage) to direct lymphatic drainage of the tracer towards the homolateral inguinal lymph nodes and/or to the demonstration of collateralization lymphatic pathways reaching lymph nodes in the ipsilateral inguinal and/or iliac area in 90 % of cases. Ipsilateral or contralateral posterior lumbo-aortic nodes were also demonstrated, as well as the opposite-contralateral inguinal lymph nodes (through lymphatic collaterals transiting in the prepubic area and/or through the genitals and rarely by transiting in the back of the patients: see Figs. 15.4 and 15.5), and more rarely, the ipsilateral axillary lymph nodes.

The results of additional injections are interesting in many respects:

- In case of lower limb lymphedemas, the demonstration of the presence of normal inguino-iliac lymph nodes (not reached by the tracer) excludes lymphadenodysplasia (associated with peripheral lymphangiodysplasia), which is associated with a worse prognosis for the lymphedema according to Kinmonth [20]
- In any case, these results specify the lymphatic status of the patients.
- These inguinal lymph nodes that are able to be visualized with the help of the injection may be used by surgeons to perform lymph node-to-vein anastomoses.
- For physical therapists, these additional injections also show the collateralization pathways present in their patients, pathways that the therapists can target for pushing the fluid of the edema. This practice could be an improvement on attempting all of the possible

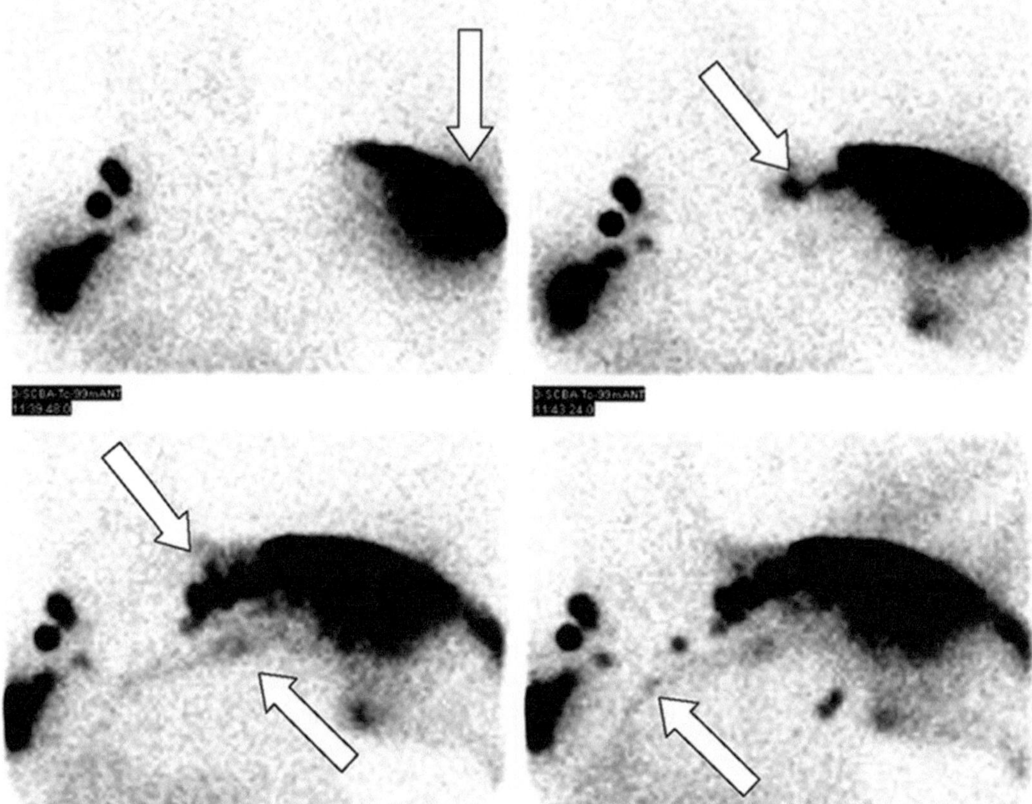

Fig. 15.3 From left to right and from top to bottom, anterior views centered on the axilla in a woman with post-therapeutic left upper limb lymphedema where the subcutaneous injection of 99mTc-HSA nanocolloid in the first interdigital space of the hands showed normal right axillary nodes, but no node in the left axilla. Intradermal injection was then performed at the level of the upper and external part of the left arm (*vertical arrow*) and the tracer was shown to spontaneously flow toward the retroclavicular lymph nodes (*left to right* *oblique arrows*) and also toward the left anterior chest wall, to cross the midline to reach the opposite axillary lymph nodes (*right to left oblique arrows*). With permission from Bourgeois P. Combined Role of Lymphoscintigraphy, X-ray Computed Tomography, Magnetic Resonance Imaging, and Positron Emission Tomography in the Management of Lymphedematous Disease. In: Lee BB, Bergan J, Rockson SG, eds. Lymphedema: A concise compendium of theory and practice © Springer 2011

collateralization pathways that physical therapists have learned but that are not systematically present in the treated patient.

Lymphoscintigraphy and Diagnosis of Lymphedema in Terms of Sensitivity and Specificity

From the previous paragraphs, it will be obvious for the readers that establishing the diagnosis of lymphedema ("edema of lymphatic origin") will depend on many factors (the tracer, the kind of injection, the materials (single-headed gamma camera, dual-headed camera, simple SPECT device, one SPECT-CT), the methodology protocol, the clinical approach or not), but also on the analytical criteria applied to the acquired imaging which will define sensitivity and specificity of the lymphoscintigraphic examination to diagnose lymphedema. Sensitivity and specificity are statistical terms, which are usually considered "simple" and easy to obtain, but only when the results of the examination can be compared to the results of

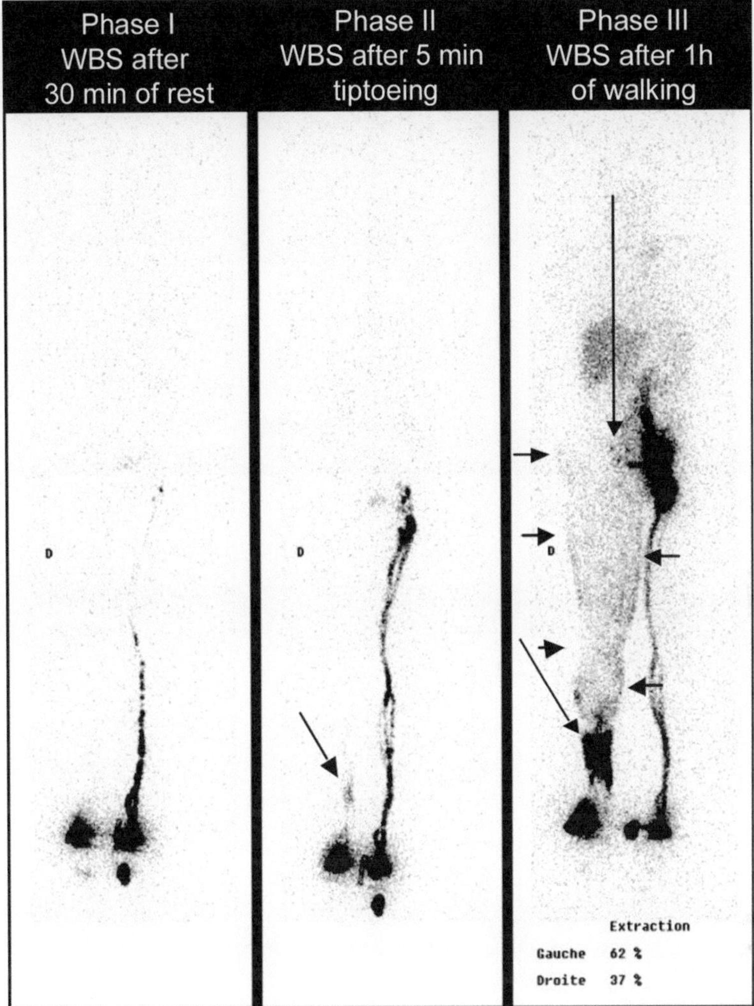

Fig. 15.4 Man with right lower limb lymphedema after resection of one distal cutaneous cancer with inguinal lymph node dissection followed by one local irradiation. From the left to the right, anterior whole-body lymphoscintigrams obtained after 30 min in resting conditions ("Phase 1"), after 5 min tip-toeing ("Phase 2") and 1 h of walking ("Phase 3"). The left lower limb is completely normal. On the right side, there is no lymphatic flow in resting conditions. After tiptoeing, lymphatic vessels are seen in the distal part of the right calf *(small oblique arrow)* and after 1 h of walking, lymphatic reflux are seen toward the superficial lymphatic network at the level of the ankle and in the distal part of the right calf *(long oblique arrow)*. Above this area, no clear lymphatic vessels are seen but one progression of the tracer through the superficial collateralization network *(small horizontal arrows)* at the level of the calf, knee, thigh and external part of the buttock and, may be, with faintly active right external iliac nodes *(long vertical arrow)*

another and/or of others viewed as the "gold standard." Table 15.7 shows the analysis made of the criteria proposed in 2003 in the literature [4, 16] and to which we added the data from another presentation in 2012, and can be summarized as:

– Based on the presence of morphological lymphoscintigraphic abnormalities, the sensitivity will range only from 70 to 78 %.

– Sensitivity of the functional parameters (considered solely) will range from 50 to 100 %. In fact, the sensitivity of a functional parameter will depend on the population studied (Table 15.7 shows the difference in the sensitivities of extraction in our first series with primary and secondary Lower Limb Edema (LLE) and in our second series with only primary LLE).

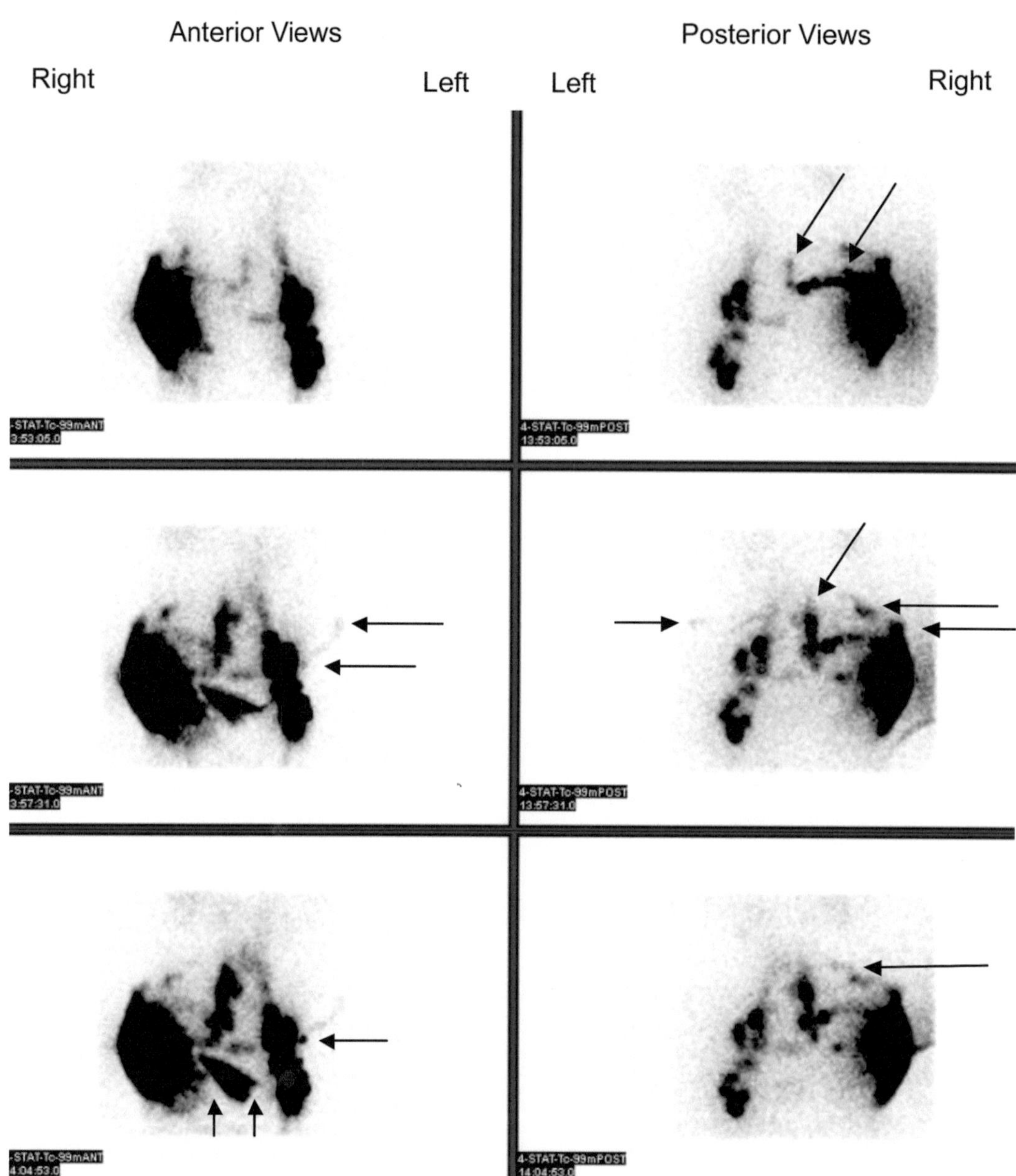

Fig. 15.5 Pictures (anterior and posterior views) obtained (in the patient described in Fig. 15.4) but after the intradermal injection of the tracer at the level of the root of the right limb in front of the great trochanter. Spontaneously (upper pictures) and quick after some massages (mid and lower pictures), we can observe (after one superficial collateralization) collecting vessels, crossing the midline under the bladder (*small vertical arrows*) to reach the opposite inguinal lymph nodes, penetrating in the buttock to reach the right common iliac lymph nodes (*oblique arrows*), ascending laterally toward the right costo-lumbar area and crossing posteriorly the midline to reach finally one left sided external inguinal lymph nodes (*horizontal arrows*)

Table 15.7 Sensitivities and Specificities of Lymphoscintigraphies for the diagnosis of Upper (ULE) and Lower (LLE) Limb Edema [14]

Authors	Year	Sensitivity based on:				Specificity based on:			
		N patients or limbs	Morphology	Function	Both	N patients	Morphology	Function	Both
Franco et al. [38]	1980	12 primary LLE		100 %[a]		48 limbs		92 %[a]	
		8 secondary LLE		75 %[a]					
Carena et al. [39]	1988	77 with LLE and 15 with ULE		90 %[b]		16 limbs		87 %[b]	
				98.2 %[c]				100 %[c]	
Golucke et al. [40]	1989	17	70–73 %						
Ter et al. [41]	1993	17				17	100 %		
Weissleider et al. [42]	1988	238 patients but 256 LLE	70 % (n=219)		100 %				
Nawaz et al. [43]	1992	164 LLE			66 %				
Cambria et al. (44)	1993	124 LLE			82 %	79 limbs			83.50 %
Bourgeois et al. [14]	1997	47 unilateral LLE	78 %	50 %[b]	98 %	47 opposite limbs	94 %	66 %	
		(primary and secondary)		68 %[a]		97 normal limbs	100 %	100 %[b]	99 %
Bourgeois et al. (personal communication, oral presentation)	2012	58 primary praecox LLE	71 %	91.4 %[b]	100 %	<35 years of age	100 %		
						Right LLE		96 %[b]	
						Left LLE		94 %[b]	
						Bilateral LLE		97.6 %[b]	

[a]Time to node
[b]Extraction
[c]Nodal uptake

Table 15.8 Cancer risk related to effective dose leading to one death per 100,000 persons in comparison with the corresponding effective doses related to other classical investigations (either of Nuclear Medicine or of Radiology) and the risks of death related to other causes

	Effective Dose (mSv)	Death per 100,000 persons
Lymphoscintigraphy	0.511	2.8[a]
CT Chest [32]	6	33.3[a]
CT Abdomen [32]	7.2	40[a]
CT head [32]	2.4	13.3[a]
CT Pelvis [32]	6.8	37.7[a]
PET-scan [33]	15	83.3[a]
Background per year [34]	2.4	13.3[a]
Cancer risk probability for a population of all ages [31]	0.18	1.0
Accident (unintentional injuries) [35]		39.4
Taxi drivers and chauffeurs (USA 2013) [36]		15.7
Deaths from road traffic accidents USA (2004) [37]		12.5–20

CT = Computed tomography; PET = positron emission tomography
[a]Adapted from ref. [31]

– Finally, optimal sensitivity is obtained using a "multi-parametric" approach combining morphological and functional criteria, as in the Transport Index proposed by Kleinhans et al. [21] ranging from 82 to 100 %. We should point out that the low value obtained by Nawaz et al. [22] is due to the fact that these authors were performing their investigations with intradermal injections of radio-colloids and thus did not acquire physiological information but only morphological.

– With regard to the term "specificity," morphological abnormalities will usually not yield false positives (when they are observed at the level of the non-edematous limb, an explanatory cause can be found in the majority of the patients).

– Well-defined functional parameters also present high values of specificity.

– The 66 % value that is shown in Table 15.7 is not an error; rather it illustrates that, when reporting the results of 47 unilateral primary or secondary LLE, in one-third of cases, the opposite limb showed functional and/or morphological abnormality that simply traduced the presence of a "clinically latent" (stage 0) lymphedematous situation at the level of the "normal" contralateral limb (which can be observed in up to half of the patients under 26 years of age with primary praecox unilateralized clinical lower limb lymphedema).

Lymphoscintigraphy and Irradiation

Regarding lymphoscintigraphy, the injection of radionuclides, of a radiolabeled tracer, and the related irradiations are a frequent concern raised in many articles in the literature, and by patients. In the case of secondary edema, it must be considered that the patients, as part of their treatment and diagnostic workup, have been frequently irradiated, with exposures that largely exceed the absorbed doses arising from radionuclide investigations. For instance, it has been calculated that the dose absorbed by one theoretical volume of distribution equal to 1 mL after the injection of 111 MBq (or 3 mCi) of 99mTc-labeled HSA nanosized colloids in the cutaneous tissue is equal to 1.23 Gy (or 1230 mJ per gram of tissue). Such a value has to be compared to the dose absorbed in the framework of classical irradiation, either of the chest wall or of the breast, that the patient will have experienced after a mastectomy or a tumorectomy and that is at least equal to 50 Gy. Even for patients with edema who have not been irradiated as a (necessary) part of their treatment(s), the irradiation risks must be placed in context. In Table 15.8, we provide some facts and compare the absorbed doses attributable to some other classical radiological

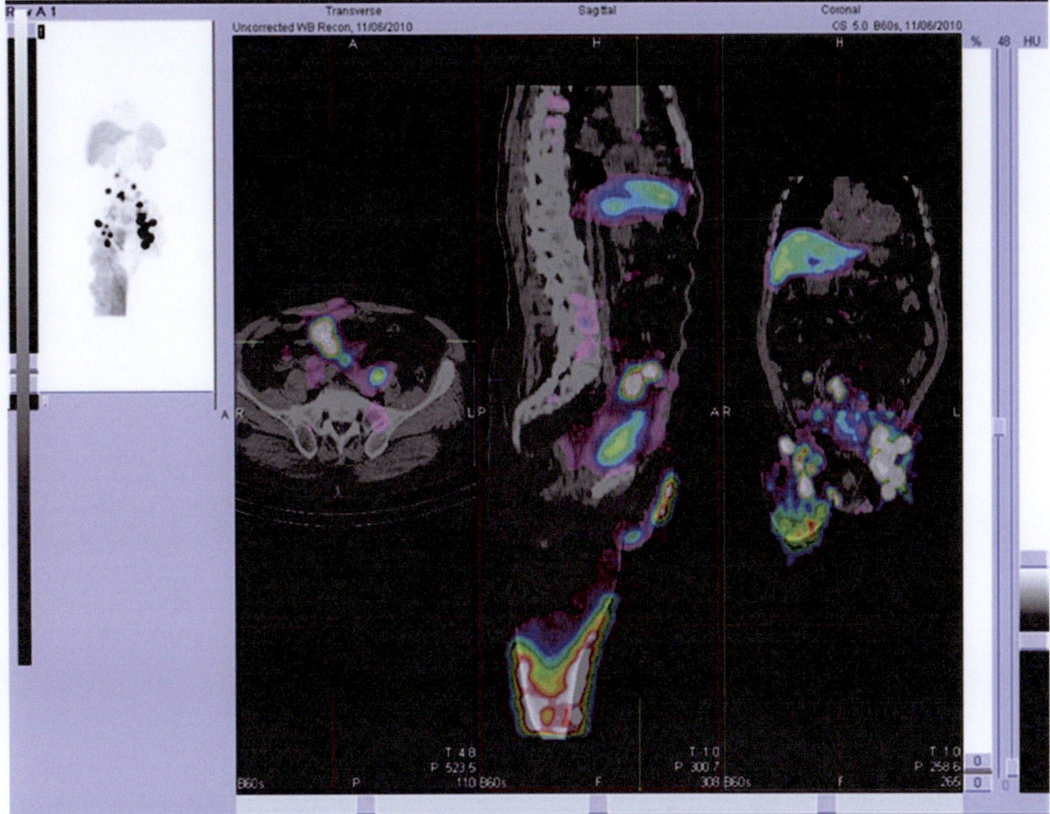

Fig. 15.6 From left to right, selected transverse, sagittal, and coronal/frontal fused slides from the SPECT-CT across the abdomen and pelvis showing nicely (1) (*top to bottom oblique arrows*) that the abnormal zone of activity seen on the planar WBS image in the mid supra-pubic part of the abdomen corresponds, in fact, to lymph flowing back from lumbo-aortic nodes in the digestive tract and (2) (*bottom to top oblique arrow*) dermal backflow in the right pre-pubic area. With permission from Bourgeois P. Combined Role of Lymphoscintigraphy, X-ray Computed Tomography, Magnetic Resonance Imaging, and Positron Emission Tomography in the Management of Lymphedematous Disease. In: Lee BB, Bergan J, Rockson SG, eds. Lymphedema: A concise compendium of theory and practice © Springer 2011.

Key Point for Figures 15.2 and 15.6:
When subsequently questioning the patient, he also complained of intermittent diarrhea

investigations (that are more frequently used than lymphoscintigraphies) to the corresponding data related to radionuclide-based investigations of the lymphatic system. Finally, it has to be emphasized that, to our knowledge and since the introduction of 99mTc-labeled pharmaceuticals for such investigations, no cutaneous radio-necrosis has been reported. Since their introduction into the medical diagnostic armamentarium, the use and related risks of the various diagnostic radionuclides are certainly the most thoroughly studied and regulated. The irradiation problem cannot to be ignored, but it also must not be exaggerated.

Thus, the second key message from this chapter for Nuclear Medicine specialists is as follows:

Key Point

Our materials that enable us to perform whole-body and/or three-dimensional imaging(s) of the lymphatic system in relation to their surrounding anatomical structures, our acquisition techniques, and our ability to quantify and dynamically analyze lymphatic system functions, and the applications of clinically based protocol(s) for investigation place our specialty at the center of the diagnosis and management of the edematous presentations. The physiological basis and limitations of our examinations have to be well known and understood. Especially with our lymphoscintigraphically based functional and morphological analysis of the lymphatic system, our results must be interpreted

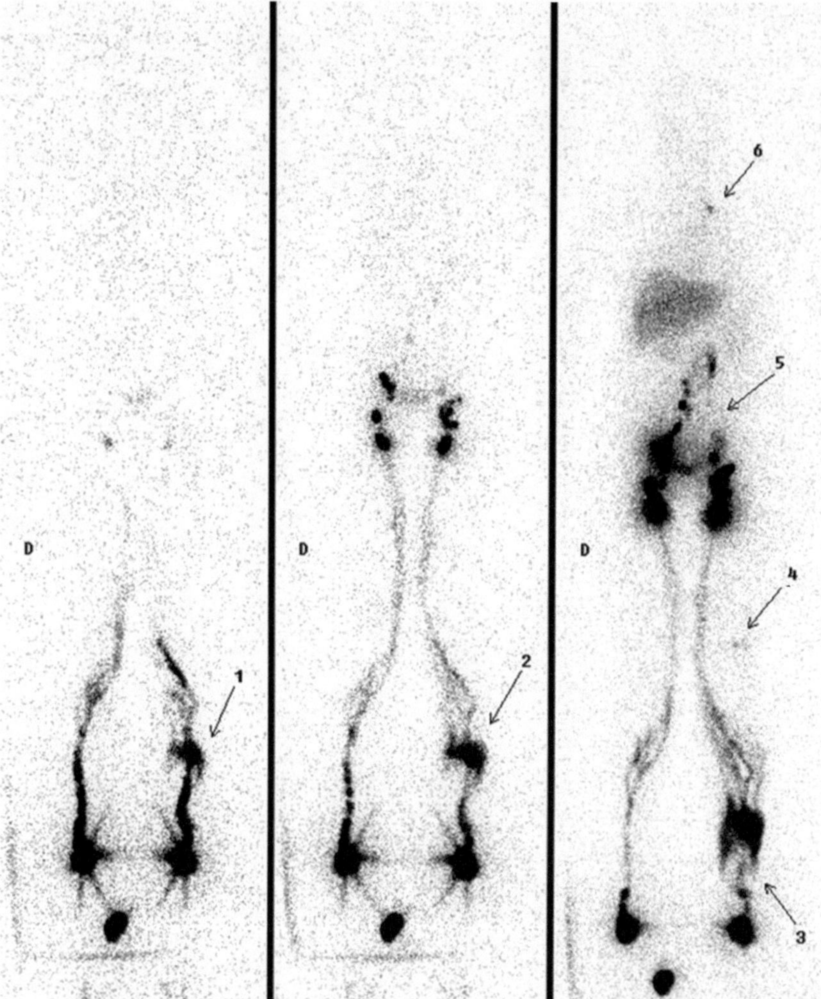

Fig. 15.7 Anterior whole-body scanning (WBS) obtained (after one subcutaneous injection of 99mTc-labeled HAS nanosized colloid in the first interdigital space of each foot, the patient lying on the table of examination), from right to left, after 30 min without movement, after 5 min of tiptoeing, and after 1 h of walking. This woman was sent for evaluation of left lower limb lymphedema. After 30 min without movement, the tracer has reached the first inferior inguinal node on both sides, but the beginning of lymphatic reflux is seen at the level of the distal part of the left calf (*arrow 1*). After 5 min of tiptoeing, lymphatic reflux in the left calf is more obvious (*arrow 2*). After 1 h of walking, the reflux of lymph in the superficial collater-alization lymphatics is obviously extended to the left ankle (*arrow 3*), one left popliteal lymph node (*arrow 4*), and one left retro-clavicular lymph node (*arrow 6*) HAS, but not the left common iliac nodes (*arrow 5*). On the basis of this lymphoscintigraphic examination, the diagnosis of primary lymphedema tarda was proposed (see Fig. 15.8). With permission from Bourgeois P. Combined Role of Lymphoscintigraphy, X-ray Computed Tomography, Magnetic Resonance Imaging, and Positron Emission Tomography in the Management of Lymphedematous Disease. In: Lee BB, Bergan J, Rockson SG, eds. Lymphedema: A concise compendium of theory and practice © Springer 2011

by taking into account the patient's clinical symptoms (see Figs. 15.2 and 15.6) *and history and also the results of other examinations* (see Figs. 15.7 and 15.8). *These investigations may seem time consuming in terms of equipment needs and human investment (they are certainly not "fast-food" medicine), but they are no more so than many other investigations now performed. These investigations must also be planned and adapted to answer clinician's questions and meet patient's expectations. If these considerations are explained to the clinicians and to the patients, you will be surprised by their adherence to and acceptance of what you propose* (Figs. 15.9, 15.10, 15.11, 15.12, and 15.13).

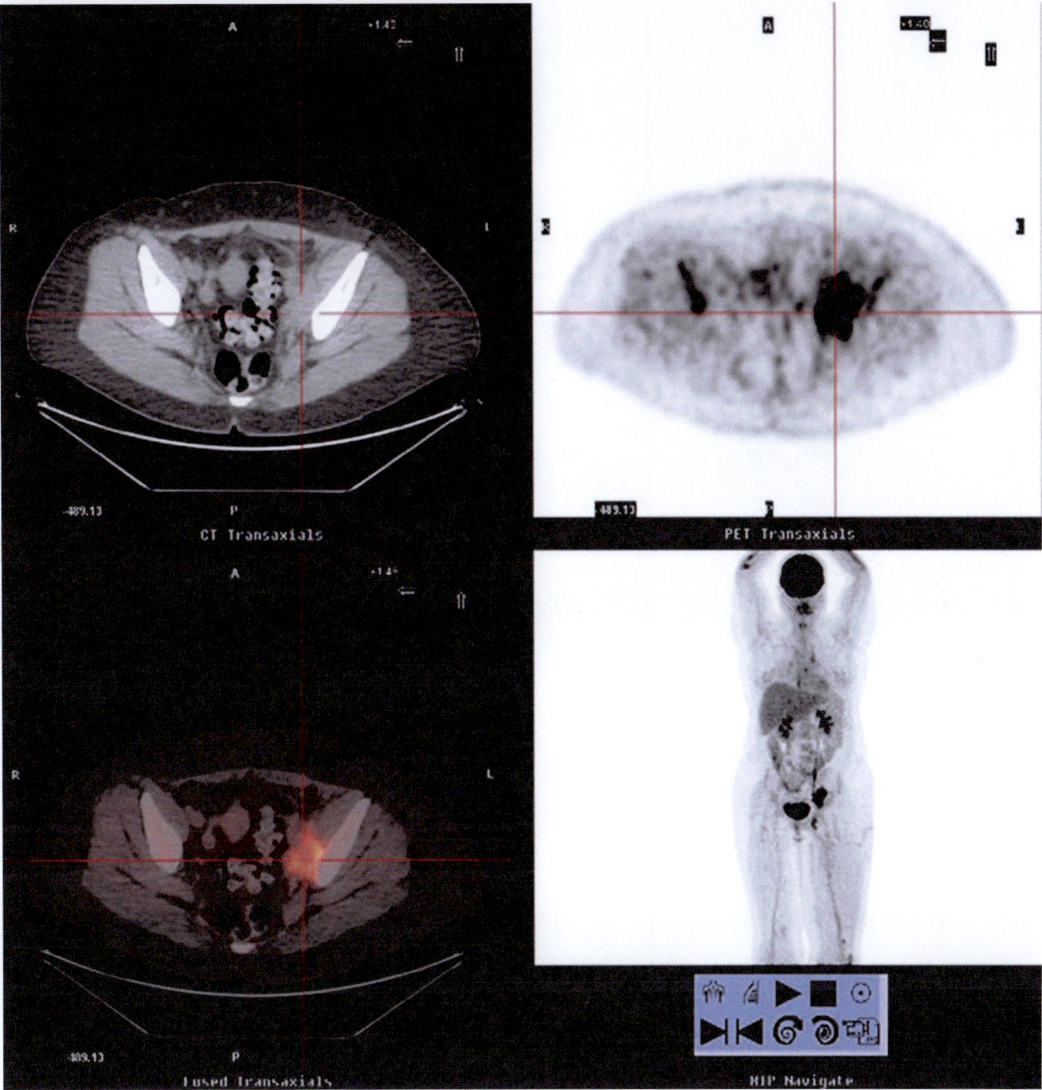

Fig. 15.8 The patient later developed left sciatica and blockage of the common iliac vein was suspected. PET-CT after IV injection of 18 F-DG was performed and demonstrated (on the selected transverse PET-CT slides) a hypermetabolic process later histologically proven to represent metastatic tumor of uterine cervix origin. With permission from Bourgeois P. Combined Role of Lymphoscintigraphy, X-ray Computed Tomography, Magnetic Resonance Imaging, and Positron Emission Tomography in the Management of Lymphedematous Disease. In: Lee BB, Bergan J, Rockson SG, eds. Lymphedema: A concise compendium of theory and practice © Springer 2011.

Key Points for Figures 15.7 and 15.8:
- False diagnosis of primary lymphedema tarda and/or a mixed situation (benign AND malignant)? The persistence of "sciatica" led to the diagnosis of the malignant disease.
- Even specialized, we remain doctors in medicine …

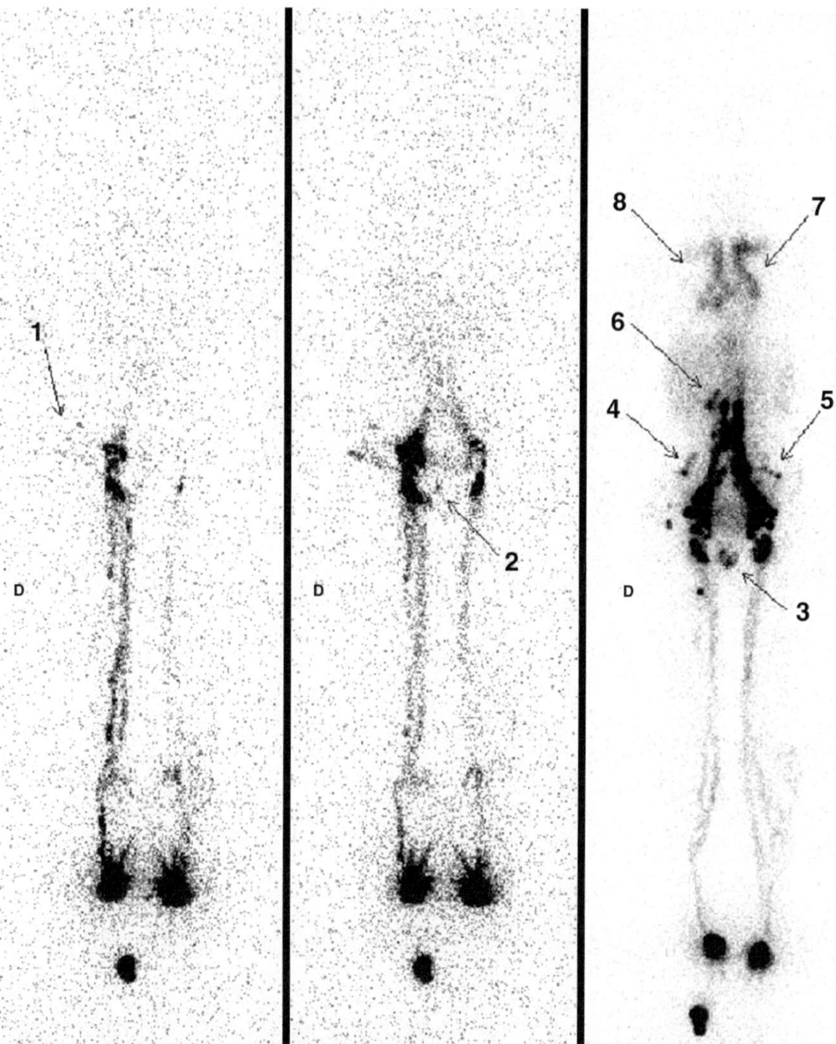

Fig. 15.9 Anterior WBS obtained (after one subcutaneous injection of 99mTc-labeled HSA nanosized colloid in the first interdigital space of each foot, the patient lying on the examination table), from right to left, after 30 min without movement, after 5 min of tiptoeing, and after 1 h of walking. This young woman did not complain of lower limb edema, but was referred for evaluation of intermittent lymph leakage at the level of her right labium majorum. After 30 min without movement, the tracer reached the first inferior inguinal node on the left side and all the inguinal nodes on the right side, but with lymphatic collaterals appearing from the inguinal nodes toward the external part of the buttock (*arrow 1*). After 5 min of tiptoeing, infra-diaphragmatic lymph nodes are now seen on both sides (and right collaterals are confirmed); the beginning of lymphatic reflux in the right labium majorum can also be observed (*arrow 2*). After 1 h of walking, the reflux of lymph in the right magna labia is now obvious (see *arrow 3*), but abnormal zones of activity are also demonstrated in the right and left lateral part of the abdomen (*arrows 4* and *5*) as well as at least two right pararenal lymph nodes (*arrow 6*) and, at the supradiaphragmatic level, there is a completely abnormal presentation of the great lymphatic thoracic duct with right and left components persisting (*arrows 7* and *8*). Coronal/frontal slide from the SPECT across the chest, the lumbar aortic nodes and the ilio-inguinal nodes showed nicely in the mediastinum, serpentine channels forming the thoracic duct and, in the abdomen, the lake of lymphatic activity in the right and left digestive tract. With permission from Bourgeois P. Combined Role of Lymphoscintigraphy, X-ray Computed Tomography, Magnetic Resonance Imaging, and Positron Emission Tomography in the Management of Lymphedematous Disease. In: Lee BB, Bergan J, Rockson SG, eds. Lymphedema: A concise compendium of theory and practice © Springer 2011

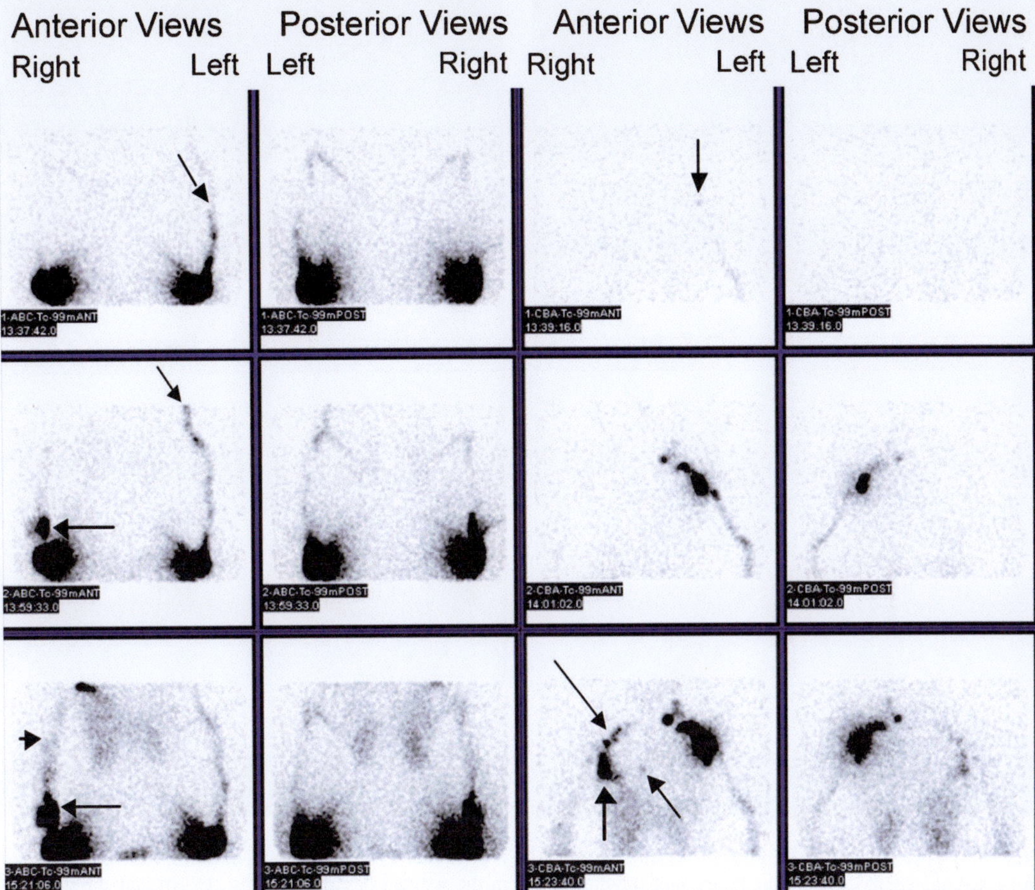

Fig. 15.10 Pictures (anterior and posterior views) centered on the hands, wrists, forearms and elbows (on the left sided part of the figure) and on the elbows, arms and axillas (on the right sided part of the figure) obtained (from up to down after 30 min without movements, after 15 min of handgripping and after 1 h of normal activities) in one woman with edema limited at the level of her right forearm 9 months after one radical mastectomy with complete axillary node dissection but who also presented one thickening of the lateral part of her right chest wall. The oblique arrows from up to down (and from your left to your right) show the normal lymphatic vascular drainage of the left interdigital injection reaching the first left axillary lymph node (faintly seen but present: *vertical arrow from up to bottom*). On the right side, one limited lymphatic reflux toward the superficial network at the level of the wrist is observed after the 15 min of exercise (*long horizontal arrow* from your right to your left). After 1 h of normal activities, lymphatic "vessels" are seen at the level of the right forearm (*small horizontal arrow* from your left to your right) and right axillary nodes are also demonstrated (*long oblique arrow* from up to down and from your left to your right). Additionally, one "lake" of activity can be observed at the level of the lateral part of the right thoracic wall (*vertical arrow* from down to up) and one focal activity median (*oblique arrow* from down to up and from your right to your left). "Conclusions of these pictures: normal situation left but lymphatic reflux and dermal backflow at the level of the right wrist with (probably deep) lymphatic drainage reaching the axillary nodes but also with one lymph leakage from the axilla toward the chest wall and drainage of this "lymphocele" into one right parasternal lymph node" (see SPECT-CT on Figs. 15.11 and 15.12)

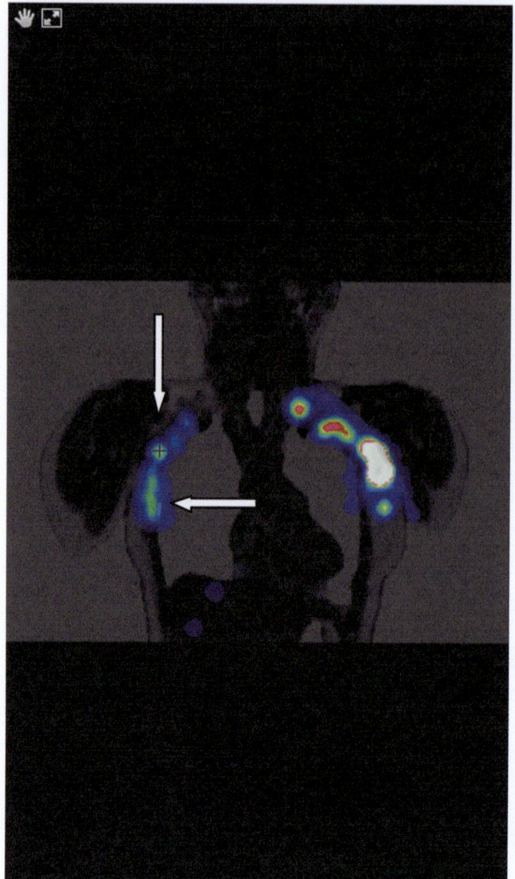

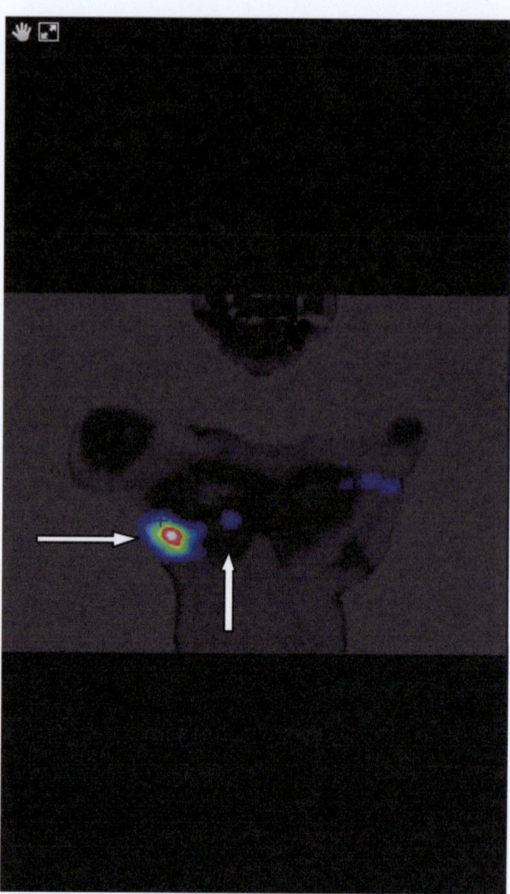

Fig. 15.11 Frontal slides from the SPECT-CT obtained in the woman (described in Fig. 15.10) and showing the right axillary nodes (*vertical arrow* up to down), the "lymphocele" at the level of the thoracic wall (*horizontal arrow*)

Fig. 15.12 Frontal slides from the SPECT-CT obtained in the woman described in Fig. 15.10) and showing the "lymphocele" at the level of the thoracic wall (*horizontal arrows*) and the right parasternal lymph node (*vertical arrow* from down to up)

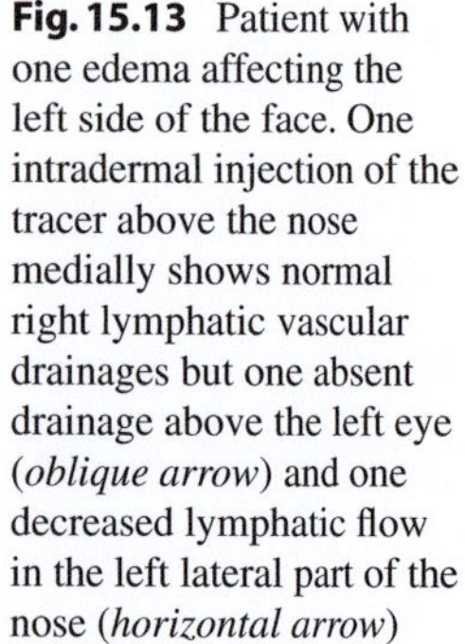

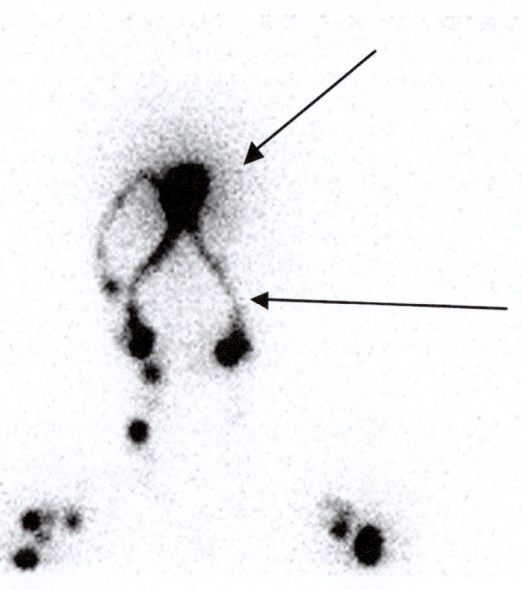

Fig. 15.13 Patient with one edema affecting the left side of the face. One intradermal injection of the tracer above the nose medially shows normal right lymphatic vascular drainages but one absent drainage above the left eye (*oblique arrow*) and one decreased lymphatic flow in the left lateral part of the nose (*horizontal arrow*)

Near-Infrared Imaging Investigations of the Lymphatic System: the "Lympho-fluoroscopies

The most fascinating novel technical method for imaging and investigating edemas of suspected lymphatic origin is Near-Infra-Red (NIR) imaging, encompassing lympho-fluoroscopies for which the published literature has grown annually. In lympho-fluoroscopic investigations, no radionuclide is used as an imaging agent, but rather a fluorescent molecule (such as indocyanine green ICG, fluorescein, or methylene blue, etc) is used as the imaging agent. When excited by light energy (i.e., photons) at the relevant wavelength (for instance 807 nm for ICG), these molecules will emit photons with a different wavelength (around 822 nm for ICG) that will be detected by the corresponding dedicated NIR camera devices. With specific excitation and emission wavelength characteristics, each of these fluorescent molecules has its unique features that define penetration of the excitation photons in tissues and the detection of the emitted photons. These characteristics will in fact determine and represent the most important limitation of lympho-fluoroscopy: the depth of the lymphatic structures (lymphatic vessels and/or lymph nodes) that can be visualized and studied (the rule of thumb is that the lower the wavelength, the more limited the depth of detection). Lympho-fluoroscopies are thus perfect for studying the superficial but not the deep lymphatic structures, although it may be hoped that technological progress will someday allow its application to deeper structures.

These fluorescent molecules can also be injected into any tissue, either coupled with another pharmaceutical (i.e., the carrier, such as dextran, immunoglobulin, albumin, HSA nano-sized colloids, etc), or free (unlabeled). In the case of a carrier, its characteristics determine what can be visualized of the lymphatic system. [23, 24] These new "fluorescent-labeled" pharmaceuticals are currently under development and if they can be expected to become available for clinical practice within the forthcoming years, it is not known at which cost.

Conversely and mainly with ICG, which is now the most commonly used, the injection of free agent into tissues (and in patients with a single edema) [25] remains associated with several open questions, including the following:

– Whereas its fate after intravenous injection (for which its use is internationally accepted) is relatively well established (rapid clearance, labeling of circulating proteins such as albumin and lipoproteins, to some cells), what happens after its injection in the interstitial spaces of one tissue has been less well studied. It is frequently hypothesized that ICG in these tissues will behave as in the blood (and that what is observed are the movements of these ICG labeled carriers from the interstitial spaces), but at what amount?

– ICG also has a low molecular weight (776 Da). It is our personal experience that just after its subcutaneous injection, ICG penetrates quickly and moves rapidly in the lymphatic vessels so that it can be supposed that it remains free (unlabeled) and that what is observed are the movements of the "lymphatic" fluids pushed into these vessels. However, this observation remains to be confirmed in controlled studies.

– The outcome of ICG injection in the cutaneous tissues is also not well established. Several users have reported that ICG fluorescence can, for instance, remain detectable up to 3 weeks after its injection.

– It has also been reported that the lymphatic vessels can remain visibly fluorescent during several days after injection. It can be hypothesized that ICG labels the cellular membranes of the lymphatic vascular walls but also that it is incorporated into these cells.

– With time, the lymphatic vessels also can sometimes lose their well-delineated aspect of simple vessels, and the fluorescence seems to diffuse into the surroundings of the lymphatic vessels.

A main question that arises and can be considered a key point of this chapter is: What are we really observing and studying after the injection of free ICG into one tissue in the framework of lympho-fluoroscopies?

These considerations lead to an additional question. Although the potential toxicity of ICG after its intravenous injection has been largely studied and its safety relatively well established

[26], few papers have been published that evaluate potential toxicity in the lymphatic structures [27, 28]. Furthermore, how the data related to the toxicity of (up to 25 mg or more of) ICG injected into the blood (with its dilution in several liters of blood and its quick hepatobiliary elimination) can be used for extrapolation to its post-injection fate and effects in the subcutaneous tissues. Even if the injected volumes and amounts are small, it has to be considered that the liquid-aqueous part of what is injected will quickly diffuse and that the injected ICG will remain concentrated in a small cutaneous volume of tissue. Another question involves the effects of this ICG on these tissues. With regard to the questions about its clearance, its time of residency in the cutaneous tissues and in the lymphatic vessels, and the potential problem of its persistence in the lymph nodes, this issue of potential toxicities of free ICG in the framework of lympho-fluoroscopies represents a matter of concern. The author is well aware that these fears might be exaggerated but remains uneasy about these uncertainties as a medical scientist who daily faces discussions about the potential toxicities of the drugs used in his institution. ICG will probably be found to be safe when injected into tissues drained by a normal lymphatic system, but what happens in patients with lymphedema, especially in the youngest ones who might be injected repeatedly?

Thus, more studies are needed evaluating its potential toxicities in such situations!

Anyway, the contributions and advantages and established limitations of the lympho-fluoroscopic approaches-investigations have to be highlighted [also in comparison with the previously presented lymphoscintigraphies (Table 15.9) and with other imaging techniques of the lymphatic system)].

Advantages and Contributions of Lympho-fluoroscopies

The following list concerns mainly the currently published data using free ICG:
- One of the main advantages of lympho-fluoroscopies is that it is not irradiating.

- The NIR camera devices cost less than gamma cameras and/or MRI imaging systems, but these other machines can be used daily to image other organs and systems. However, we are also aware of and studying other fields of great medical interest in which these NIR cameras might be and are already being used.
- The resolution of these NIR cameras is unique and superior to what can currently be acquired with conventional gamma cameras and can be compared only to what is today obtained with lympho-MRI approaches (presented in another chapter).
- The lymphatic vessels can be nicely visualized and studied at a fine-grained resolution. The contractility of the lymphatic vessels, their density, the pulses of the lymphatic liquids in these vessels, and the lymphatic speeds can be precisely analyzed. However, this information is somewhat sparse and limited to date (and sometimes not easily applied to clear diagnostic conclusions). Nevertheless, they are interesting for surgeons and physical therapists, and these approaches allow us to very precisely study some previously less well-known parameters of the lymphatic system and even the effects of some therapies.
- In general, lympho-fluoroscopies yield images of the so-far superficial aspects of the lymphatic system (lymphatic vessels, reflux, dermal backflows, collateralization pathways) that can be compared with those derived using lympho-MRI techniques and (less precisely) by lymphoscintigraphies.

Disadvantages and Limitations of Lympho-fluoroscopies

The lympho-fluoroscopies are, to date, merely descriptive, which is sufficient in several indications but not in patients with functional lymphedemas.

One of the main disadvantages of lympho-fluoroscopies is that they currently only allow visualization and study of the superficial lymphatic structures.

Table 15.9 Comparison of the respective advantages and drawbacks of the classical planar lymphoscintigraphic examination (LySc); of LySc when combined with a SPECT-CT acquisition (SPECT-CT-LySc) and of the Lympho-fluoroscopies (Ly-Fluo)

	Ly-Sc	SPECT CT LySc	Ly-Fluo	Comments
Overall anatomical contribution				
Superficial lymphatic vessels	++	+++	+++	
Deep lymphatic vessels	+++	++	?[b]	
Superficial lymph nodes	++	+++	+?	
Deep lymph nodes	+++	+++	?[b]	
Intra-abdominal and/or intra-thoracic lymphatic LV and/or LN	++	++	/–/[ab]	
Existing hardware to perform imaging?				
Planar and dynamic acquisitions	**Yes**		**Yes**	
Field of view	**Large**		**Limited (a)**	(a) In development
Resolution	++	+	+++++	
Whole-Body-Scanning?	**Yes**	Possible	**?**	
Acquisitions technically "operator"?	**Independent**	Independent	**Dependent (a)**	(a) In development?
Functional imaging of the lymphatic system				
Superficial lymphatic vessels	+++	+++	+++	
Deep lymphatic vessels	++	++	?	
Existing "Software" to perform quantifications and analysis of dynamic acquisitions	**Yes**	**Yes**	In development	
Value established on large series?	++++	+	++	
Potential patient limitations	**Pregnant women** Obese, Claustro		**Allergy?**[ab]	
Irradiation	+	++	/–/	
Potential toxicity of the imaging agent	/–/	/–/	**Unknown**	
Cost	+	++	**Unknwon**	

SPECT, single photon emission computed tomographic
[a]Except if performed with the patient "opened" in the operating room
[b]Some ICG formulations contain iodine

The fields of view of the proposed NIR imaging devices are also limited in that they do not allow easy visualizations of long lymphatic structures, as do MRI lymphographies and whole-body scanning lymphoscintigraphies. In practice, the implication, especially in the infra-diaphragmatic lymphedematous situation, is that lympho-fluoroscopies are operator-dependent and time-consuming, with the related costs in terms of human resources implied in their achievement.

Lympho-fluoroscopic images are also now mainly bidimensional with a limited third dimension (i.e., the depth of the lymphatic structures) and cannot be put in perspective relative to the surrounding tissues and structures.

Finally, the software packages that would allow analysis of the acquired images remain to be developed.

It can, however, be hoped that technological progress will eventually allow for the study of deeper structures, although probably not the intra-abdominal and intra-thoracic lymphatic vessels and nodes, and that more sophisticated (but likely more expensive) hardware systems (perhaps hybrids, for instance combining NIR-acquired information with ultrasonographic devices) and software [29] will be developed that will overcome these limitations.

These limitations could be considered relatively minor, but some more major limitations also exist. For example, the most frequently used fluorescent molecule, ICG, is officially approved in the USA (and other countries in the Americas) and in the European Community as an imaging agent after its intravenous injection. It is not, however, approved for other intra-tissue injections such as intradermal or subcutaneous routes. In practice, lympho-fluoroscopies with subcutaneous or intradermal injection of free ICG can be performed only in the framework of clinical studies, after submission to local or national ethics committees, with the approval of the national regulatory and control services for the use of new pharmaceuticals. Furthermore, adequate insurance coverage is required, as well as informed consent from patients (taking into account the uncertainties regarding ICG toxicity), and the study must be undertaken without cost to the patients.

But the main problem with the NIR imaging of the lymphatic system with injection of free ICG will be—probably—related to the difficulties to perform some exact quantification. Quantitative parameters such as analyzing the frequency of the contractility of the lymphatic vessels, the speed of the lymph in the studied lymphatics, and numeration of the lymphatic vessels will be relatively easy and are ICG-independent; but we fear that many other quantitative approaches (and quantitative parameters used in lymphoscintigraphies) will raise and meet many difficulties. Quantifying the fluorescence with free ICG is possible, but it implies:

1. To apply strict conditions for the acquisitions (light in the room where the acquisition is performed, distance between the camera of the studied fluorescent area, the studied area has to be well centered)
2. To eventually adapt the characteristics of the NIR camera system (intensity of the light emitted) to obtain the best images of the studied structures.
3. To know what is measured, what are the exact amounts of ICG measured. A fixed concentration of ICG may be measurable with some acquisitions parameters of the camera but not with other parameters. Too high ICG concentration may be unmeasurable and too low, if these ICG concentrations are decreasing, may also become unmeasurable).
4. To keep in mind (a) that parameters "adequate" for very superficial structures might not be applicable for the (also of interest) surrounding fluorescent structures as far as they will be more deeply located and (b) that the deeper the fluorescent structures, the more attenuated the fluorescence,
5. To keep in mind that the quantification of the fluorescence in one lymphatic vessel does not correspond to the volume in the vessel (within the same volume, the fluorescence of the ICG will vary with its concentration).

Conclusion and Final Key Message

Lymphoscintigraphies have, until now, occupied a central place in the management of edema of suspected lymphatic origin. These imaging approaches have to be well understood by clinicians who request these exams, the specialists who perform them, and patients for whom they are proposed. Lymphoscintigraphy must be performed with care and thought, using available materials in the most appropriate ways, with the best applied methodological approaches, and always analyzed and interpreted taking into account the specific patient's situation and expectations and the clinician's demands. The specialist in Nuclear Medicine who performs lymphoscintigraphy also must integrate lymphoscintigraphic investigations into the growing field of other imaging techniques now proposed for investigating patients with edema, while never forgetting that the primary duty of a doctor of medicine is service to the patients.

Acknowledgements The author gratefully acknowledges Thomas-Baptiste De Brouwer for his "radio-physical" contribution for this article.

Declaration of conflict of interest: The author declares no conflict of interest (except may be in the "regard" of some, to be "specialist" in Nuclear Medicine …).

References

1. Bourgeois P, Leduc O, Belgrado JP, Leduc A. Imaging techniques in the prevention and management of post-therapeutic upper limb edemas? Cancer. 1998;83:2805–13.
2. Bourgeois P. Combined role of Lymphoscintigraphy, X-ray Computed Tomography, Magnetic Resonance Imaging and Positron Emission Tomography in the management of lymphadem013atous diseases. In: Lee BB, Bergan JJ, Rockson SG, editors. Lymphedema: a concise compendium of theory and practice. London: Springer; 2011;56–60.
3. Bourgeois P. Imaging the lymphatic system in 2011-2012. Lymphology. 2012;45(suppl):56–60.
4. Bourgeois P, Munck D, Leduc O, Leduc A. Oedème des membres et lymphoscintigraphies. Rev Med Brux. 2003;24(1):20–8. Review. French.
5. Szuba A, Shin WS, Strauss HW, Rockson S. The third circulation: radionuclide lymphoscintigraphy in the evaluation of lymphedema. J Nucl Med. 2003;44:43–57.
6. Scarsbrook AF, Ganeshan A, Bradley KM. Pearls and pitfalls of radionuclide imaging of the lymphatic system. Part 2: evaluation of extremity lymphoedema. Br J Radiol. 2007;80:219–26.
7. Pecking AP, Albérini JL, Wartski M, Edeline V, Cluzan RV. Relationship between lymphoscintigraphy and clinical findings in lower limb lymphedema: towards a comprehensive staging. Lymphology. 2008;41:1–10.
8. Baulieu F, Bourgeois P, Maruani A, Belgrado JP, Tauveron V, Lorette G, Vaillant L. Contributions of SPECT/CT Imaging to the lymphoscintigraphic investigations of the lower limb lymphedema. Lymphology. 2013;46:106–19.
9. Mortimer PS, Simmonds R, Rezvani M, Robbins R, Hopewell JW, Ryan TJ. The measurement of skin lymph flow by isotope clearanc: reliability, reproducibility, and the effect of massage. J Invest Dermatol. 1990;95:677–82. doi:10.1111/1523-1747.ep12514347.
10. Modi S, Stanton AWB, Svensson WE, Peters AM, Mortimer PS, Levick JR. Human lymphatic pumping measured in healthy and lymphedematous arms by lymphatic congestion lymphoscintigraphy. J Physiol. 2007;583:271–85.
11. Modi S, Stanton AW, Mortimer PS, Levick JR. Clinical assessment of human lymph flow using removal rate constants of interstitial macromolecules: a critical review of lymphoscintigraphy. Lymphat Res Biol. 2007;5(3):183–202. Review.
12. Fowler JC, Britton TB, Provenzano E, Ravichandran D, Lawrence D, Solanki CK, Ballinger JR, Douglas-Jones A, Mortimer PS, Purushotham AD, Peters AM. Measurement of lymph node function from the extraction of immunoglobulin in lymph. Scand J Clin Lab Invest. 2010;70(2):112–5. doi:10.3109/00365510903572040.
13. Burnand KM, Glass DM, Mortimer PS, Peters AM. Lymphatic dysfunction in the apparently clinically normal contralateral limbs of patients with unilateral lower limb swelling. Clin Nucl Med. 2012;37(1):9–13. doi:10.1097/RLU.0b013e31823931f5.
14. Bourgeois P, Munck D, Becker C, Leduc O, Leduc A. Evaluation of a three-phase lymphoscintigraphic investigation protocol of the lower limbedemas. Eur J Lymphol Related Problems. 1997;VI/21:22–8.
15. Belnuc. How I do it…. Procédures détaillées. http://www.belnuc.be/index.php?option=com_content&task=view&id=66&Itemid=74, accessed, 11/2014.
16. Bourgeois P. Critical analysis of the literature on lymphoscintigraphic investigations of limbedemas. Eur J Lymphol Related Problems. 1997;VI/21:1–21.
17. Bourgeois P, Leduc O, Belgrado JP, Leduc A. Scintigraphic investigations of the superficial lymphatic system: quantitative differences between intradermal and subcutaneous injections. Nucl Med Commun. 2009;30(4):270–4.
18. Bourgeois P. Scintigraphic investigations of the lymphatic system: the influence of the injected volume and quantity of labeled colloidal tracer. J Nucl Med. 2007;48:693–5.
19. Bräutigam P, Hogerle S, Reunhardt M, Otte A, Van Scheidt W, Föedli E, Moser E. The quantitative Two-Compartment Lymphoscintigraphy for evaluation of the lower limb edema. Eur J Lymphol Related Problems. 1997;VI/21:47–51.
20. Wolfe JHN, Kinmonth JB. The prognosis of primary lymphedema of the lower limbs. Arch Surg. 1981;116(9):1157–60. doi:10.1001/archsurg.1981.01380210037007.
21. Kleinhans E, Baumeister RGH, Hahn D, Siuda S, Büll U, Moser E. Evaluation of transport kinetics in lymphoscintigraphy: Follow-up study in patients with transplanted lymphatic vessels. Eur J Nucl Med. 1985;10:349–52.
22. Nawaz MK, Hamad MM, Abdel-Dayem HM, Sadek S, Eklof BG. Lymphoscintigraphy in lymphedema of the lower limbs using 99mTc-HSA. Angiology. 1992;43(2):147–54.

23. Davies-Venn CA, Angermiller B, Wilganowski N, Ghosh P, Harvey BR, Wu G, Kwon S, Aldrich MB, Sevick-Muraca EM. Albumin-binding domain conjugate for near-infrared fluorescence lymphatic imaging. Mol Imaging Biol. 2012;14(3):301–14. doi:10.1007/s11307-011-0499-x.

24. Heuveling DA, Visser GWM, de Groot M, de Boer JF, Baclayon M, Roos WH, Wuite GJL, Leemans CR, de Bree R, van Dongen GAMS. Nanocolloidal albumin-IRDye 800CW: a near-infrared fluorescent tracer with optimal retention in the sentinel lymph node. Eur J Nucl Med Mol Imaging. 2012;39(7):1161–8.

25. Marshall MV, Rasmussen JC, Tan IC, Aldrich MB, Adams KE, Wang X, Fife CE, Maus EA, Smith A, Sevick-Muraca EM. Near-infrared Fluorescence Imaging in Humans with Indocyanine Green: a Review and Update. Open Surg Oncol J. 2010;2(2):12–25.

26. Gandorfer A, Haritoglou C, Kampik A. Toxicity of Indocyanine Green in vitro-retinal surgery. Dev Ophtalmol. 2008;42:69–81.

27. Weiler M, Dixon JB. Differential transport function of lymphatic vessels in the rat tail models and the long-term effects of Indocyanine Green as assessed with near-infrared imaging. Front Physiol. 2013;4:1–10.

28. Gashev AA, Nagai T, Bridenbaugh EA. Indocyanine Green and lymphatic imaging: current problems. Lymphat Res Biol. 2010;8:127–30.

29. Zhang J, Zhou SK, Xiang X, Bautista ML, Niccum BA, Dickinson GS, Tan IC, Chan W, Sevick-Muraca EM, Rasmussen JC. Automated analysis of investigational near-infrared fluorescence lymphatic imaging in humans. Biomed Opt Express. 2012;3(7):1713–23. doi:10.1364/BOE.3.001713. Epub 2012 Jun 22.

30. Bourgeois P, Belgrado JP, Aerens C. La lymphoscintigraphie dans la prise en charge thérapeutique des œdèmes des membres par les soins de santé en Belgique. Médecine Nucléaire. 2010;34(12):675–82.

31. The 2007 Recommendations of the International Commission on Radiological Protection, ICRP Publication 103. Ann ICRP 2007;37(2-4). http://www.icrp.org/publication.asp?id=ICRP%20Publication%20103

32. Rapport UNSCEAR 2000, Annex D: Medical Radiation Exposures. http://www.unscear.org/docs/reports/annexd.pdf, Table 19, p385.

33. Safety Reports Series No. 58, Radiation Protection in Newer Medical Imaging Techniques: PET/CT, IAEA, pg 17. http://www.irsn.fr/FR/Larecherche/publications-documentation/collection-ouvrages-IRSN/Documents/CIPR_103.pdf, pg 53, 2007.

34. Rapport UNSCEAR 2000: Annex B: Exposures from natural radiation sources

35. U.S. Department of Labor, Bureau of Labor Statistics (BLS)-Census of Fatal Occupational Injuries 2014. Deaths: Preliminary Data for 2011. Donna L. Hoyert and Jiaquan Xu, National Vital Statistics Reports, October 2012;61(6):4 (Table B).

36. Census of Fatal Occupational Injuries 2014. U.S. Department of Labor, Bureau of Labor Statistics (BLS). www.cfoi_rates_2013hb.pdf.

37. WHO Disease and injury country estimates. World Health Organization, 2004. http://www.who.int/healthinfo/global_burden_disease/estimates_country/en/ Retrieved November 11, 2009

38. Carena M, Campini R, Zelaschi G, Rossi G, Aprile C, Paroni G. Quantitative lymphoscintigraphy. Eur J Nucl Med. 1988;14(2):88–92.

39. Golucke PJ, Montgomery RA, Petronis JD, Minken SL, Perler BA, Williams GM. Lymphoscintigraphy to confirm the clinical diagnosis of lymphedema. J Vasc Surg. 1989;10(3):306–12.

40. Ter SE, Alavi A, Kim CK, Merli G. Lymphoscintigraphy. A reliable test for the diagnosis of lymphedema. Clin Nucl Med. 1993;18(8):646–54.

41. Weissleder H, Weissleder R. Lymphedema: evaluation of qualitative and quantitative lymphoscintigraphy in 238 patients. Radiology. 1988;167(3):729–35.

42. Nawaz MK, Hamad MM, Abdel-Dayem HM, Sadek S, Eklof BG. Lymphoscintigraphy in lymphedema of the lower limbs using 99mTc HSA. Angiology. 1992;43(2):147–54.

43. Cambria RA, Gloviczki P, Naessens JM, Wahner HW. Noninvasive evaluation of the lymphatic system with lymphoscintigraphy: a prospective, semiquantitative analysis in 386 extremities. J Vasc Surg. 1993;18(5):773–82.

Differential Diagnosis of Lymphedema

16

Arin K. Greene

Key Points

- "Lymphedema" is a specific condition and should not be used as a generic term to describe any patient with extremity overgrowth.
- Lymphoscintigraphy should be used to differentiate lymphedema from other causes of extremity overgrowth.
- Lymphedema is isolated to the skin and subcutis; if structures below the muscle fascia are involved, then the patient has a condition other than lymphedema.
- It is important to determine whether or not a patient has lymphedema so that they receive proper counseling and treatment.

Introduction

The term "lymphedema" often is used to describe overgrowth of an extremity, regardless of the underlying etiology. Lymphedema is a much more prevalent condition than other causes of limb overgrowth, and thus, physicians are most familiar with the term "lymphedema." A similar paradigm occurs in the field of vascular anomalies, where any type of lesion frequently is labeled as a "hemangioma"

[1]. Lymphedema, however, is a specific disease that causes chronic progressive swelling because of inadequate lymphatic function. Lymphedema may result from anomalous lymphatic development (*primary*) or injury to lymph nodes or lymphatic vessels (*secondary*).

Because various disorders can appear clinically similar, lymphedema often is confused with other etiologies that may cause limb overgrowth. For example, in a review of 170 pediatric patients referred to our vascular anomalies center with a diagnosis of "lymphedema," 27 % had another condition (Table 16.1) [2]. In the pediatric population 70 % of conditions mistaken for lymphedema are other types of vascular anomalies (i.e., micro/macrocystic lymphatic malformation, non-eponymous combined vascular malformation, diffuse capillary malformation with overgrowth, Klippel–Trénaunay syndrome, Parkes Weber syndrome, venous malformation, infantile hemangioma, kaposiform hemangioendothelioma [2]. Other conditions mistaken for lymphedema in children include: hemi-hypertrophy, posttraumatic swelling, lipedema, rheumatologic disease, and lipofibromatosis [2]. In another study of both children and adults referred to a Lymphedema Center, we found that 25 % of the patients had another condition [3]. In the adult population, conditions that were confused with lymphedema included: venous stasis disease, lipedema, obesity, systemic diseases (e.g., cardiac, renal, hepatic, rheumatological), and trauma (Table 16.2) [3].

A.K. Greene, M.D., M.M.Sc. (✉)
Department of Plastic and Oral Surgery,
Boston Children's Hospital, Harvard Medical School,
300 Longwood Avenue, Boston, MA 02115, USA
e-mail: arin.greene@childrens.harvard.edu

A.K. Greene et al. (eds.), *Lymphedema: Presentation, Diagnosis, and Treatment*,
DOI 10.1007/978-3-319-14493-1_16, © Springer International Publishing Switzerland 2015

Table 16.1 Diagnosis of an overgrown limb referred to a vascular anomalies center incorrectly labeled as "lymphedema"

Micro/macrocystic lymphatic malformation	19.6 %
Non-eponymous combined vascular malformation	13.0 %
Klippel–Trénaunay syndrome	10.9 %
Capillary malformation	10.9 %
Hemihypertrophy	8.7 %
Posttraumatic swelling	8.7 %
Parkes Weber syndrome	6.5 %
Lipedema	6.5 %
Venous malformation	4.3 %
Rheumatologic disease	4.3 %
Infantile hemangioma	2.2 %
Kaposiform hemangioendothelioma	2.2 %
Lipofibromatosis	2.2 %

With permission from Schook CC, Mulliken JB, Fishman SJ, Alomari AI, Grant FD, Greene AK. Differential diagnosis of lower extremity enlargement in pediatric patients referred with a diagnosis of lymphedema. Plast Reconstr Surg 2011;127:1571–1581 © Wolters Kluwer in 2011 [2]

Table 16.2 Diagnosis of patients referred to a lymphedema center with an enlarged extremity (n=217)

		≤21 years (n=61) (%)	>21 years (n=156) (%)
Total (%)			
Lymphedema	75	90	69
Venous stasis	7	0	10
Lipedema	6	0	8
Obesity	4	0	6
Injury	4	4	4
Rheumatological disease	3	3	3
Vascular malformation	1	3	0

With permission from Maclellan RA, Couto RA, Sullivan JE, Grant FD, Slavin SA, Greene AK. Management of primary and secondary lymphedema: analysis of 225 referrals to a center. Ann Plast Surg 2014 Apr 8 [Epub ahead of print] © Wolters Kluwer in 2014 [3]

Accurately diagnosing a patient with lymphedema is necessary in order to be able to counsel the individual and family about the prognosis and treatment of the disease. As we previously have shown for infantile hemangioma, if a disease is called by the incorrect name, the patient is more likely to receive erroneous (and potentially harmful) treatment [1]. Consequently, the burden is on the health care provider to determine whether an individual with an overgrown extremity does, in fact, have lymphedema. The prognosis and management of lymphedema can be very different than for other conditions. For example, a patient with diffuse capillary malformation is not at risk for infection and may have a leg-length discrepancy (in contrast to an individual with lymphedema).

Diagnosis of Lymphedema

History

Ninety percent of patients with lymphedema may be diagnosed by history and physical examination. In the pediatric population, at least 97 % of children have idiopathic, primary disease (Fig. 16.1); only 3 % have secondary lymphedema from injury to axillary or inguinal lymph nodes [4]. Primary lymphedema affects approximately 1/100,000 children [5]. Boys are most likely to present during infancy and have bilateral lower extremity disease [4]. Girls usually develop swelling in adolescence; typically only one lower extremity is involved [4]. Males most commonly present with lymphedema in infancy (68.0 %), compared to childhood (12.0 %) or adolescence (20.0 %) [4]. The median age when males and females develop lymphedema is <12 months and 10 years, respectively [4]. Boys and girls are equally at risk for developing primary lymphedema, and thus, the gender of the patient does not heighten the suspicion for lymphedema [4]. Idiopathic upper extremity or generalized lymphedema is rare. Children with primary lymphedema have an 11 % chance of having hereditary and/or syndromic lymphedema (e.g., Milroy, Noonan, Meige, lymphedema–distichiasis, Turner, Hennekam) [4]. If a child has a parent with lymphedema, it is very likely that the patient also has the condition because many syndromic causes of lymphedema are hereditary.

In the adult population, secondary lymphedema accounts for approximately 99 % of cases (Fig. 16.2). Adult-onset primary lymphedema is rare. Patients are asked about a history of injury to the axillary or inguinal nodes (e.g., lymphadenopathy, radiation, operations). If they have had a significant trauma to the axillary or

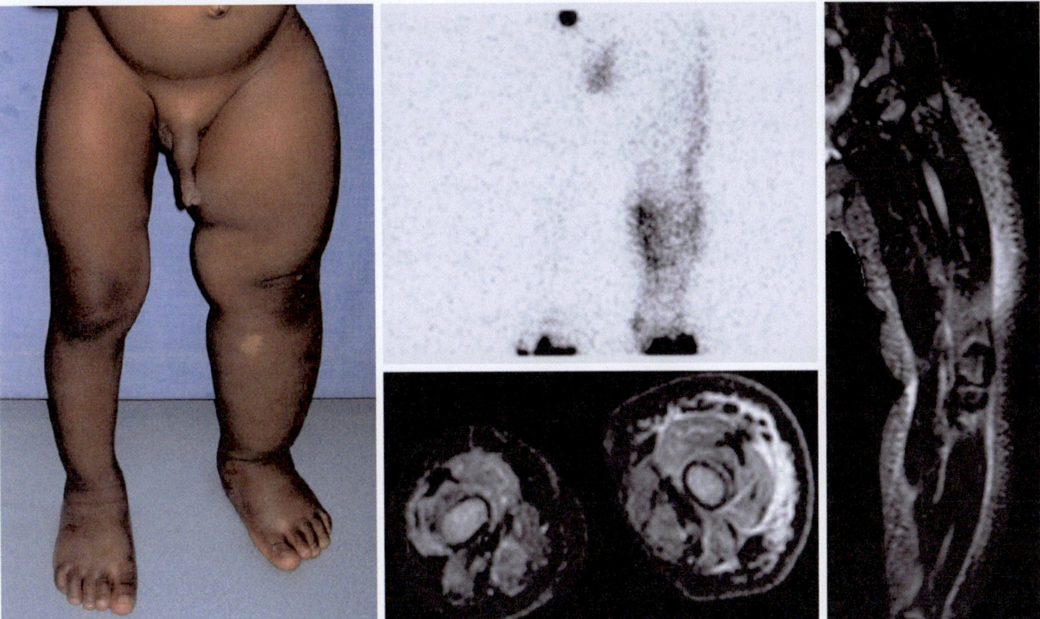

Fig. 16.1 Primary lymphedema. 2-year-old male with left lower extremity swelling since birth. Lymphoscintigram demonstrates dermal backflow and absent inguinal node drainage 2.5 h after injection. Axial T2-weighted MR with fat saturation shows a hyperintense reticular network of dilated subcutaneous channels between the dermis and fascial plane. With permission from Schook CC, Mulliken JB, Fishman SJ, Alomari AI, Grant FD, Greene AK. Differential diagnosis of lower extremity enlargement in pediatric patients referred with a diagnosis of lymphedema. Plast Reconstr Surg 2011;127:1571–1581 © Wolters Kluwer in 2011 [2]

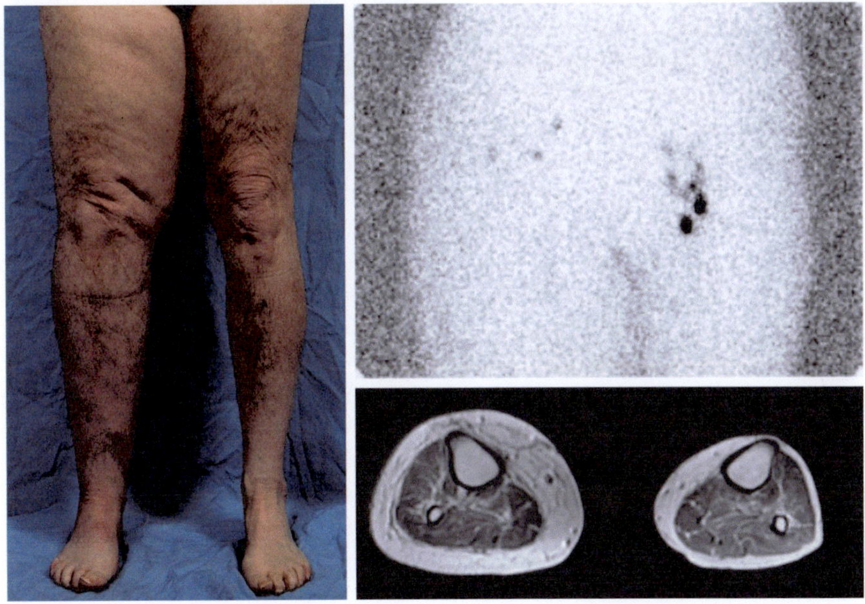

Fig. 16.2 Secondary lymphedema. Adult male with a history of right inguinal lymphadenectomy for cancer. Lymphoscintigram shows minimal drainage on the right side 1 h after injection. MRI illustrates thickening of the subcutaneous fat with edema

inguinal nodes, then the likelihood that they have lymphedema is increased. Adults are also queried about systemic diseases (e.g., congestive heart failure, renal failure, hepatic dysfunction, rheumatological disorders) and history of extremity trauma. Patient body mass index (BMI) is recorded; if it is greater than 60, then it is probable that the individual has obesity-induced lymphedema [6, 7].

If a patient has a history of infections involving the extremity, then it is more likely that he/she has lymphedema because individuals with lymphedema have a significantly increased risk of infection in the affected limb. Because the most common cause of lymphedema worldwide is a parasitic infection, families are queried about a history of travel to areas endemic for filariasis. If the patient has resided in an area endemic for filariasis, then the probability that the individual has lymphedema is increased.

Physical Examination

Primary lymphedema affects an extremity in 95.7 % of children [4]. The lower limb is most often involved (91.7 %), and 9.4 % have both upper and lower extremity swelling [4]. Bilateral disease is more likely in patients presenting in infancy (62.9 %) or childhood (66.7 %), versus adolescence (30.8 %) [4]. There is no difference in bilateral lymphedema between the upper extremities (63.6 %) or lower extremities (52.9 %), or in females (49.4 %) compared to males (49.0 %) [4]. Bilateral disease is more common in patients presenting in infancy (62.9 %) or childhood (66.7 %), versus adolescence (30.8 %) [4]. Genital lymphedema occurs in 18.1 % of patients with primary lymphedema; 4.3 % of males have isolated involvement and 13.8 % have genital and lower extremity lymphedema [4]. Males are more likely than females to have genital lymphedema (36.8 % versus 4.9 %) [4].

Lymphedema almost universally affects the distal extremity and then migrates proximally. If a patient does not have distal limb swelling, it is very unlikely that he/she has lymphedema. A fairly sensitive and specific sign for lymphedema is the Stemmer sign. If the examiner is unable to pinch the skin on the dorsum of the hand or foot (positive Stemmer sign), then it is likely the patient has lymphedema [8]. Chronic swelling, inflammation, and adipose deposition cause the skin to thicken which reduces the ability to lift and pinch the integument of the distal extremity. Patients also are examined for scars in the axillary or inguinal regions, which may represent injury to lymph nodes in these regions. Lymphedema is typically a painless condition and cutaneous ulceration is uncommon. Overlying skin discoloration can occur, but is unusual. Lymphedema does not affect the underlying bone, and thus, patients do not have a leg-length discrepancy. Over time, individuals with lymphedema can develop lymphatic vesicles, usually involving the toes, which can bleed and leak lymph fluid (lymphorrhea).

Imaging

Because lymphedema easily can be confused with other causes of extremity overgrowth, we have a low threshold to obtain a lymphoscintigram to: (1) confirm or rule-out the disease, and (2) assess the degree of lymphatic dysfunction in patients who have a high likelihood of having the condition. Lymphoscintigraphy is 92 % sensitive and 100 % specific for lymphedema [9]. Although MRI and CT are non-diagnostic for lymphedema, findings consistent with the condition include: (1) subcutaneous adipose tissue overgrowth, (2) edema, (3) thickened skin, and (4) findings isolated to soft-tissue above the muscle fascia [2]. Typically, subcutaneous adipose hypertrophy and fluid findings are symmetrical and circumferential. A key finding is that lymphedema does not affect structures beneath the muscle fascia. If a patient has a normal lymphoscintigram and/or their disease involves muscle or bone, then it is very unlikely the patient has lymphedema.

Differential Diagnosis of Lymphedema

Capillary Malformation

A diffuse capillary malformation of an extremity can cause circumferential and longitudinal limb enlargement (Fig. 16.3) [4, 10]. These children have diffuse capillary malformation with overgrowth (DCMO). Capillary malformation is caused by a somatic mutation in *GNAQ*. Unlike lymphedema, the underlying bone is involved and patients are monitored for a leg-length discrepancy [2]. The capillary malformation causes progressive overgrowth of the underlying subcutaneous adipose tissue which generally results in circumferential and symmetrical growth. Occasionally, hypertrophy of tissues beneath the stain can be localized. Patients have normal lymphatic function by lymphoscintigraphy and do not have an increased risk of infection. Patients are managed using pulsed-dye laser to lighten the cutaneous stain, liposuction to debulk the subcutaneous adipose hypertrophy, and orthopedic procedures to address the bony overgrowth.

CLOVES Syndrome

CLOVES syndrome (*C*ongenital *L*ipomatosis, *O*vergrowth, *V*ascular malformations, *E*pidermal nevi, and *S*coliosis/*S*keletal/*S*pinal anomalies) is a non-familial condition caused by a *PIK3CA* mutation. Major features include: (1) a truncal lipomatous mass, (2) a slow-flow vascular malformation (typically a capillary malformation overlying the lipomatous mass), and (3) hand/foot anomalies (increased width, macrodactyly, first web-space sandal gap) [11]. Less common

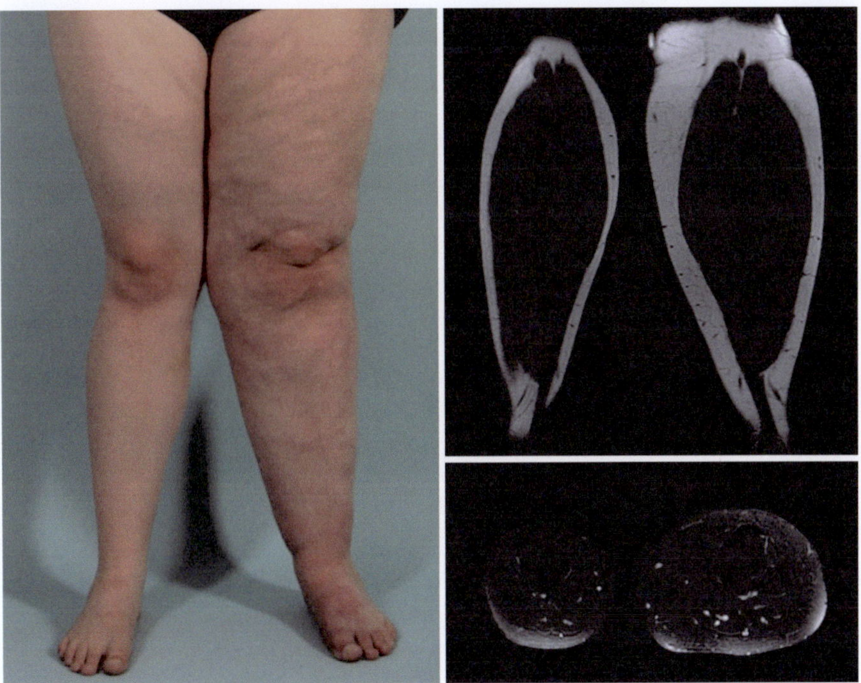

Fig. 16.3 Capillary malformation. 24-year-old female with a diffuse capillary malformation of the skin and subcutaneous adipose overgrowth of the left lower extremity. MRI shows thickening of the subcutaneous fat without edema

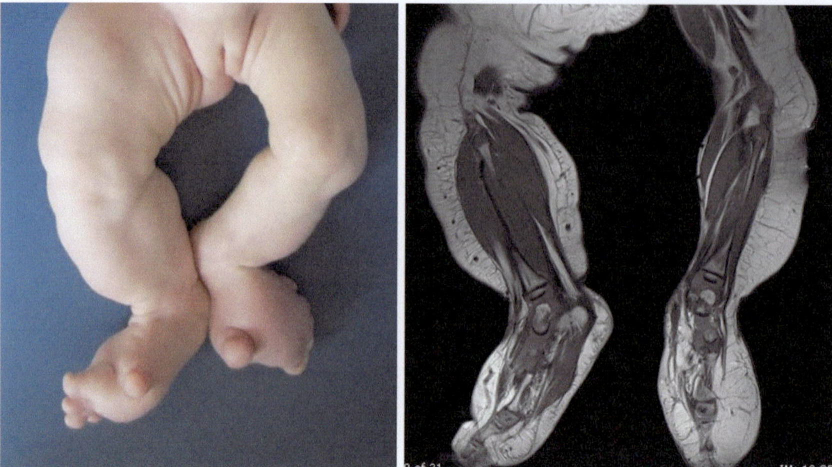

Fig. 16.4 CLOVES syndrome. In contrast to lymphedema, the right leg has asymmetrical overgrowth of all structures (skin, subcutis, muscle, and bone) and the patient has bilateral foot anomalies

findings include paraspinal fast-flow malformations, linear epidermal nevus, and hemihypertrophy. Children are at risk for developing Wilms tumor and thus require renal ultrasound examination every 3 months until they reach 8 years of age. Central and thoracic phlebectasia can cause pulmonary embolism. Extremity overgrowth is typically hemihypertrophy affecting all tissues of the extremity (skin, subcutis, muscle, and bone) (Fig. 16.4). Orthopedic consultation is obtained to determine whether a leg-length discrepancy is present. Patients may require soft-tissue debulking or amputations to facilitate shoewear and/or ambulation.

Hemihypertrophy

Hemihypertrophy is the idiopathic enlargement of an area compared to the contralateral side (Fig. 16.5). It is a rare condition that is present at birth [2, 12]. All components of an extremity are overgrown (i.e., bone, muscle, subcutis, skin). Imaging studies do not exhibit pathological findings other than enlarged structures [2]. Lymphatic function and lymphoscintigraphy are normal. Hemihypertrophy is usually a diagnosis of exclusion. Because the bone may be involved, children can have a leg-length discrepancy that necessitates orthopedic intervention. Circumferential

overgrowth can be improved by removing subcutaneous adipose tissue using suction-assisted lipectomy. Because patients are at risk for Wilms tumor, they must undergo renal ultrasound screening.

Infantile Hemangioma

Rarely, an infantile hemangioma can be diffuse and cause overgrowth of an extremity (Fig. 16.6). These lesions are differentiated from lymphedema because they grow rapidly during the first few months of life, then stabilize, and regress after 12 months of age [13]. "Reticular" hemangioma involves the lower extremity and can be infiltrative and involve fascia or muscle [14]. These children are at risk for underlying urogenital anomalies, and thus, ultrasound and/or MRI is considered. Infantile hemangiomas may ulcerate and/or cause congestive heart failure. Large, symptomatic tumors are managed with prednisolone or propranolol. Residual telangiectasias are treated with pulsed-dye laser.

Kaposiform Hemangioendothelioma

Kaposiform hemangioendothelioma is a rare vascular neoplasm that is locally aggressive, but

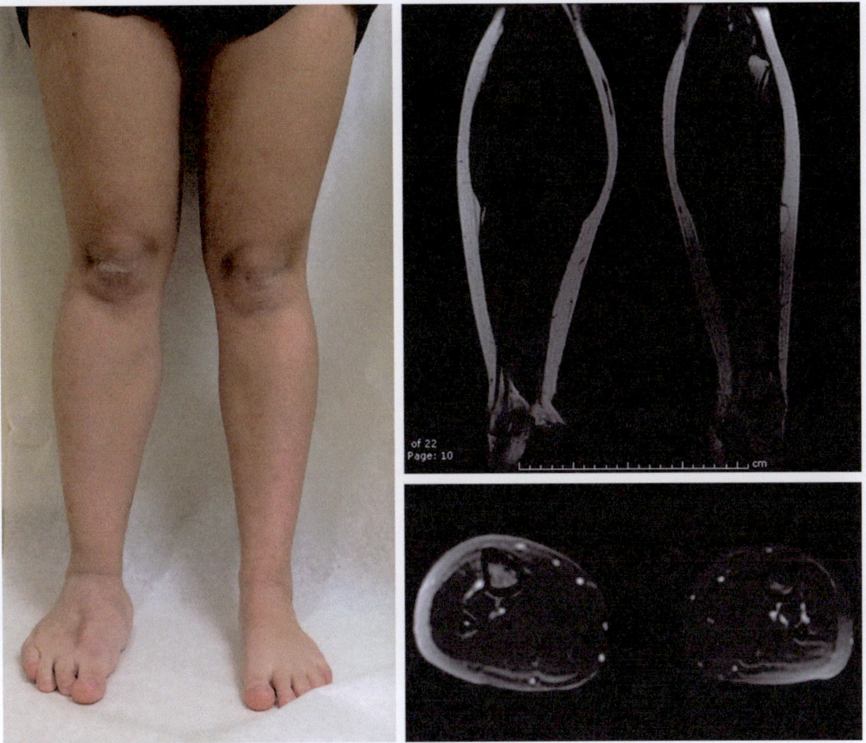

Fig. 16.5 Hemihypertrophy. 15-year-old female with right lower extremity hemihypertrophy diagnosed at birth. She was screened for Wilms tumor and had a ray amputa- tion to facilitate her ability to wear shoes. MRI demonstrates overgrowth of the subcutaneous fat, muscle, and bone

does not metastasize (Fig. 16.7). It affects approximately 1/100,000 persons (similar to primary lymphedema) [15]. Sixty percent are present at birth, and 93 % are diagnosed during infancy [15]. The tumor is often diffuse, and an extremity is affected in approximately one-third of patients. The lesion slowly enlarges during the first 2 years of life and then partially regresses. Kaposiform hemangioendothelioma frequently persists long-term and can cause chronic pain, stiffness, and contractures. The skin is reddish-purple, and pain is common. Seventy percent of patients have Kasabach–Merritt phenomenon (KMP) (thrombocytopenia <25,000/mm, [3] petechiae, bleeding), which is pathognomonic for the condition [15]. Kaposiform hemangioendothelioma also has a lymphatic component, which stains positive for the lymphatic markers D240 and PROX1. Most patient with kaposiform hemangioendothelioma are treated to prevent life-threatening complications from Kasabach–Merritt phenomenon and to minimize long-term pain and contractures. Management includes either vincristine or sirolimus [13]. Resection is rarely possible because the tumor involves multiple tissue planes and important structures.

Klippel–Trénaunay Syndrome

Like "lymphedema" and "hemangioma," Klippel–Trénaunay syndrome is often used mistakenly to label many types of overgrowth conditions. Patients with Klippel–Trénaunay syndrome typically have: (1) lower extremity overgrowth, (2) a cutaneous stain, (3) lymphatic malformations, and (4) venous malformations (Fig. 16.8) [16]. Rarely, the upper extremity is involved (5 %) and a limb may be hypoplastic (10 %). The contralateral extremity may be enlarged and

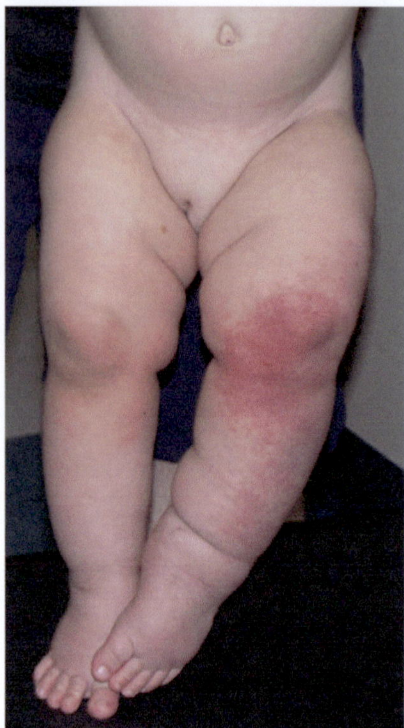

Fig. 16.6 Infantile hemangioma. 3-month-old with a reticular infantile hemangioma of the left lower extremity that appeared shortly after birth. The red appearance of the skin and rapid postnatal progression was inconsistent with lymphedema, but typical for infantile hemangioma. With permission from Schook CC, Mulliken JB, Fishman SJ, Alomari AI, Grant FD, Greene AK. Differential diagnosis of lower extremity enlargement in pediatric patients referred with a diagnosis of lymphedema. Plast Reconstr Surg 2011;127:1571–1581 © Wolters Kluwer in 2011 [2]

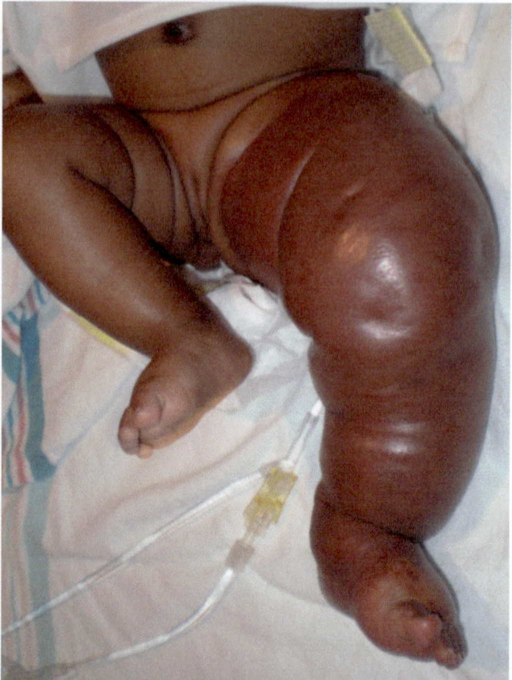

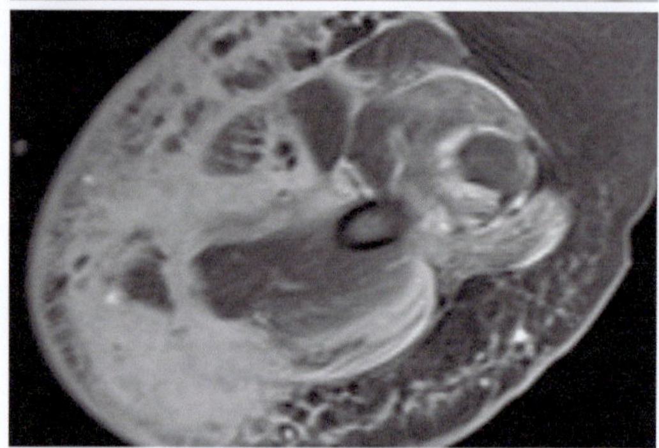

Fig. 16.7 Kaposiform hemangioendothelioma. 3-month-old with kaposiform hemangioendothelioma diagnosed by history, physical examination, and laboratory findings. The patient suffered from diffuse discoloration of the extremity, bruising, and thrombocytopenia which do not occur with lymphedema. With permission from Schook CC, Mulliken JB, Fishman SJ, Alomari AI, Grant FD, Greene AK. Differential diagnosis of lower extremity enlargement in pediatric patients referred with a diagnosis of lymphedema. Plast Reconstr Surg 2011;127:1571–1581 © Wolters Kluwer in 2011 [2]

exhibit macrodactyly. The venous component of Klippel–Trénaunay syndrome manifests as phlebectasia and abnormal drainage. An embryonal vein of Servelle in the subcutaneous tissue or the lateral calf and thigh is pathognomonic for the condition. On MRI a deep venous system typically is not illustrated. The lymphatic malformation usually is microcystic in the extremity and involves the skin. Klippel–Trénaunay syndrome is not isolated to the subcutis, but involves tissues below the muscle fascia (including muscle and bone). Patients are at risk for a pulmonary embolus from the embryonal vein, which is usually ablated. Staged subcutaneous resections of circumferentially overgrown tissues may be needed to facilitate wearing clothes and ambulation. A shoe-lift or epiphysiodesis is often necessary to correct leg-length discrepancy. Selective amputations may be required to permit footwear and to facilitate ambulation. Children are not at risk for Wilms tumor, and thus do not require screening [17].

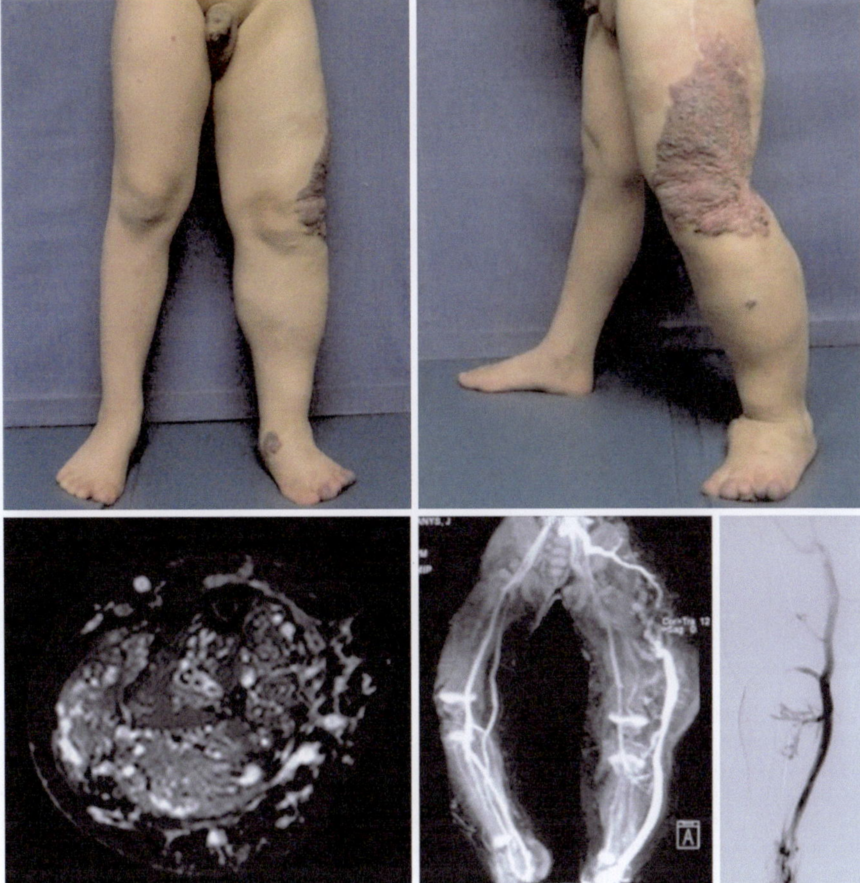

Fig. 16.8 Klippel–Trénaunay syndrome. 6-year-old male with a capillary–venous–lymphatic malformation of the left lower extremity causing overgrowth. MR image shows a diffuse vascular malformation involving tissues above and below the muscle fascia. MR venogram illustrates a lateral embryonic vein. Venography delineates the anatomy of the marginal vein of Servelle. With permission from Greene AK. Vascular Anomalies: Classification, Diagnosis, and Management. © CRC Press, Boca Raton, FL in 2013 [26]

Lipedema

Although lipedema is often used to describe lower extremity overgrowth in obese patients, it is a specific disease (Fig. 16.9). Lipedema is a disorder that begins in adolescence and affects both lower limbs of females [18]. The condition is often familial. Unlike obese patients who have excess subcutaneous adipose tissue throughout their body (including their legs), females with lipedema have a lipodystrophy that is isolated to their legs (the rest of their body does not have adipose overgrowth and is normally proportioned). Unlike morbid obesity, weight loss does not significantly improve the lower extremity adipose hypertrophy. In contrast to lymphedema, lipedema is painful. Patients with lipedema have a key physical examination; the adipose overgrowth stops at the ankle (the feet are normal) and patients have a negative Stemmer sign. MRI shows increased subcutaneous adipose tissue without stranding or thickened skin; lymphoscintigraphy is normal [2]. The condition may be improved using suction-assisted lipectomy.

Lipofibromatosis

Lipofibromatosis is a rare, benign neoplasm that, when diffuse, can cause enlargement of the upper

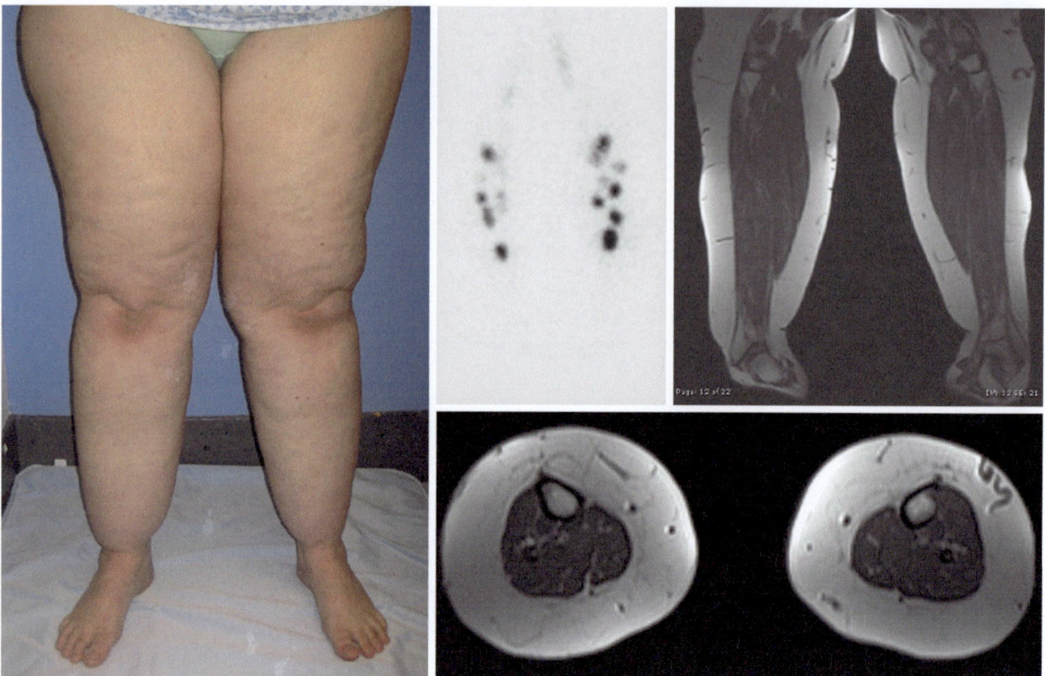

Fig. 16.9 Lipedema. Example of a patient with lipedema referred with a mistaken diagnosis of "lymphedema." 34-year-old female with enlarged lower extremities since adolescence. Because the feet were not involved, it was diagnosed as lipedema by physical examination and confirmed with imaging. Lymphoscintigram was normal (prompt tracer uptake into abdominal nodes bilaterally), and coronal T1-weighted MR showed circumferential overgrowth of the subcutaneous fat. With permission from Schook CC, Mulliken JB, Fishman SJ, Alomari AI, Grant FD, Greene AK. Differential diagnosis of lower extremity enlargement in pediatric patients referred with a diagnosis of lymphedema. Plast Reconstr Surg 2011;127:1571–1581 © Wolters Kluwer in 2011 [2]

or lower extremity (Fig. 16.10) [19, 20]. It is not aggressive and does not metastasize. The limb usually is enlarged at birth or by early childhood; subcutaneous fatty overgrowth is the predominant finding. Lipofibromatosis can involve the subfascial compartments and cause bony overgrowth; the distal extremity may be spared. Diagnosis is confirmed by histopathologic examination showing abundant adipose tissue, spindled fibroblasts, focal fascicular growth, and limited mitotic activity. Patients with lower extremity involvement are monitored for a leg-length discrepancy. Suction-assisted lipectomy can improve limb contour [19, 20].

Lymphatic Malformation

Lymphatic malformation results from an error in embryogenesis of the lymphatic system. There are four major phenotypes: macrocystic, microcystic, primary lymphedema, and generalized [21]. Macrocystic lymphatic malformation contains cysts that are able to be treated with sclerotherapy. Microcystic lymphatic malformation has small cysts that are not able to be treated with sclerotherapy. Primary lymphedema is a type of lymphatic malformation because the lymphatics in the extremity were malformed at birth, and are usually hypoplastic. Primary lymphedema differs from microcystic, macrocystic, and combined lymphatic malformations because it is not cystic, and only involves the subcutaneous tissues. Micro/macrocystic lymphatic malformation can be infiltrative and affect all structures of the extremity, including muscle and bone (Fig. 16.11). Microcystic lymphatic malformation is a localized lesion that may or may not affect the distal extremity. Unlike lymphedema, microcystic

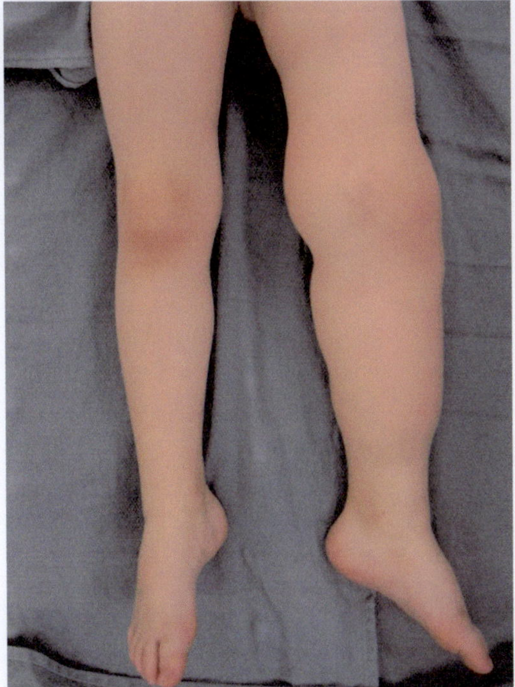

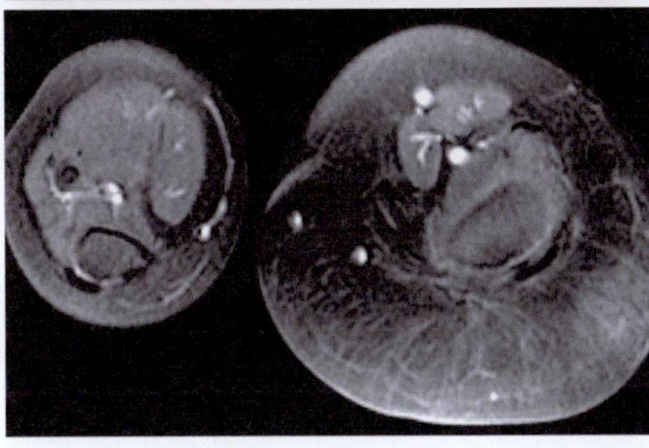

Fig. 16.10 Lipofibromatosis. 5-year-old with lipofibromatosis. Because history, physical examination, and MRI were inconclusive, biopsies were obtained. The diagnosis was made histopathologically. With permission from Schook CC, Mulliken JB, Fishman SJ, Alomari AI, Grant FD, Greene AK. Differential diagnosis of lower extremity enlargement in pediatric patients referred with a diagnosis of lymphedema. Plast Reconstr Surg 2011;127:1571–1581 © Wolters Kluwer in 2011 [2]

lymphatic malformation does not cause symmetrical involvement of only the subcutaneous tissue. Several germ-line mutations cause primary lymphedema (*VEGFR3, FOXC2, SOX18, CCBE1*). In contrast, micro/macrocystic lymphatic malformations result from a somatic mosaic mutation in *PIK3CA*. Symptomatic micro/macrocystic lymphatic malformations of the lower extremity are managed by compression, sclerotherapy, and/or resection.

Non-eponymous Combined Vascular Malformation

Non-eponymous combined malformations include lesions that contain more than one type of vascular anomaly, but do not fit a syndromic designation such as Klippel–Trénaunay Syndrome or Parkes Weber Syndrome. The two most common examples are capillary–venous malformation and lymphatic–venous malformation (Fig. 16.12). Like single vessel vascular malformations, these lesions can cause extremity overgrowth [2]. Typically, non-eponymous combined malformations affect the integument as well as tissues below the muscle fascia. Diagnosis is made by physical examination and MRI. Treatment is similar to single vessel vascular malformations, and is based on the predominant/symptomatic component.

Obesity

Morbidly obese patients have extra subcutaneous adipose deposition throughout their body, including their legs. Enlargement of the legs in individuals with morbid obesity differs from patients with lipedema, who have a true lipodystrophy that only affects the legs (and begins in puberty when the patient is not obese). Unlike lymphedema, which can affect only one limb, obesity affects both lower extremities. Patients with a body mass index less than 50 have normal lymphatic function and lymphoscintigram findings (Fig. 16.13) [6, 7]. Morbid obesity does not affect lymphatic function until the body mass index reaches a threshold between 54 and 60 [6, 7]. Once the body mass index reaches 60, secondary lymphedema occurs [6, 7]. The mechanism by which extreme obesity can cause lymphedema still remains to be elucidated. Treatment for leg overgrowth from obesity is weight loss.

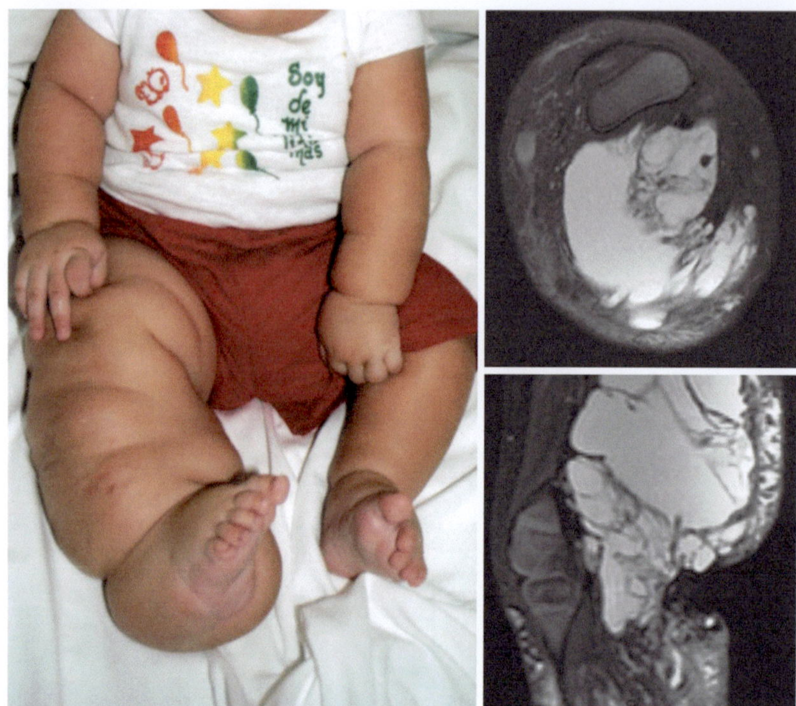

Fig. 16.11 Lymphatic malformation. 12-month-old male with a lymphatic malformation of the right lower limb. Macrocystic lymphatic malformation was diagnosed based on MR findings. Sagittal T2-weighted MR with fat saturation demonstrates fluid-filled lymphatic macrocysts within the intermuscular space. With permission from Schook CC, Mulliken JB, Fishman SJ, Alomari AI, Grant FD, Greene AK. Differential diagnosis of lower extremity enlargement in pediatric patients referred with a diagnosis of lymphedema. Plast Reconstr Surg 2011;127:1571–1581 © Wolters Kluwer in 2011 [2]

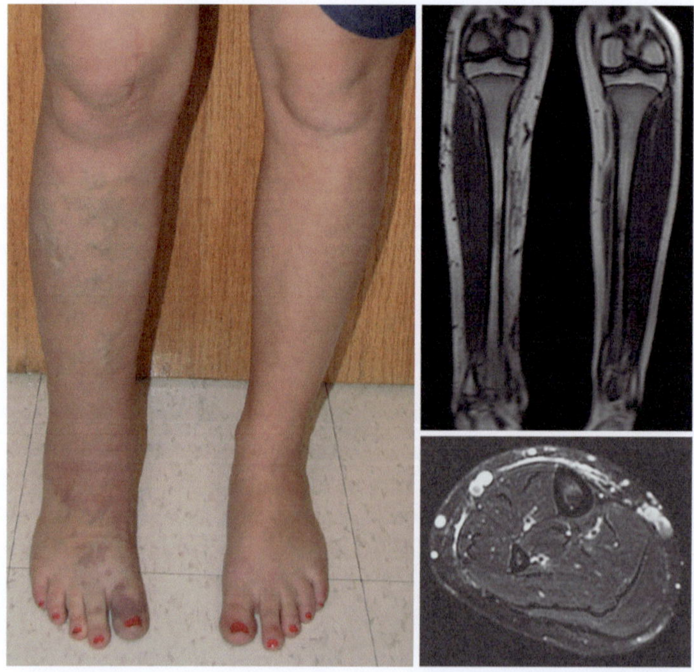

Fig. 16.12 Non-eponymous combined vascular malformation referred with a diagnosis of "lymphedema." 15-year-old female with a capillary–venous malformation of the right lower limb. Axial T2-weighted MR shows dilated veins within the subcutaneous fat underlying the capillary stain. With permission from Schook CC, Mulliken JB, Fishman SJ, Alomari AI, Grant FD, Greene AK. Differential diagnosis of lower extremity enlargement in pediatric patients referred with a diagnosis of lymphedema. Plast Reconstr Surg 2011;127:1571–1581 © Wolters Kluwer in 2011 [2]

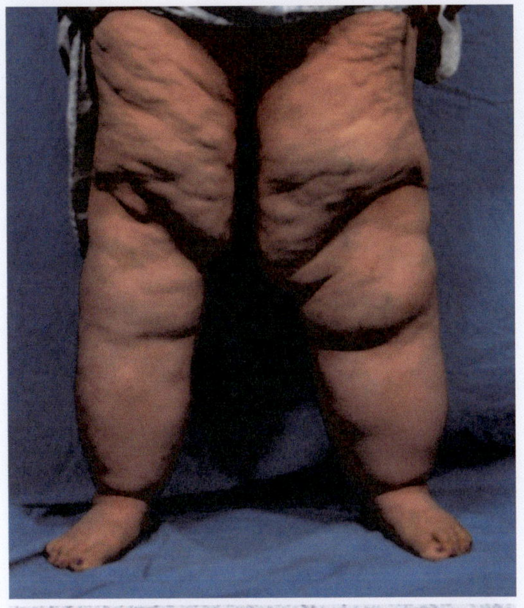

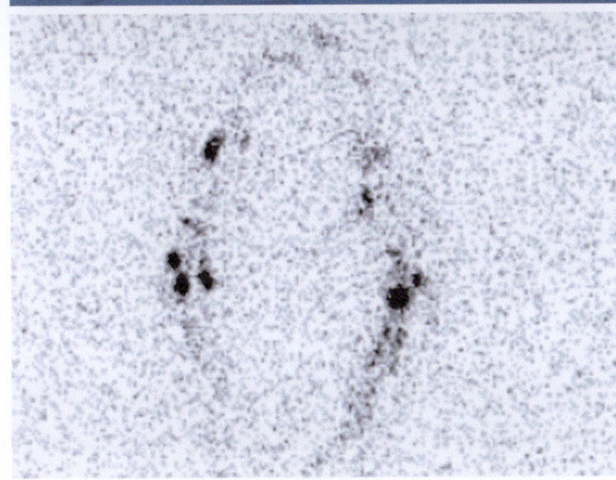

Fig. 16.13 Obesity. 56-year-old female with bilateral lower extremity overgrowth and a body mass index of 58. Her lymphoscintigram shows normal lymphatic function with tracer accumulation in the inguinal nodes 45 min following injection

Parkes Weber Syndrome

Parkes Weber syndrome consists of a diffuse arteriovenous malformation of an extremity causing soft-tissue and/or bony overgrowth (Fig. 16.14) [22]. A capillary malformation involves the skin of the affected limb. The condition most commonly involves one lower extremity. The malformation is evident at birth. The limb exhibits symmetric enlargement and the cutaneous stain is warmer than a typical capillary malformation. Parkes Weber syndrome can be sporadic, or familial due to a mutation in *RASA1* (capillary malfor-

mation–arteriovenous malformation) [23]. Parkes Weber syndrome caused by a *RASA1* mutation affects the upper limb (1/3) or lower extremity (2/3). The overlying capillary malformation is heterogeneous (e.g., single, multiple, localized, or diffuse). Fast-flow is present on handheld Doppler examination. Patients have subcutaneous and intramuscular microshunting and can develop congestive heart failure (6 %) [23]. On MRI all components of the extremity are typically overgrown (i.e., subcutis, muscle, bone). The enlarged limb muscles and bones exhibit abnormal signal and enhancement, arteriovenous fistulas are illustrated as flow voids [4]. Most children are observed until symptoms necessitate intervention. If a patient has high-output congestive heart failure embolization is performed to reduce shunting. Children are monitored annually by an orthopedic surgeon for axial overgrowth. If the discrepancy is more than 1.5 cm, a shoe-lift for the shorter limb can prevent limping and scoliosis. Epiphysiodesis of the distal femoral growth plate is typically performed around 11 years of age. Occasionally, amputation is necessary.

Systemic Diseases

Several systemic illnesses can cause extremity swelling, such as congestive heart failure, renal disease, hepatic disease, and rheumatological disorders (Fig. 16.15). Systemic conditions typically cause bilateral lower limb edema. Patients are queried about illnesses and medications. Lymphedema can be ruled-out by lymphoscintigraphy. Other pathological conditions can be excluded by MRI. If the patient is thought to have a systemic cause of their swelling, then they are referred for appropriate consultation (e.g., cardiology, gastroenterology, nephrology, and rheumatology).

Trauma

Posttraumatic swelling is erroneously labeled "lymphedema" in some patients (Fig. 16.16). Prolonged edema of the lower extremity can occur following injury, particularly after a severe sprain or fracture. Unlike lymphedema, the

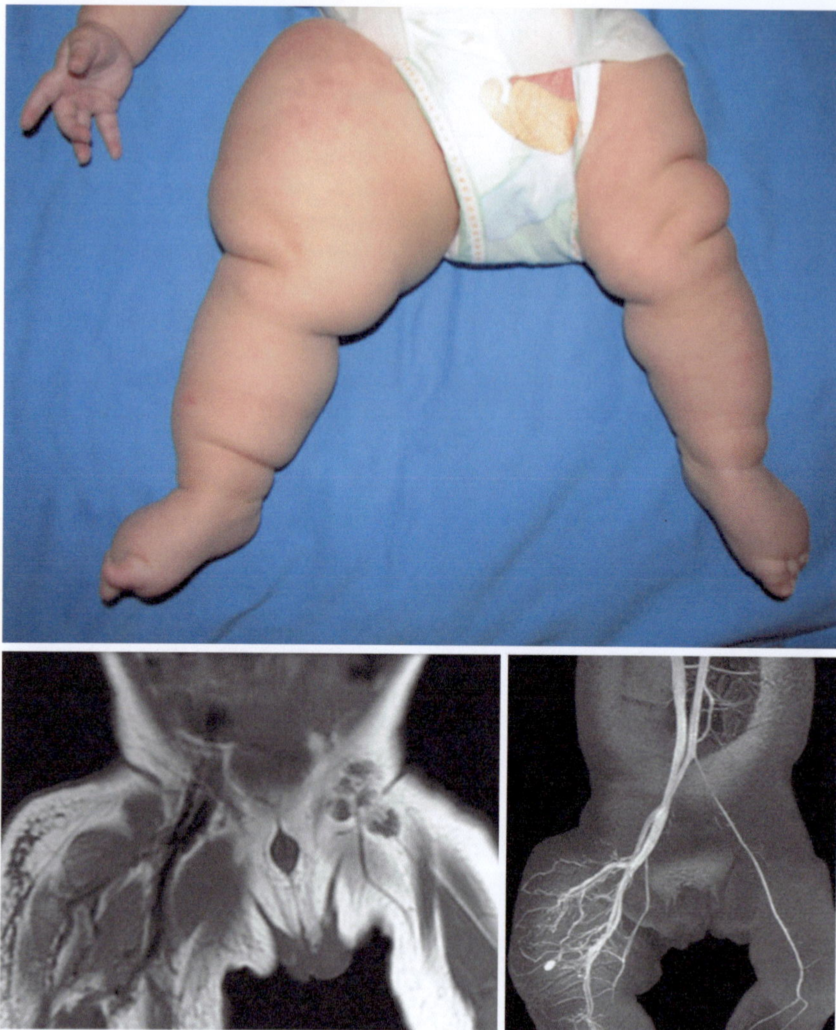

Fig. 16.14 Parkes Weber syndrome. 6-month-old with a cutaneous stain and warm extremity indicating a fast-flow malformation. Diagnosis was confirmed by MR angiography demonstrating enlargement of the arteries and early opacification of the dilated veins. With permission from Schook CC, Mulliken JB, Fishman SJ, Alomari AI, Grant FD, Greene AK. Differential diagnosis of lower extremity enlargement in pediatric patients referred with a diagnosis of lymphedema. Plast Reconstr Surg 2011;127:1571–1581 © Wolters Kluwer in 2011 [2]

lymphatic function of the extremity is normal. If the diagnosis is equivocal, lymphoscintigraphy will demonstrate intact lymphatic flow. Some patients will have a ligament tear or small fracture that can be identified by plain film and/or MRI.

Venous Malformation

Venous malformations are usually localized, but also can affect deep structures (e.g., muscle, bone, joints, viscera). One-half of sporadic venous malformations have a somatic mutation in the *TIE2* receptor. Venous malformations of the lower limb typically involve the skin and/or muscles (Fig. 16.17) [2]. If all tissues, including bone, are affected, the disorder is called *phlebectasia of Bockenheimer.* Extremity venous malformation can cause leg-length discrepancy, hypoplasia due to disuse atrophy, fibrosis, pain, pathologic fracture, hemarthrosis, and degenerative arthritis [24]. A large venous malformation involving the deep venous system is at risk for thrombosis and pulmonary embolism. Stagnation

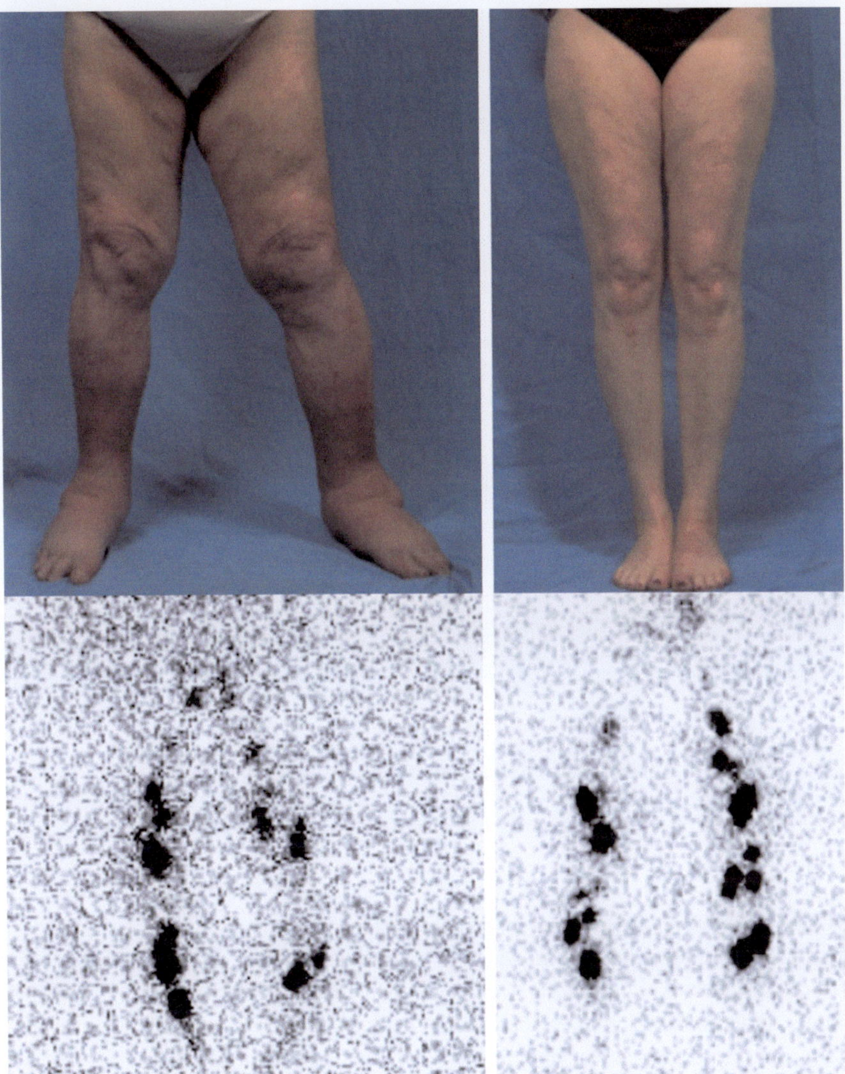

Fig. 16.15 Systemic cause of lower extremity edema. (*Left*) 66-year-old female with congestive heart failure and lower extremity swelling. Lymphoscintigram shows normal transit time to the inguinal nodes 45 min after injection. (*Right*) 59-year-old female with a rheumatological disorder and lower extremity swelling. She has normal lymphatic function with inguinal node uptake of tracer 1 h following injection

within a lesion can cause localized intravascular coagulopathy and painful phlebothromboses. Treatment of lower extremity venous malformation includes compression garments, sclerotherapy, and/or resection [24].

Venous Insufficiency

Venous insufficiency is the most common cause of lower extremity swelling in the adult popula-tion (Fig. 16.18). The risk of venous insufficiency increases with age, and women are more com-monly affected. As many as 2.8 % of females and 1.5 % of males suffer from the condition [25]. Obesity, hypertension, and a sedentary lifestyle are risk factors. The primary etiopathogenesis of the condition is valvular incompetence that causes reflux of venous blood. Symptoms begin with leg heaviness, followed by telangiectasias, varicose veins, edema, trophic skin changes, and ultimately ulceration. Unlike patients with

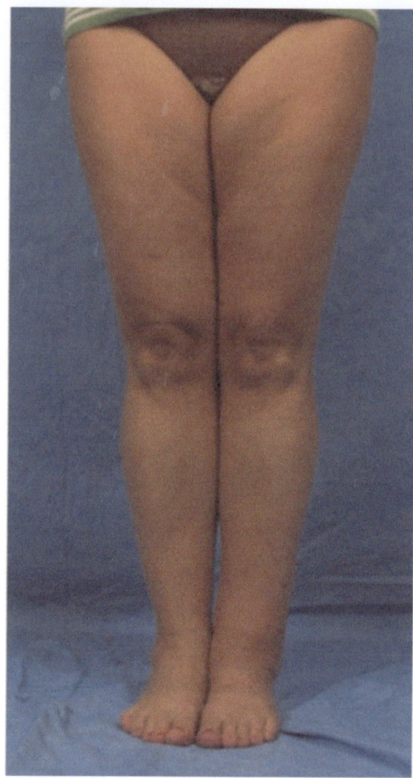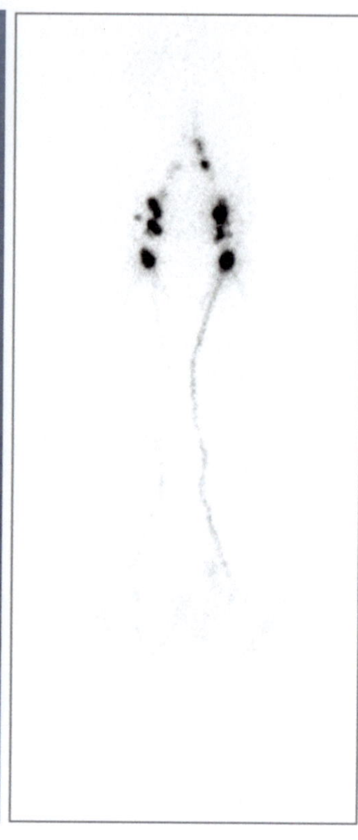

Fig. 16.16 Trauma. 51-year-old female who developed periodic left lower extremity swelling 1 year following open reduction and internal fixation of a fibula fracture. Lymphoscintigraphy shows normal lymphatic function with tracer uptake into the inguinal nodes 30 min following injection

lymphedema, individuals with venous insufficiency have normal lymphatic function. In addition, venous stasis causes secondary skin changes (i.e., lipodermatosclerosis, dermatitis, ulceration). Patients undergo ultrasound examination to document incompetent valves and reflux. Treatment includes compression garments, pneumatic compression, and treatment of the varicose veins using thermal ablation, sclerotherapy, or surgical stripping.

Conclusions

Approximately one-fourth of patients with an enlarged lower extremity are misdiagnosed as having "lymphedema." The most commonly confused etiologies are vascular anomalies, lipedema, obesity, and venous diseases. Although lymphedema is almost always an isolated condition, a patient can have lymphedema as well as another lesion of the extremity. For example, primary lymphedema can occur with capillary, lymphatic, venous, or arteriovenous anomalies. In adults, lymphedema can occur with obesity or venous disease.

Lymphedema typically can be differentiated from other conditions by history and physical examination (Table 16.3). If the diagnosis remains unclear, then the extremity is imaged using lymphoscintigraphy and/or MRI (Fig. 16.19). If lymphedema is suspected, a lymphoscintigram is the first test ordered. A patient thought to have a condition other than lymphedema on history and physical examination usually undergoes MRI evaluation to confirm the suspected diagnosis and/or to define the extent of disease. MRI also is commonly used as a secondary imaging study if lymphoscintigraphy is negative. Correct diagnosis is important because the natural history and management of lymphedema are very different compared to that of other extremity diseases.

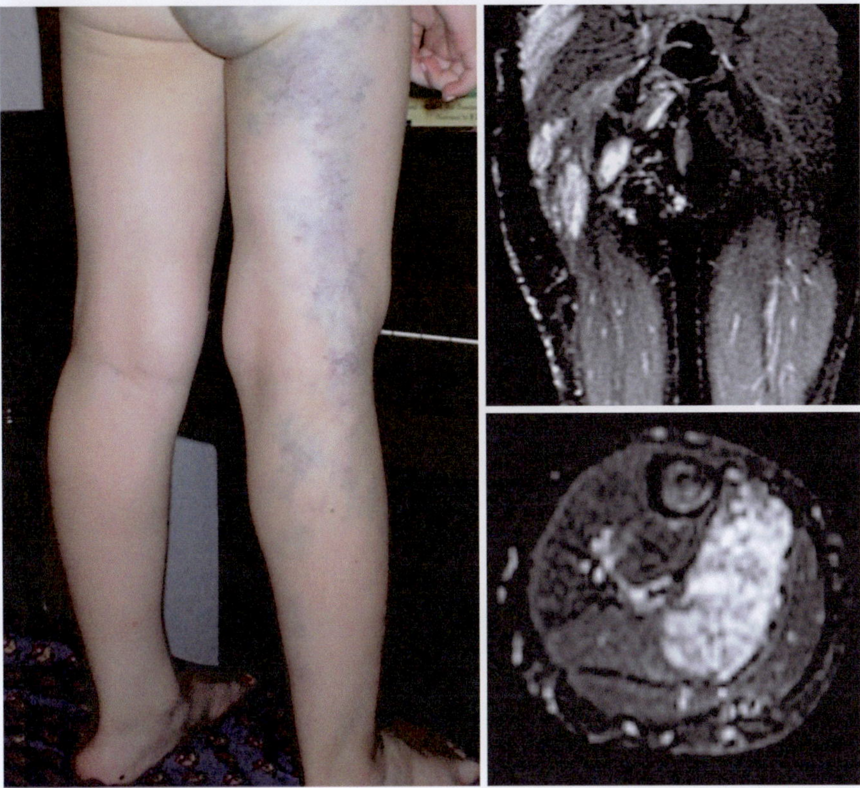

Fig. 16.17 Venous malformation. 8-year-old female with a venous malformation of the right lower extremity. Coronal T2-weighted MR shows deep intramuscular and cutaneous venous anomalies. With permission from Schook CC, Mulliken JB, Fishman SJ, Alomari AI, Grant FD, Greene AK. Differential diagnosis of lower extremity enlargement in pediatric patients referred with a diagnosis of lymphedema. Plast Reconstr Surg 2011;127:1571–1581 © Wolters Kluwer in 2011 [2]

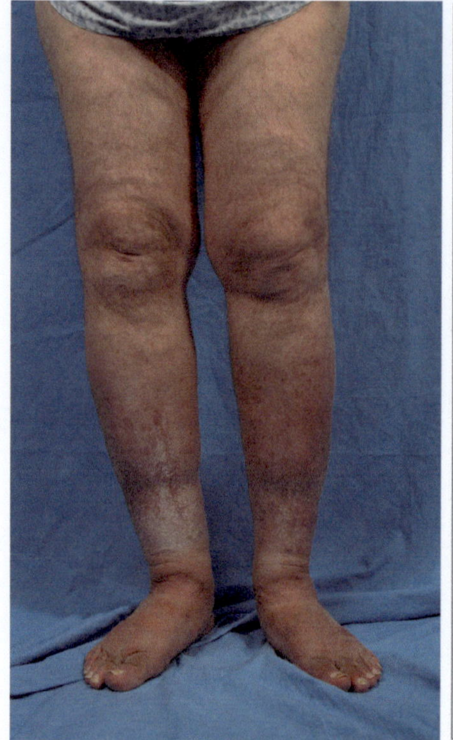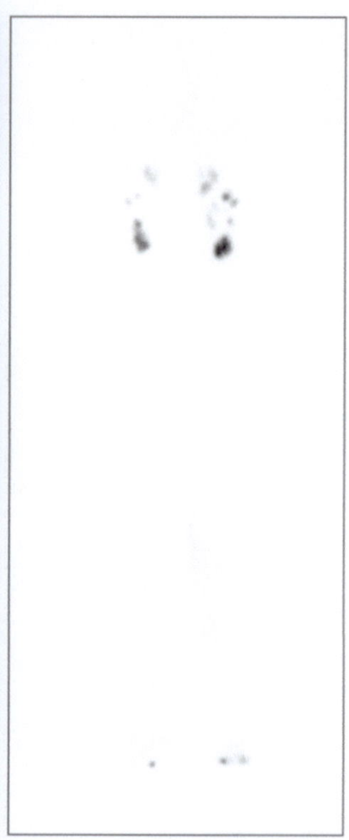

Fig. 16.18 Venous insufficiency. 57-year-old male with cutaneous changes consistent with venous stasis. He has normal lymphatic transit of tracer to the inguinal nodes 25 min following the injection

Table 16.3 Characteristics of conditions causing lower extremity overgrowth

	Lymphedema	Hemi-hypertrophy	Lipedema	Obesity	Posttraumatic Edema	Systemic Edema Cardiac Renal Hepatic Rheumatologic	Tumor Hemangioma Kaposiform Hemangioendothelioma Lipofibromatosis	Vascular Malformation Capillary Lymphatic Venous Combined CLOVES Klippel–Trénaunay Parkes Weber	Venous Insufficiency
Male–female	M=F	M=F	F	M=F	M=F	M=F	M=F	M=F	M=F
Onset	Infancy Adolescence Adulthood	Infancy	Adolescence	Adulthood	Infancy Childhood Adolescence Adulthood	Infancy Childhood Adolescence Adulthood	Infancy	Infancy Childhood Adolescence	Adulthood
Familial transmission	+/−	−	+/−	−	−	−	−	−	−
Unilateral/bilateral	U/B	U	B	B	U/B	U/B	U	U	B
Foot/hand involvement	+	+/−	−	+/−	+/−	+/−	+/−	+/−	+/−
Cutaneous changes	+/−	−	−	−	−	−	+	+	+
Abnormal blood tests	−	−	−	−	+/−	+/−	+/−	+/−	−
Wilms tumor	−	+	−	−	−	−	−	−	−
Lymphoscintigram	+	−	−	−	−	−	−	−	−
MRI	↑ Subcutaneous adipose/edema	↑ Adipose, muscle, bone	↑ Subcutaneous adipose	↑ Subcutaneous adipose	↑ Subcutaneous subfascial edema	↑ Subcutaneous subfascial edema	Tumor-specific (enhancing lesion)	Abnormal vasculature	Varicosities Subcutaneous Edema
Diagnostic histopathology	−	−	−	−	−	−	+	+	−
Management	Compression Operative	Wilms screening Operative	Operative	Weight loss	Treat underlying condition	Treat underlying condition	Drugs Operative	Sclerotherapy Embolization Operative	Compression Treat Varicosities

With permission from Schook CC, Mulliken JB, Fishman SJ, Alomari AI, Grant FD, Greene AK. Differential diagnosis of lower extremity enlargement in pediatric patients referred with a diagnosis of lymphedema. Plast Reconstr Surg 2011;127:1571–1581 © Wolters Kluwer in 2011 [2]

Fig. 16.19 Algorithm to differentiate lymphedema from other causes of extremity overgrowth

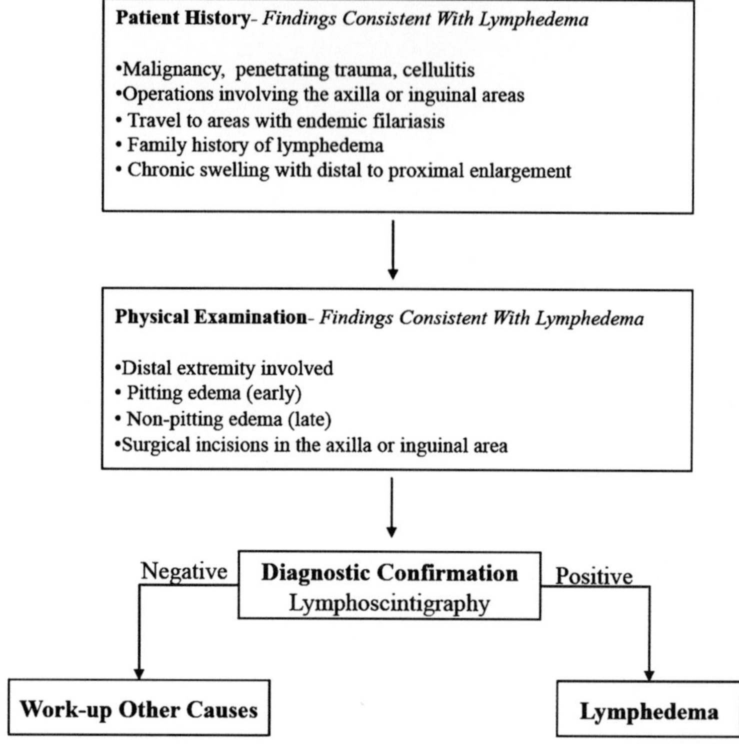

References

1. Hassanein AH, Mulliken JB, Fishman SJ, Greene AK. Evaluation of terminology for vascular anomalies in current literature. Plast Reconstr Surg. 2011;127:347–51.
2. Schook CC, Mulliken JB, Fishman SJ, Alomari AI, Grant FD, Greene AK. Differential diagnosis of lower extremity enlargement in pediatric patients referred with a diagnosis of lymphedema. Plast Reconstr Surg. 2011;127:1571–81.
3. Maclellan RA, Couto RA, Sullivan JE, Grant FD, Slavin SA, Greene AK. (2014) Management of primary and secondary lymphedema: analysis of 225 referrals to a center. Ann Plast Surg (in press).
4. Schook CC, Mulliken JB, Fishman SJ, Grant FD, Zurakowski D, Greene AK. Primary lymphedema: clinical features and management in 138 pediatric patients. Plast Reconstr Surg. 2011;127:2419–31.
5. Smeltzer DM, Stickler GB, Schirger A. Primary lymphedema in children and adolescents: a follow-up study and review. Pediatrics. 1985;76:206–18.
6. Greene AK, Grant FD, Slavin SA. Lower-extremity lymphedema and elevated body-mass index. N Engl J Med. 2012;366:2136–7.
7. Greene AK, Grant F, Slavin SA, Maclellan RA. Obesity-induced lymphedema: clinical and lymphoscintigraphic features. Plast Reconstr Surg (in press)
8. Stemmer R. A clinical symptom for the early and differential diagnosis of lymphedema. Vasa. 1976;5:261–2.
9. Gloviczki P, Calcagno D, Schirger A, et al. Noninvasive evaluation of the swollen extremity: experiences with 190 lymphoscintigraphic examinations. J Vasc Surg. 1989;9:683–9.
10. Lee MS, Liang MG, Mulliken JB. Diffuse capillary malformation with overgrowth: a clinical subtype of vascular anomalies with hypertrophy. J Am Acad Dermatol. 2013;69:589–94.
11. Alomari AI. Characterization of a distinct syndrome that associates complex truncal overgrowth, vascular, and acral anomalies: a descriptive study of 18 cases of CLOVES syndrome. Clin Dysmorphol. 2009;18:1–7.
12. Ballock RT, Wiesner GL, Myers MT, et al. Hemihypertrophy. Concepts and controversies. J Bone Joint Surg Am. 1997;79:1731–8.
13. Greene AK. Management of hemangiomas and other vascular tumors. Clin Plast Surg. 2011;38:45–63.
14. Mulliken JB, Marler JJ, Burrows PE, Kozakewich HP. Reticular infantile hemangioma of the limb can be associated with ventral-caudal anomalies, refractory

ulceration, and cardiac overload. Pediatr Dermatol. 2007;24:356–62.

15. Croteau SE, Liang MG, Kozakewich HP, Alomari AI, Fishman SJ, Mulliken JB, Trenor 3rd CC. Kaposiform hemangioendothelioma: atypical features and risks of Kasabach-Merritt phenomenon in 107 referrals. J Pedatr. 2013;162:142–7.

16. Kulungowski AM, Fishman SJ. Management of combined vascular malformations. Clin Plast Surg. 2011;38:107–20.

17. Greene AK, Kieran M, Burrows PE, Mulliken JB, Kasser J, Fishman SJ. Wilms tumor screening is unnecessary in Klippel-Trenaunay syndrome. Pediatrics. 2004;113:e326–9.

18. Rudkin GH, Miller TA. Lipedema: a clinical entity distinct from lymphedema. Plast Reconstr Surg. 1994;94:841–7.

19. Greene AK, Karnes J, Padua HM, Schmidt BA, Kasser JR, Labow BI. Diffuse lipofibromatosis of the lower extremity masquerading as a vascular anomaly. Ann Plast Surg. 2009;62:703–6.

20. Greene AK, Labow B. Diffuse lipofibromatosis of the extremity. Lymphology. 2012;45(suppl):105–8.

21. Greene AK, Perlyn C, Alomari AI. Management of lymphatic malformations. Clin Plast Surg. 2011;38:75–82.

22. Greene AK, Orbach DB. Management of arteriovenous malformations. Clin Plast Surg. 2011;38:95–106.

23. Revencu N, Boon LM, Mulliken JB, Enjolras O, Cordisco MR, Burrows PE, Clapuyt P, Hammer F, Dubois J, Baselga E, Brancati F, Carder R, Quintal JM, Dallapiccola B, Fischer G, Frieden IJ, Garzon M, Harper J, Johnson-Patel J, Labrèze C, Martorell L, Paltiel HJ, Pohl A, Prendiville J, Quere I, Siegel DH, Valente EM, Van Hagen A, Van Hest L, Vaux KK, Vicente A, Weibel L, Chitayat D, Vikkula M. Parkes Weber syndrome, vein of Galen aneurysmal malformation, and other fast-flow vascular anomalies are caused by RASA1 mutations. Hum Mutat. 2008;29:959–65.

24. Greene AK, Alomari AI. Management of venous malformations. Clin Plast Surg. 2011;38:83–93.

25. Brown KR, Rossi PJ. Superficial venous disease. Surg Clin N Am. 2013;93:963–82.

26. Greene AK. Vascular Anomalies: Classification, Diagnosis, and Management. Boca Raton, FL: CRC Press; 2013.

Part IV

Non-Operative Management of Lymphedema

Arin K. Greene

Key Points

- Patient behaviors can influence morbidity caused by lymphedema.
- Individuals may eat any type of food, but should maintain a normal body mass index.
- Exercise of a lymphedematous extremity is not harmful, but improves the condition.
- Extremities with lymphedema should be protected from incidental trauma.
- Patients with lymphedema should avoid sauna use, but can be in other warm environments.

Introduction

Lymphedema can result from the anomalous development of the lymphatic system (primary) or from injury to lymph nodes/vessels (secondary). Independent of the cause of lymphedema, the subsequent pathophysiology is the same. Over time high-protein interstitial fluid causes subcutaneous adipose hypertrophy and the lymphedematous area enlarges. Some patients have minimal morbidity from the disease, while most have problems from the condition: lowered self-esteem, infections, skin changes, and/or difficulty using the limb.

Patient behavior can significantly affect the course of lymphedema. If an individual with lymphedema adheres to favorable activities of daily living, he/she will have a more benign course compared to a patient who engages in unfavorable activities. This paradigm is similar to any disease. For example, a patient with diabetes who becomes obese, smokes, and does not maintain glucose control will have more complications and a shorter life span than a diabetic individual with a healthy lifestyle.

The field of lymphedema suffers from a paucity of randomized, prospective evidence regarding patient behaviors that positively or negatively affect disease progression. Consequently, most recommendations are based on case series and expert opinion. A principle of recommending a behavior for a patient to follow is that strong evidence should exist if the advice will negatively affect the patient's quality of life. For example, before suggesting that a patient drive across the country instead of taking an airplane, evidence about the negative effects of air travel must outweigh the inconvenience for the patient driving such a long distance (flying is not harmful to patients with lymphedema) [1]. The following activities of daily living that are listed were chosen because they have the best evidence available to communicate to patients.

A.K. Greene, M.D., M.M.Sc. (✉)
Department of Plastic and Oral Surgery, Boston
Children's Hospital, Harvard Medical School,
300 Longwood Avenue, Boston, MA 02115, USA
e-mail: arin.greene@childrens.harvard.edu

A.K. Greene et al. (eds.), *Lymphedema: Presentation, Diagnosis, and Treatment*,
DOI 10.1007/978-3-319-14493-1_17, © Springer International Publishing Switzerland 2015

Diet

No evidence exists that a certain diet is beneficial or harmful to patients with lymphedema. Consequently, individuals are educated that they may eat any type of food as well as drink alcohol. However, diet might indirectly affect lymphedema because obesity can cause the disease and worsen the condition [2, 3]. Patients are advised to maintain a normal body mass index because obesity causes inflammation, which damages lymphatic vessels and worsens lymphedema [4, 5]. Obese patients, or individuals at risk for obesity, are referred to a dietician or surgical weight loss center.

Heat

Patients at risk for lymphedema, or who have the condition, have been advised to avoid heat to the lymphedematous area because increased blood flow might worsen the condition [1, 6]. Prospective, randomized evidence has shown that exercise, hot weather, and sunburn are not harmful to the lymphatic system [1]. Sauna use, in contrast, does increase the risk of lymphedema sixfold in women at risk for the disease following breast cancer treatment [1]. Unlike other sources of heat, however, patients who reported sauna use also had an increased risk of having a cut on the extremity which might confound the cause for the increased risk of lymphedema [1]. We currently recommend that patients with lymphedema avoid sauna use, but they may be in other warm environments (e.g., bath, hot-tube, sun). Allowing patients to engage in warm activities benefits their mental health and improves their quality of life.

Protection of the Limb

Patients with lymphedema are advised to protect their limb from incidental trauma. A lymphedematous extremity has a significantly increased risk for infection; a break in the skin can lead to cellulitis. Keeping the limb clean by washing it daily with mild soaps is recommended [7]. Applying a moisturizer to prevent dry skin minimizes the risk of skin injury from desiccation and trauma that could lead to infection [7]. Patients with lower extremity lymphedema are counseled not to walk barefoot in areas where they are at risk for trauma (e.g., beach, forest, garden). The leg should be covered with clothing when the individual is in an environment at risk for incidental trauma (e.g., gardening, walking through bushes). A break in the skin of a lymphedematous extremity can cause an infection, which further damages lymphatic vessels and worsens the disease [8, 9]. Patients with lower extremity disease should elevate their leg when sleeping. Lying on a lymphedematous extremity is not harmful to the limb and does not worsen the condition [1].

Use of the Lymphedematous Extremity

Historically, individuals with lymphedema were counseled to avoid vigorous use of the affected extremity because it might worsen the condition [6]. This myth, however, has been disproven with prospective, randomized evidence. Patients at risk for cancer-related lymphedema who exercise their extremity with weight lifting and/or physical activity have a lower risk of lymphedema compared to controls who do not exercise [10, 11]. Not only does weight lifting and exercise not worsen lymphedema in patients with the condition, but it improves their disease (i.e., reduces exacerbations and symptoms, increases strength) [12]. Although the mechanism by which exercise benefits a limb with lymphedema is unknown, muscle action likely promotes proximal transport of lymphatic fluid.

In addition to being directly beneficial to a lymphedematous extremity, physical activity has other advantages for the patient as well. Because obesity worsens lymphedema, exercise helps the patient maintain a normal body mass index. Patients with excellent health have a better prognosis and less risk of injury to the lymphatic system, compared to individuals with fair/poor

Table 17.1 Recommended activities of daily living for patients with lymphedema

May eat any type of food
Maintain a normal body mass index
Exercise
Can perform heavy activity with lymphedematous extremity
Keep the limb clean and wash with mild soap twice a day
Moisturize the extremity to avoid desiccation and incidental trauma
Wear clothing to protect the limb to prevent incidental trauma
Avoid sauna use, but other warm environments are not harmful (e.g., bath, sun)

health [13]. Physical activity also provides significant psychological benefits which improves quality of life [14].

Conclusions

Activities of daily living can affect the natural course of lymphedema (Table 17.1). Patients who protect their limb, maintain a normal body mass index, and exercise will improve their prognosis and quality of life. Individuals should avoid sauna use but may be in other warm environments. Health care providers must educate patients about favorable and unfavorable behaviors that will influence their disease.

References

1. Showalter SL, Brown JC, Cheville AL, Fisher CS, Sataloff D, Schmitz KH. Lifestyle risk factors associated with arm swelling among women with breast cancer. Ann Surg Oncol. 2013;20:842–9.
2. Helyer LK, Varnic M, Le LW, Leong W, McCready D. Obesity is a risk factor for developing postoperative lymphedema in breast cancer patients. Breast J. 2010;16:48–54.
3. Greene AK, Grant FD, Slavin SA. Lower-extremity lymphedema and elevated body-mass index. N Engl J Med. 2012;366:2136–7.
4. Weitman ES, Aschen SZ, Farias-Eisner G, Albano N, Cuzzone DA, Ghanta S, et al. Obesity impairs lymphatic fluid transport and dendritic cell migration to lymph nodes. PLoS One. 2013;8:e70703.
5. Savetsky IL, Torrisi JS, Cuzzone DA, Ghanta S, Albano NJ, Gardenier JC, Joseph WJ, Mehrara BJ. Obesity increases inflammation and impairs lymphatic function in a mouse model of lymphedema. Am J Physiol Heart Circ Physiol. 2014;15;307:H165–72.
6. Cemal Y, Pusic A, Mehrara BJ. Preventative measures for lymphedema: separating fact from fiction. J Am Coll Surg. 2011;213:543–51.
7. The diagnosis and treatment of peripheral lymphedema: 2013 consensus document of the international society of lymphology. Lymphology 2013;46:1–11.
8. McLaughlin SA, Wright MJ, Morris KT, Sampson MR, Brockway JP, Hurley KE, et al. Prevalence of lymphedema in women with breast cancer 5 years after sentinel lymph node biopsy or axillary dissection: patient perceptions and precautionary behaviors. J Clin Oncol. 2008;26:5220–6.
9. Ugur S, Arici C, Yaprak M, Mesci A, Arici GA, Dolay K, et al. Risk factors of breast cancer-related lymphedema. Lymphat Res Biol. 2013;11:72–5.
10. Schmitz KH, Ahmed RL, Troxel AB, Cheville A, Lewis-Grant L, Smith R, et al. Weight lifting for women at risk for breast cancer-related lymphedema: a randomized trial. JAMA. 2010;304:2699–705.
11. Brown JC, John GM, Segal S, Chu CS, Schmitz KH. Physical activity and lower limb lymphedema among uterine cancer survivors. Med Sci Sports Exerc. 2013;45:2091–7.
12. Schmitz KH, Ahmed RL, Troxel A, Cheville A, Smith R, Lewis-Grant L, et al. Weight lifting in women with breast-cancer-related lymphedema. N Engl J Med. 2009;361:664–73.
13. Ahmed RL, Schmitz KH, Prizment AE, Folsom AR. Risk factors for lymphedema in breast cancer survivors, the Iowa women's health study. Breast Cancer Res Treat. 2011;130:981–91.
14. Schook CC, Mulliken JB, Fishman SJ, Grant F, Zurakowski D, Greene AK. Primary lymphedema: clinical features and management in 138 pediatric patients. Plast Reconstr Surg. 2011;127:2419–31.

Controlled Compression Therapy and Compression Garments

18

Karin Ohlin, Barbro Svensson, and Håkan Brorson

Key Points

There are several ways to increase compression.

- Decrease circumferential measurements of garments
- Increase compression class
- Multilayer
- Amount of garments
- Take in existing garments

Introduction

The most important factor to maintain the effect of any therapy is the use of compression garments. Garments should be prescribed in such a number so that the edema does not recur. A common mistake is that the patient receive one, or if lucky two garments, after treatment. When the arm or leg is swollen again the patient comes back to the therapist and treatment starts again, and so on. Instead the patient must be followed up at regular intervals during the first year in order to find out the exact number of garments that the patient needs in order to prevent recurrence. This means that treatment must be individualized. An elderly woman may need two garments every 6 months, while a young active patient with a heavy work may need two garments every month. One can draw a parallel to the dosage of insulin to a patient with diabetes that in the same way must be individualized. You do not prescribe two vials of insulin for 6 months, when the patient needs that same amount for one month.

The purpose of compression therapy is to increase the interstitial pressure so that the capillary filtration is decreased. When treated with standard compression garments a study showed a reduction of the excess volume (1,680 ml; range 670–3,320) after 2 weeks with 20 % (range 5–37) corresponding to 338 ml (range 95–1,225) [1]. Studies of treatment for 6 months have shown a reduction of excess volume of 17 % (range 16–52), corresponding to a volume of 139 ml (range 150–345) [2].

Compression garments can be used at the onset of symptoms to possibly prevent the development of lymphedema. Garments that are used throughout the day (15 years' follow-up) [3] as well as only daytime (6 months follow-up) [2] prevent the lymphedema to recur.

Compression garments must be ordered by a qualified and experienced lymphedema team consisting of a lymph therapist with a basic edu-

K. Ohlin, B.S., O.T. • B. Svensson, B.S., P.T.
H. Brorson, M.D., Ph.D.(✉)
The Lymphedema Unit, Department of Clinical Sciences, Lund University, Plastic and Reconstructive Surgery, Jan Waldenströms gata 18, 2nd floor, Skåne University Hospital, Malmö SE-205 02, Sweden
e-mail: hakan.brorson@med.lu.se

A.K. Greene et al. (eds.), *Lymphedema: Presentation, Diagnosis, and Treatment*,
DOI 10.1007/978-3-319-14493-1_18, © Springer International Publishing Switzerland 2015

cation in physiotherapy or occupational therapy and a physician. The team should have vast knowledge regarding various compression trademarks and how to take measurements for ordering of garments. In order to increase compliance and feedback the team should never let the patient have the measurements for ordering of garments taken by a retailer outside of the team.

Ordering of Garments

When ordering for compression garments the following must be considered:
- Compression class
- Material
- Size
- Design
- The patient's ability to take on/off the garment and the ability to care for it

Compression Class

Table 18.1 shows the compression classes that are provisionally adopted by the European Standardization Committee [4].

Compression garments for the arm and hand are usually ordered in CCL 2. When only incipient symptoms are present, CCL 1 can be sufficient. Garments for the leg often require CCL 3 or more. If the lymphedema requires higher compression a combination with an additional garment on top on the first one can be used. This increases the compression further and can be easier to put on than just one garment in very high compression

Table 18.1 Compression classes that are provisionally adopted by the European Standardization Committee [4]

CCL I:	Mild	15–21	mmHg[a]
CCL II:	Moderate	23–32	mmHg
CCL III:	Strong	34–46	mmHg
CCL IV:	Very strong	49–	mmHg

[a]Compression at the ankle. The values indicate the compression exerted by the compression garments at a hypothetical cylindrical ankle

class. In severe cases another leg long garment may be needed, either round knitted or flat knitted.

Material

Materials and production methods vary between different manufacturers. There are circular knitted garments without a seam and flat knitted with a seam. The higher compression classes are usually flat knitted. It should be noted that each class is within a compression interval, and within the compression class different materials may have higher or lower compression. Verify how long the manufacturer guarantees that the garment lasts for the specified compression. Garments in softer materials have a shorter durability and must be replaced more often, even though the compression is the same as that of a more rigid garment.

Patients with sensitive skin may need to try different brands. If the patient encounters irritation at the elbow or at the back of the knee, a soft lining can be sewn into the sock. There are also modifications in the knitting technique that decreases skin irritation at these locations. There are also different brands of silicone or hydrogel plates, to be put under the garment that will relieve irritated skin.

Size

Compression stockings are produced in different standard sizes or made to measure.

Standard size garments—advantage
- The patient receives the garment at once
- Measuring is simpler

Standard Size Garments: Disadvantage

- Do not have enough widths and lengths to suit all
- Smaller selection of materials
- Smaller selection of models

Made to Measure Garments: Advantages

- Optimal fit
- Greater possibility when remeasuring in order to gradually reduce the size of the garment as the edema is reduced

Made to Measure Garments: Disadvantages

- More extensive measuring
- Delivery time
- The cost

If made to measure is selected after treatment, the patient must either use a standard garment or bandage the extremity until the custom-made garment has been delivered. Later on, when measuring for the next garment the measurements must be compared with the previous order to check that the garment gives the intended effect. The technique when measuring varies from brand to brand. See the instructions of each manufacturer.

Design

Compression stockings are available in various models (Fig. 18.1). You can also choose various fasteners, such as silicone ribbon at the top of the

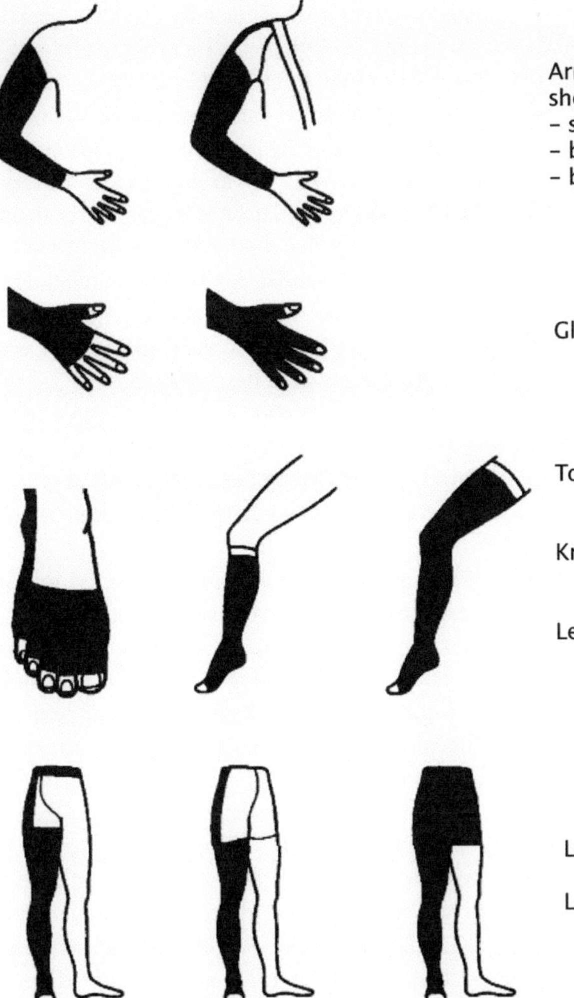

Fig. 18.1 Compression garments are available in various models. © Karin Ohlin

garment or a band around the waist. Each manufacturer provides information about the different varieties available. Which one you choose depends on:

- Edema location
- The patient's body constitution
- The patient's wishes
- How compression stocking works in daily activities

Taking On and Off the Garment and Maintenance of the Garment

Check that the patient can maintain and manage to take on and off the garment. If the patient has problems one must arrange for someone to help out, such as a relative or home care/district nurse, who also may need instructions. At follow-up, check that this has worked. The manufacturers provide different types of aids that facilitate the procedure.

Use

The various alternatives depend on the severity of the edema:

- Continuously throughout the day
- Continuously during daytime (the garment must be taken on in the morning)
- Only use it when performing strenuous labor (prolonged static or heavy work, where patients experience that the extremity gets swollen) and at long journeys by plane or car

After a few weeks, it is important to verify that compression stockings have the intended effect. Rash after use may be due to an allergic reaction to detergents, or to the garment material, which is very uncommon. If the excess volume has increased at follow-up, this can be due to several factors:

- Bad patient compliance; check the patient's motivation and every day routines
- The patient has not understood how the garment must be taken care of or has taken it on in the wrong way (for example not pulled it high enough)
- Incorrect measurements have been taken—check them

- Insufficient compression class—increase compression class at the next order
- Progress of underlying malignancy

Costs

The life span of a compression garment varies between 3 and 6 months, provided that the patient has two garments to switch between. Two garments are required so that the patient every day can take on a newly washed garment. At the first time only one garment is ordered to evaluate the fit and to be able to make any corrections. Then the second garment is promptly ordered. Henceforth two garments should be ordered at each occasion. The minimum amount of compression garments for an arm lymphedema is two every 6 months. If gloves/gauntlets are needed, 2–3 garments every 6 months may be needed since they wear out faster. For legs new garments may need to be reordered every 3–6 months depending on activity level. Very active patients and children may need up to six stockings every 6 months. There should be no upper limit to how many garments that need to be ordered. Additional garments may be needed at the start of treatment.

Funds must be set aside anyway so that patients can obtain sufficient numbers of compression garments as described above.

Controlled Compression Therapy: Gradually Increasing Compression

When an untreated edema is subjected to compression, the excess volume is reduced and compression must be adapted continuously. This can be done with bandaging or controlled compression therapy. The methods can be used individually or in combination. It is very important that treatment outcome is checked regularly with excess volume measurements and that treatment continues until there is no or minimal or no pitting. No manual lymph drainage is needed so the treatment is less time consuming and concerning CCT the patient does not need to be on sick leave. Also manual lymph drainage lacks evidence in reduction of the excess volume [5–7].

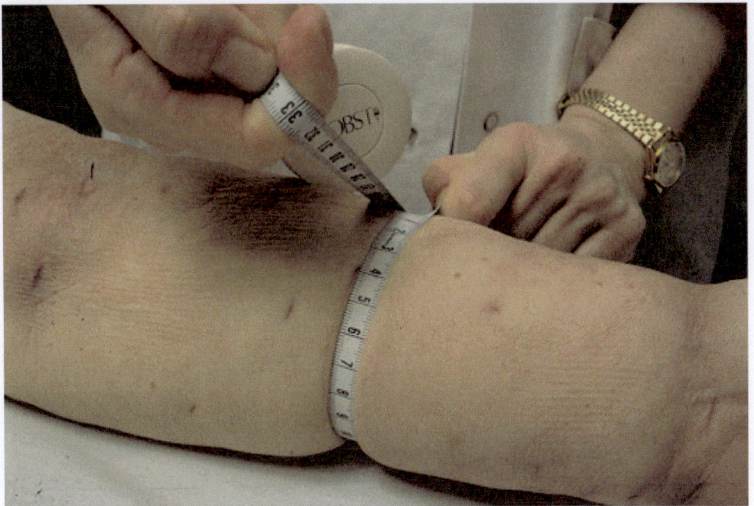

Fig. 18.2 Compression can be increased by taking firm measurements in order to decrease the circumference. © Håkan Brorson

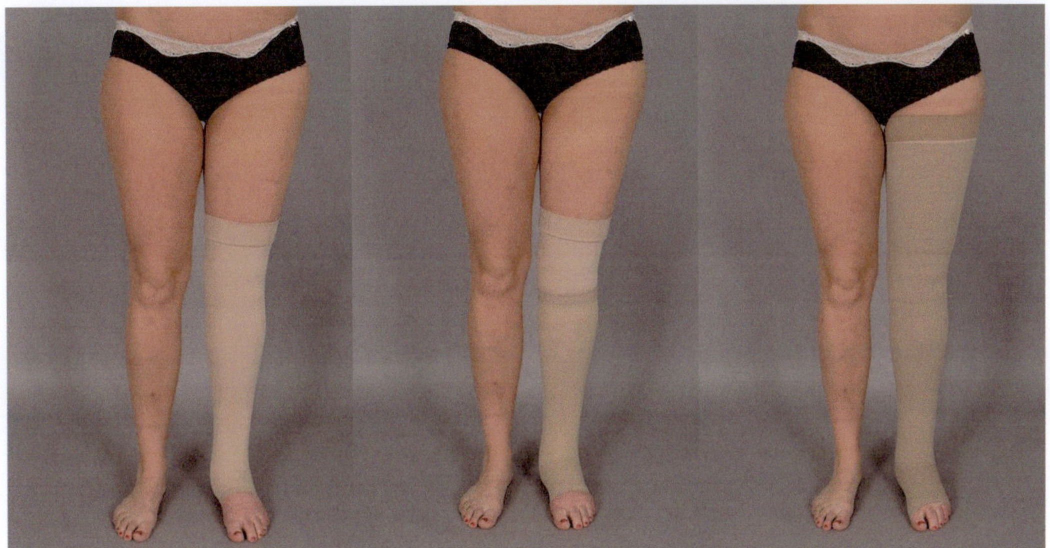

Fig. 18.3 Compression can be increased by using various garments on top of each other (multilayer). © Håkan Brorson

How Can Compression Be Increased?

There are several ways to increase compression
- Decrease circumferential measurements of garments (Fig. 18.2)
- Increase compression class
- Multilayer (Fig. 18.3)
- Amount of garments
- Take in existing garments (Fig. 18.4)

As long as the extremity shows pit on pressure the garment can be reduced in size by using a sewing machine. The circumference can be decreased at 0.5–1 cm increments at regular controls and can also be easily made by the patient when necessary. After 3–4 times the patient needs new garments in a smaller size. Every time new garments are ordered they are ordered in a smaller size than last time, if ordering made to measure garments. The method is an alternative to bandaging in connection with the initial edema reduction [1].

Controlled compression therapy can be used as the only treatment. It can also be used while

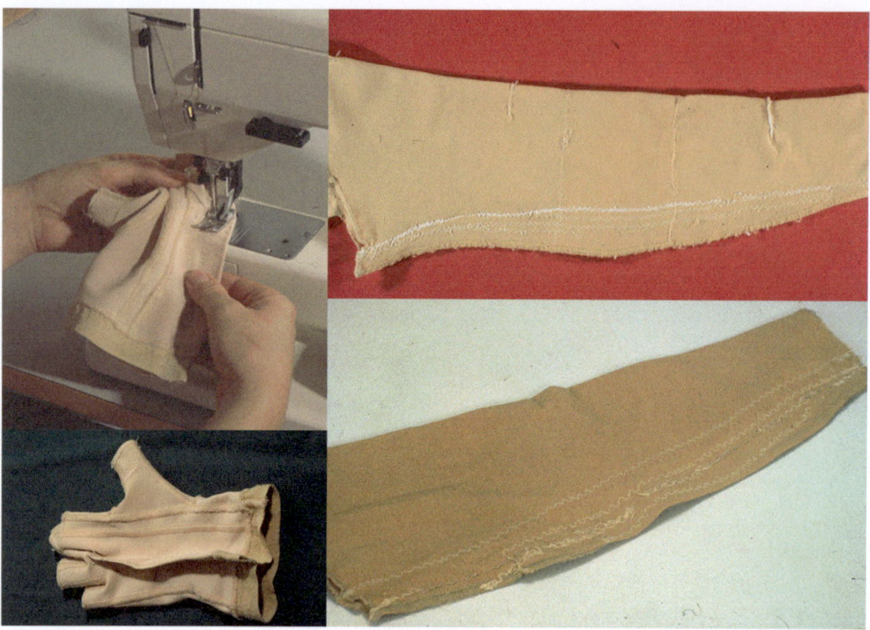

Fig. 18.4 Compression can be increased by taking in existing garments by the use of a sewing machine. © Håkan Brorson

waiting for other physical-medical methods or surgical treatment as may be indicated.

Treatment and Results

For arm lymphedema CCL 2 is mostly used. Occasionally CCL 3 may be necessary. The glove can be of the same material or thinner material (glove for burns) if the patient's hand edema is not as pronounced. At follow-up, measurements for garments are taken much "tighter" (Fig. 18.2) than the recommendations specified by the manufacturer in order to increase compression and to get sufficient compression for a longer time. The same also goes for leg lymphedema when CCL 3 (leg long) and CCL 2 (knee long) are used. This particular measuring requires an experienced therapist.

Further follow-up and reduction of the compression garments is made when needed and at scheduled visits at 1 and 3 months. Up to the 3-month control—when new garments are ordered in smaller size—3–4 reductions (using a sewing machine) have been made by the patient when she/he notices that the compression decreases. Further follow-up with ordering of new garments is done every 3 months until the maximum edema reduction is achieved, i.e., when there is no minimal pitting (3–4 mm for arms and 5–6 mm for legs). This is usually achieved after 6–12 months of treatment. The excess volume is measured at each control.

If the excess volume is stable at 1 year, the patient is provided with garments for the next 6 months. If still stable at 1.5 years the patients is seen at 2 years. Then, if stable, the patient needs only to be seen once a year and is provided with all the garments for the following year, and so on.

Controlled Compression Treatment with compression garments show an excess volume reduction of 47 % (range 2–80) after 1 year. Already after 2 weeks with a standard garment a reduction of 20 % (340 ml) is achieved. The results are permanent after 2 years. These results have been achieved with excess volumes of on average 1.7 l (0.7–3.3 l), the relative volume of 1.6 (range 1.3–2.7) and long duration (mean duration 8 years, range 1–19) [1, 8]. Lymphoscintigraphy shows signs of increased mobilization of lymph after

3 months of compression therapy. After 12 months there is no difference compared with values before treatment [9]. This is consistent with findings from combined physiotherapy [10].

Follow-Up (Summary)

Initial follow-up visits are made with a few weeks apart and can then, at steady state, be reduced to 1–2 times per year. Treatment is lifelong.

The control procedures must be included:

- Measurement and calculation of absolute and relative excess volume
- Review of the compression garments' fit and elasticity. When necessary it is reduced in size by the use of a sewing machine and/or new garments are ordered
- At steady state with persistent troublesome excess volume and minimal or no pitting liposuction can further reduce the excess volume (see Chap. 28)

Case Studies

Case 1 (Figs. 18.5 and 18.6)

This patient was treated for penis cancer. He had suffered from lymphedema for 27 years. He was retired but still very physically active working on his house, doing sports. The excess volume was 4,655 ml before treatment. After 1 year he was below zero, i.e., the lymphedematous leg was smaller than the healthy one. The postoperative treatment with CCT is showed by the arrows in different colors, one color for each method to increase compression. At some follow-up controls the circumferential measurements were decreased when ordering new garments, but at some visits several strategies were combined. There is always a possibility for the patient to take an active part in the discussion in which way to go. All the time the compression is gradually increased, step by step, so that the patient can

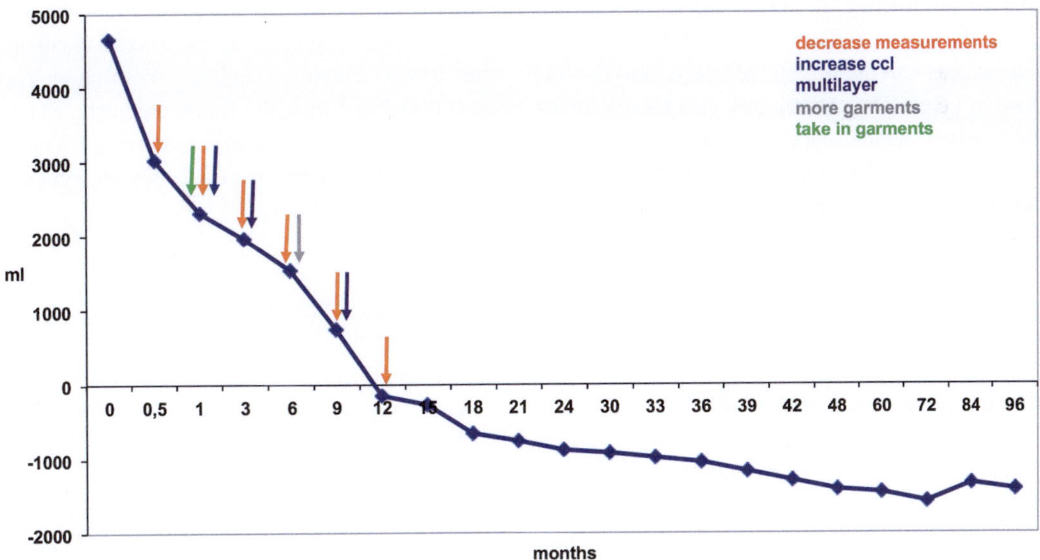

Fig. 18.5 Case 1: Notice the decrease in excess volume during the postoperative treatment and that complete reduction was achieved at 12 months. © Karin Ohlin

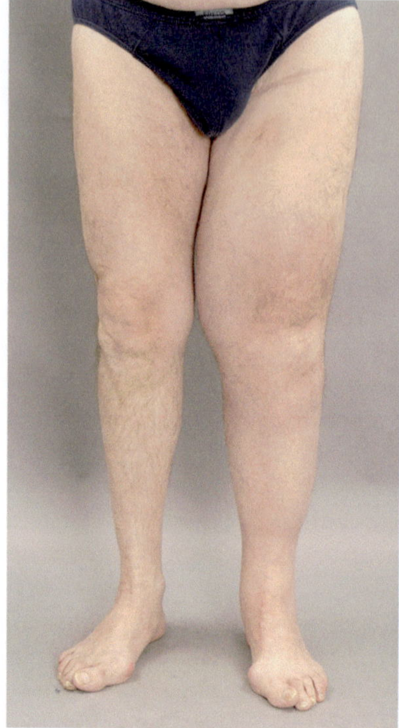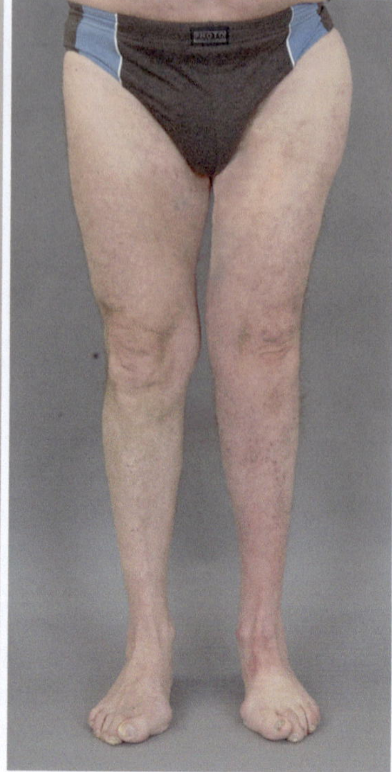

Fig. 18.6 Case 1: Preoperative excess volume 4,655 ml (*left*). Postoperative excess volume after 4 years is – (minus) 1,420 ml, i.e., the treated leg is smaller than the unaffected leg. © Håkan Brorson

adapt and tolerate it. After the first year the patient's excess volume was completely reduced. The excess volume was stable below zero the following years. The patient now gets the garments he needs at annual check-ups and garments are ordered in the same size every time. At the 4 year follow-up the excess volume is −1,420 ml, i.e., an over-correction, partly depending on that the patient had gained weight after surgery and partly on the liposuction.

Case 2 (Figs. 18.7 and 18.8)

This patient was a retired woman treated for uterine cancer. She had had her lymphedema for 9 years. She had many intellectual interests and was not very physically active. Before surgery her excess volume was 5,925 ml. In spite of her large preoperative excess volume, postoperative CCT consisted only of decreasing the measurements when ordering garments every time and

adding a knee compression garment. Complete reduction was achieved at the 1-year checkup, when it was −280 ml, a slight overcorrection. The result is stable during the following years. She is only seen once a year when leg volumes are measured and all garments for the following year are ordered.

Case 3 (Figs. 18.9 and 18.10)

This patient is a middle-aged woman with primary lymphedema since 23 years. She works full time and lives a very active life. She had a preoperative excess volume of 2,555 ml. She was below zero already at the 4-week checkup, but when she took up her work and sports the excess volume increased again. We used different combinations to increase the compression, in a quite tough and active way, in order to again get control over the edema. One year after surgery the legs were equal in size. The following year the

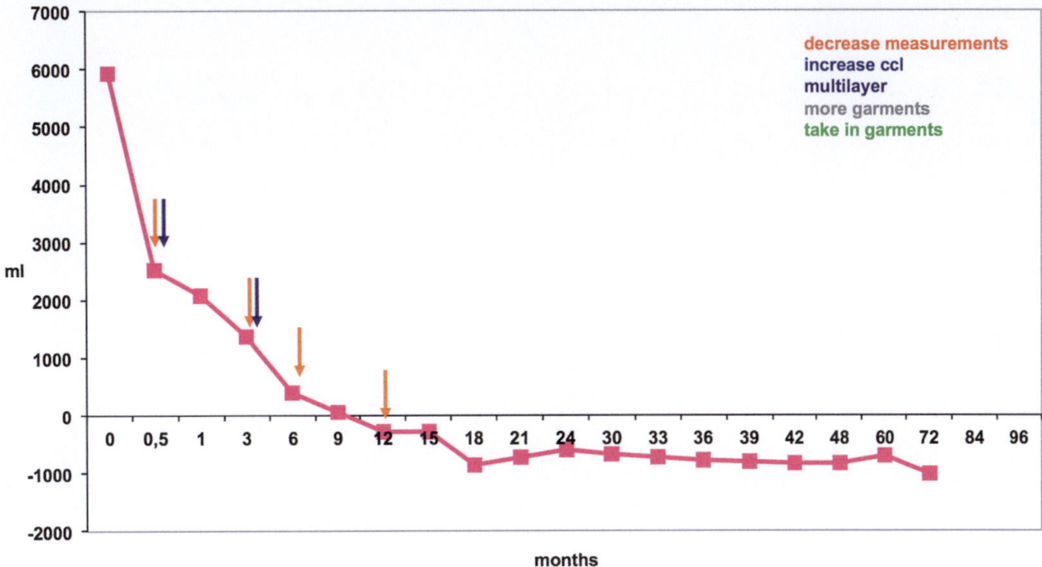

Fig. 18.7 Case 2: Notice the decrease in excess volume during the postoperative treatment and that complete reduction was achieved at 12 months. © Karin Ohlin

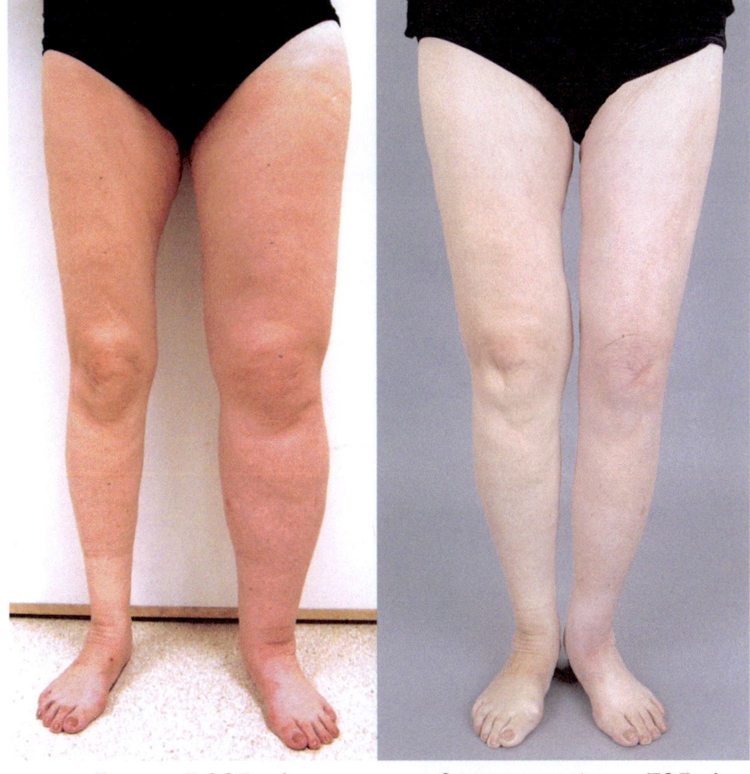

Fig. 18.8 Case 2: Preoperative excess volume 5,925 ml (*left*). Postoperative excess volume after 3 years is – (minus) 795 ml, i.e., the treated leg is smaller than the unaffected leg. © Håkan Brorson

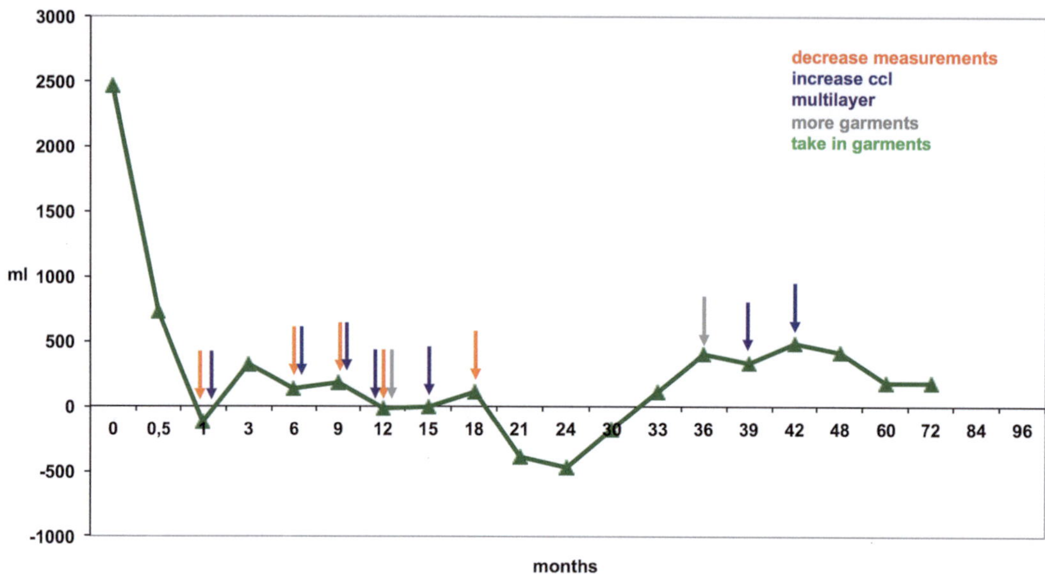

Fig. 18.9 Case 3: Notice the decrease in excess volume during the postoperative treatment and that complete reduction was achieved at 1 month and the variations during the postoperative 6 years due to very high activity level. © Karin Ohlin

Fig. 18.10 Case 3: Preoperative excess volume 2,555 ml (*left*). Postoperative excess volume after 6 years is 180 ml. © Håkan Brorson

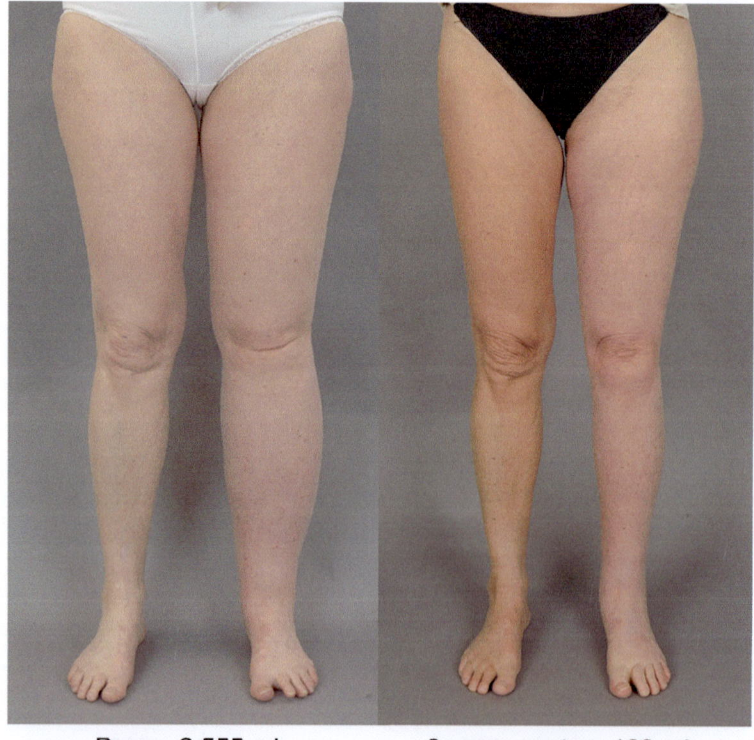

lymphedematous leg was even a little smaller. Then something happened: The patient had problems in sleeping with a thigh high stocking and she was even more active than before, challenging herself in running and golf so we needed to find a combination of garments that worked better for her. We worked very actively with this the following year and saw her every third month again to be able to evaluate the measures we took. At the last checkup she was down at 180 ml in excess volume. We continue to see her every third month to keep control [10].

Case 4 (Figs. 18.11 and 18.12)

This patient is a girl in her teens suffering from primary lymphedema since 2 years. She is a student and likes to ride and care for her horse. Her preoperative excess volume was 2,900 ml. During the first year we were very active with different combinations in order to increase compression. The patient's excess volume never reached zero. One of the reasons for this was that the girl at the same time wanted to lose weight, so we were always a little behind, chasing the volume of the healthy leg. When it was possible we decreased measurements of the garments and two and a half year ago we changed compression class to CCL 4 daytime. Her excess volume has been more and more stable around zero, at 4 years postoperatively it was −40 ml, Now there is only need for seeing her on checkups once a year when all compression garments for the following year is ordered.

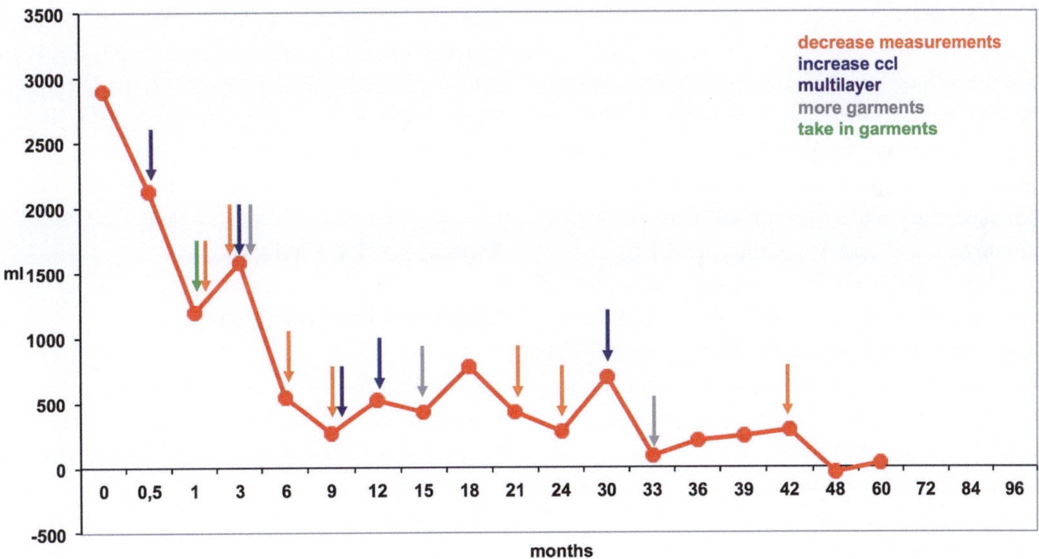

Fig. 18.11 Case 4: Notice the decrease in excess volume during the postoperative treatment and that complete reduction was finally achieved at 4 years due to high activity level with horse riding and at times increasing the volume of the operated leg, and also weight loss, leading to decrease of the volume of the control leg. © Karin Ohlin

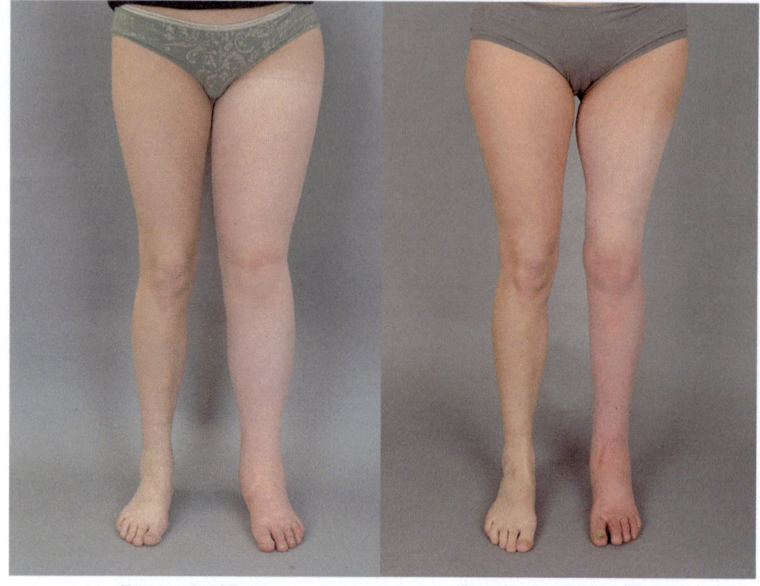

Fig. 18.12 Case 4: Preoperative excess volume 2,900 ml (*left*). Postoperative excess volume after 4 years is – (minus) 40 ml, i.e., the treated leg is smaller than the unaffected leg. © Håkan Brorson

Conclusion

All five strategies of increasing compression can be combined to treat leg lymphedema. Three of the strategies are useful also when you want to shape specific parts of the leg. You localize the parts needing extra compression by comparing circumferences and by estimating pitting.

These four cases illustrate the importance of providing the correct amount of garments. Case 3 and 4 need more garments to keep control. This can depend on both the severity of the lymphedema and the activity level of the patient.

Case 1: 8 set/12 months

Case 2: 6 set/12 months

Case 3: 14 set/12 months

Case 4: 18 set/12 months

One set = one thigh high garment and one knee long garment

Finally most important is to involve the patient in the decisions. It is the patient that has to do the job, putting on the garments every day and keep them on day and night. If they feel they have a choice in which way to go, they will most likely do their part.

We used different combinations of increasing compression, the patients needed different amount of garments and different interval between checkups, but the important thing is to help them never lose control over their lymphedema and help them back on track if the edema temporarily gets worse.

Advice to the Patient

Taking on the Garment

See the manufacturers' instructions.

- Rubber gloves can be used for better grip.
- Easy Slide is a simple pull-on tool for both leg and arm.
- Anti-slip mat on the floor can make it easier to brace against and herd up the sock over the heel.
- The material should be distributed evenly over the limb so that pleats are avoided. Pleats lead to folds and increased pressure.
- It is important that the arm garment is pulled high enough so that the elbow marking is at the right level. The elbow and the terminations need to be at the correct level. Poorly fitted garment leads to lower pressure and risk of chafing.

Care

- To maintain the garment's properties during 3–6 months it must be handled according to the manufacturer's instructions.
- The garment is washed daily to restore its compression and shape and to remove the salt precipitations from perspiration. The salt dries the skin and increases the risk of skin irritation.
- The garment should be left to dry horizontally to avoid stretch. It dries faster if you first roll it in a towel and gently squeeze the water.
- Soaking, use of fabric softener, and tumbling harm the compression garments.
- Fat, oil-based skin creams should not be used because they can dissolve the rubber thread in rubber-based garments. Use moisturizing lotions instead.

Miscellaneous

- Skin rash after using the garment may be due to allergic reaction to detergent or the material used.
- If a new garment feels too tight, it can be stretched over an object while drying after washing, for example a bottle that is somewhat wider the extremity for a few hours.
- Taking in the garment can be made between scheduled visits if it is too loose or as part of the treatment for controlled compression therapy. The patient can be instructed to do it by herself.
- Thick seams, for example on the fingers, may need to be stretched somewhat before use to prevent chafing.

- During hot summer days, it is wise to bathe or shower with compression garment on and let it dry on the skin. This provides a cooling effect.

References

1. Brorson H, Svensson H. Liposuction combined with controlled compression therapy reduces arm lymphedema more effectively than controlled compression therapy alone. Plast Reconstr Surg. 1998;102(4):1058–67. discussion 68.
2. Swedborg I. Effects of treatment with an elastic sleeve and intermittent pneumatic compression in postmastectomy patients with lymphoedema of the arm. Scand J Rehabil Med. 1984;16(1):35–41.
3. Brorson H. From lymph to fat: liposuction as a treatment for complete reduction of lymphedema. Int J Low Extrem Wounds. 2012;11(1):10–9.
4. European Committee for Standardisation (CEN/TC 205WG2). Medical compression hoisery. European Standard CEN/ENV 12718, 2001.
5. Andersen L, Hojris I, Erlandsen M, Andersen J. Treatment of breast-cancer-related lymphedema with or without manual lymphatic drainage–a randomized study. Acta Oncol. 2000;39(3):399–405.
6. Dayes IS, Whelan TJ, Julian JA, Parpia S, Pritchard KI, D'Souza DP, et al. Randomized trial of decongestive lymphatic therapy for the treatment of lymphedema in women with breast cancer. J Clin Oncol. 2013;31(30):3758–63.
7. Javid SH, Anderson BO. Mounting evidence against complex decongestive therapy as a first-line treatment for early lymphedema. J Clin Oncol. 2013;31(30):3737–8.
8. Brorson H, Svensson H. Complete reduction of lymphoedema of the arm by liposuction after breast cancer. Scand J Plast Reconstr Surg Hand Surg. 1997;31(2):137–43.
9. Brorson H, Svensson H, Norrgren K, Thorsson O. Liposuction reduces arm lymphedema without significantly altering the already impaired lymph transport. Lymphology. 1998;31(4):156–72.
10. Ketterings C, Zeddeman S. Use of the C-scan in evaluation of peripheral lymphedema. Lymphology. 1997;30(2):49–62.

19

Stéphane Vignes

Key Points
- Complex decongestive therapy comprises two successive stages: an intensive phase to reduce lymphedema volume and a maintenance phase to stabilize lymphedema volume.
- Compression (low-stretch bandage, elastic garment) is the cornerstone of lymphedema treatment.
- Patient-education programs, including self-management, aim to improve patient autonomy.

Introduction

Lymphedema is a chronic debilitating pathological disorder, with lymph stagnation inducing tissue modifications, including adipose deposition, increased fibrosis (responsible for Stemmer's sign), and elastic fiber disruption. It requires long-term specific treatment.

Complete decongestive therapy (CDT), also called complex or multimodal decongestive physiotherapy, is the term proposed by Michael Földi in the 1980s to define lymphedema treatment.

His approach is divided into two separate phases (Table 19.1) [1]. The first, intended to obtain the most important reduction of lymphedema volume, is comprised of several components: low-stretch bandage, manual lymph drainage (MLD), skin/nail care, and exercises, each having its own specific objective and role in limiting the impact of this disorder. The intensive strategy of this stage aims to achieve a 30–40 % lymphedema-volume reduction [2–4], eliminating only the fluid component of lymphedema. The second phase of CDT helps stabilize lymphedema volume over the long-term and is based on wearing an elastic garment, exercises, skin care, and, sometimes, MLD [5].

Low-Stretch Bandage

Each of the four CDT components has a different goal and those objectives are not of equal importance. Low-stretch bandage is the major element of CDT. It is able to achieve important and significant lymphedema-volume reduction. A low-stretch bandage is wrapped in multiple—2 to 4 (even 5 when lymphedema volume is huge)—layers after covering the affected limb with padding composed of foam and/or cotton batting (Figs. 19.1, 19.2, and 19.3). A low-stretch bandage is defined as having an elongation below 100 %, as previously described by Partsch et al. [6]. The bandage should be wrapped around the affected limb by a trained physiotherapist

S. Vignes, M.D. (✉)
Department of Lymphology, Centre National de Référence des Maladies Vasculaires Rares (Lymphoedèmes Primaires), Hôpital Cognacq-Jay, 15, rue Eugène-Millon, 75015 Paris, France
e-mail: stephane.vignes@cognacq-jay.fr

A.K. Greene et al. (eds.), *Lymphedema: Presentation, Diagnosis, and Treatment*,
DOI 10.1007/978-3-319-14493-1_19, © Springer International Publishing Switzerland 2015

Table 19.1 Two phases of CDT to treat lymphedema [1]

Phase I. Intensive phase (volume reduction)	Phase II. Maintenance phase (volume stabilization)
Low-stretch bandages worn 24 h/24, for 1–3 weeks	Elastic garments, every day, from morning to evening
Manual lymph drainage	Low-stretch bandages overnight (3 or more per week)
Exercises	Exercises
Skin care	Skin care
	Manual lymph drainage, if necessary

CDT complete decongestive therapy

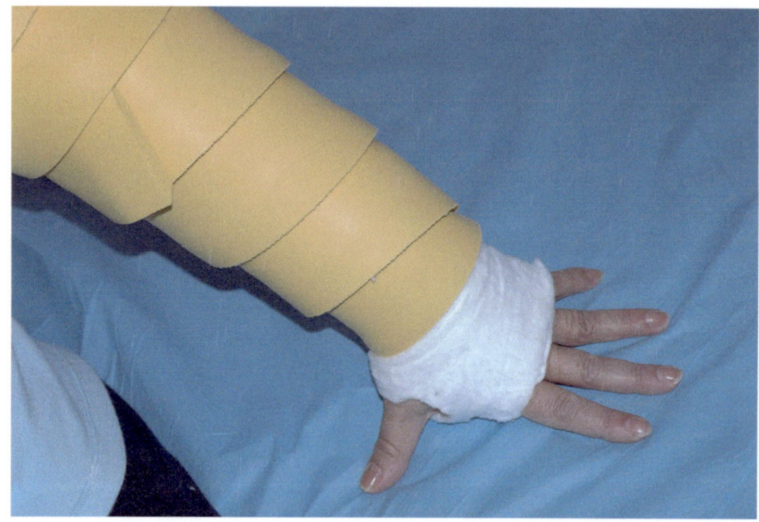

Fig. 19.1 Upper-limb lymphedema: bandage with foam

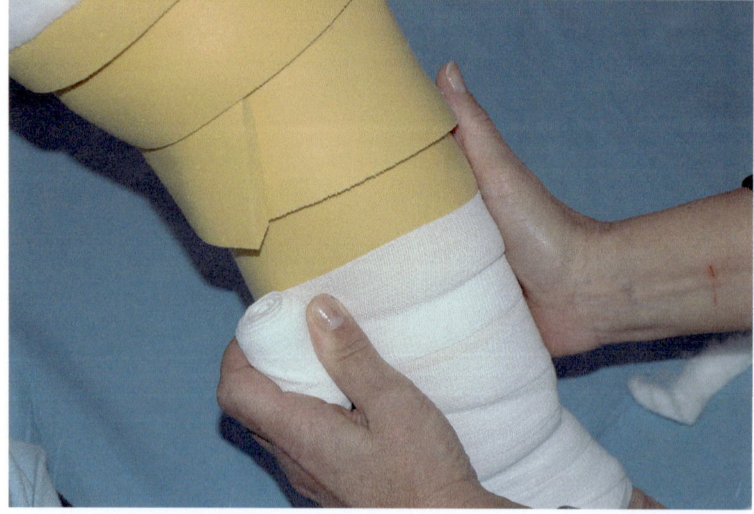

Fig. 19.2 Upper-limb lymphedema: foam padding partially covered with a first layer of low-stretch bandage

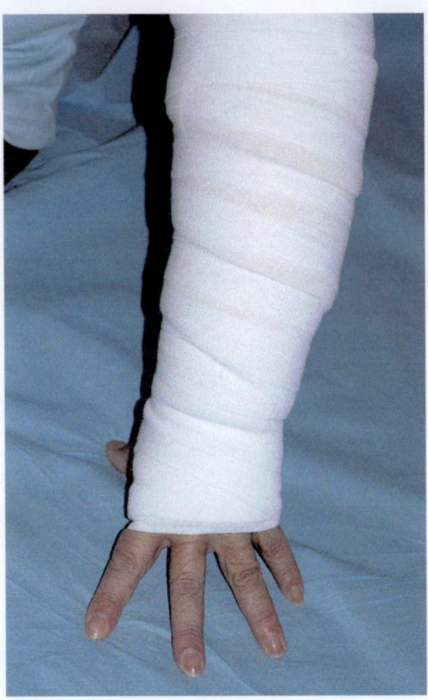

Fig. 19.3 Complete upper-limb low-stretch bandage for lymphedema

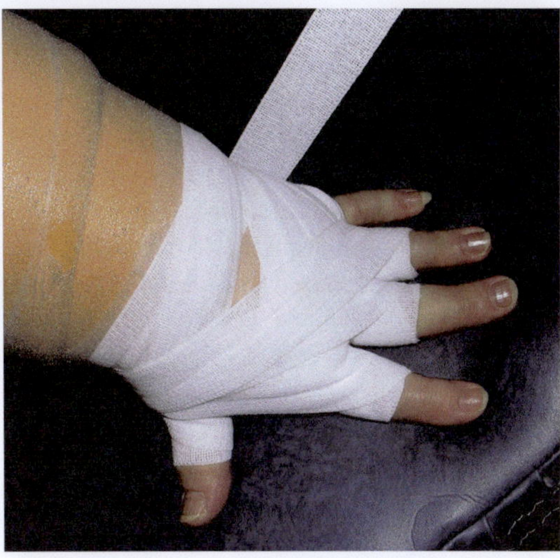

Fig. 19.4 Finger bandage for lymphedema

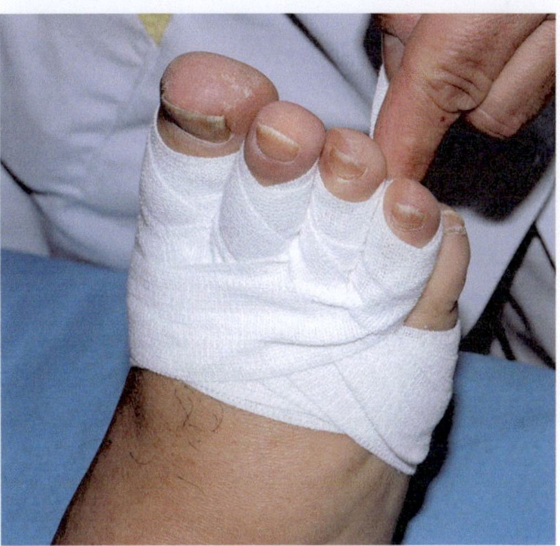

Fig. 19.5 Toe bandage with low-stretch bandage

or nurse (depending on the various practices in different countries), applying pressure with the hand without pulling the band and squeezing the limb, which causes pain and makes it impossible for the patient to keep the bandage in place, especially during the night. Bandages are applied progressively, starting from the distal extremity (hand, foot, sometimes toe or finger) and gradually placed more proximally until reaching the axilla or groin (knee if lymphedema only concerns the lower leg). The low-stretch bandage exerts a low but not non-existent pressure that increases with muscular activity (exercise) that is recommended while wearing it. It may be kept in place for 24 h and reapplied every day or 48–72 h for the weekend. Bandaging may include finger/hand or toes/feet if they are affected by lymphedema (Figs. 19.4 and 19.5).

Because bandages are the cornerstone of the first phase, the patient (self-bandaging technique) and/or family members are sometimes taught the technique during the intensive phase under the supervision of the physiotherapist or nurse.

Each patient should be proposed several training sessions in validated specific patient-education programs to master the wrapping procedure and verify good understanding and implementation. At least three overnight bandages per week are recommended during the long-term maintenance phase. The aim of learning self-bandaging is to improve the patient's autonomy to manage his/her own lymphedema.

During the maintenance phase, follow-up visits are scheduled at 6 and 12 months, and then annually to ensure lymphedema-volume stability and the patient's motivation to pursue treatment. Workshops to reinforce the ability to pursue the self-bandaging technique are probably useful for patients having technical difficulties. Pertinently, because it must be maintained lifelong, lymphedema treatment is constraining.

After the intensive phase of treatment, most patients' lymphedema volume tends to increase, often moderately, without reaching the pretreatment volume. The degree of adherence to regular low-stretch bandage strapping and wearing an elastic garment are the two predictors of whether or not the volume will increase [7]. Other types of bandages are currently not recommended for lymphedema management but some promising data are available on low-stretch cohesive bands [8].

Manual Lymph Drainage

MLD is a specific technique practiced by physiotherapists specialized in lymphatic-drainage techniques. The theoretical goal of MLD is to increase the lymphokinetic activity of normal lymphatics or stimulate the functional units of lymph vessels (lymphangion) to contract more frequently to channel lymph towards adjacent lymphatics. Several MLD technical variants (Casley-Smith, Vodder, Földi, Leduc) have been described, with or without node pumping, using more or less cutaneous pressure, and beginning on the proximal or distal side [9]. MLD usually lasts 30–45 min, or even longer for some authors. Classically, it begins by manual stimulation of the lymph nodes in adjacent drainage regions (neck, subclavicular, contralateral axilla, back, ipsilateral groin) and is followed by manual decongestion of the involved trunk, shoulder, arm, forearm and, if necessary, hand and fingers for the upper limb or back, abdomen, thigh, calf, and foot and, if necessary, toes. Several physiotherapists proposed not doing the first step of manual stimulation and retaining only manual decongestion; others suggest exerting greater pressure on the skin, especially when it is firm or hard.

MLD is recommended during the CDT intensive phase, just before applying the low-stretch bandage, and procures an additive effect, particularly for patients with moderate lymphedema [10]. MLD is not considered a stand-alone treatment for lymphedema to reduce volume but is advocated for breast, thoracic, mons pubic, face, or neck lymphedema, as these zones are difficult to compress or inaccessible to compression with bandages or an elastic garment, or in a palliative care context that is inconducive to compression [9, 11].

MLD is not consistently recommended during the maintenance phase. However, patients may learn self-lymphatic drainage (SLD), also called modified lymphatic drainage, to be performed while in a decubitus position. SLD is easy to do for breast, upper limb, or mons pubic lymphedema but more difficult for the lower limb. The patient must be highly motivated to learn and practice self-drainage.

In any case, MLD also assures regular followup by the physiotherapist and may help encourage some patients to find the necessary motivation to pursue and comply with long-term treatment (bandage, elastic garment). Notably, MLD may also improve their quality of life by reducing psychosocial and lymphedema-related symptoms [9].

Exercises

Exercises are considered another major component of CDT. Most of the proposed exercises concern upper-limb lymphedema occurring after breast-cancer treatment; much fewer deal with primary or secondary lower-limb lymphedema. Different types of exercises have been devised: against/without resistance, isometric, aerobic, including the lymphedematous limb, with repetitive, progressive, and therapist-guided movements. Various types of soft and remedial exercises are used, always associated with posture correction, abdominal breathing, including neck (stretches), shoulder (shrugs, rotations, stretches), arm (isometric biceps curl), elbow (circles), forearm, wrist (rotations), and fingers (opening/closing) [2]. During the CDT intensive phase, ideally with the short-stretch bandage or elastic garment in place, these exercises are intended to facilitate lymph resorption into remaining functional lymph channels. However, muscular activity may more difficult while wearing an elastic garment (recommended) that nonetheless appears essential in this situation [12, 13]. During the maintenance phase, patients are encouraged to continue regular daily exercises at home.

Speaking more generally, physical activity is always recommended for lymphedema patients, whose disease and/or comorbidities do not impose medical restrictions, especially when the upper limb is affected and even outside the CDT setting. Importantly, exercises, even intensive, such as weight lifting, Dragon Boat racing or pole walking, do not trigger or worsen lymphedema, and might even prevent it [14–16]. Physical activity greatly improves the quality of life after breast-cancer treatment and reduces the risk of breast-cancer recurrence and mortality due to it [17]. In conclusion, exercising is strongly recommended for lymphedema patients but the movements should be progressive in intensity and repeated, under the supervision of a trained therapist, and ideally done while wearing an elastic garment and guided by the patient's sensations.

Skin and Nail Care

Meticulous skin and nail care is mandatory for patients with lymphedema. Patients with limb lymphedema are confronted with various cutaneous complications, most of which can represent a site of entry for infections, particularly cellulitis (erysipelas). Notably, lower-limb lymphedema increases the risk of cellulitis 70-fold, in comparison to a non-lymphedematous limb [18]. Moreover, skin care is also essential to prevent worsening of the condition and infections. Cutaneous disorders predominate in the lower limb and include different types of lesions, whose treatments are specific:

- Nail deformation: nail plates are shortened and hypercurved, with possible raised toenails, with the risk of ingrown toenails (pedicure, eventually nail surgery);
- Toe-web fungal infections, especially due to dermatophytes (topical treatment with antifungal agents) (Fig. 19.6);
- Hyperkeratosis: the skin is thickened, with risk of skin cracking (heel) (regular daily moisturizing, pedicure) (Fig. 19.7);
- Papillomatosis: lymphedema induces skin proliferation, sometimes pseudotumoral (untreated and surgery can be considered if the lesions are voluminous);
- Skin dryness with risk of skin cracking (regular daily moisturizing);
- Lymphatic vesicles, essentially located on the toe, frequently with oozing lymph, sometimes very abundantly, increasing skin maceration (untreated, localized compression to effectively stop lymph oozing, laser coagulation with the risk of recurrence).

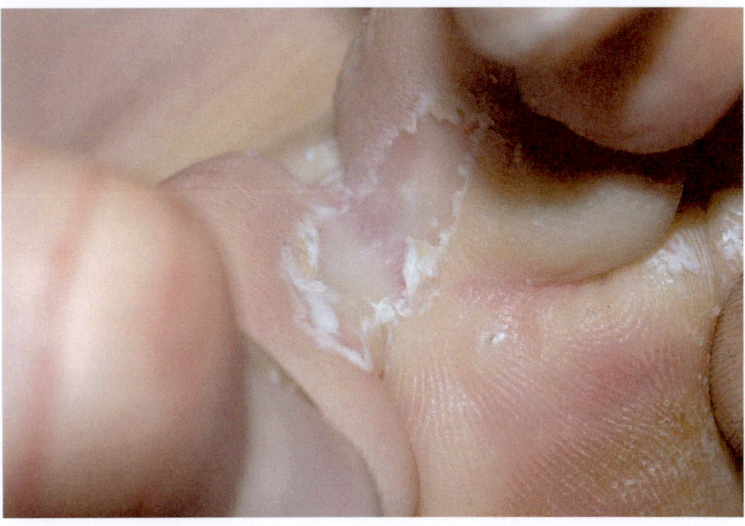

Fig. 19.6 Toe-web intertrigo

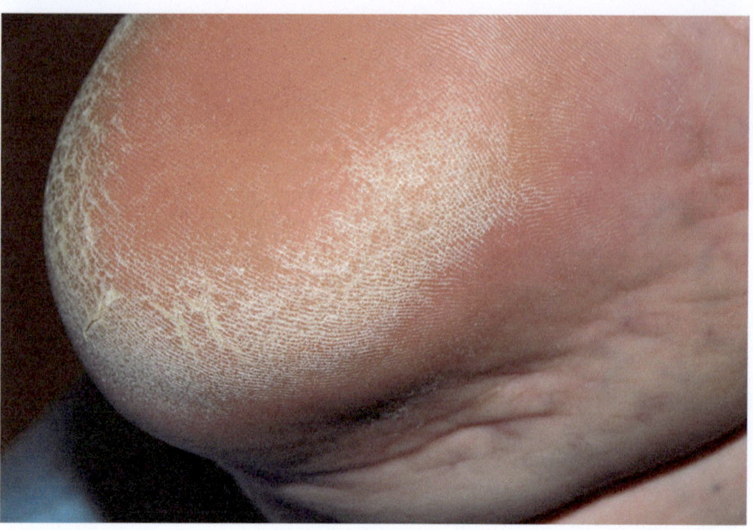

Fig. 19.7 Heel hyperkeratosis

Simultaneously, patients are instructed to avoid cutaneous abrasions (e.g., cuts, burns, insect bites, cat scratches, cracks in dry skin) and to protect their skin during daily activities (e.g., wearing gloves for gardening, a thimble when sewing).

Elastic Garment

Practitioners should encourage long-term and consistent wearing of an elastic garment. Their own motivation is a major driving force to stoke the patient's motivation. Wearing an elastic garment is the foundation of the CDT maintenance phase to stabilize lymphedema volume after the intensive phase. An elastic garment may be also the first-line treatment for patients with recent-onset moderate lymphedema after breast-cancer treatment. Indeed, the results of a recent randomized study demonstrated that CDT was unable to achieve significantly better lymphedema-volume reduction than elastic compression for patients after breast-cancer treatment [19].

The elastic sheath is worn from morning to evening every day, and the garment model is adapted to the lymphedema localization: sleeve including or not the hand and the finger (gantlet for lymphedema that extends to the hand or the fingers) (Figs. 19.8, 19.9, and 19.10), below-the-knee sock or stocking (ideally closed-toe to avoid toe lymphedema with its risk of vesicles and oozing lymph) (Fig. 19.11). Pressures delivered by compression garments have to attain 20–60 mmHg, with the possibility of stocking superposition for lower-limb lymphedema. Two weaving techniques are used to make the elastic garments, flat and circular knitting, each of which has its own advantages or disadvantages, and also depending on the practices in each country. The ideal compression garment should be custom-made, fitted by trained personnel and replaced every 4–6 months. Use of specific devices (donning tool) may be recommended to facilitate the accurate positioning of the elastic garment.

Other Components Not Included in CDT

Although CDT is composed of low-stretch bandage, MLD, skin care, exercises and wearing an elastic garment, some other major factors contribute importantly to managing lymphedema. Obesity is a predictor of upper-limb lymphedema after breast-cancer treatment [20]. High body mass index (BMI) is also associated with the severity of lymphedema, i.e., its volume [21]. Overweight and obese patients should be oriented towards specific consultation with a dietician or nutritionist to incite them to lose weight because weight control

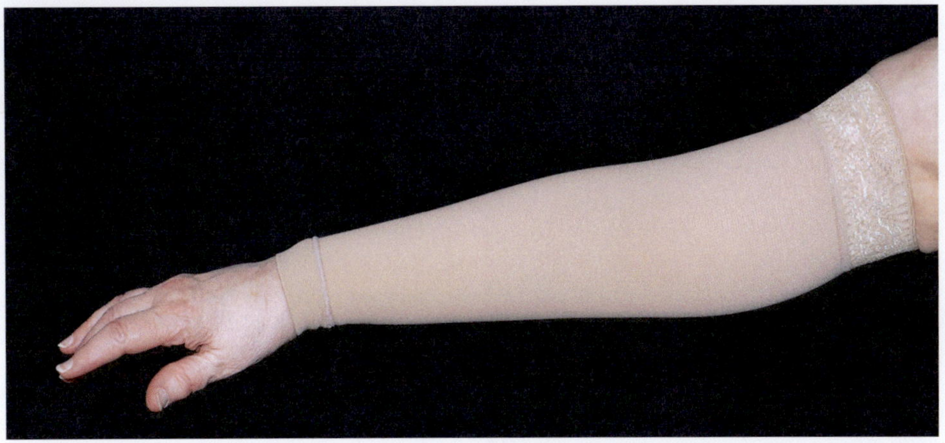

Fig. 19.8 Elastic sleeve not including the hand for upper-limb lymphedema

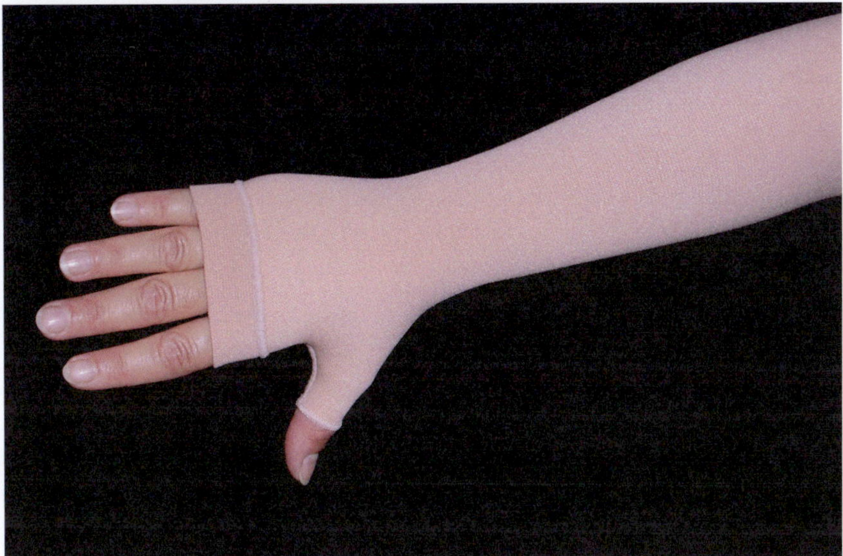

Fig. 19.9 Elastic sleeve including hand for lymphedema

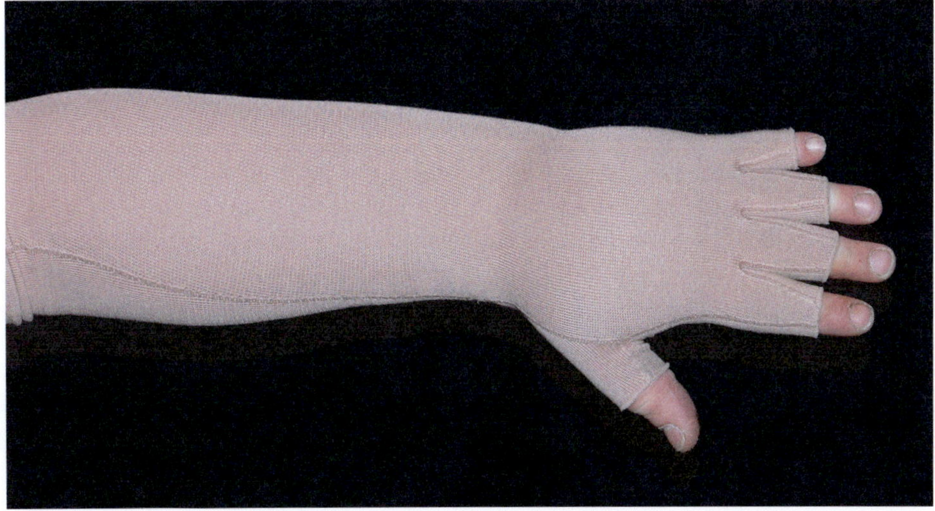

Fig. 19.10 Elastic sleeve including the hand and fingers (gantlet) for upper-limb lymphedema

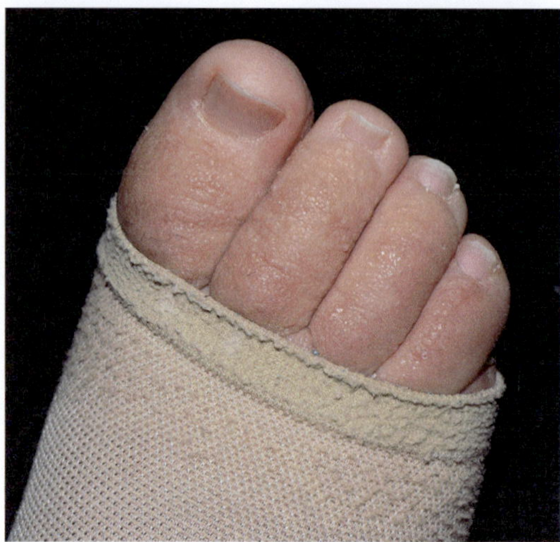

Fig. 19.11 Lower-limb lymphedema: papillomatosis and lymphatic vesicles with oozing worsened by wearing an open-toe stocking

is a major component of lymphedema management [22]. Pneumatic compression is not included in CDT but is sometimes associated with bandaging during the first intensive phase [23].

Alternative techniques (electrostimulation, acupuncture, elastic taping, laser, endermology (mechanical cellulite massage therapy), extracorporeal shock wave, deep oscillation, hyperbaric oxygen, ultrasound) are sometimes used but weakness of their evaluations does not allow us to recommend these techniques before further well-defined studies are conducted [24]. Other medical therapies, including diuretics, benzopyrones, selenium, or tocopherol, are not recommended [23].

Treatment Indications

No clear indication exists to prescribe CDT for patients with lymphedema. Several questions should be considered before deciding with the patient what therapeutic approach to pursue.

- Is the aim of the CDT to reduce lymphedema volume, improve limb shape/appearance, soften the skin or to attenuate symptoms (heaviness)? What is the patient's motivation? Is an elastic garment alone sufficient?

- Are the infections (cellulitis) recurrent? In this context, lymphedema management should be based on prevention of infections: antibiotic prophylaxis, recommendations to avoid creating sites of entry.

- Finally, the essential question is: what are the therapeutic objectives, for the patient and the practitioner and/or nurse and/or the physiotherapist? The different parameters to consider before prescribing CDT include the patient's age, lymphedema characteristics (duration, volume, skin hardness, topography (e.g., hand lymphedema), status: stability/worsening), complications such as cellulitis, association with other limb problems (pain, radiation-induced plexopathy, limited shoulder mobility range), and the patient's motivation.

Importantly, the patient must be fully informed that lymphedema remains a chronic disease whose management is also lifelong and constraining.

Conclusion: Future Perspectives

CDT is the recommended reference standard for lymphedema treatment, but its different components have not been evaluated separately. Each one has its proper main objective that contributes to managing the disorder. Therapeutic goals should be defined with the patient and the different therapists implicated in the patient's management. A multidisciplinary meeting for each patient is required to define the personalized treatment program and adapt the role of each CDT component: excluding MLD, emphasizing skin care or exercises, wearing a compression garment alone. Although randomized trials on self-management are sorely lacking, it seems important to include, as part and parcel of lymphedema management, a patient-education program with specific and evaluated workshops to give to the patients the expertise (self-techniques) and knowledge about lymphedema they need to self-manage their chronic pathology and maintain long-term motivation [25].

References

1. Cheville AL, McGarvey CL, Petrek JA, Russo SA, Taylor ME, Thiadens SR. Lymphedema management. Semin Radiat Oncol. 2003;13:290–301.
2. Ko DS, Lerner R, Klose G, Cosimi AB. Effective treatment of lymphedema of the extremities. Arch Surg. 1998;133:452–8.
3. Szuba A, Cooke JP, Yousuf S, Rockson SG. Decongestive lymphatic therapy for patients with cancer-related or primary lymphedema. Am J Med. 2000;109:296–300.
4. Vignes S, Porcher R, Champagne A, Dupuy A. Predictive factors of response to intensive decongestive physiotherapy in upper limb lymphedema after breast cancer treatment: a cohort study. Breast Cancer Res Treat. 2006;98:1–6.
5. International Society of Lymphology. The diagnosis and treatment of peripheral lymphedema: 2013 consensus document of the International Society of Lymphology. Lymphology. 2013;46:1–11.
6. Partsch H, Clark M, Bassez S, Benigni JP, Becker F, Blazek V, et al. Measurement of lower leg compression in vivo: recommendations for the performance of measurements of interface pressure and stiffness: consensus statement. Dermatol Surg. 2006;32:224–32.
7. Vignes S, Porcher R, Arrault M, Dupuy A. Factors influencing breast cancer-related lymphedema volume after intensive decongestive physiotherapy. Support Care Cancer. 2011;19:935–40.
8. Moffatt CJ, Franks PJ, Hardy D, Lewis M, Parker V, Feldman JL. A preliminary randomized controlled study to determine the application frequency of a new lymphoedema bandaging system. Br J Dermatol. 2012;166:624–32.
9. Lasinski BB, McKillip Thrift K, Squire D, Austin MK, Smith KM, Wanchai A, et al. A systematic review of the evidence for complete decongestive therapy in the treatment of lymphedema from 2004 to 2011. PM R. 2012;4:580–601.
10. McNeely ML, Magee DJ, Lees AW, Bagnall KM, Haykowsky M, Hanson J. The addition of manual lymph drainage to compression therapy for breast cancer related lymphedema: a randomized controlled trial. Breast Cancer Res Treat. 2004;86:95–106.
11. Jeffs E. Treating breast cancer-related lymphoedema at the London Haven: clinical audit results. Eur J Oncol Nurs. 2006;10:71–9.
12. Johansson K, Tibe K, Weibull A, Newton RC. Low intensity resistance exercise for breast cancer patients with arm lymphedema with or without compression sleeve. Lymphology. 2005;38:167–80.
13. Brennan MJ, Miller LT. Overview of treatment options and review of the current role and use of compression garments, intermittent pumps, and exercise in the management of lymphedema. Cancer. 1998;83(12 (Suppl American)):2821–7.
14. Schmitz KH, Ahmed RL, Troxel AB, Cheville A, Lewis-Grant L, Smith R, et al. Weight lifting for women at risk for breast cancer-related lymphedema: a randomized trial. JAMA. 2010;304:2699–705.
15. Schmitz KH, Ahmed RL, Troxel A, Cheville A, Smith R, Lewis-Grant L, et al. Weight lifting in women with breast-cancer-related lymphedema. N Engl J Med. 2009;361:664–73.
16. Harris SR. "We're All in the Same Boat": a review of the benefits of Dragon Boat racing for women living with breast cancer. Evid Based Complement Alternat Med. 2012;2012:167651.
17. Ibrahim EM, Al-Homaidh A. Physical activity and survival after breast cancer diagnosis: meta-analysis of published studies. Med Oncol. 2011;28:753–65.
18. Dupuy A, Benchikhi H, Roujeau JC, Bernard P, Vaillant L, Chosidow O, et al. Risk factors for erysipelas of the leg (cellulitis): case–control study. BMJ. 1999;318:1591–4.
19. Dayes IS, Whelan TJ, Julian JA, Parpia S, Pritchard KI, D'Souza DP, et al. Randomized trial of decongestive lymphatic therapy for the treatment of lymphedema in women with breast cancer. J Clin Oncol. 2013;31:3758–63.
20. Ridner SH, Dietrich MS, Stewart BR, Armer JM. Body mass index and breast cancer treatment-related lymphedema. Support Care Cancer. 2011;19:853–7.
21. Vignes S, Arrault M, Dupuy A. Factors associated with increased breast cancer-related lymphedema volume. Acta Oncol. 2007;46:1138–42.
22. Shaw C, Mortimer P, Judd PA. Randomized controlled trial comparing a low-fat diet with a weight-reduction diet in breast cancer-related lymphedema. Cancer. 2007;109:1949–56.
23. Harris SR, Schmitz KH, Campbell KL, McNeely ML. Clinical practice guidelines for breast cancer rehabilitation: syntheses of guideline recommendations and qualitative appraisals. Cancer. 2012;118(8 Suppl):2312–24.
24. Rodrick JR, Poage E, Wanchai A, Stewart BR, Cormier JN, Armer JM. Complementary, alternative, and other noncomplete decongestive therapy treatment methods in the management of lymphedema: a systematic search and review. PM R. 2014;6:250–74.
25. Ridner SH, Fu MR, Wanchai A, Stewart BR, Armer JM, Cormier JN. Self-management of lymphedema: a systematic review of the literature from 2004 to 2011. Nurs Res. 2012;61:291–9.

Pneumatic Compression

Reid A. Maclellan

Key Points

- Intermittent pneumatic compression aids in reducing lymphedematous extremities by recapitulating physiologic lymphatic flow
- Models are single or multichambered and have a wide range of therapeutic options.
- Pumps should be used as an adjunct treatment for patients with lymphedema; however, patients should concurrently use pressure gradient garments.

Introduction

Lymphedema is a chronic disease that requires lifetime maintenance. Protein-rich fluid accumulates in the interstitial space resulting in limb swelling, impaired extremity function, unsatisfactory cosmesis, and psychosocial morbidity. Conservative treatments consist of compression garments, massage, multilayered bandages, and intermittent pneumatic compression. The goal of these interventions is to decrease fluid production and promote lymph clearance. Pneumatic compression has been a beneficial adjunct therapy for lymphedema for over 60 years [1, 2].

R.A. Maclellan, M.D. M.M.Sc. (✉)
Lymphedema Program, Department of Plastic and Oral Surgery, Boston Children's Hospital,
Harvard Medical School, 300 Longwood Avenue,
Boston, MA 02115, USA
e-mail: Reid.Maclellan@childrens.harvard.edu

Intermittent Pneumatic Compression

Pneumatic compression devices administer intermittent pressure via a wide variety of inflation and deflation patterns. They are hypothesized to aid in delivering retained fluid to functional lymphatics that can then remove the lymph. The mechanical factors involved in decreasing a lymphedematous extremity are the compression cycle, pressure gradient, and distribution of pressure. The phenotypic characteristics of the diseased extremity also influence the efficacy of the pump. Intermittent pneumatic compression has been shown to be less effective in patients with increased subcutaneous fibrosis causing poor tissue compliance [3]. Devices can be fitted for either the upper or lower extremity (Fig. 20.1); custom designs also can be made for scrotal lymphedema.

Pump variables include: (1) single or multiple chambers; (2) sequential or nonsequential compression; and (3) gradient or non-gradient options (Table 20.1). Single compartment models were initially used to treat lymphedema. The entire limb receives a constant level of compression as the cuff expands and contracts in a rhythmic fashion. The pressure is delivered both centripetally and centrifugally. There is no sequential distribution or gradient of pressure given to the extremity. When comparing single and multi-compartment pumps, subcutaneously injected radioisotope has a more rapid transit to the inguinal lymph nodes with a multi-cell device [4]. Single chamber intermittent pneumatic compression pumps currently are not recommended for

A.K. Greene et al. (eds.), *Lymphedema: Presentation, Diagnosis, and Treatment*,
DOI 10.1007/978-3-319-14493-1_20, © Springer International Publishing Switzerland 2015

Fig. 20.1 Inflated upper extremity pneumatic pump

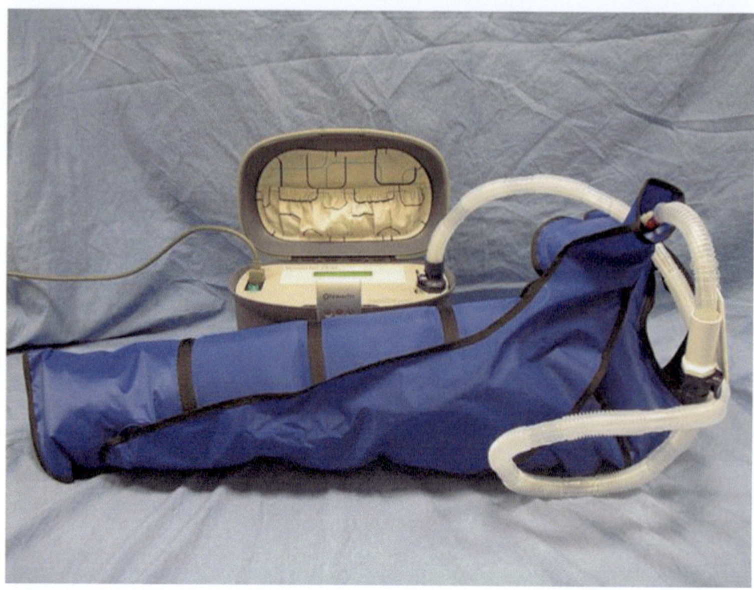

Table 20.1 Pneumatic compression pumps currently available for the treatment of lymphedema

Device	Compartment design	Sequential inflation	Gradient
Presion	Single	No	No
Eureduc	Multiple	Yes	No
Hadomer	Multiple	Yes	No
Huntleigh Flowpress	Multiple	Yes	No
Flexitouch	Multiple	Yes	Yes
KCI JOBST System	Multiple	Yes	Yes
Lymphapress	Multiple	Yes	Yes
NormaTec	Multiple	Yes	Yes
Petite Basic System	Multiple	Yes	Yes
Sequential Circulator	Multiple	Yes	Yes
Ventipress	Multiple	Yes	Yes
Wright Linear Pump	Multiple	Yes	Yes

patients because superior machines with multiple cells have been developed [5, 6].

There are two types of multichamber devices that were developed in the 1970s. One pump sequentially inflates up to four individual cells beginning distally and moving proximally. Once all chambers are inflated for a set time, the cuff deflates. This creates a wave of compression that ascends the limb. The other type of pump delivers a gradient of pressure with higher force in the distal chambers and lower pressure in the proximal ones. Unlike the 4-chamber device, this pump may have up to 36 small individual cells with at least three separate zones of compression [5]. The primary difference between each type of system is the amount of pressure delivered to the diseased limb, the pattern of delivery, and the total time of compression. Timed cycles range from a few seconds to several minutes.

Pressure of Compression

There is a large array of settings for intermittent pneumatic compression pumps. The pressure of lymphatic vessels in normal skin ranges from 4 to 8 mmHg, while patients with lymphedema have measurements between 15 and 18 mmHg in the absence of fibrosis [7, 8]. The therapeutic compression must be sufficient to overcome the resistive forces present within diseased tissue, but not so high that it collapses the superficial lymphatics.

Muscle contraction normally is required to aid in lymph returning to the heart because of the extremely low pressures in the lymphatics. Intermittent pneumatic compression devices recapitulate the pumping action of muscles.

In addition to possibly collapsing lymphatic vessels, sustained elevated force for a prolonged time period also can lead to ischemic skin damage. Pressures >60 mmHg for an extended time can reduce blood flow [9, 10]. Several studies recommend a peak inflation pressure range of 25–60 mmHg [11–13]. A few authors have demonstrated volume reduction with higher pressures (110–150 mmHg) [14–16].

Time and Frequency of Compression

Unlike manual lymphatic drainage that requires the assistance of a physical therapist, intermittent pneumatic compression therapy can be performed at the convenience of the patient in his/her home. Scientific evidence for the appropriate amount of time and frequency of treatment is sparse. Therapy may range from 30 minutes to 8 hours depending on the device and condition of the patient. One study evaluated self-reported data from patients who were asked to use their pump 2 hours per day for a month, then 1 hour per day thereafter [17]. More than half of individuals surveyed used the pump for the recommended duration; approximately 10 % did not attempt pneumatic compression therapy at all. Patients who followed the prescribed protocol reported a higher satisfaction [17]. We recommend that an individual pump for 2 hours per day at his/her convenience.

Volume Reduction from Compression

The primary goal of intermittent pneumatic compression is to reduce the excess volume in diseased limbs. Patients with upper extremity lymphedema secondary to breast cancer treatment had a 29 % reduction in volume in a randomized controlled trial after receiving pneumatic compression therapy for 12 weeks [6]. In another prospective study of individuals with upper extremity lymphedema, the experimental arm had a 45 % reduction in volume after undergoing decongestive lymphatic therapy and pneumatic compression therapy for 2 weeks compared to a decrease of 26 % for individuals who only had decongestive lymphatic therapy [18]. Patients with upper extremity lymphedema had a 3-3.5-fold reduction in volume when intermittent pneumatic compression was added to their self-administered maintenance therapy [12, 18]. Individuals who wear a standard compression sleeve for maintenance therapy had an additional volume reduction when sequential pneumatic compression was added to their treatment for 2 h per day [13, 19]. Patients with lymphedema of the lower extremity also benefit from intermittent pneumatic compression therapy. One-third had >10 % reduction in limb volume with the addition of pneumatic compression to their therapy; the mean reduction was 8 % [20]. In another prospective study 80 % of patients maintained a reduced limb size at 2-year follow-up [21].

Complications

Worsening of genital lymphedema has been reported from pneumatic compression. In a retrospective series of 53 patients with lower extremity lymphedema prescribed pump compression, 43 % had worsening genital edema [22]. However, a review of the literature from 2004 to 2011 found no reports of genital lymphedema development associated with intermittent pneumatic compression [5]. Worsening genital lymphedema also was not appreciated in a study following patients treated for 3 years with pneumatic compression [15]. Patients should abstain from pump therapy if they have an infection or deep vein thrombosis in the limb, local malignancy, or are anticoagulated [23].

Conclusion

The 2013 Consensus Document of the International Society of Lymphology supports the use of intermittent pneumatic compression as an adjunct treatment for patients with lymphedema; however, patients should concurrently use pressure gradient garments [24]. The primary purpose of compression is to facilitate a reduction in edema. Patients tolerate the therapy well. We recommend patients undergo treatment for 2 h per day at their convenience. Although most US insurance companies cover the cost of a pneumatic pump, patients occasionally are required to purchase their device at a cost of $1,000–$5,000 [25].

Acknowledgement *Disclosure*: The author has no disclosures.

References

1. Brush BE, Heldt TJ. A device for relief of lymphedema. J Am Med Assoc. 1955;158(1):34–5.
2. Brush BE, Wylie JH, Beninson J, Block MA, Heldt TJ. The treatment of postmastectomy lymphedema. AMA Arch Surg. 1958;77(4):561–7.
3. Raines JK, O'Donnell Jr TF, Kalisher L, Darling RC. Selection of patients with lymphedema for compression therapy. Am J Surg. 1977;133(4):430–7.
4. Partsch H, Mostbeck A, Leitner G. [Experimental studies on the efficacy of pressure wave massage (Lymphapress) in lymphedema]. Journal Lymphol. 1981;5(1):35–9.
5. Feldman JL, Stout NL, Wanchai A, Stewart BR, Cormier JN, Armer JM. Intermittent pneumatic compression therapy: a systematic review. Lymphology. 2012;45(1):13–25.
6. Fife CE, Davey S, Maus EA, Guilliod R, Mayrovitz HN. A randomized controlled trial comparing two types of pneumatic compression for breast cancer-related lymphedema treatment in the home. Support Care Cancer. 2012;20(12):3279–86.
7. Spiegel M, Vesti B, Shore A, Franzeck UK, Becker F, Bollinger A. Pressure of lymphatic capillaries in human skin. Am J Physiol. 1992;262(4 Pt 2):H1208–10.
8. Zaugg-Vesti B, Dorffler-Melly J, Spiegel M, Wen S, Franzeck UK, Bollinger A. Lymphatic capillary pressure in patients with primary lymphedema. Microvasc Res. 1993;46(2):128–34.
9. Xakellis GC, Frantz RA, Arteaga M, Meletiou S. Dermal blood flow response to constant pressure in healthy older and younger subjects. J Gerontol. 1993;48(1):M6–9.
10. Mayrovitz HN. Compression-induced pulsatile blood flow changes in human legs. Clin Physiol. 1998;18(2):117–24.
11. Mayrovitz HN. Interface pressures produced by two different types of lymphedema therapy devices. Phys Ther. 2007;87(10):1379–88.
12. Szolnoky G, Lakatos B, Keskeny T, Varga E, Varga M, Dobozy A, et al. Intermittent pneumatic compression acts synergistically with manual lymphatic drainage in complex decongestive physiotherapy for breast cancer treatment-related lymphedema. Lymphology. 2009;42(4):188–94.
13. Johansson K, Lie E, Ekdahl C, Lindfeldt J. A randomized study comparing manual lymph drainage with sequential pneumatic compression for treatment of postoperative arm lymphedema. Lymphology. 1998;31(2):56–64.
14. Moseley AL, Carati CJ, Piller NB. A systematic review of common conservative therapies for arm lymphoedema secondary to breast cancer treatment. Ann Oncol. 2007;18(4):639–46.
15. Zaleska M, Olszewski WL, Durlik M. The effectiveness of intermittent pneumatic compression in long-term therapy of lymphedema of lower limbs. Lymphat Res Biol. 2014;12(2):103–9.
16. Zelikovski A, Manoach M, Giler S, Urca I. Lymphapress A new pneumatic device for the treatment of lymphedema of the limbs. Lymphology. 1980;13(2):68–73.
17. Ridner SH, McMahon E, Dietrich MS, Hoy S. Home-based lymphedema treatment in patients with cancer-related lymphedema or noncancer-related lymphedema. Oncol Nurs Forum. 2008;35(4):671–80.
18. Szuba A, Achalu R, Rockson SG. Decongestive lymphatic therapy for patients with breast carcinoma-associated lymphedema. A randomized, prospective study of a role for adjunctive intermittent pneumatic compression. Cancer. 2002;95(11):2260–7.
19. Swedborg I. Effects of treatment with an elastic sleeve and intermittent pneumatic compression in post-mastectomy patients with lymphoedema of the arm. Scand J Rehabil Med. 1984;16(1):35–41.
20. Muluk SC, Hirsch AT, Taffe EC. Pneumatic compression device treatment of lower extremity lymphedema elicits improved limb volume and patient-reported outcomes. Eur J Vasc Endovasc Surg. 2013;46(4):480–7.
21. Pappas CJ, O'Donnell TF. Long-term results of compression treatment for lymphedema. J Vasc Surg. 1992;16(4):555–62. discussion 62-4.
22. Boris M, Weindorf S, Lasinski BB. The risk of genital edema after external pump compression for lower limb lymphedema. Lymphology. 1998;31(1):15–20.
23. Brennan MJ, Miller LT. Overview of treatment options and review of the current role and use of compression garments, intermittent pumps, and exercise in the management of lymphedema. Cancer. 1998;83(12 (Suppl American)):2821–7.
24. The diagnosis and treatment of peripheral lymphedema: 2013 Consensus Document of the International Society of Lymphology. Lymphology. 2013;46(1):1–11.
25. Cheville AL, McGarvey CL, Petrek JA, Russo SA, Taylor ME, Thiadens SR. Lymphedema management. Semin Radiat Oncol. 2003;13(3):290–301.

Operative Management of Lymphedema

Arin K. Greene, Sumner A. Slavin, and Håkan Brorson

Key Points
- Placing alloplastic materials to drain lymphatic fluid has not proved effective.
- The Kondoleon operation has been replaced by staged skin/subcutaneous excisional procedures.
- The Thompson operation does not offer advantages to staged skin/subcutaneous excisional procedures and is more complicated.
- The morbidity and efficacy of omental transposition are outweighed by current operations.
- Muscle flaps have not been popularized because the procedures are more complicated and have not shown superior efficacy compared to other procedures.

A.K. Greene, M.D., M.M.Sc. (✉)
Department of Plastic and Oral Surgery,
Boston Children's Hospital, Harvard Medical School,
300 Longwood Avenue, Boston, MA 02115, USA
e-mail: arin.greene@childrens.harvard.edu

S.A. Slavin, M.D.
Department of Plastic and Oral Surgery, Boston
Children's Hospital, Harvard Medical School,
300 Longwood Avenue, Boston, MA 02115, USA

Division of Plastic Surgery, Beth Israel Deaconess
Medical Center, Boston, MA, USA

H. Brorson, M.D., Ph.D.
Esculera de Graduasos, Asociación Médica
Argentina, Buenos Aires, Argentina

Plastic and Reconstructive Surgery, Skåne University
Hospital, Scania, Sweden

Department of Clinical Sciences, Lund University,
Malmö, Sweden

Introduction

A standard operation for the treatment of lymphedema does not exist. Some surgeons prefer physiological procedures, which attempt to restore lymphatic flow, while others use excisional operations to remove diseased tissue. The most common physiological procedures currently performed include lymphatic–venous anastomosis and vascularized lymph node transfer. The most widely practiced excisional operations are liposuction and staged skin/subcutaneous excision. This chapter highlights other surgical treatments for lymphedema that are not commonly used (Table 21.1).

Physiologic Procedures Using Alloplastic Materials

In 1908, Handley attempted to drain a lymphedematous lower extremity by placing silk threads subcutaneously along the length of the limb [1]. He hypothesized that lymph might be transported proximally by capillary action, but found that his technique did not work [2]. Similar attempts using other substances to drain the limb also have failed (e.g., fascia, gelfoam, nylon, polythene, polyvinyl chloride) [2]. These techniques were not successful because of infection, extrusion, and movement of lymph against gravity with valveless materials.

A.K. Greene et al. (eds.), *Lymphedema: Presentation, Diagnosis, and Treatment*,
DOI 10.1007/978-3-319-14493-1_21, © Springer International Publishing Switzerland 2015

Table 21.1 Operations for lymphedema that are no longer commonly performed

Alloplastic materials
Kondoleon
Thompson
Intraabdominal flaps
Muscle flaps

Kondoleon Procedure

In 1912, Kondoleon recognized that lymphedema only affects the tissues above the muscle fascia; the muscle compartment and deeper areas of the limb were not affected. He hypothesized that the muscle fascia was a barrier between the superficial and deep lymphatic systems. Consequently, he made long incisions along the extremity and removed strips of muscle fascia in an effort to allow superficial lymph drain into deeper lymphatics [3–5]. He removed subcutaneous tissue beneath the skin excision so that a path existed between skin and muscle.

Kondoleon's procedure had minimal efficacy and no evidence of physiologic benefit. Reasons for the lack of improvement were hypothesized to be as follows: (1) the deep lymphatics are also abnormal and unable to drain superficial tissues, and/or (2) a neo-fascia reforms that again blocks superficial to deep drainage [2]. Although the Kondoleon procedure was abandoned, it served as the basis for the staged-skin/subcutaneous excisional procedures that are used today.

Thompson Procedure

In 1962 Thompson described an operation based on the work of Kondoleon (1912), Sistrunk (1918), and Homans (1936) [2]. Because Kinmonth showed that lymphedema also has abnormal deep lymphatics, it was hypothesized that the muscle compartment is not swollen because lymph is propelled by muscle contraction and pulsation of blood vessels [2, 6]. Sistrunk modified the physiologic Kondoleon operation by removing deeper fascia and adding the excision of skin and more subcutaneous fat [4–7]. Homans furthered Sistrunk's excisional procedure to include removal of all deep fascia and subcutaneous fat by raising thin vascularized skin flaps and applying them to the underlying muscle in staged procedures [8].

Thompson modified Homans' procedure by de-epithelializing his thin skin flap, which he then buried into an intramuscular area along the entire extremity [2]. He hypothesized that by burying the flap into the muscle he would facilitate superficial drainage into the deep compartment as well as prevent fibrosis/neo-fascial formation that may re-separate the superficial and deep systems. In 1970, Thompson reviewed his experience using the procedure on 79 limbs (56 legs, 23 arms) [9]. He found that 61 % of his patients had "good" results and 33 % had "satisfactory" outcomes; all subjects had a reduced risk of infection [9]. Patients with secondary lymphedema of the lower extremity had a greater chance of having "good" results (83 %), compared to patients with primary disease (58 %) [9]. Thompson hypothesized that patients with primary lymphedema do not benefit as much from his technique because their deep lymphatics are more abnormal compared to patients with secondary disease [9].

Although there is evidence that Thompson's procedure may improve lymphatic flow [10, 11], any physiologic benefit likely is based on the wide excisional component because skin/subcutaneous excisions (without a buried dermal flap) also have been shown to potentially improve lymphatic function [12–14]. Currently, the Thompson procedure does not appear to offer any additional benefit compared to staged skin/subcutaneous excision without burying a skin flap into muscle. In contrast to the Homans procedure, the Thompson operation is more complicated, and patients are at risk for epithelial sinuses and skin necrosis at the site where the de-epithelialized flap is sutured to the native skin (1/3 of patients in Thompson's series) [9].

Intraabdominal Flaps

Pedicled transposition of omentum was first described by Goldsmith and De Los Santos as a treatment for lymphedema in 1966 [15]. They hypothesized that the lymphatics in the omentum would be able to bridge the lymphedematous extremity and allow drainage of lymph from the limb. In 1974, Goldsmith published his long-term evaluation of the technique [16]. He performed the procedure in 22 patients (13 legs, 9 arms) [16]. Only ten patients (45 %) were thought to have benefit based on the following criteria: decreased size of the extremity, reduced infections, increased function, or reduction of tissue turgor [16]. One-third of the patients had major complications: hernia, infection, wound dehiscence, pulmonary embolus, gastric ulcer, adhesions causing bowel obstruction, and death from intestinal necrosis [16]. After Goldsmith reviewed his experience with omental transposition he questioned "whether the clinical results of omental transposition justify its continued performance…. I have been impressed with favorable reports of simpler operations such as the Thompson operation or the subcutaneous excision of lymphedematous tissue… if I were asked to recommend an operation… I would suggest that one of these two procedures be performed since neither operation violates the peritoneal cavity as does omental transposition" [16].

Hurst et al. described an enteromesenteric bridge procedure in eight patients [17]. A segment of ileum and its mesentery was transected and transferred to the inguinal area. After removing the mucosa, the bridge was sutured over the inguinal nodes that had been bisected or unroofed. The authors stated that six patients had improvement and two failed the procedure and required excisional operations [17]. Lymphoscintigraphy showed clearance of tracer in three out of four limbs. One patient had a bowel obstruction requiring lysis of adhesions [17].

Strong evidence that omental flap transposition or an enteromesenteric bridge improves lymphatic drainage or reduces the size of an extremity does not exist. The procedures require an intraabdominal operation that exposes the patient to significant risks, including the lifelong chance of adhesions and bowel obstructions. Currently performed physiologic (lymphatic–venous anastomosis, lymph vessel transplantation, lymph node transfer) and excisional (liposuction, staged skin/subcutaneous excision) have superior efficacy and are safer that intraabdominal flap transpositions.

Consequently, these flaps are rarely performed at this time and are not recommended by the International Society of Lymphology [18].

Muscle Flaps

Similar to the omental flap, extraabdominal flaps have been used as a physiological procedure to drain a lymphedematous extremity. Muscle flaps have not gained wide acceptance because of the morbidity of the procedure and equivocal benefit. Current excisional procedures offer better, more consistent results and have less morbidity.

Latissimus dorsi flap transposition has been reported as a treatment for upper extremity lymphedema in two patients who were felt to have improvement in their disease; although improved lymph drainage was not shown [19]. A case report of a free muscle flap for upper extremity lymphedema showed lymphatic drainage through the flap [20].

Lower extremity lymphedema has been managed with tensor fascia lata flaps in 13 patients who were reported to have some improvement [21]. However, follow-up was short and evidence of improved lymphatic drainage was not studied. More recently, a contralateral rectus abdominis musculocutaneous flap has been used to treat groin wounds in patients who also had lower extremity lymphedema; a cutaneous pedicle containing dermal lymphatics was maintained [22]. Improvement in limb volume and episodes of cellulitis were reported, although the effects of the flap in patients with lymphedema but without groin wounds are unknown. Also, sacrificing a rectus muscle in a patient with moderate/severe lower extremity lymphedema that may have difficulty ambulating could further inhibit the patient's function.

Conclusions

Several types of operations may be used to treat lymphedema. A consensus about the best procedure for the disease does not exist. Physiologic procedures using alloplastic materials have been shown to be ineffective and are no longer used. The Kondoleon procedure was the foundation for the current staged skin/subcutaneous excision operation. The Thompson procedure is more complicated and associated with greater morbidity than staged skin/subcutaneous excision and does not provide any added benefit. Although omentum and muscle flaps might have efficacy, the morbidity of these procedures do not favor their use compared to liposuction, staged skin/subcutaneous excision, lymphatic–venous anastomosis, and/or lymph node transfer.

References

1. Handley WS. Lymphangioplasty: a new method for the relief of the brawny arm of breast cancer and for similar conditions of the lymphatic oedema. Preliminary note. Lancet. 1908;171:783–5.
2. Handley WS. Hunterian lectures on the surgery of the lymphatic system. Br Med J. 1910;1:922–8.
3. Kondoleon E. Die operative Behandlung der elephantiastischen Odeme. Zentralbl Chir. 1912;30:1022–5.
4. Sistrunk WE. Further experiences with the Kondoleon operation for elephantiasis. JAMA. 1918;71:800–6.
5. Weinstein M, Roberts M. Elephantiasis and the Kondoleon operation. Am J Surg. 1950;79:327–31.
6. Kinmonth JB, Taylor GW. The lymphatic circulation in lymphedema. Ann Surg. 1954;139:129–36.
7. Sistrunk WE. Contribution to plastic surgery: removal of scars by stages; an open operation for extensive laceration of the anal sphincter; the Kondoleon operation for elephantiasis. Ann Surg. 1927;85:185–93.
8. Homans J. The treatment of elephantiasis of the legs: a preliminary report. N Eng J Med. 1936;24:1097–104.
9. Thompson N. Buried dermal flap operation for chronic lymphedema of the extremities. Ten-year survey of results in 79 cases. Plast Reconstr Surg. 1970;45:541–8.
10. Thompson N. The surgical treatment of chronic lymphedema of the extremities. Surg Clin North Am. 1967;47:445–503.
11. Harvey RF. The use of I 131-labelled human serum albumin in the assessment of improved lymph flow following buried dermis flap operation in cases of postmastectomy lymphedema of the arms. Br J Radiol. 1969;42:260–5.
12. Miller TA, Harper J, Longmire Jr WP. The management of lymphedema by staged subcutaneous excision. Surg Gynecol Obstet. 1973;136:586–92.
13. Miller TA, Wyatt LE, Rudkin GH. Staged skin and subcutaneous excision for lymphedema: a favorable report of long-term results. Plast Reconstr Surg. 1998;102:1486–98.
14. Fines NR. The surgical management of 324 children and young adults with lymphedema. Surg Rounds. 1997;1997:63–72.
15. Goldsmith HS, De Los Santos R. Omental transposition for the treatment of chronic lymphedema. Rev Surg. 1966;23:303–4.
16. Goldsmith HS. Long term evaluation of omental transposition for chronic lymphedema. Ann Surg. 1974;180:847–9.
17. Hurst PA, Stewart G, Kinmonth JB, Browse NL. Long-term results of the enteromesenteric bridge operation in the treatment of primary lymphedema. Br J Surg. 1985;72:272–4.
18. International Society of Lymphology. The diagnosis and treatment of peripheral lymphedema: 2013 consensus document of the international society of lymphology. Lymphology. 2013;46:1–11.
19. Kambayashi J, Ohshiro T, Mori T. Appraisal of myocutaneous flapping for treatment of postmastectomy lymphedema. Case report. Acta Chir Scand. 1990;156:175–7.
20. Classen DA, Irvine L. Free muscle flap transfer as a lymphatic bridge for upper extremity lymphedema. J Reconstr Microsurg. 2005;21:93–9.
21. Chitale VR. The role of tensor fascia lata musculocutaneous flap in lymphedema of the lower extremity and external genitalia. Ann Plast Surg. 1989;23:297–305.
22. Parrett BM, Sepic J, Pribaz JJ. The contralateral rectus abdominis musculocutaneous flap for treatment of lower extremity lymphedema. Ann Plast Surg. 2009;62:75–9.

Ruediger G.H. Baumeister

Key Points
- Lymphatic vessel transplantation uses the patient's own lymphatic collectors for bypasses within the lymphatic vascular system.
- Lymphatic vessel transplantation restores with the help of advanced operating microscopes the lymphatic vessel continuity by anastomosing main lymphatic collectors in front and behind a discontinuity of the lymphatic transporting system.
- Edemas due to a locally interrupted lymphatic system, e.g., after a medical intervention or a trauma can be treated by lymphatic vessel transplantation.
- Specific indications for lymphatic vessel transplantation exist for penile and scrotal edemas and specific primary lymphedemas due to a localized lymphatic atresia.
- Follow-up studies after lymphatic vessel transplantation show a long time patency of grafts and scintigraphically a significant improvement or even normalization of the lymphatic transport.

R.G.H. Baumeister, Prof., Dr., Dr., med., Habil. (✉)
Plastic-, Hand-, Microsurgery Department of Surgery,
Ludwig Maximilians University Munich,
Campus Grosshadern, Marchioninistr.15,
Muenchen 81375, Germany
e-mail: baumeister@lymphtransplant.com

Introduction

Different approaches have been described for the surgical treatment of lymphedemas. One approach corrects the outer form of the enlarged lymphedematous extremities. Resections of the epifascial tissue have been performed using large incisions, whereas modern approaches minimize the scars using liposuction techniques [1].

Enhancing the outflow of lymph by creating new pathways is the aim of another group of surgeries. These methods performed resections of the fascia to facilitate the drainage to the subfascial compartment, inserted pediculated tissue compartments, like skin flaps, omentum majus flaps, and pedunculated parts of ileum into the edematous extremities or performed connections to the lymphatic system of the edematous and the peripheral venous system, like lymph node–venous and lymphatic–venous anastomoses [2–5]. Microsurgical lymph-node transplantations combine the flap procedure which is dependent on the spontaneous connections of lymphatic capillaries and the peripheral venous connection via intra-nodal lymphatic venous shunts and the outflow through the micro-surgical created venous anastomoses [6].

Lymphatic vessel transplantation aims at the direct restoration the lymphatic vessel continuity by anastomosing main lymphatic collectors in front and behind a discontinuity of the lymphatic transporting system, which is often due to resection procedures at narrow passes of the lymphatic system like in the axilla and the inguinal region [7, 8].

A.K. Greene et al. (eds.), *Lymphedema: Presentation, Diagnosis, and Treatment*,
DOI 10.1007/978-3-319-14493-1_22, © Springer International Publishing Switzerland 2015

Since lymphedema has its origin in an excess of lymphatic fluid in comparison to the number of functioning lymphatic draining vessels [9], it is important to correct this imbalance. If this is not the case, lymphedema may recur after the different procedures if no additional continuous treatment is performed.

Indication

Lymphatic vessel transplantation is designed to overcome regional interruptions of the lymphatic transporting system. This is the case in most lymphedemas in Europe and the USA. Arm edemas after axillary dissection are there the most frequent lymphedemas. Resection of lymph nodes at the inguinal or the pelvic region is also a frequent reason to develop lymphedema. Another bottleneck of the lymphatic transporting system is the inner aspect of the knee region. Surgeries, but also a trauma, often complicated by an infection are other reasons to locally impede the lymph transport.

A specific form of primary lymphedemas of the lower extremities which is due to a local unilateral atresia of lymph nodes and vessels at the inguinal and/or pelvic region has been described by Kinmonth [10] and may be treated therefore also by this method.

Like in other vascular areas, e.g., at the arteries of the heart, a bypass procedure is useful only in cases of a defined vascular interruption. Also there is a need of an undisturbed vascular outflow at the end of the bypass. Furthermore, it needs an appropriate possibility for harvesting the grafts.

In lymphatic vessel transplantation lymphatic grafts may be taken form the so-called ventromedial lymphatic bundle at the inner side of the thigh. Without touching the lymphatic bottlenecks at the groin and the knee is possible to harvest grafts at a length up to about 30 cm.

This is enough to overcome the axillary region and to reach the opposite thigh in case of a lymphedema of the lower extremity.

Outflow of lymph into an undisturbed lymphatic vascular system in the cases bypassing an axilla is no problem, since at the neck enough untouched lymphatic vessels exist.

In cases of lymphedemas of lower extremities due to blockades at the inguinal and the pelvic region, one side with normal lymphatic transport has to be present since only than the lymph can flow via the bypasses into a normal draining system. This means that only unilateral edemas of the lower extremities can be treated by lymphatic vessels grafting.

Prerequisites

There are different types of prerequisites. They are dependent of the addressee: the surgeon, the equipment, and the patient.

The surgeon has to be aware, that microlymphatic surgery is the most demanding type of microsurgery. The reason for that is the tininess of the vessels, their ultrathin wall and the difficulty about discriminating lymphatic vessels from small nerves, veins, and fibrous tissue cords. It is helpful to search through the operating microscope during other procedures first to healthy and undisturbed lymphatic vessels before dealing with the partly fibrous and altered lymphatic vessels in lymphedema patients.

Also trained microsurgeons should be aware to go back to the lab to get used to handling lymphatic vessels. The rat model with the easy accessible abdominal thoracic duct or with major lymphatic vessels in the pelvic area can serve as training objects [11]. Because of the fragile vessel wall tension in an oblique direction has to be avoided. Only a limited number of single stitches are necessary to prevent a leakage (Fig. 22.1).

Also because of the tininess of the vessels high magnifying microscopes have to be used. The finest instruments should be used and also the threads should be accustomed as much as possible to the needs of the lymphatic vessels. In the rat experiments it was found, that absorbable suture material showed less disturbance in the vicinity of the lymphatic anastomoses compared to non-absorbable material, where in relation to the vessels extended foreign body material has been observed [12].

Anastomoses between lymphatic vessels have a great advantage compared to anastomoses

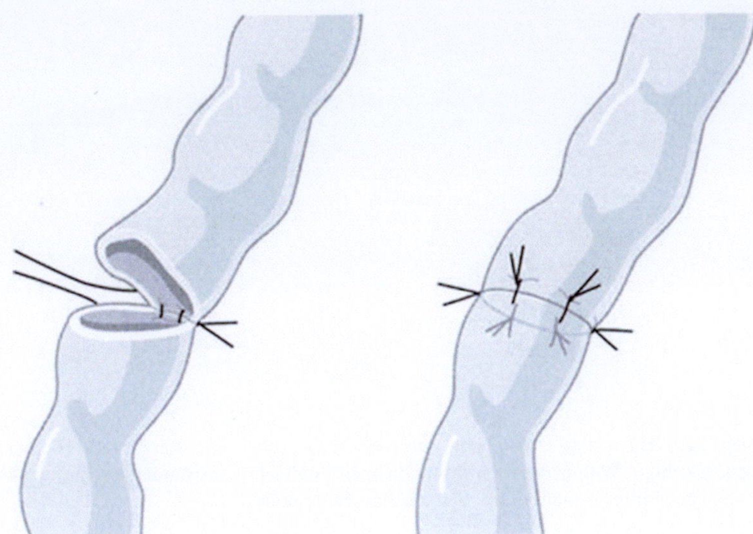

Fig. 22.1 Tension-free lymphatic–lymphatic end-to-end anastomosis technique. With permission from Baumeister RGH. Mikrochirurgie peripherer Lymphgefäße. In: Berger A, Hierner, R eds. Plastische Chirurgie: Band I Grundlagen Prinzipien Techniken. Springer © 2003, pp 213–217

between lymphatic vessels and blood containing vessels. The coagulation abilities of lymphatic fluid are much lower compared to these of blood. Occlusion of anastomoses between lymphatic vessels is therefore rare.

Furthermore, lymphatic vessels showed in the experiments performed by Danese [13] the ability of building connection by themselves if lying next to each other. These effects may be one of the explanations about the high patency rate in lymphatico-lymphatic experimental anastomosing procedures. When anastomosing within the lymphatic transporting system there is no danger of an adverse pressure gradient which may be the fact by connecting lymphatic vessels to the peripheral venous system.

Patients should get the full range of conservative treatment consisting of manual lymphatic drainage and elastic stockings for at least half a year because during this time period also transient edemas are known. By that way he additionally got to know what is possible for him by the non-operative treatment. He may make up his mind whether this procedure fits for him or if it does not fulfill his expectations. He now is better willing to take a risk which is especially immanent to all invasive treatment options.

The most important factor for lymphatic vessel grafting is the possibility of harvesting lymphatic grafts. At least one lower extremity has to

be edema free clinically. Additionally a normal lymphatic outflow prior to the harvest should be documented by a lymphatic scintigraphy.

The patient has to be ready for only a limited burden. This is a general anesthesia which lasts for about 2–4 h. The intervention itself takes place only within the subcutaneous tissue and a minimal blood loss has to be expected.

Harvesting of the Grafts

At the inner aspect of the thigh exists the ventromedial bundle. There up to 16 lymphatic collectors run in an almost parallel manner between the two narrowing areas of the lymphatic vascular system in the lower extremity: the knee region and the groin [14]. They are connected with side branches. This allows harvesting grafts with peripheral side branches giving the possibility to perform a greater number of peripheral lymphatic anastomoses than taking out lymphatic main collectors. Two to three collectors are mostly used (Fig. 22.2).

In order to alleviate harvesting the grafts, patent blue™ is injected subdermally within the first and second web space. Within about 15 min lymphatic vessels at the thigh get stained. It is easy therefore to follow the vessels starting with an incision underneath the groin between the

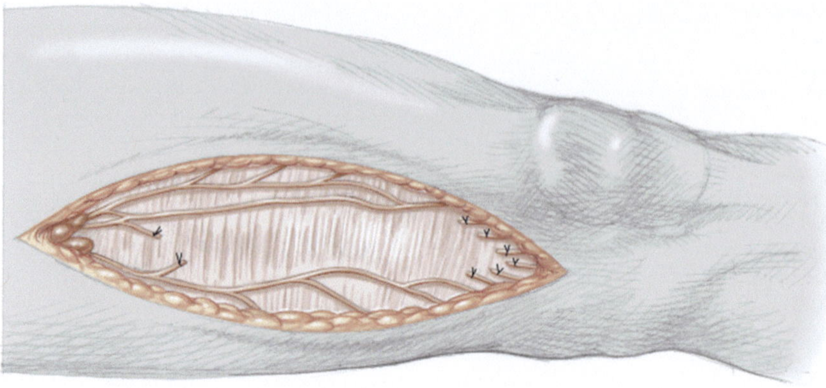

Fig. 22.2 Harvesting lymphatic vessels from the patient's thigh. With permission from: Baumeister RGH. Lymphgefäßtransplantation an der oberen Extremität. In: Berger A, Hierner R, Eds. Plastische Chirurgie Extremitäten. Springer © 2009

femoral artery and the greater saphenous vein. The incision ends proximal to the knee region. Care is taken to leave untouched stained lymphatic vessels behind in order to ensure a sufficient remaining lymphatic transport.

In order to reach ascending lymphatic vessels at the opposite leg the lymphatic grafts remain attached to the inguinal lymph nodes at the harvesting side. The peripheral endings of the grafts are occluded with a 6–0 thread with long endings. The grafts can be easily manipulated and pulled via an artificial tunnel above the symphysis to the opposite leg. The transected lymphatic collectors are sealed either by coagulation or by suturing to avoid lymphatic leakage.

For free transfers the lymphatic grafts are cut through beneath the inguinal lymph nodes and also occluded with a 6–0 thread providing long endings for further manipulation. In this case the peripheral openings of the grafts remain open. The grafts are freed from bigger fat lumps to reduce friction later on by gliding through artificial tunnels provided by silicone tubes.

Arm Edemas

Arm edemas are mostly caused by interference with the content of the axilla by surgery or irradiation, mostly in women suffering from mammary carcinomas. However, also treatment of male mammary carcinomas and lymph node resections in cases of Hodgkin disease are reasons for the development of edemas.

In these cases the axillary region has to be bypassed.

In front of the obstacle for the lymphatic transport an oblique incision is made above the vascular bundle. Ascending lymphatic main collectors run just above the fascia. The search starts by blunt meticulous dissection of the subcutaneous tissue. Small lymphatic vessels will be seen superficially. However, it should be looked for the greater vessels running more deeply. In contrast to small nerves, which are bright white and show oblique stripes, lymphatic vessels a grey looking and found between the fat tissue and also in the neighborhood of greater veins.

The next undisturbed lymphatic vessels are found at the neck. Below the sternocleoid muscle major lymphatic vessels transport lymph from the head to the venous angulation. The lymphatic vessels and the lymph nodes are imbedded in the fat tissues lateral to the internal jugular vein. They can be approached via a small oblique incision. An injection of patent blue™ subdermally behind the ear may facilitate to find the thin-walled lymphatic vessels. Alternatively lymphatic–lymph nodal anastomoses may be performed [15].

Between the incisions at the upper arm and the neck, a tunnel is created by blunt preparation using a long forceps. A silicone tube Charrier 18

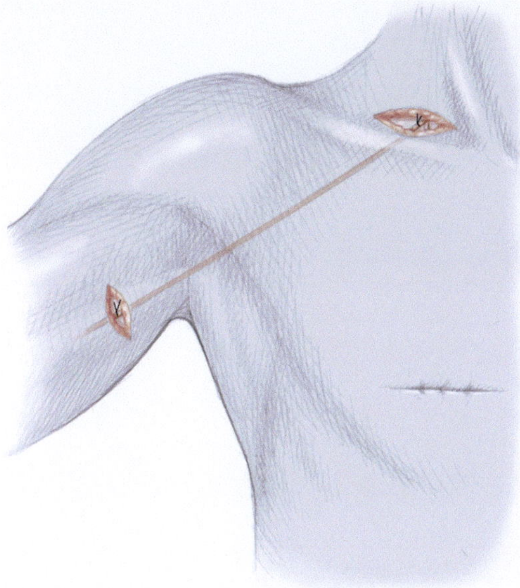

Fig. 22.3 Bridging a lymphatic gap at the axilla with autologous lymphatic vessels: lympho-lymphatic anastomoses at the upper arm and the neck. With permission from: Baumeister RGH. Lymphgefäßtransplantation an der oberen Extremität. In: Berger A, Hierner R, Eds. Plastische Chirurgie Extremitäten. Springer © 2009

with an appropriate length to exceed the length of the tunnel is prepared containing a long thread. The tube is inserted and the thread on the peripheral ending of the grafts is connected to the peripheral part of the thread within the tube. The graft is now pulled within tube until it appears at the neck. The graft is fixed manually at the neck and the tube is retracted towards the upper arm incision. Now the graft lies in place within the subcutaneous tissue. The proximal part is directed towards the neck, which means that the graft is situated in the appropriate direction to transport lymph from the peripheral ones towards the central anastomoses (Fig. 22.3).

The anastomoses between the lymphatic vessels are performed mostly in an end-to-end fashion, sometimes also in an end-to-side version. Experimental data have shown that also anastomoses between lymphatic vessels and lymph nodes are possible and show also a high patency rate [16]. In this case the capsule is opened, giving access to the outer sinus close to the efferent lymphatic vessels. The anastomosis is performed with about four single stitches using smallest available suture material.

Unilateral Edemas of Lower Extremities

In unilateral lymphedemas of the lower extremities the option for the outflow of the lymphatic fluid consists in a diversion into the lymphatic vascular system of the opposite extremity.

The harvest is performed at the normal leg. Prior to surgery a normal lymphatic outflow should be demonstrated with the help of a lymphatic scintigraphy.

The grafts remain in these cases connected to the inguinal lymph nodes. The peripheral endings are occluded by a thread with long endings. At the affected limb ascending lymphatic main collectors are searched from an oblique incision distally to the inguinal area or distally to an existing scar formation. The main vessels will be found between the axis of the femoral artery and the greater saphenous vein just above the fascia.

A tunnel is created between the two incisions above the symphysis and a tube is inserted. With the help of an additional thread within the tube the lymphatic grafts are pulled through and the tube thereafter is removed. The anastomoses are performed microsurgically between the ascending lymphatic collectors and the peripheral endings of the grafts. Lymph from the edematous extremity may now flow in the right direction towards the inguinal nodes of the healthy side (Fig. 22.4).

Scrotal and Penile Lymphedemas

Scrotal and penile edemas are difficult to treat conservatively. If at least one leg shows a normal lymphatic outflow lymphatic transport may be provided by short lymphatic grafts, transposed to the root of the penis or scrotum. Lymphatic vessels can be found there just under the skin. If however in severe cases all the tissue is heavily fibrosed, it may be impossible to find lymphatic collectors. Than only a resectional procedure may be an option.

When lymphatic collectors, however, are found, then short lymphatic grafts can be transposed. Preferentially lymphatic vessels approaching the lateral lymph nodes at the groin region should be used because medially located lymph nodes may be

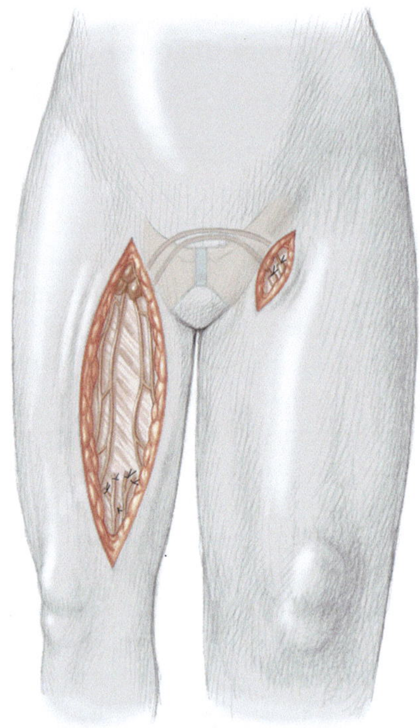

Fig. 22.4 Lymphatic grafting in unilateral lymphedema of lower extremities; the grafts remain attached to the inguinal lymph nodes at the harvesting side. With permission from: Baumeister RGH. Lymphgefäßtransplantation an der oberen Extremität. In: Berger A, Hierner R, Eds. Plastische Chirurgie Extremitäten. Springer © 2009

altered and are a possible reason for the edema. Again, between the two incisions, a tunnel is created and the grafts pulled through. End-to-end anastomoses are performed leading the lymph towards the lateral undisturbed lymph nodes (Fig. 22.5).

Peripheral Localized Interruptions

Traumas and peripheral surgical interventions especially on bottlenecks of the lymphatic system may lead to a diminished transport of lymph resulting in a local lymphedema. Sometimes a lymphocele is formed, marking the area of the problem.

It is helpful to get a better knowledge of the single lymphatic collectors with the help of a 3T MRI Lymphography. It allows exact three-dimensional localization of the entrance of the lymphatic vessels into the lymphocele [17].

To overcome such a blockade lymphatic vessels are dissected in front and behind the blockade

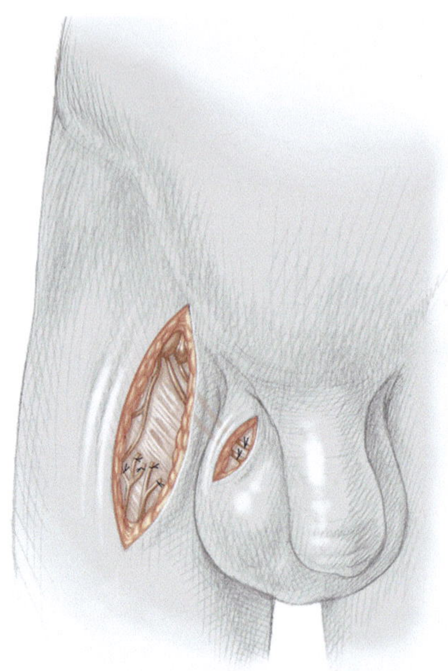

Fig. 22.5 Transposition of short lymphatic grafts to the root of the penis and scrotum. With permission from: Baumeister RGH. Lymphgefäßtransplantation an der oberen Extremität. In: Berger A, Hierner R, Eds. Plastische Chirurgie Extremitäten. Springer © 2009

(Fig. 22.6). *If* necessary a lymphocele is resected. The short grafts are interposed and anastomosed in an end-to-end fashion.

Primary Lymphedemas

Primary lymphedemas show a broad variety of malformations within the lymphatic system. Kinmonth [10] describes one form of a unilateral local atresia at the inguinal and pelvic region by undisturbed peripheral lymphatic vessels. The patients show a unilateral edema of one leg until the groin area. In MRI lymphographies the lymphatic vessels peripheral to the groin appear normal. Especially in primary lymphedemas the opposite side has to be checked and a preexisting lymphatic abnormality excluded carefully by lymphatic scintigraphy and MRI lymphography since a later development of lymphedema in the other leg is known. In these cases it is possible to conduct the lymph from the affected leg towards the normal one via transposed grafts as performed in unilateral secondary lymphedema of the lower extremity.

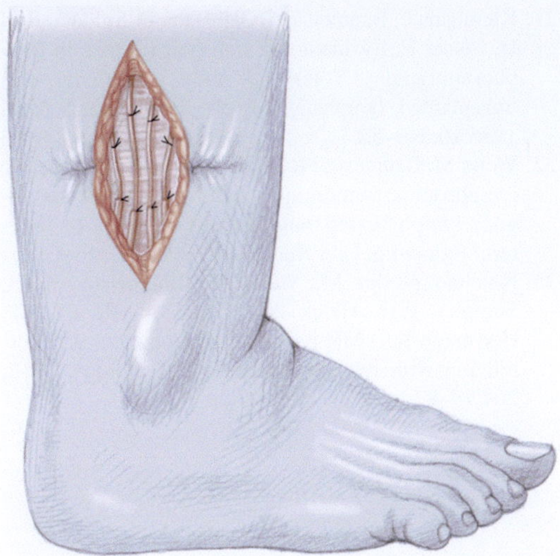

Fig. 22.6 Lymphatic grafts for bypassing an interruption of lymphatic vessels distally, lymphatico-lymphatic anastomoses in front and behind the blockade. With permission from: Baumeister RGH. Lymphgefäßtransplantation an der oberen Extremität. In: Berger A, Hierner R, Eds. Plastische Chirurgie Extremitäten. Springer © 2009

Objective of Results

For lymphedema treatment by microsurgical lymphatic vessel transplantation, besides own measurements of volumes and quality of life analysis [18–20] results have been proved also by others [21–23].

The Department of Nuclear Medicine followed patients after lymphatic grafting for more than 7 years. They found a significant improvement of the transport index also 7 years after the surgery. In a subgroup with clear visible lymphatic transport along the route of the grafts the transport came in the range of normal transport figures. Long-term patency of autologous lymphatic grafts was proved by the Department of Clinical Radiology.

Conclusion

Lymphatic vessel transplantation is able to reconstruct a locally interrupted lymphatic vascular system using an autologous bypass with lymphatic vessels. The method has been proved experimentally and clinically. Long-term follow-up studies showed long-term patency of the grafts and a significant improvement of lymphatic flow via the grafts up to normal values.

References

1. Brorson H, Svensson H. Complete reduction of lymphedema of the arm by liposuction after breast cancer. Scand J Plast Reconstr Surg Hand Surg. 1997;1997:137–43.
2. Nielubowicz J, Olszewski W. Surgical lymphaticovenous shunts in patients with secondary lymphedema. Br J Surg. 1968;55:440–2.
3. Degni M. New technique of lymphatico-venous anastomosis for the treatment of lymphedema. J Cardiovasc Surg. 1978;19:577.
4. O'Brien B, Sykes PJ, Threlfall GN, Browning FSC. Microlymphaticovenous anastomoses for obstructive lymphedema. Plast Reconstr Surg. 1977;60:197–211.
5. Koshima I, Inagawa K, Urshibara K, Moriguchi T. Supermicrosurgical lymphaticovenular anastomosis for the treatment of lymphedema in the upper extremities. J Reconstr Microsurg. 2000;16:437–42.
6. Becker C, Hidden G, Godart S, Maurage H, Pecking A. Free lymphatic transplant. Eur J Lymphol. 1991;2:75–7.
7. Baumeister RG, Seifert J, Wiebecke B. Transplantation of lymph vessels on rats as well as a first therapeutic application on the experimental lymphedema of the dog. Eur Surg Res. 1980;12 Suppl 2:7.
8. Baumeister RG, Seifert J, Wiebecke B, Hahn D. Experimental basis and first application of clinical lymph vessel transplantation of secondary lymphedema. World J Surg. 1981;5:401–7.
9. Földi M. Physiologie des Lymphgefäßsystems. Angiologica. 1971;8:212.
10. Kinmonth JB. The lymphatics. London: Arnold; 1982.
11. Baumeister RGH, Seifert J, Wiebecke B. Homologous and autologous experimental lymph vessel transplantation: initial experience. Int J Microsurg. 1981;3:19–24.
12. Baumeister RGH, Seifert J, Wiebecke B. Untersuchungen zum Verhalten von resorbierbarem und nichtresorbierbarem Nahtmaterial bei der Lymphgefäßnaht. Handchir Mikrochir Plast Chir. 1982;14:87–91.
13. Danese C, Bower R, Howard J. Experimental anastomosis of lymphatics. Arch Surg. 1982;84:24.
14. Kubik S. Zur klinischen Anatomie des Lymphsystems. Verh Anat Ges. 1975;69:109–16.
15. Wallmichrath J, Baumeister RGH, Giunta R, Frick A. Lymphgefäßtransplantation mit Anastomosierung der Transplantate an regionale Lymphknoten zur Therapie von Lymphödemen. LymphForsch. 2011;15:68–71.
16. Wallmichrath J, Baumeister RG, Deglmann CJ, Greiner A, Heim S, Frick A. Technique and proof of patency of microsurgical lympho-lymphonodular anastomoses: a study in the rat model. Microsurgery. 2009;29:303–12.

17. Notohamiprodjo M, Baumeister RGH, Jakobs TF, Bauner K, Boehm H, Horng A, Reiser MF, Glaser C, Herrmann KA. MR-lymphangiography at 3.OT – a feasibility study. Eur Radiol. 2009;19:2771–8.
18. Baumeister RGH, Siuda S. Treatment of lymphedema by microsurgical lymphatic grafting: what is proved? Plast Reconstr Surg. 1990;85:64–75.
19. Baumeister RGH, Frick A. Die mikrochirurgische Lymphgefässtransplantation. Handchir Mikrochir Plast Chir. 2003;35:202.
20. Springer S, Koller R, Baumeister RGH, Frick A. Changes in quality of life of patients with lymphedema after lymphatic vessel transplantation. Lymphology. 2012;44:65.
21. Kleinhans E, Baumeister RGH, Hahn D, Siuda S, Büll U, Moser E. Evaluation of transport kinetics in lymphoscintigraphy: follow-up study in patients with transplanted lymphatic vessels. Eur J Nucl Med. 1985;10:349–52.
22. Weiss M, Baumeister RGH, Hahn K. Post-therapeutic lymphedema: scintigraphy before and after autologous lymph vessel transplantation 8 years of long-term follow-up. Clin Nucl Med. 2002;27:788–92.
23. Notohamiprodjo M, Weiss M, Baumeister RGH, Sommer WH, Helck A, Crispin A, Reiser MF, Herrmann KA. MR lymphangiography at 3.0.T: correlation with lymphoscintigraphy. Radiology. 2012;264:78–87.

Jiro Maegawa

Key Points

- Lymphoscintigraphy is used to identify the indications for lymphatic–venous anastomosis.
- ICG fluorescence lymphography is helpful in detecting functional lymph vessels in the subcutaneous layer during surgery; selection of suitable veins for anastomosis is also essential to obtaining good patency.
- Postoperative patency of anastomoses in relatively shallow subcutaneous layers can be examined by ICG fluorescence lymphography
- Preoperative CDP improves the condition of the surgical site, which would facilitate detection of the lymph vessels during surgery.
- Lymphatic–venous anastomosis reduces the volume of lymph edema to some extent and enables decrease of the contents of postoperative CDP in some patients.

Introduction

The possibility of decompressing high pressure in the lymph system distal to areas of obstruction by performing lymphovenous shunts was suggested by Edwards and Kinmonth [1]. Experimental lymphatic–venous anastomosis in dogs was reported by Yamada in 1969 [2]. Since then, clinical reports of lymphatic–venous anastomosis have been published by O'Brien et al. in 1977 [3], and Huang [4], Campisi [5], and Koshima [6], who reported the long-term results of this procedure [4–7].

Two types of techniques are used for lymphatic–venous anastomosis: invagination, which involves suturing the lymphatics onto a vein, and a vein graft with one or two stitches and edge-to-edge approximation of the intima, including end-to-end, end-to-side, and side-to-side anastomosis. The Campisi group in Italy adopts the former technique, while the others perform the latter.

Although advancements in instruments and microscopes for microsurgery have resulted in improved technical results of lymphatic–venous anastomosis, patency rates and the duration for which the anastomosis remains patent following the different anastomotic techniques are still unclear. One of the reasons for this is the difficulty in visualization and evaluation of lymph flow in real time.

In this chapter, I address the protocols, procedures, and outcomes of lymphaticovenous side-to-end anastomosis and stress the importance of imaging studies in evaluating the results of the anastomosis.

J. Maegawa, M.D., Ph.D. (✉)
Plastic and Reconstructive Surgery, Yokohoma City
University Hospital, 3-9 Fukuura, Kanazawa-ku,
Yokohoma 236-0004, Japan
e-mail: jrmaegawa@gmail.com

A.K. Greene et al. (eds.), *Lymphedema: Presentation, Diagnosis, and Treatment*,
DOI 10.1007/978-3-319-14493-1_23, © Springer International Publishing Switzerland 2015

Surgical Indications

Preoperative Imaging and Indications

Lymphoscintigraphy is the standard method of evaluating the severity of lymph edema and dysfunction of the lymphatic system. There are several reports on evaluation of the lymphatic system by lymphoscintigraphy [8–12]. These are helpful for classifying the indications of lymphatic–venous anastomosis.

Obstructive lymphedema is one of the main indications for lymphatic–venous anastomosis. Preoperative lymphoscintigraphy images enable determination of the area where suitable lymphatic vessels exist. Referring to Maegawa's classification [11], lymphographic imaging can

be used to identify suitable lymphatics in both the thigh and leg. In type I images, obvious inguinal lymph nodes and lymphatics along the great saphenous vein, and/or lymph stasis in the collateral lymphatics can be identified. However, the number of visible inguinal lymph nodes is reduced, since they are slightly affected (Fig. 23.1a). In type II images, few or no inguinal lymph nodes can be seen. Lymph stasis in the lymphatics and collateral lymphatics are observed in the thigh and leg. Small dermal backflow may be seen in the thigh (Fig. 23.1b). In type III images, no inguinal lymph nodes are detected. Dermal backflow can be seen in the thigh and/ or leg. Lymph stasis in the lymphatics and/or collaterals is observed (Fig. 23.1c). The inguinal lymph nodes and lymphatics in the thigh are affected. In type IV images, dermal backflow and

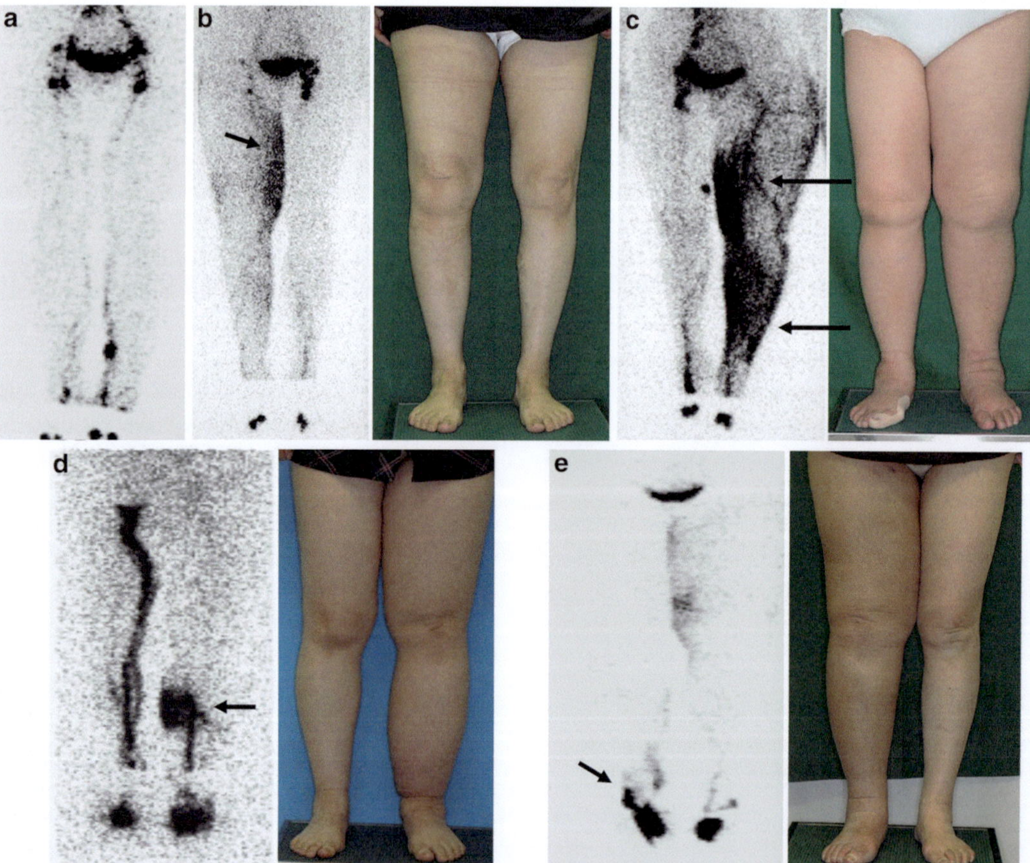

Fig. 23.1 Classification of lymphoscintigraphy images of the lower limbs. (**a**) Type I. There are obvious regional lymph nodes and no dermal backflow. (**b**) Type II. Dermal backflow (*arrow*) in the thigh is visible. (**c**) Type III. Dermal backflow can be seen in both the thigh and leg (*arrows*). (**d**) Type IV. Dermal backflow is visible in the leg (*arrow*). (**e**) Type V. Dermal backflow remains at the ankle and foot (*arrow*)

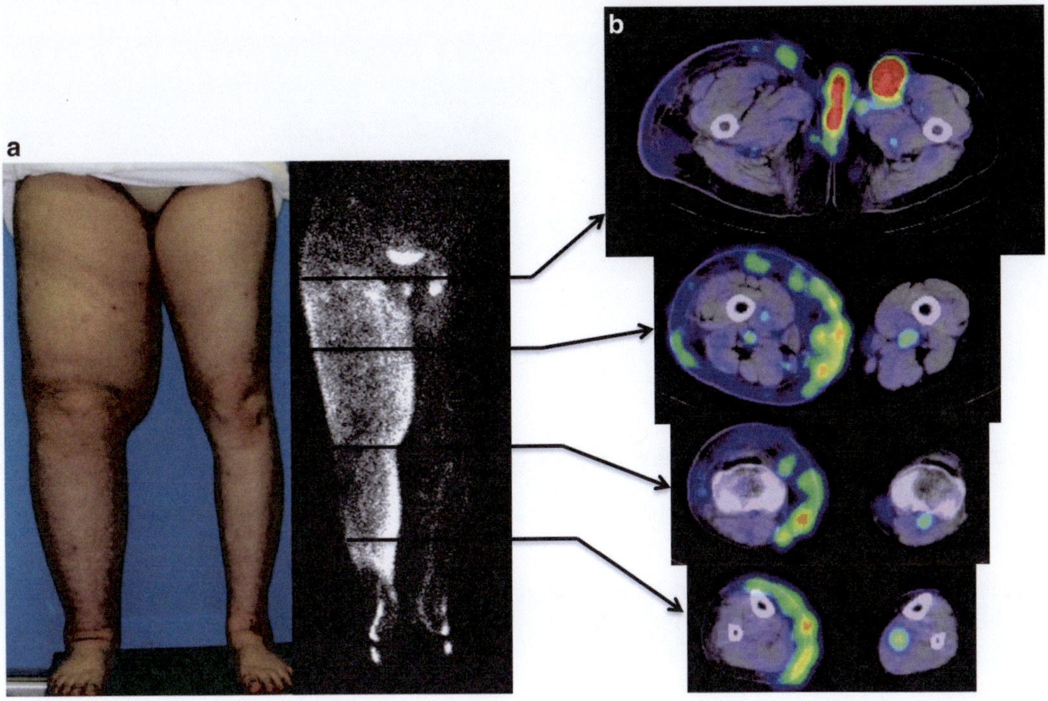

Fig. 23.2 SPECT-CT lymphoscintigraphy in secondary lymphedema in a 50-year-old woman. Secondary lymphedema of the right lower limb. (**a**) Clinical photo and plain lymphoscintigraphy of a patient with secondary lymphedema of the right leg. Lymphoscintigraphy demonstrated type III images. (**b**) SPECT-CT images in the same patient. *Green*, *yellow*, and *red* marks indicate stasis of lymph and the lymphatics in the subcutaneous, inter-muscular and perivascular layers of the thigh to lower leg

lymph stasis in the lymphatics in the leg can be recognized (Fig. 23.1d). The inguinal lymph nodes and lymphatics in the thigh and leg are affected. In type V images, no dermal backflow in the thigh and leg can be seen (see Fig. 23.1e). The inguinal lymph nodes and lymphatics in the thigh and leg are severely affected.

In secondary obstructive lymphedema, types II, III, and IV lymphoscintigraphic images are good indications for lymphatic–venous anastomosis, because superficial collecting lymph vessels can be easily found in the affected limb and it is relatively easy to anastomose the lymph vessels and veins together due to dilatation of the lymph vessels. In type V images, it is sometimes difficult to identify the lymph vessels because lymph fluid does not flow sufficiently. Patients with type I lymphoscintigraphic images may only require observation for a while, because their clinical symptoms are not as advanced, although the lymph vessels in the affected limb of such patients may already be dilated to some degree because of mild stenosis of the lymphatics at a proximal site.

Primary lymphedema is also an indication for lymphatic–venous anastomosis if the patient has Type I, II, III, and IV lymphographic images, although it is difficult to identify suitable lymphatics in cases with hypoplasia of the lymphatic system.

Near-infrared ICG fluorescence lymphography has recently been introduced for real time imaging of the lymphatic system [13, 14]. The equipment for this diagnostic modality is compact and easy to handle. Classification of the severity of lymphedema based on fluorescence lymphographic images has been reported [15]. Visualization of linear patterns on images enables easy determination of functional lymph vessels, but if the patient has thick skin or fibrous subcutaneous tissue, locating functional vessels by lymphography is not easy.

SPECT-CT lymphoscintigraphy has the potential to determine the indications for surgery and predict the sites of lymph vessels that are difficult to find by ICG fluorescence lymphography or plain lymphoscintigraphy (Fig. 23.2a) [16–18]. Recently, SPECT-CT has been used preoperatively, because

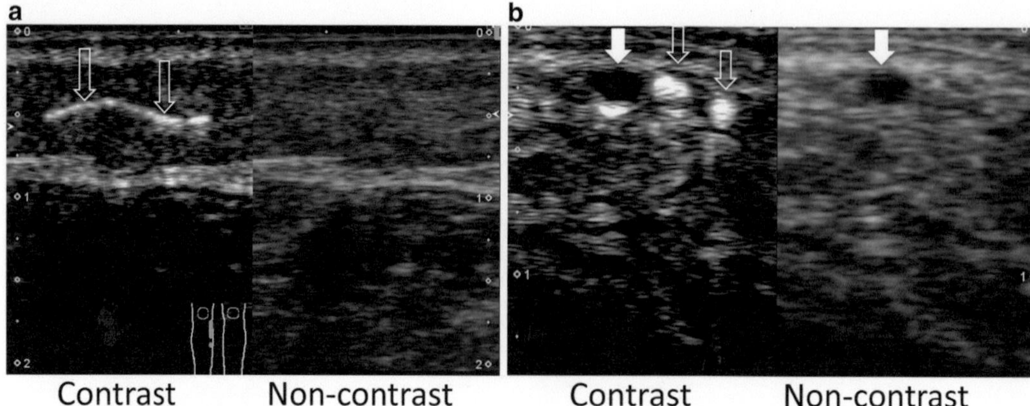

Fig. 23.3 Contrast-enhanced and non-contrast enhanced ultrasonography on the medial side of the leg in secondary lymphedema. (**a**) Longitudinal sections in contrast-enhanced (*left*) and non-contrast enhanced modes (*right*). (**b**) Axial sections in contrast-enhanced (*left*) and non-contrast enhanced modes (*right*). *Courtesy of Dr. Shinobu Matsubara*

locations of the lymph vessels can be detected precisely even in the thigh area (Fig. 23.2b). In the figure, the green, yellow, and red marks indicate stasis of lymph and the lymphatics in the subcutaneous, intermuscular, and perivascular layers of the thigh to lower leg.

Contrast-enhanced ultrasonography may also be useful in detecting lymphatic vessels. This technique has been reported by several authors for sentinel lymph node biopsy [19–21]. This diagnostic modality can visualize lymph vessels and lymph flow in real time and identify the locations of lymph vessels even in the thigh area where ICG fluorescence lymphography cannot easily identify vessels in severe cases (Fig. 23.3).

Contraindications

A recent attack of dermato-lymphangio-adenitis (DLA) is a contraindication for lymphatic–venous anastomosis, which should only be performed more than 3 months after DLA. In such cases, fatty tissue around the lymphatic vessels adheres to the lymphatics, which, according to my clinical experience, makes them difficult to find. Patients with lymphatic hypoplasia should also not undergo lymphatic–venous anastomosis because suitable lymphatics can rarely be detected. Patients with venous diseases, such as deep vein thrombosis or severe varicose veins of more than C2 severity according to the CEAP classification [22] are not indicated for anastomosis, because venous pressure in the leg is probably higher than that in the lymphatics in such patients. Although Huang

[23] reported the relationship between the pressure in the lymphatic vessels and veins, attention should be paid to the presence of venous diseases before attempting lymphatic–venous anastomosis.

Preoperative Treatment

Preoperative Complex Decongestive Physiotherapy (CDP)

O'Brien reported a percentage decrease in volume after lymphatic–venous anastomosis of 36 % in patients with preoperative CDP and 29 % in those without preoperative CDP [7]. Hence, his report did not clearly highlight the importance of CDP.

If preoperative CDP is not applied appropriately to patients with lymphedema, the presence of a significant amount of interstitial fluid in the subcutaneous layer of the affected limb makes it difficult to locate the superficial lymph vessels for anastomosis. The presence of thinner subcutaneous tissue facilitates the detection of functional lymph vessels by ICG fluorescence lymphography. Hence, the purpose of preoperative CPD is to prepare the surgical site and to create the best possible conditions for surgery by drainage of the excess interstitial fluid, thus, also leading the patient toward the maintenance phase [24]. The duration for which preoperative CDP is performed depends on the severity of edema and compliance of the patient [25], ranging from a few months to half a year.

Procedures

Equipment

An operating microscope is essential for performing lymphatic microsurgery. Since the outer diameters of the targeted lymphatic vessels mainly range from 0.25 to 0.5 mm in Japanese female patients, in my experience, magnification of 20–25 times is required for anastomosis. For dissection in the subcutaneous layer, micro-scissors and mosquito forceps with fine tips are useful. A micro-knife, forceps with 0.1 mm tips, and scissors with small blades are needed for cutting, and suturing of vessels is performed with 11-0 suture and an 80 μ needle.

Anesthesia

General anesthesia is the preferred anesthesia method during surgical anastomosis in a thick subcutaneous layer and when many anastomoses need to be performed in many parts of the affected limb. On the other hand, local anesthesia is preferable if few anastomoses are planned in the upper extremity, the lower leg, or the dorsum of the foot.

Position

In most cases of lower limb lymphedema, the anastomosis can be performed in the supine position. However, if the lymphatic vessels along the short saphenous vein are targeted, the prone position is preferable. If suitable lymph vessels and veins for anastomosis are present in the medial thigh, the knee of the affected side should be bent at about 90°, together with abduction of the hip. Vessels in the thigh can be anastomosed with the surgeon sitting on the affected side of the patient while using a microscope.

Locating the Sites for Anastomosis

Two dyes, ICG and Patent Blue, are injected into the dermal and subdermal tissue of the interdigital spaces. Five percent Patent Blue is useful for visualization of the lymph vessels in the surgical field. If the skin of the patient is not very thick and darkly colored, ICG fluorescence lymphography using a near-infrared camera system is helpful to pinpoint the sites for anastomosis, because lymph vessels can be detected as linear fluorescence and the subcutaneous veins as black lines due to nonfluorescence. The areas where linear fluorescence and black lines cross each other are determined as the sites for anastomosis. However, we sometimes encounter cases in which we cannot detect the subcutaneous veins by the camera system. In such cases, we shortlist one or two sites for anastomosis on each lymph vessel.

Detection of Suitable Lymphatic Vessels

As mentioned above, ICG fluorescence lymphography, which uses the near-infrared camera system, makes suitable lymphatics visible through the skin in the surgical field as linear fluorescence (Fig. 23.4a) [13, 14]. However, using this method, lymphatics cannot be detected in the thigh area or in cases with thickened skin, because the maximum depth that near-infrared rays can reach is between 1 and 2 cm. Lines can be marked on the skin along the linear fluorescence, to highlight the lymphatics (Fig. 23.4b).

Selection of Suitable Veins

As mentioned above, subcutaneous veins for lymphatic–venous anastomosis are identified as black lines during ICG fluorescence lymphography. Selection of the veins for anastomosis is quite important for obtaining good patency. In cases with breast cancer-related lymphedema, intravenous infusion of an anticancer agent on the affected arm as preoperative chemotherapy may damage the subcutaneous vein. The integrity of the vein can be confirmed by washing out of saline through the vein using a syringe with a fine plastic needle.

From a technical point of view, veins with an outer diameter of 1–2 times that of the lymphatic vessel are suitable for anastomosis. Further, it is essential that the vein be sufficiently mobilized by dissection to reach the lymphatic vessel without tension and torsion, to ensure easy passage of lymph through the anastomosis.

Fig. 23.4 Preoperative ICG fluorescence lymphography. (**a**) Linear fluorescence on the dorsum of the foot. (**b**) Markings on the skin along the lines

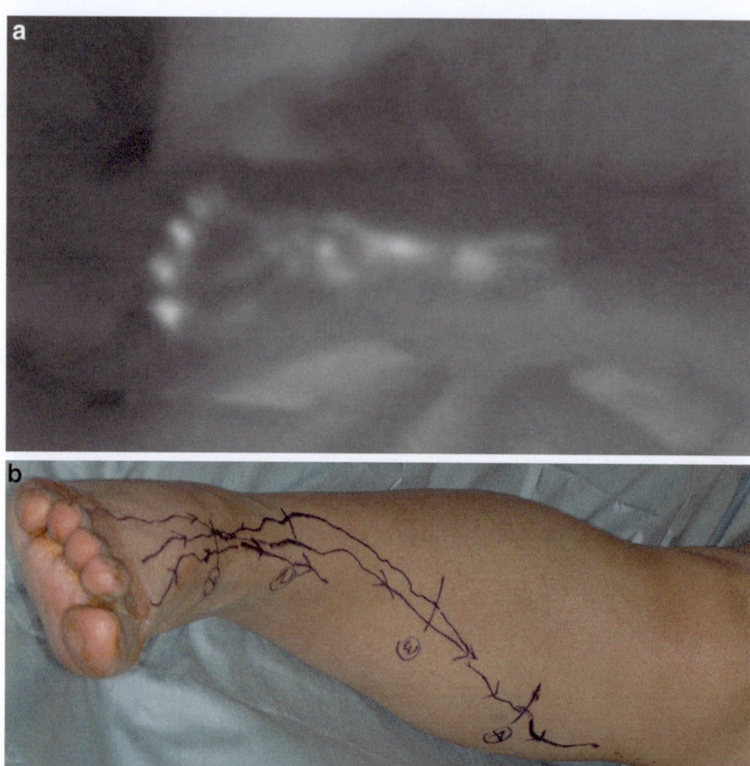

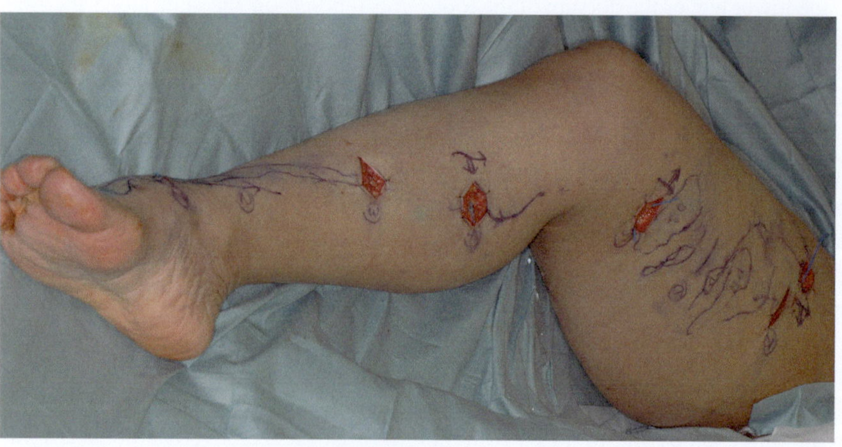

Fig. 23.5 Skin incisions for anastomosis in the lower limb

Anastomosis

Skin incisions 2–3 cm in length are made at each selected anastomotic site (Fig. 23.5). The subcutaneous fat layer is carefully dissected with mosquito forceps with fine tips (Fig. 23.6a). A vessel loop (blue) is introduced beneath the lymph vessel to stretch the wall of the lymphatic vessel (Fig. 23.6b, c). For side-to-end anastomosis, the side of the lymphatic vessel is incised

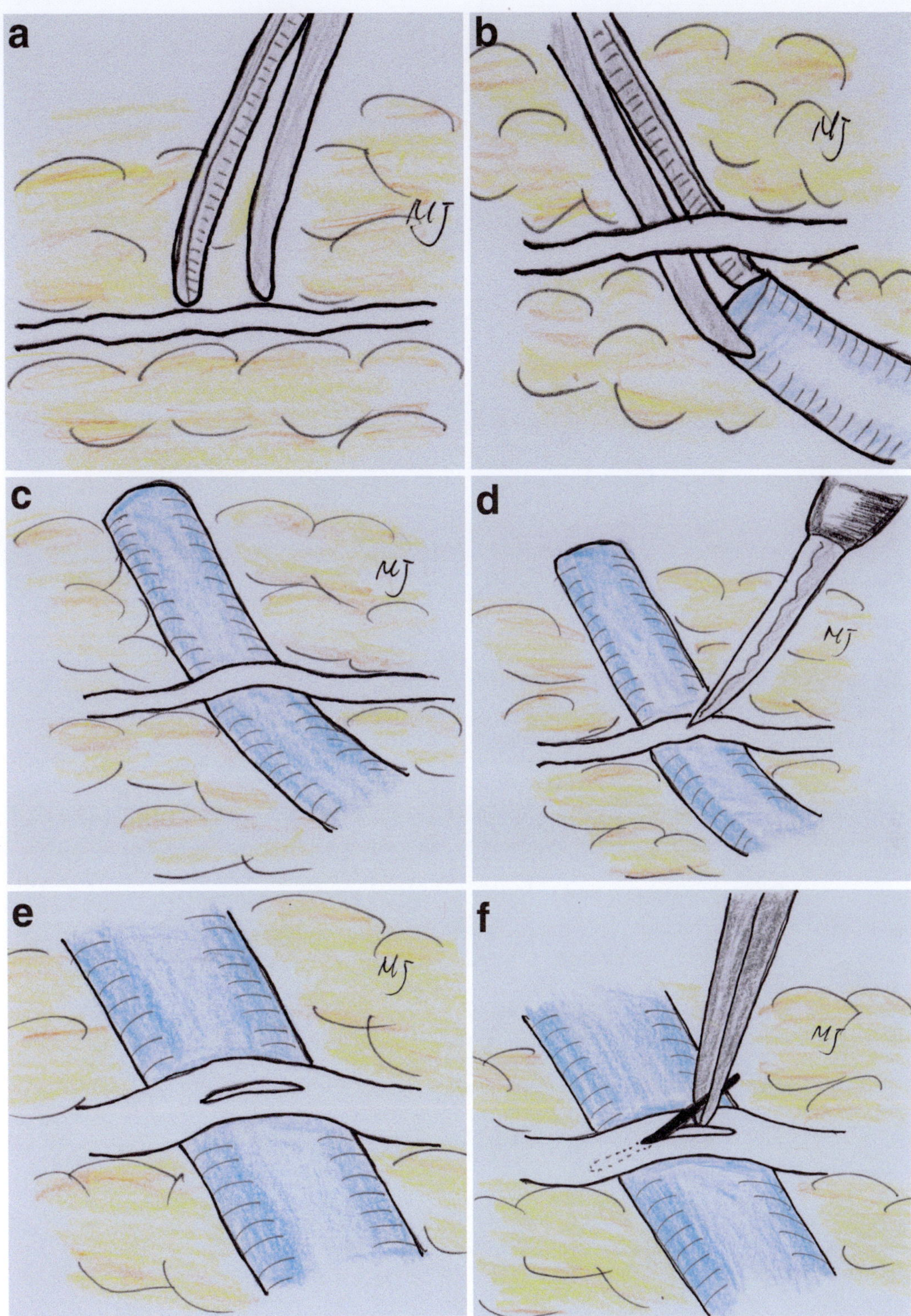

Fig. 23.6 Operative steps of lymphatic–venous side-to-end anastomosis

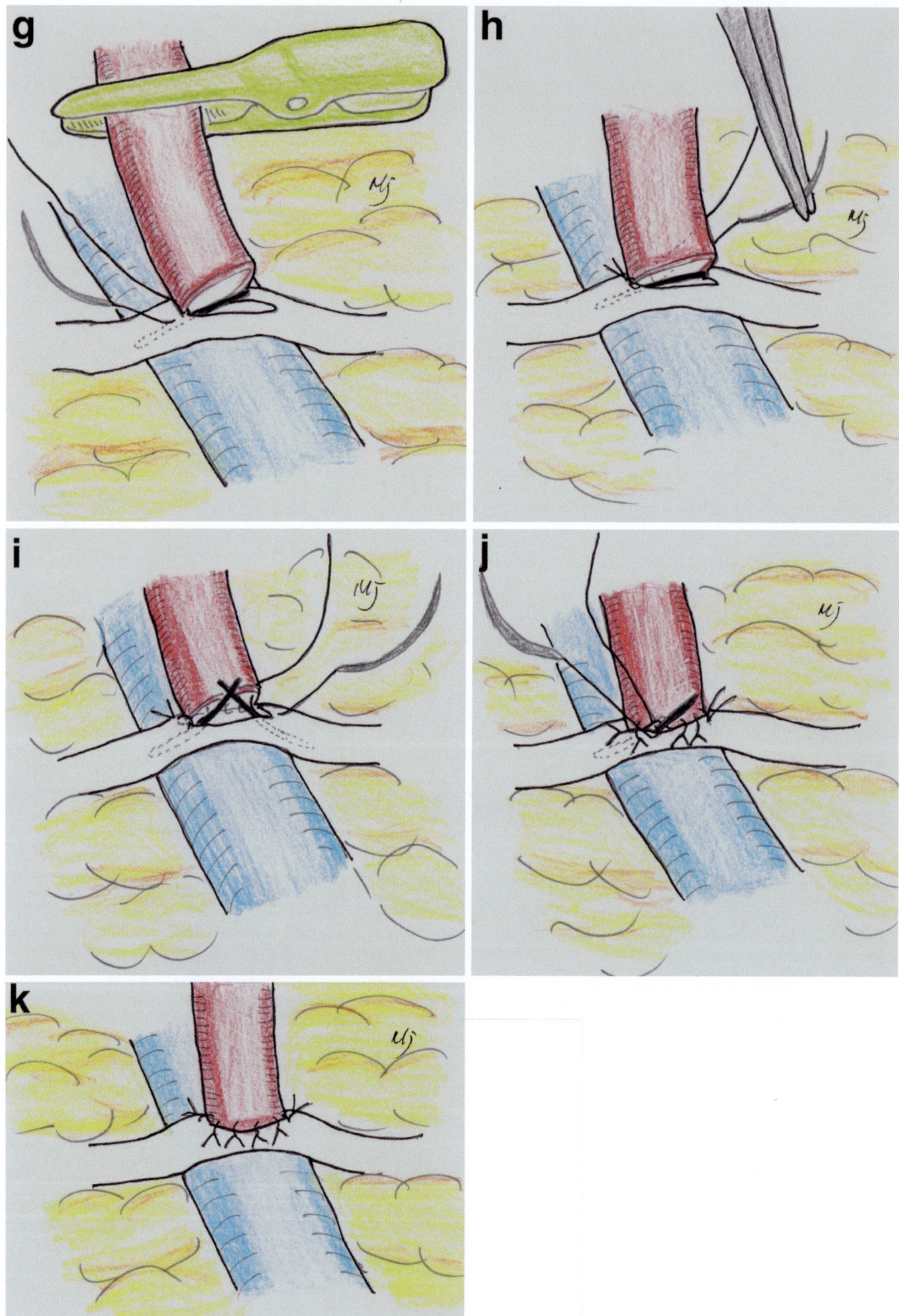

Fig. 23.6 (continued)

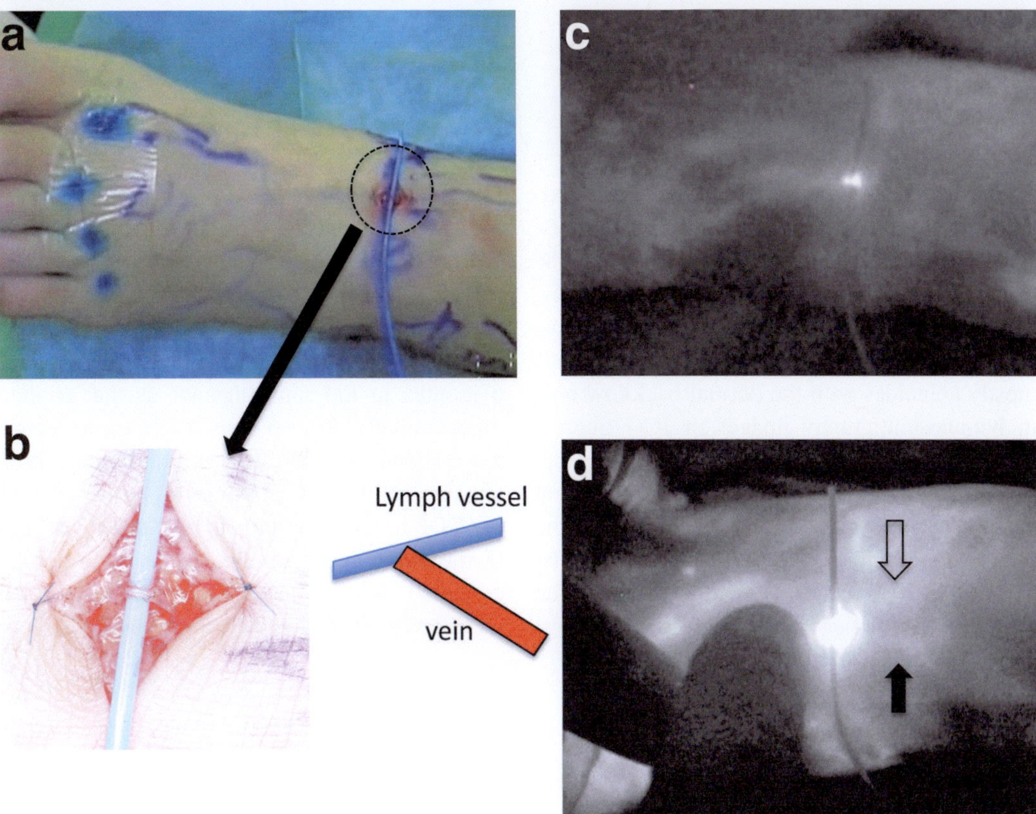

Fig. 23.7 Intraoperative confirmation of patency. (**a**) and (**b**), *left*: Operative photos of lymphatic–venous side-to-end anastomosis. (**b**) *right*: Schema of lymphatic–venous side-to-end anastomosis. (**c**) Intraoperative ICG fluorescence lymphography shows patency of the anastomosis and positive run-off from the lymphatics to the vein by massage. (**d**) The open arrow indicates lymphatic vessels and the closed *arrow* indicates the vein

with a micro-knife (Fig. 23.6d). When the tip of the knife reaches the lumen of the lymphatic vessel, lymph flows out through the incision. The length of the incision on the lymphatic vessel should be shorter than the outer diameter of the vein (Fig. 23.6e). Stents (6-0 nylon stitch of 3 mm length) are inserted to secure the lumen of the lymph vessel (Fig. 23.6f) [26, 27]. The first stitch should be placed at the left edge of the incision and appropriate stitches are placed according to the size of the vein (Fig. 23.6g–k). Another stent should be inserted to the lymph vessels to secure to put the stitches at the other end. So, two stents are usually required for anastomosis. If the outer diameter of the venous end is less than 0.3 mm, another stent should be inserted into the venous end to secure the anastomosis.

Three stents are required totally. These stents are removed from the vein and lymph vessel at the end of anastomosis.

Confirmation of Patency

After completion of the anastomosis, patency can be confirmed by direct visualization through the microscope (Fig. 23.7a, b) and by ICG fluorescence lymphography. If the anastomosis is technically well done, lymph passes from the lymph vessel to the vein and the vein becomes puffed up by massage. In cases that have good flow of lymph to the vein, the vein can be observed through the skin, which is called a good "run off test" (Fig. 23.7c, d).

Complications

Early Postoperative Complications

Ecchymosis may be observed in the area proximal to the anastomotic sites the day after surgery, because blood flows in a reverse direction via the anastomoses, from the vein to the lymphatic vessels, in cases with higher venous pressure relative to lymphatic pressure. The area of ecchymosis mostly coincides with the dermal backflow area in lymphoscintigraphy images or ICG fluorescence lymphography (Fig. 23.8). Nonsteroidal anti-inflammatory medication taken for several days usually result in disappearance of the ecchymosis within 1 week postoperatively. Lymphorrhea sometimes occurs through the closed wound after removal of the stitches, although this usually resolves spontaneously.

Late Postoperative Complications

Hypertrophic scar formation is a rare complication of lymphatic–venous anastomosis. Prevention of bulging scars is recommended in patients who have a tendency to hypertrophic scar formation.

Postoperative Treatment

Immediately After Surgery

Intermittent pneumatic compression (IPC) helps to maintain lymph flow from the lymphatic vessels to the veins at the anastomotic sites. The patient can put on compressive garments a few days after surgery. About 1 week after surgery, CDP is commenced and continued for at least 6 months in the same manner as that applied preoperatively. After 6 months, we try to reduce the contents of CDP, and if the affected limb remains stable, we continue to further reduce the CDP to improve the patient's quality of life. If the limb again swells up or the patient's condition worsens subjectively, the initial CDP is recommenced.

Postoperative Evaluations

The primary surgical outcome of lymphatic–venous anastomosis is patency of the anastomosis, with volume reduction of the affected limb and improvement in the patient's activities of daily living (ADL) being secondary and tertiary outcomes, respectively [28]. Patency can be

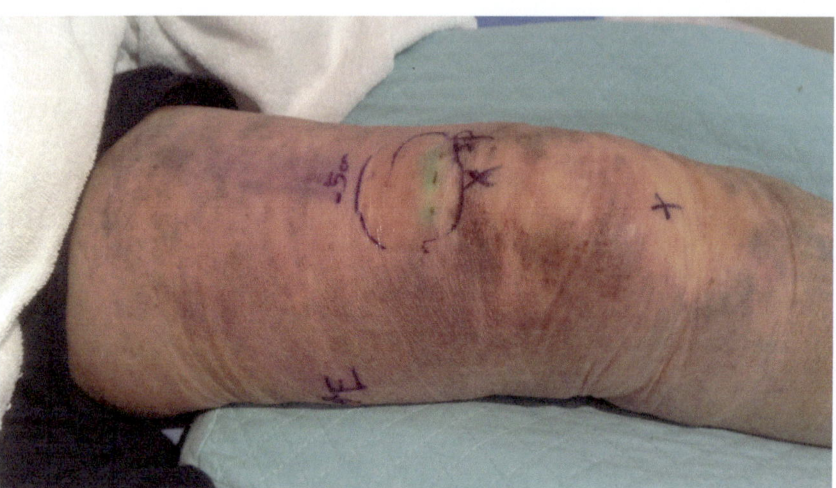

Fig. 23.8 Postoperative ecchymosis in the lower limb

assessed by ICG fluorescence lymphography, decrease in volume by circumferential and length measurements, and ADL by a questionnaire.

Physical Evaluations

In my clinical practice, the patient comes to the outpatient clinic every few months after surgery. Volume and/or circumference of both the affected limb and the contralateral limb are measured. In most cases with lymphatic–venous side-to-end anastomosis, volumes and circumferences of the affected limb decrease slightly in the first few months and remain stable thereafter.

Subjective Evaluations

In my experience, the frequency of dermato-lymphangio-adenitis (DLA) decreases after surgery in most cases. The contents of CDP can also be decreased in some patients, which improves their ADL. The total duration and frequency of wearing compressive garments and the size and class of compression garments can also be reduced by anastomotic surgery.

Evaluation of Patency by Imaging

Direct Method by ICG Fluorescence Lymphography

Evaluation by ICG fluorescence lymphography is performed 6 months or more after surgery. As described in this chapter, ICG fluorescence lymphography is limited in its ability to detect the lymphatics and veins selected for anastomosis. If the anastomoses are performed in a relatively superficial layer of subcutaneous tissue, this method can evaluate the patency of the anastomoses. In my study, out of 223 anastomoses in the lower limb, only 79 (35 %) could be evaluated by ICG lymphography. The remaining 144 anastomoses could not be evaluated because the subcutaneous layer was too thick to allow detection of the lymph vessels. In the 79 anastomoses that could be evaluated, cumulative patency rates of lymphatic–venous side-to-end anastomosis

(LVSEAs) were 75 ± 7.1 % at 12 months and 36 ± 9.4 % at 24 months after surgery [26]. The patency rates, thus, gradually decreased over time. Gloviczki reported in animal experiments that 8 of 19 anastomoses were patent at 2–6 weeks and 2 of 6 anastomoses were patent at 8 months [29]. We have seen some patients who showed relatively long-term patency (Fig. 23.7d).

In my clinical experience of postoperative ICG lymphography, we sometimes observe new pathways of superficial lymph flow created near the anastomosis sites where obvious patency could not be observed. This indicates that it may be possible to create new lymph pathways via surgical stimulation. On the other hand, the status of the anastomosis at sites that cannot be evaluated due to thickness of the skin and subcutaneous fat or masking by dermal backflow is unknown. In the thigh of patients with type III lymphoscintigraphy images, for example, lymphatic collectors exist relatively deep in the subcutaneous layer. These collectors are expected to be patent because the lymphatic vessels are large in diameter and there is a greater amount of lymph flow here than in the foot. If we perform five or six anastomoses from the foot to the thigh, about two can be expected to remain patent.

Indirect Method by Lymphoscintigraphy

Postoperative lymphoscintigraphy sometimes shows disappearance of dermal backflow in the affected limb. This is because patent anastomoses may reduce internal pressure in the lymph vessels, which improves the dermal backflow of lymph.

Results of Surgery

Several reports have addressed the long-term results after lymphatic–venous anastomosis [5–7]. The results seem to include those of CDP. Although O'Brien et al. divided patients with lymphatic–venous anastomosis into two groups, with and without preoperative CDP, they did not mention the reduction effects of CDP alone [7]. Surgical effects and efficacy of CDP should be assessed separately in order to provide a clear picture of the efficacy of anastomotic surgery. In a study by our group, the true efficacy of LVSEA in terms of volume reduction was about 100 ml in the affected limb in all patients. On the other hand, preoperative CDP reduced patients' lower limb volume by up to 600 ml [24]. Hence, in terms of volume reduction, the efficacy of CDP seems better than that of lymphatic–venous shunt operations.

Additional LVSEA

If the patient exhibits objective deterioration, obvious absence of patency at the anastomotic sites, no remarkable subjective improvement, and has detectable lymphatics by ICG fluorescence lymphography, additional lymphatic–venous anastomosis can be recommended.

A Typical Case

A 59-year-old woman complaining of left lower limb edema for 6 years came to our hospital for surgical treatment because of worsening of edema despite CDP for several years (Fig. 23.9a, upper row). She had no history of cancer therapy.

Lymphoscintigraphy showed dermal backflow in the left lower leg, with no obvious lymph nodes in the left inguinal and pelvic regions (Fig. 23.9a, *lower row*). Hence, we diagnosed her as primary type IV lymphedema, which is an indication for lymphaticovenous shunt. Five LVSEAs were then performed under general anesthesia, one at the foot and four in the lower leg. Postoperative ICG fluorescence lymphogra-

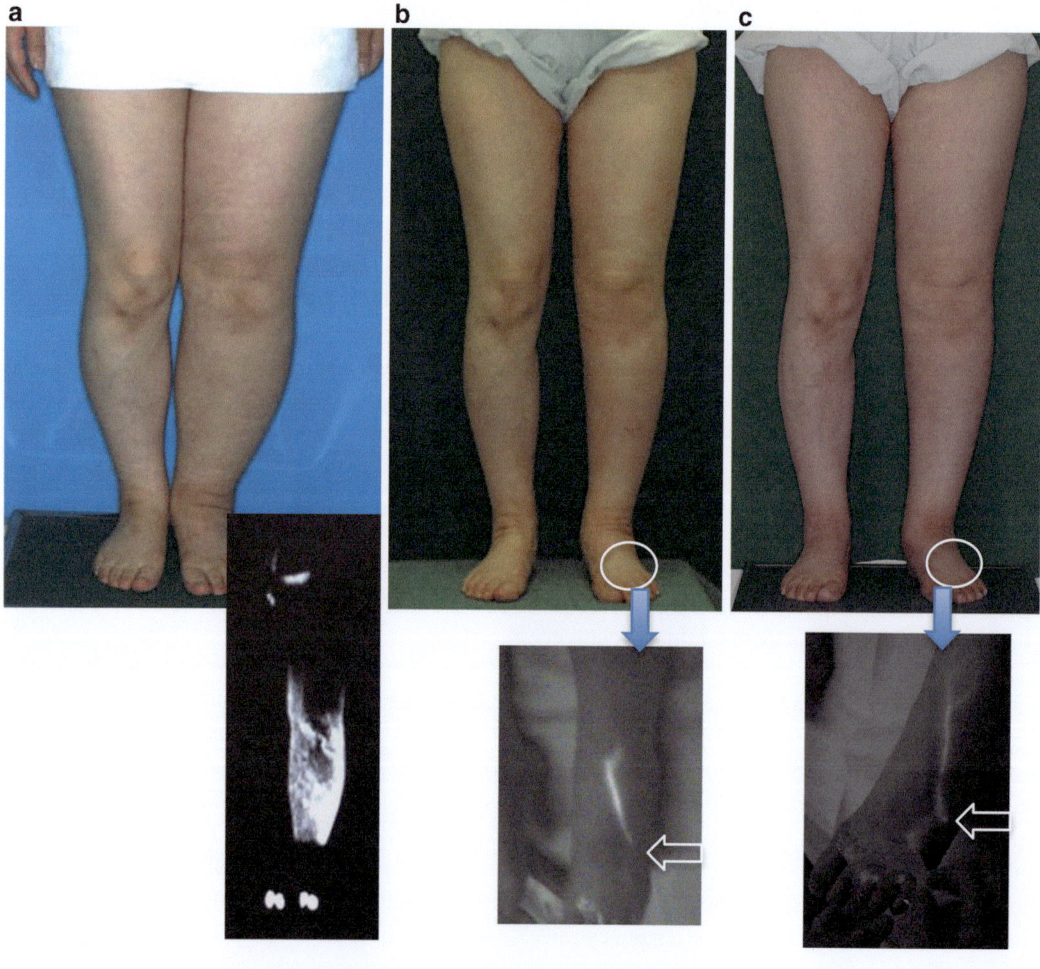

phy was performed 10 months after surgery, which indicated that only two of the five anastomoses could be evaluated, only one (the foot anastomosis) of which was patent (Fig. 23.9b, *lower row*). The arrow indicates the site of anastomosis. The volume of the affected leg had reduced by about 500 ml after surgery (Fig. 23.9b, *upper row*). Postoperative ICG fluorescence lymphography was again repeated 4 years and 2 months after surgery. The foot anastomosis was still seen to be patent (Fig. 23.9c, *lower row*; the arrow indicates the site of anastomosis) and edema of the affected limb had remained stable for more than 4 years (Fig. 23.9c, *upper row*).

Conclusion

The introduction of ICG fluorescence lymphography has made real-time visualization of lymph flow possible. Although there are still limitations to the evaluation of patency at all anastomotic sites, the patency rate is about 40 % 2 years postoperatively. Patients are able to subjectively appreciate anastomotic patency by a sense of softness in the leg, and quick improvement of the edema if it once again deteriorates with prolonged standing or walking Lymphatic–venous anastomosis does not produce much improvement in terms of volume reduction, because the amount of lymph drained via the anastomosis is not significant, and the function of the contractile muscles of the lymph vessels worsens after surgery. Therefore, postoperative CDP is required in most cases, although if patients have some patent anastomoses and maintain contractile function of the lymph vessels, it is possible for them to become free from CDP after surgery. Another problem during lymphatic–venous anastomosis is visualization of deep lymph vessels. SPECT-CT lymphoscintigraphy, MR lymphangiography, and contrast-enhanced ultrasonography may help resolve this issue.

Lymphatic–venous anastomosis is a less invasive and more physiological treatment option for peripheral lymphedema. Improved accuracy in detecting functional lymph vessels using new diagnostic modalities for evaluating lymph flow will produce better surgical results. Postoperative evaluations provide feedback for improvement of surgical skills and methods.

References

1. Edwards JM, Kinmonth JB. Lymphovenous shunts in man. Br Med J. 1969;4:579–81.
2. Yamada Y. The studies on lymphatic venous anastomosis in lymphedema. Nagoya J Med Sci. 1969;32:1–21.
3. O'Brien BM, Sykes P, Threlfall GN, Browning FS. Microlymphaticovenous anastomoses for obstructive lymphedema. Plast Reconstr Surg. 1977;60:197–211.
4. Huang GK, Hu RQ, Liu ZZ, Shen YL, Lan TD, Pan GP. Microlymphaticovenous anastomosis in the treatment of lower limb obstructive lymphedema: analysis of 91 cases. Plast Reconstr Surg. 1985;76:671–85.
5. Campisi C, Boccardo F, Zilli A, Macciò A, Napoli F. Long-term results after lymphatic-venous anastomoses for the treatment of obstructive lymphedema. Microsurgery. 2001;21:135–9.
6. Koshima I, Nanba Y, Tsutsui T, Takahashi Y, Itoh S. Long-term follow-up after lymphaticovenular anastomosis for lymphedema in the leg. J Reconstr Microsurg. 2003;19:209–15.
7. O'Brien BM, Mellow CG, Khazanchi RK, Dvir E, Kumar V, Pederson WC. Long-term results after microlymphaticovenous anastomoses for the treatment of obstructive lymphedema. Plast Reconstr Surg. 1990;85:562–72.

Fig. 23.9 Lymphedema of the left leg after treatment of uterine cancer in a 59-year-old woman. Out of five anastomoses in the foot and leg, two could be evaluated, one of which was patent. (**a**) Before surgery. Clinical photo at the first visit and lymphoscintigraphy at the same time (Type III). (**b**) 10 months after surgery. Clinical photo and ICG fluorescence lymphography at the anastomotic site in the foot 10 months after surgery. The *open arrow* indicates the site of anastomosis and the white line indicates the anastomosed vein. The patient underwent five lymphatic–venous side-to-end anastomoses in the foot and leg. Of these, only one of the two that could be evaluated was patent. (**c**) 4 years 2 months after surgery. A clinical photo and ICG fluorescence lymphography at the anastomotic site in the foot. The *open arrow* indicates the site of anastomosis, while the *white line* indicates the same vein that was visualized at 10 months after surgery

8. Szuba A, Strauss W, Sirsikar SP, Rockson SG. Quantitative radionuclide lymphoscintigraphy predicts outcome of manual lymphatic therapy in breast cancer-related lymphedema of the upper extremity. Nucl Med Commun. 2002;23:1171–5.

9. Pecking AP, Albérini JL, Wartski M, Edeline V, Cluzan RV. Relationship between lymphoscintigraphy and clinical findings in lower limb lymphedema (LO): toward a comprehensive staging. Lymphology. 2008;41:1–10.

10. Vaqueiro M, Gloviczki P, Fisher J, Hollier LH, Schirger A, Wahner HW. Lymphoscintigraphy in lymphedema: an aid to microsurgery. J Nucl Med. 1986;27:1125–30.

11. Maegawa J, Mikami T, Yamamoto Y, Satake T, Kobayashi S. Types of lymphoscintigraphy and indications for lymphaticovenous anastomosis. Microsurgery. 2010;30:437–42.

12. Mikami T, Hosono M, Yabuki Y, Yamamoto Y, Yasumura K, Sawada H, et al. Classification of lymphoscintigraphy and relevance to surgical indication for lymphaticovenous anastomosis in upper limb lymphedema. Lymphology. 2011;44:155–67.

13. Ogata F, Narushima M, Mihara M, Azuma R, Morimoto Y, Koshima I. Intraoperative lymphography using indocyanine green dye for near- infrared fluorescence labeling in lymphedema. Ann Plast Surg. 2007;59:180–4.

14. Unno N, Inuzuka K, Suzuki M, Yamamoto N, Sagara D, Nishiyama M, et al. Preliminary experience with a novel fluorescence lymphography using indocyanine green in patients with secondary lymphedema. J Vasc Surg. 2007;45:1016–21.

15. Yamamoto T, Narushima M, Doi K, Oshima A, Ogata F, Mihara M, et al. Characteristic indocyanine green lymphography findings in lower extremity lymphedema: the generation of a novel lymphedema severity staging system using dermal backflow patterns. Plast Reconstr Surg. 2011;27:1979–86.

16. Blum KS, Radtke C, Knapp WH, Pabst R, Gratz KF. SPECT-CT: a valuable method to document the regeneration of lymphatics and autotransplanted lymph node fragments. Eur J Nucl Med Mol Imaging. 2007;34:1861–7.

17. Cheville AL, Brinkmann DH, Ward SB, Durski J, Laack NN, Yan E, et al. The addition of SPECT/CT lymphoscintigraphy to breast cancer radiation planning spares lymph nodes critical for arm drainage. Int J Rad Oncol Biol Phys. 2013;85:971–7.

18. Fairbairn N, Munson C, Ali Khan Z, Butterworth M. The role of hybrid SPECT/CT for lymphatic mapping in patients with melanoma. J Plast Reconstr Aesthet Surg. 2013;66(9):1248–55.

19. Petralia G, Conte G, De Fiori E, Alessi S, Bellomi M. Contrast-enhanced ultrasound sonography optimises the assessment of lymph nodes in oncology. Ecancer. 2013;7:328.

20. Rubaltelli L, Beltrame V, Scagliori E, Bezzon E, Frigo AC, Rastrelli M, et al. Potential use of contrast-enhanced ultrasound (CEUS) in the detection of metastatic superficial lymph nodes in melanoma patients. Ultraschall Med. 2014;35:67–71.

21. Dudau C, Hameed S, Gibson D, Muthu S, Sandison A, Eckersley RJ, et al. Can contrast-enhanced ultrasound distinguish malignant from reactive lymph nodes in patients with head and neck cancers? Ultrasound Med Biol. 2014;40:747–54.

22. Eklöf B, Rutherford RB, Bergan JJ, Carpentier PH, Gloviczki P, Kistner RL, et al. Revision of the CEAP classification for chronic venous disorders: consensus statement. J Vasc Surg. 2004;40:1248–52.

23. Huang GK, Hsin YP. Relationship between lymphatic and venous pressure in normal and lymphedematous rabbit ears. Microsurgery. 1984;5:36–9.

24. Maegawa J, Hosono M, Tomoeda H, Tosaki A, Kobayashi S, Iwai T. Net effect of lymphaticovenous anastomosis on volume reduction of peripheral lymphoedema after complex decongestive physiotherapy. Eur J Vasc Endovasc Surg. 2012;43:602–8.

25. Yamamoto R, Yamamoto T. Effectiveness of the treatment-phase of two-phase complex decongestive physiotherapy for the treatment of extremity lymphoedema. Int J Clin Oncol. 2007;12:463–8.

26. Shaper NJ, Rutt DR, Browse NL. Use of Teflon stents for lymphovenous anastomosis. Br J Surg. 1992;79:633–6.

27. Narushima M, Mihara M, Yamamoto Y, Iida T, Koshima I, Mundinger GS. The intravascular stenting method for treatment of extremity lymphedema with multiconfiguration lymphaticovenous anastomoses. Plast Reconstr Surg. 2010;125:935–43.

28. Maegawa J, Yabuki Y, Tomoeda H, Hosono M, Yasumura K. Outcomes of lymphaticovenous side-to-end anastomosis in peripheral lymphedema. J Vasc Surg. 2012;55:753–60.

29. Gloviczki P, Hollier LH, Nora FE, Kaye MP. The natural history of microsurgical lymphovenous anastomoses: an experimental study. J Vasc Surg. 1986;4:148–56.

Lymph Node Transfer to Proximal Extremity

24

Heli Kavola, Sinikka Suominen, and Anne Saarikko

Key Points

- In the lymph node transfer method lymphatic vessels are not anastomosed since they are expected to form spontaneously after the scar release and transfer of lymphatic tissue.
- Wide scar release is an essential step when preparing the recipient site.
- Lymph node transfer can be conveniently combined with microvascular abdominal wall breast reconstruction.
- To date we do not know what the clinical benefit of VLNT surgery is in the long run. All lymph node transfer patients need to be followed in order to detect any clinical symptoms in the donor site.

Introduction

In industrialized countries, the populations primarily affected by lymphedema are patients undergoing treatment of malignancy, particularly breast cancer and melanoma [1, 2]. According to a recent review, the incidence of breast cancer related arm lymphedema is 19.9 % after axillary dissection [3]. In patients with sentinel node biopsy the incidence is smaller, from 4 to 10 %. The incidence of lymphedema after inguinal lymph node dissection in melanoma varies from 20 to 64 % [4–6].

Vascularized lymph node transfer (VLNT) is a microsurgical method, in which lymph nodes from a healthy lymph basin are transferred to a lymphedematous extremity and the artery and vein of this lymph node flap are anastomosed to local vessels to maintain vascularity. Lymph vessels are not anastomosed since they are expected to form spontaneously from the transferred lymph nodes. This procedure aims to restore physiological lymphatic flow where lymphatic system is damaged, e.g., due to previous surgery.

Since 1979, several animal and anatomical studies have shown promising results for vascularized lymph node transfers [7–9]. In 2006, Becker at al. published a series of 24 patients treated with vascularized lymph node transfer for postmastectomy lymphedema [10]. During recent years this technique has gained popularity.

The exact mechanism by which VLNT improves lymphatic flow is still unclear.

It is hypothesized that scar tissue release opens the obstructed lymphatic vessels and replacing the scar with a well-vascularized flap bridge the distal lymphatics with the healthy proximal system. Experimental studies have demonstrated that

H. Kavola, M.D., Ph.D.
Department of Plastic Surgery,
Helsinki University Hospital, Helsinki, Finland

S. Suominen, M.D., Ph.D.
Department of Plastic Surgery, Helsinki University,
Helsinki, Finland

A. Saarikko, M.D., Ph.D. (✉)
Department of Plastic Surgery, Toolo Hospital,
Topeliuksen katu 5, Helsinki 00260, Finland
e-mail: anne.saarikko@hus.fi

A.K. Greene et al. (eds.), *Lymphedema: Presentation, Diagnosis, and Treatment*,
DOI 10.1007/978-3-319-14493-1_24, © Springer International Publishing Switzerland 2015

lymphatic vessels have an enormous capacity to regenerate after tissue transfer by regrowth of lymphatic vessels and spontaneous reconnections of existing lymphatics [11, 12]. Transplanted lymph nodes produce vascular endothelial growth factor C (VEGF-C) that stimulates lymphangiogenesis and new lymph vessels are formed to reconnect the lymphatic pathways [13]. There is also direct connection with lymph nodes and veins inside the flap to allow drainage directly to venous system [14]. Is also proposed that lymph node flap acts as a "pump" that draws fluid from surrounding interstitium to the transferred lymphatics by gradient between arterial inflow and venous outflow [15]. Obstruction in the venous outflow might be one factor in postoperative lymphedema sequelae. It is our clinical observation that releasing the compressing scar around the axillary vein sometimes provide immediate relief of symptoms well before the lymphatics have, even theoretically, regenerated.

Indications

At the moment lymph node transfer is still considered as experimental surgery. We do not know what the effect of this method is on the lymphedema limb volume in the long run. VLNT is considered to be most effective in early stages of lymphedema when adipose tissue hypertrophy and fibrosis have not yet developed.

The main indication for VLNT is secondary lymphedema where complete blockade of lymphatic drainage is caused by surgical removal of lymph nodes or damage to lymphatic pathways and this is diagnosed by lymphoscintigraphy, magnetic resonance lymphography or indocyanine green lymphography. Some groups have suggested that lymphedema patients with impaired lymphatic drainage who do not respond to conservative treatment can also be considered for VLNT [15, 16].

A large number of mastectomy patients suffer from lymphedema, and mastectomy is an independent risk factor for post-breast-cancer lymphedema [3]. For these patients combined autologous breast reconstruction and inguinal axillary lymph node transfer is a tempting option.

In cases of chronic infections or recurrent episodes of erysipelas related to lymphedema VLNT might be useful since transplanted healthy lymph nodes are expected to improve the local immune response [16]. VLNT seems to be beneficial in treatment of chronic pain, neuromas and brachial plexus neuropathies associated with breast cancer surgery [17, 18]. This is possibly due to wide scar release combined with VLNT and vascularized soft tissue with active lymph nodes might prevent recurring fibrosis and scar tissue.

VLNT has also been proposed as a treatment option in cases of primary/congenital lymphedemas, but mainly in lower limb lymphedema [19]. However, especially in this patient population it is of utmost important to estimate the risk of postoperative lymphedema problem in the flap donor area.

Donor Sites

Inguinal

The most common donor site for a lymph node flap is the inguinal area (Fig. 24.1). Superficial lymph nodes are harvested based in the superficial circumflex vessels. Superficial inferior epigastric vessels can be used as a secondary vascular pedicle. Exact flap design varies among authors [10, 13, 15, 16, 20–22]. Dr. Becker starts the flap harvest by incision along the line between iliac crest and the pubis bone and the lymph nodes between muscular aponeurosis and the superficial fascia are harvested above the inguinal ligament. Superficial circumflex iliac vessels (SCIA/V) and superficial inferior epigastric vessels (SIEA/V) are isolated with vessel loops. It is emphasized not to dissect beyond the deep (muscular aponeurosis) and the caudal (inguinal ligament) border to avoid harvesting lymph nodes draining the leg.

Saaristo et al. used similar inguinal lymphatic flap design, with the modification of avoiding harvesting SIEA as a second vascular pedicle. It hypothesized that surgical trauma to this central area might interfere with lymphatic drainage of the lower limbs [13, 23]. In most patients lymph node transfer was combined with the lower

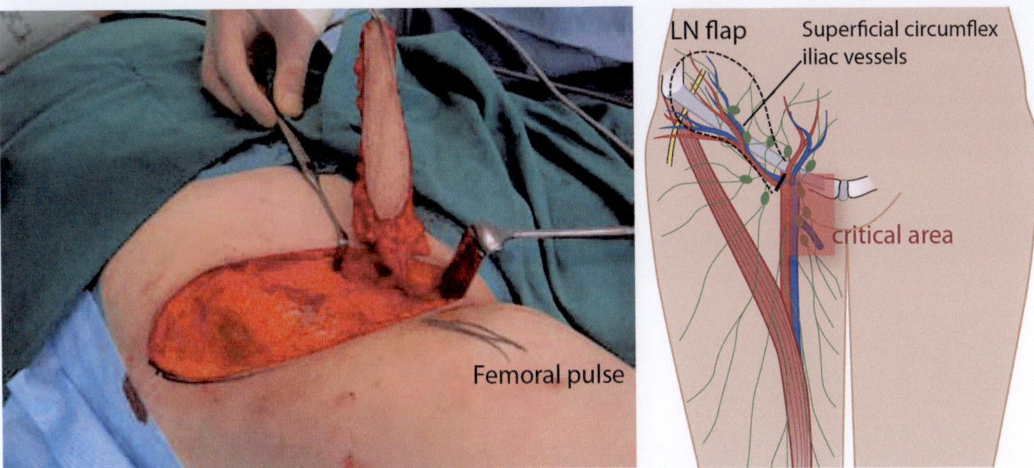

Fig. 24.1 Inguinal lymph node (LN) flap. Superficial lymph nodes are harvested based in the superficial circumflex vessels. Lymph nodes draining lower limb are located medially and centrally to the femoral artery, and should therefore be left intact

abdominal breast reconstruction. They emphasize limiting the lymphatic flap dissection to the lateral border of the femoral artery. Lymph nodes draining lower limb are located medially and centrally to the femoral artery [24], and should therefore be left intact. This is recommended also by Tourani et al. [25].

Dayan et al. describe a slightly more distal flap design. The landmarks for flap are the pubic tubercle, the anterior superior iliac spine, and the line 3 cm below inguinal ligament where the targeted lymph nodes are located based on the magnetic resonance angiography. They also advocate the use of intraoperative indocyanine lymphography to confirm the nodes of interest and reverse lymphatic mapping to avoid harvesting lymph nodes draining the lower extremity [21]. Some other authors report similar below inguinal ligament flap design [15, 20, 22]. Gharb et al. describe a modified technique of harvesting the flap with only the superficial branch of SCIA [26].

Thoracic

The thoracic lymph node flap consists lymph nodes from the lower axilla along the anterior border of latissimus dorsi muscle (Fig. 24.2).

According to studies by Suami et al. axillary lymph nodes have separate groups for drainage of the thorax and the arm [27]. Therefore, the lymph nodes of the lower part of axilla could be used for lymph node transfer. The nodes are vascularized either by lateral thoracic vessels or braches of thoracodorsal vessels [16, 28]. The incision is made at the anterior axillary line and dissection is continued through subcutaneous tissue to the lateral border of the pectoralis minor. The lateral thoracic and thoracodorsal vessels are identified and lymph nodes around the appropriate vessels are harvested. According to Dr. Becker, in 60 % of the cases the nodes are supplied by lateral thoracic vessels and these are preferred. In remaining 40 % of the cases the nodes are harvested with the thoracodorsal vessels. It is important to keep the level of harvest inferior to the lateral border of pectoralis minor (level I) to avoid damaging nodes draining upper extremity and breast (level II–III). Reverse sentinel node mapping can be used to identify lymph node draining the arm in order to avoid these during the flap harvest. Prolonged local edema at the donor site has been reported [28] and we have also experienced a postoperative lymphedema of the breast after harvesting the thoracic lymph node flap.

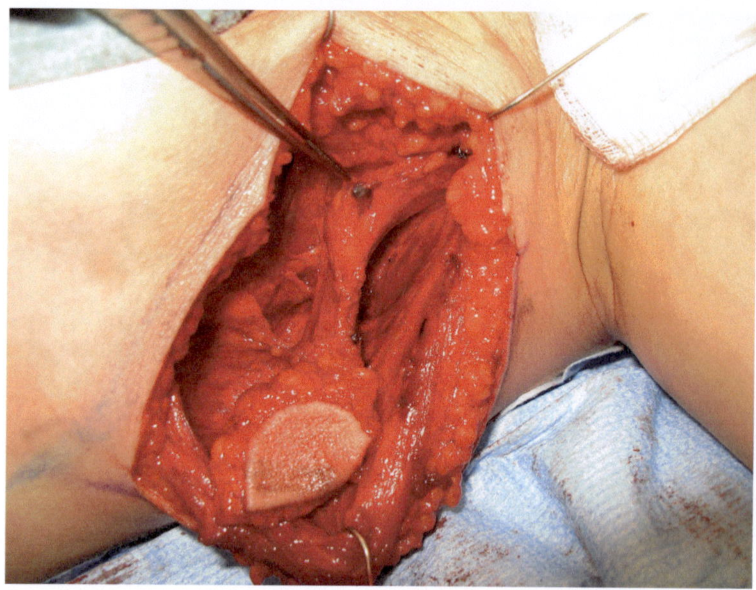

Fig. 24.2 The thoracic lymph node flap containing lymph nodes from the lower axilla along the anterior border of latissimus dorsi muscle

Cervical/Supraclavicular

The cervical lymph node flap [29, 30] is based on the transverse cervical artery and its concomitant transverse cervical vein. External jugular vein is included in the flap to improve venous outflow. It is recommended to be harvested at the right side of the neck to avoid potential damage to the main lymphatic duct. The landmarks of the flap are the clavicle inferiorly, the sternocleidomastoid muscle anteriorly, the trapezius muscle posteriorly, and the external jugular vein. The incision made 1.5 cm above the clavicle and through the platysma. The omohyoid muscle is retracted and deep to this muscle the TCA and the surrounding lymph nodes are identified and harvested. There are anatomical variations in the origin of TCA. It most often originates from the thyrocervical branch (80 %) or directly from the subclavian artery (20 %), but it may arise as a branch of the internal mammary artery [30]. The main advantage of the cervical lymph node flap is that there is less risk of developing lymphedema at the donor site.

Submental

Submental lymph node flap [31] is based on the submental artery arising from the facial artery. The flap is harvested with an elliptical skin paddle with its upper margin along the lower border of mandible. The facial artery and its junction with the submental artery are identified and the soft tissue around this area containing the lymph nodes is included. The flap is raised along the axis of the submental artery from proximal end to the distal end. The marginal mandibular nerve must be carefully preserved. The anterior belly of the digastricus muscle can be included in the flap for easier harvest.

Lymph Node Transfer to Axilla

Wide scar release is an essential step when preparing the recipient site. All scarred and fibrotic tissue around vessels and nerves is excised and removed if possible. The axillary vein should be completely released to allow free venous outflow (Fig. 24.3).

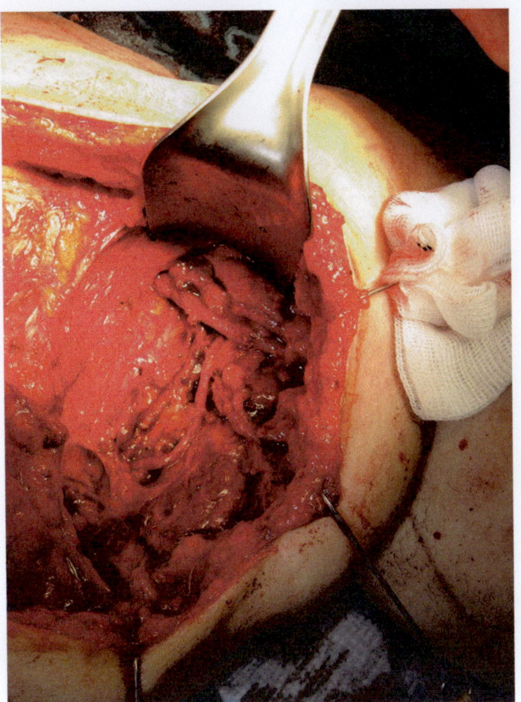

Fig. 24.3 In the upper limb lymphedema patients wide scar release is an essential step when preparing the recipient site for the lymph node flap in the axilla

It is recommended to start dissection from the healthy area to identify normal anatomy and avoid injury to the vital structures within the axilla. Dissection should be continued until healthy tissue is again reached. If the patient has chronic pain or symptoms of brachial plexus neuropathy or neuroma is encountered external neurolysis of the brachial plexus should be performed.

Recipient vessels, either thoracodorsal or circumflex scapular, are prepared and anastomosed with the flap pedicle using microsurgical technique. Also the lateral thoracic vessels can be used if still available. The lymph node flap is positioned along the axillary vein extending into the proximal brachium.

Lymph Node Transfer to Groin

At the moment there is very few publications about the use lymph node transfer in the inguinal area. Unlike in the breast cancer related lymphedema, the lymphatic vascular problem in the lower extremity is rarely localized only to the proximal area of the limb. According to Becker et al., the principles of lymph node transfer to groin are similar as for that in axilla [16]. Wide scar release is considered important and should be continued until healthy tissue is reached. The superficial circumflex iliac vessels or any local vessels available are used for anastomosis. A pocket just caudal to the inguinal ligament is created to accommodate the lymph node flap.

Some authors favor distal recipient sites (knee or ankle) advocating that "pumping" mechanism of the lymph node flap works better at the distal sites due to gravitational forces [31]. So far, there are no comparative studies of the efficacy of proximal versus distal recipient site. The method is chosen according to the patient's situation and surgeon's personal preferences [32].

Combined with Breast Reconstruction

Lymph node transfer can be conveniently combined with microvascular abdominal wall breast reconstruction (Fig. 24.4). For postmastectomy patients suffering from upper extremity lymphedema, breast reconstruction with lymph node transfer is an optimal choice. Any soft tissue flap from the lower abdominal wall, either based on the deep inferior epigastric vessels (traditional TRAM-flap, muscle spearing TRAM-flap or DIEP flap) or superficial ineferior epigastric vessels (SIEA flap) can be used as a carrier of lymph node flap. The superficial lateral lymph nodes are located just caudal to this flap, and therefore, the skin incision in the combined flap is placed slightly lower (in a W-fashion) than when performing only abdominal flap (Fig. 24.4). The dissection starts with identification of SCIA and SIEA/V. The lymph node flap is dissected from lateral to medial following SCIA or its perforator and the pedicle vessel are ligated at their origin. The lymph node flap stays in connection to the abdominal flap at this level. Dissection should be limited to the lateral border of the femoral artery not to damage lymphatic tissue draining the lower limb, and SIEA and SIEV should be dissected

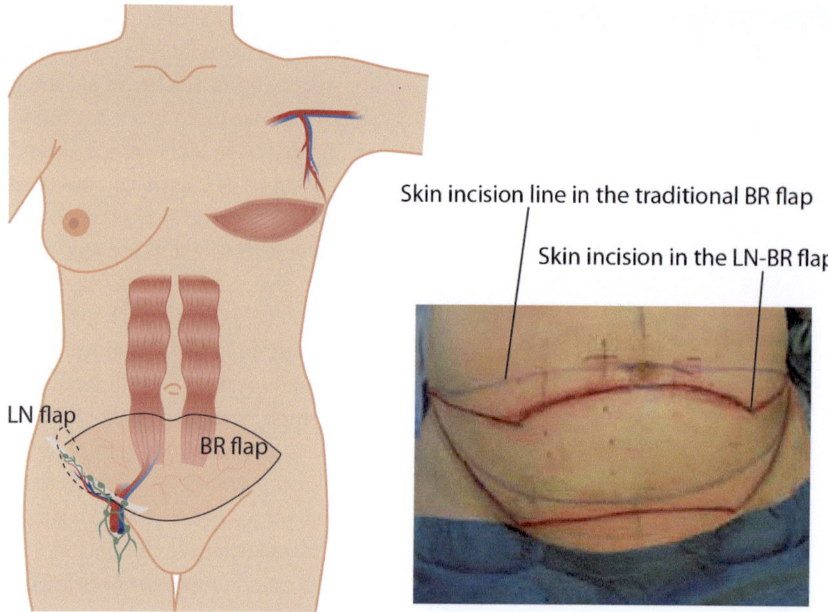

Fig. 24.4 Lymph node transfer can be conveniently combined with microvascular abdominal wall breast reconstruction (a TRAM, msTRAM, DIEP, or SIEA flap reconstruction). The superficial lateral lymph nodes are located just caudal to the lower abdominal wall breast reconstruction flap, and therefore, the skin incision in the combined flap is placed slightly lower (in a W-fashion) than when performing only abdominal flap

with care. Abdominal flap is then elevated as TRAM flap, ms-DIEP, DIEP or SIEA flap depending on the patient's anatomy and surgeon's preference. Before ligating the main pedicle vessels, blood flow to the tip of the lymph node flap is assessed. Perioperative ICG angiography can be useful when evaluating the blood perfusion to the lymph node flap. Axillary recipient site is prepared as described earlier. The main pedicle of the abdominal flap in anastomosed to the thoracodorsal vessels [13] or the internal mammary vessels [16]. If blood perfusion to the lymph node flap is not adequate, the SCIA/V are anastomosed to the retrograde thoracodorsal vessels or to circumflex scapulae vessels [12, 33] or to intact thoracodorsal vessels in case of internal mammary vessels were used for the main anastomosis [16]. The lymph node flap is the placed into the pocket along the axillary vein extending to the proximal brachium and the abdominal flap is shaped to reconstruct the missing breast.

Postoperative Care

There is no clear consensus of the optimal postoperative treatment.

Becker et al. start physiotherapy on the first postoperative day and continue it daily up to 3 months. After that physiotherapy is done two times a week for the next 3 months and then discontinued. Compression therapy is not used postoperatively [10].

It is our practice to start manual lymphatic drainage as soon as possible postoperatively to theoretically support the spontaneous regrowth of the lymphatic vasculature in the axilla. From the experimental studies we know that lymphatic vascular growth and maturation process may take 2 to 6 months after surgical operation [34]. However, there are no clinical studies to support this practice. The compression therapy is always continued minimum 6 months after the surgery.

After 6 months we encourage patients to stop using the compression garments. However, most patients still need to use compression also after that at least in physically strenuous situations. Depending on the extent and duration of preoperative lymphedema, compression may be needed up to 2 to 3 years, or permanently.

Complications

When using the groin area as a donor site, the risk of developing postoperative iatrogenic lower limb lymphedema is a major concern. Iatrogenic upper limb lymphedema is a potential risk also when using thoracic lymph nodes.

Postoperative seroma seems to be a common problem in the inguinal area after the lymphatic flap harvesting. However, that problem can usually be managed by local compression and repeated needle aspirations. Vignes et al. report a series of 26 patients who underwent VLNT for treatment of upper or lower limb lymphedema. Thirty-eight percent of them developed complications including chronic lymphedema at the donor site, lymphocele, testicular hydrocele, and persistent donor-site pain [35]. In a study by Viitanen et al. 4 of 13 patients complained postoperative numbness or pain in the superficial femoral cutaneous nerve area [23]. Pons et al. report a case of donor-site thigh lymphedema after lymph node–superficial circumflex iliac artery perforator flap transfer among 42 patients of VLNT operation [36].

Viitanen et al. evaluated the donor-site lymphatic function in the lower limb after microvascular lymph node transfer by postoperative lymphoscintigraphy. In six of ten patients, the lymphatic flow was slightly slower in a donor-site limb compared with non-operated limb, although none of these patients had clinical symptoms of lymphedema [23]. This emphasizes the importance of postoperative follow-up to detect possible developing postoperative lymphedema. Azuma et al. recommend ICG lymphography for following donor-site lymphatic function [37, 38].

Sound knowledge of anatomy and meticulous surgery are the cornerstone of safe surgery. Additional methods can be used to avoid damaging the essential structures. Patent Blue dye (Guerbert, France) injected intradermally into lower lateral abdominal wall may help identifying the lymph nodes to be harvested in the groin area. However, anaphylactic reactions to Patent Blue are possible although rare and must be taken into account [39].

Intraoperative indocyanine green lymphography has become more popular to detect lymph nodes to be harvested within the lymph node flap. Indocyanine green fluorescence is injected intradermally to lower abdominal areas. By illuminating the lymph node area with near-infrared light the lymph nodes draining from the injection site, i.e., the nodes meant to be harvested are visualized.

Reverse lymphatic mapping is another useful method of identifying the nodes of interest. Technetium99 is injected to ipsilateral foot or hand and by gamma probe the lymph node draining lower or upper extremity, respectively, are identified and avoided. All these abovementioned methods can be useful when starting lymph node transfer practice but they are neither substitutes for meticulous surgery nor absolute necessities.

Patient Outcomes

There is paucity of studies on long-term results from VLNT to proximal extremity of lymphedema patients. In addition to that, the methods of evaluating the results vary among authors, which makes it difficult to compare different studies. Becker et al. reported VLNT to 24 patients having postmastectomy lymphedema and they found upper limb perimeter returning to normal in 10 out of those 24 patients, decreasing in 12 and remaining unchanged in 2. In 31 % of the cases the postoperative lymphoscintigraphy showed activity in transplanted lymph nodes. Physiotherapy was discontinued in 15 patients (62 %) during 1-year follow up. The most remarkable was the effect on infectious episodes: 17 patients did not experience any lymphedema related infections and among the remaining 7 patients only one infectious episode for each patient was reported during the follow-up period of 5–11 years [10].

Dr. Becker's personal experience of 1,500 patients over a period of 20 years stated that 98 % of the patients with stage 1–3 (ISL staging) had some degree of improvement during minimum of 3-year follow-up [16]. Becker et al. discovered that VLNT is effective in postmastectomy neuropathic pain. Six patients with chronic regional neuropathic pain and upper limb lymphedema after breast surgery underwent VLNT from inguinal area to axilla. Lymphedema was resolved in five out of six patients, and neuropathic pain disappeared in all patients [18].

In our own previously published patient material (including 19 patients), one third of the lymph node transfer patients showed improvement of the lymphatic flow function in postoperative lymphoscintigraphy [13, 17]. In most patients the lymph node transfer was combined with breast reconstruction [13]. Half of the patients seem to show some reduction in arm circumferences after the lymph node transfer surgery [17]. However, the amount of edema varies during the day and it is dependent on temperature, amount of physical work, the quality of the compression garment used on the day of the examination, and several other factors. Most of the erysipelas patients (6/7) have not had upper limb infections during 15–67 months follow-up and all patients with neuropathic pain reported significant relieve of pain postoperatively (5/5).

Vignes et al. used a volumetric calculation measuring the effect of VLNT in 26 patients of whom 14 were operated for upper limb and 12 for lower limb lymphedema. They found no statistically significant difference between preoperatively and postoperative lymphedema volumes [35].

Dancey et al. studied the effect of VLNT in continuity with a DIEP flap in 18 patients by a quality of life measure for limb lymphedema (LYMQOL). According to their study, the patients experienced significant improvement in appearance, function, symptoms, and mood, and the quality of life significantly increased postoperatively [33].

More specific and objective outcome measures are needed to evaluate the true benefit of VLNT. In a compliant patient wearing pressure garment preoperatively the volume decrease postoperatively may not be striking and cannot be guaranteed. Despite this, the patient may have improvement in quality of life, for example being able to leave out daily use of pressure garment.

Conclusion

Autologous microsurgical lymph node transfer in human patients was first introduced by Dr. Corinne Becker in 2006 [10]. To date, there have been seven published studies with a total of 82 patients reporting the outcomes of lymph node transfer into the axilla [10, 13, 17, 18, 33, 35, 36]. These preliminary results suggest that lymph node transfer may be beneficial for lymphedema patients. Especially patients with recurrent erysipelas infections or neuropathic pain of the arm seem to benefit from the lymph node transfer. However, larger randomized studies are needed to clarify the therapeutical effect of lymph node transfer. To date, it is still considered as experimental surgery and the patient should be informed that complete cure cannot be promised. In addition, all lymph node transfer patients need to be followed in order to detect any clinical symptoms in the donor lower limb, and it is of utmost important to emphasize to the patients that there might be a risk of donor-area swelling.

References

1. Suami H, Chang DW. Overview of surgical treatments for breast cancer-related lymphedema. Plast Reconstr Surg. 2010;126:1853–63.
2. Warren AG, Brorson H, Borud LJ, Slavin SA. Lymphedema: a comprehensive review. Ann Plast Surg. 2007;59:464–72.
3. DiSipio T, Rye S, Newman B, Hayes S. Incidence of unilateral arm lymphoedema after breast cancer: a systematic review and meta-analysis. Lancet Oncol. 2013;14:500–15.
4. de Vries M, Vonkeman WG, van Ginkel RJ, Hoekstra HJ. Morbidity after inguinal sentinel lymph node biopsy and completion lymph node dissection in

patients with cutaneous melanoma. Eur J Surg Oncol. 2006;32:785–9.

5. Karakousis CP, Driscoll DL, Rose B, Walsh DL. Groin dissection in malignant melanoma. Ann Surg Oncol. 1994;1:271–7.

6. Baas PC, Schraffordt Koops H, Hoekstra HJ, van Bruggen JJ, van der Weele LT, Oldhoff J. Groin dissection in the treatment of lower-extremity melanoma. Short-term and long-term morbidity. Arch Surg. 1992;127:281–6.

7. Shesol BF, Nakashima R, Alavi A, Hamilton RW. Successful lymph node transplantation in rats, with restoration of lymphatic function. Plast Reconstr Surg. 1979;63:817–23.

8. Becker C, Hidden G. Transfer of free lymphatic flaps. Microsurgery and anatomical study. J Mal Vasc. 1988;13:119–22.

9. Chen HC, O'Brien BM, Rogers IW, Pribaz JJ, Eaton CJ. Lymph node transfer for the treatment of obstructive lymphoedema in the canine model. Br J Plast Surg. 1990;43:578–86.

10. Becker C, Assouad J, Riquet M, Hidden G. Postmastectomy lymphedema: long-term results following microsurgical lymph node transplantation. Ann Surg. 2006;243:313–5.

11. Yan A, Avraham T, Zampell JC, Aschen SZ, Mehrara BJ. Mechanisms of lymphatic regeneration after tissue transfer. PLoS One. 2011;6:e17201.

12. Aschen SZ, Farias-Eisner G, Cuzzone DA, et al. Lymph node transplantation results in spontaneous lymphatic reconnection and restoration of lymphatic flow. Plast Reconstr Surg. 2014;133:301–10.

13. Saaristo AM, Niemi TS, Viitanen TP, Tervala TV, Hartiala P, Suominen EA. Microvascular breast reconstruction and lymph node transfer for postmastectomy lymphedema patients. Ann Surg. 2012;255:468–73.

14. Cheng MH, Huang JJ, Wu CW, et al. The mechanism of vascularized lymph node transfer for lymphedema: natural lymphaticovenous drainage. Plast Reconstr Surg. 2014;133:192e–8.

15. Cheng MH, Chen SC, Henry SL, Tan BK, Lin MC, Huang JJ. Vascularized groin lymph node flap transfer for postmastectomy upper limb lymphedema: flap anatomy, recipient sites, and outcomes. Plast Reconstr Surg. 2013;131:1286–98.

16. Becker C, Vasile JV, Levine JL, et al. Microlymphatic surgery for the treatment of iatrogenic lymphedema. Clin Plast Surg. 2012;39:385–98.

17. Viitanen TP, Visuri MT, Hartiala P, et al. Lymphatic vessel function and lymphatic growth factor secretion after microvascular lymph node transfer in lymphedema patients. Plast Reconstr Surg Glob Open. 2013;1:1–9.

18. Becker C, Pham DN, Assouad J, Badia A, Foucault C, Riquet M. Postmastectomy neuropathic pain: results of microsurgical lymph nodes transplantation. Breast. 2008;17:472–6.

19. Becker C, Arrive L, Saaristo A, et al. Surgical treatment of congenital lymphedema. Clin Plast Surg. 2012;39:377–84.

20. Sapountzis S, Ciudad P, Lim SY, et al. Modified Charles procedure and lymph node flap transfer for advanced lower extremity lymphedema. Microsurgery. 2014;34:439.

21. Dayan JH, Dayan E, Kagen A, et al. The use of magnetic resonance angiography in vascularized groin lymph node transfer: an anatomic study. J Reconstr Microsurg. 2014;30:41–5.

22. Lin CH, Ali R, Chen SC, et al. Vascularized groin lymph node transfer using the wrist as a recipient site for management of postmastectomy upper extremity lymphedema. Plast Reconstr Surg. 2009;123:1265–75.

23. Viitanen TP, Maki MT, Seppanen MP, Suominen EA, Saaristo AM. Donor-site lymphatic function after microvascular lymph node transfer. Plast Reconstr Surg. 2012;130:1246–53.

24. van der Ploeg IM, Kroon BB, Valdes Olmos RA, Nieweg OE. Evaluation of lymphatic drainage patterns to the groin and implications for the extent of groin dissection in melanoma patients. Ann Surg Oncol. 2009;16:2994–9.

25. Tourani SS, Taylor GI, Ashton MW. Anatomy of the superficial lymphatics of the abdominal wall and the upper thigh and its implications in lymphatic microsurgery. J Plast Reconstr Aesthet Surg. 2013;66:1390–5.

26. Gharb BB, Rampazzo A, Spanio di Spilimbergo S, Xu ES, Chung KP, Chen HC. Vascularized lymph node transfer based on the hilar perforators improves the outcome in upper limb lymphedema. Ann Plast Surg. 2011;67:589–93.

27. Suami H, O'Neill JK, Pan WR, Taylor GI. Superficial lymphatic system of the upper torso: preliminary radiographic results in human cadavers. Plast Reconstr Surg. 2008;121:1231–9.

28. Barreiro GC, Baptista RR, Kasai KE, et al. Lymph fasciocutaneous lateral thoracic artery flap: anatomical study and clinical use. J Reconstr Microsurg. 2014;30:389–96.

29. Althubaiti GA, Crosby MA, Chang DW. Vascularized supraclavicular lymph node transfer for lower extremity lymphedema treatment. Plast Reconstr Surg. 2013;131:133e–5.

30. Sapountzis S, Singhal D, Rashid A, Ciudad P, Meo D, Chen HC. Lymph node flap based on the right transverse cervical artery as a donor site for lymph node transfer. Ann Plast Surg. 2014;73:398.

31. Cheng MH, Huang JJ, Nguyen DH, et al. A novel approach to the treatment of lower extremity lymphedema by transferring a vascularized submental lymph node flap to the ankle. Gynecol Oncol. 2012;126:93–8.

32. Raju A, Chang DW. Vascularized lymph node transfer for treatment of lymphedema: a comprehensive literature review. Ann Surg. 2014, Jun 19.

33. Dancey A, Nassimizadeh A, Nassimizadeh M, Warner RM, Waters R. A chimeric vascularised groin lymph node flap and DIEP flap for the management of lymphoedema secondary to breast cancer. J Plast Reconstr Aesthet Surg. 2013;66:735–7.

34. Tammela T, Saaristo A, Holopainen T, et al. Therapeutic differentiation and maturation of lymphatic vessels after lymph node dissection and transplantation. Nat Med. 2007;13:1458–66.

35. Vignes S, Blanchard M, Yannoutsos A, Arrault M. Complications of autologous lymph-node transplantation for limb lymphoedema. Eur J Vasc Endovasc Surg. 2013;45:516–20.

36. Pons G, Masia J, Loschi P, Nardulli ML, Duch J. A case of donor-site lymphoedema after lymph node-superficial circumflex iliac artery perforator flap transfer. J Plast Reconstr Aesthet Surg. 2014;67:119–23.

37. Azuma S, Yamamoto T, Koshima I. Donor-site lymphatic function after microvascular lymph node transfer should be followed using indocyanine green lymphography. Plast Reconstr Surg. 2013;131:443e–4.

38. Yamamoto T, Matsuda N, Doi K, et al. The earliest finding of indocyanine green lymphography in asymptomatic limbs of lower extremity lymphedema patients secondary to cancer treatment: the modified dermal backflow stage and concept of subclinical lymphedema. Plast Reconstr Surg. 2011;128:314e–21.

39. Bezu C, Coutant C, Salengro A, Darai E, Rouzier R, Uzan S. Anaphylactic response to blue dye during sentinel lymph node biopsy. Surg Oncol. 2011;20:e55–9.

Lymph Node Transfer to Distal Extremity

Jung-Ju Huang

Key Points

- Selection of appropriate flap with sizable lymph nodes and better donor vessels based on preoperative evaluation.
- Recipient vessels preparation requires complete resection of the surrounding fibrotic tissue to prevent complications.
- A tension-free wound closure.
- Transfer the flap to distal extremity, especially when the edema is more severe in the distal limb.

Introduction

With earlier cancer detection and multi-modality cancer treatment, the prognosis of cancer is improving. On the other hand, complications from cancer treatment present and are becoming a daily inconvenience after free from disease. Lymphedema, either primary or secondary from cancer surgery, causes pain, recurrent infection, and cosmetic problems. Conservative treatments, static compression, intermittent pneumatic compression, and multilayer lymphedema banding, cannot provide constant results, especially in advanced stage. Debulking surgeries, including suction-assisted lipectomy and excision, can only be applied in patients with earlier stage lymphedema. Lymphaticovenous anastomosis and vascularized lymph node transfers have been introduced for patients with advanced lymphedema with better results. The lymphaticovenous anastomosis is technically demanding and the anastomosis becomes occluded with time. Vascularized lymph node transfer becomes the one with the most constant results for advanced stage lymphedema.

There remains controversy regarding recipient site selection for transferring a vascularized lymph node flap to treat lymphedema. In earlier literatures, most of the lymph flaps were transferred to post-mastectomy upper extremity and surgeons put the flaps in the axillary area [1]. This is considered especially important when the lymph node transfer is done together with autologous breast reconstruction [2]. However, Cheng compared different recipient sites for flap transfer and associated the most distal recipient sites with better results [3]. Since the authors prefer to transfer the vascularized lymph node flap to the distal end of the affected limb, the wrist and the ankle are the preferred recipient sites for vascularized lymph node flap transfer for upper and lower extremity lymphedema, respectively.

In an earlier publication by Becker, groin lymph node flap was transferred to the axilla for lymphedema post mastectomy. Although 42 % of the cases return to normal status and 50 % presented with improvement in Becker's series,

J.-J. Huang, M.D. (✉)
Chang Gung Memorial Hospital,
No 5 Fu-Shing St. Kweishan, Taoyuan,
Taiwan (R. O. C.)
e-mail: jungjuhuang@gmail.com

A.K. Greene et al. (eds.), *Lymphedema: Presentation, Diagnosis, and Treatment*,
DOI 10.1007/978-3-319-14493-1_25, © Springer International Publishing Switzerland 2015

continuous postoperative compression is required [4]. The axilla was also used as recipient site for simultaneous breast reconstruction and lymph node flap transfer for postmastectomy breast reconstruction and lymphedema management. Putting the flap in axilla for upper extremity lymphoma generally provides better cosmesis of the flap. However, Cheng demonstrated a better overall outcome with putting the flap in more distal, dependent site of the edematous extremity [3, 5].

Mechanism of Vascularized Lymph Node Transfer

For more advanced-staged lymphedema, vascularized lymph node transfer has been proved to be effective in terms of reducing the limb circumference and reducing infection episodes. However, the exact mechanism was rarely addressed. Cheng and colleagues did a mechanism study using both animal model and clinical cases. ICG (indocyanine green dye), which binds to large plasma proteins and emits fluorescence that could be detected, was used in their study with a near-infrared source [6]. Both lymph node carrying and non-lymph node carrying flaps were evaluated. In an animal study, the ICG was injected subcutaneously in both lymph node-carrying flaps and non-lymph node carrying flaps. Direct lymph node injection was also performed in some of the lymph-node carrying flaps. In lymph node flaps, the dye drained into the pedicle vein 153 ± 129 s. The drainage time shortened to 12.8 ± 8.1 s if the ICG was injected directly into the lymph node. Contrast to lymph node flaps, the fluorescent dye did not drain into the pedicle vein in non-lymph node carrying flaps. Similar findings were found in clinical cases. Since the ICG could be detected in the pedicle vein of the lymph node-carrying flaps with either subcutaneous injection or direct injection into the lymph nodes, they proved the existence of the natural lymphaticovenous connection and the "pumping" effect of vascularized lymph node on draining the lymphatic fluid into the vein after vascularized lymph node flap transfer. Besides, spontaneous lymphatic reconnection and restoration of lymphatic flow have been noticed by Aschen and colleagues [7] after lymph node transfer, which helps the "catchment" and "pumping" mechanism of the flap with drainage of the lymphatic fluid back into venous system.

Preoperative Evaluation

Since the vascularized lymph node transfer is a microsurgery with a long operation time, the patient's medical history should be carefully reviewed before surgery. Patients with many medical diseases are not encouraged to receive the surgery for surgical and anesthesia risks. Based on the proposed mechanism of lymphatic drainage by the venous system, patients who have unhealthy, obstructed recipient superficial vein or congestive heart disease that limits venous return are not good candidates for vascularized lymph node transfer.

Before surgery, evaluation of the potential donor site and recipient vessels is equally important. The authors prefer a preoperative lymphoscintigraphy to document the presentation of lymphedema before proceeding to more aggressive surgical treatment for lymphedema [8].

Preoperative Duplex Ultrasonography is used for preoperative lymph node mapping and evaluation of both the donor and recipient vessels. The author prefers to choose vascularized submental lymph node flap for lower extremity lymphedema and either vascularized submental lymph node flap or groin flap for upper extremity lymphedema based on preoperative Duplex Ultrasonography evaluation. Both sides of the flaps are evaluated before surgery. Flaps with more sizable lymph nodes (greater than 5 mm in diameter) and larger caliber of the donor vessels are preferred. Potential recipient artery and vein are both are preferred surgery as well. Both the upper and lower extremity presents with two main potential recipient arteries: the radial and ulnar arteries in upper and dorsalis pedis artery and posterior tibial artery in lower extremities. The patency, flow, and size of the recipient arteries should be carefully evaluated. Beside, venous insufficiency is not uncommon, especially in lower extremity lymphedema. Many of the patients receive stent implantation in the venous system before they visit for vascularized lymph node transfer. The patency and adequate venous flow should be confirmed before surgery.

Duplex Ultrasonography is an easily performed yet experience-dependent diagnostic tool. Recently, Dayan and colleagues used MRA to evaluate the donor site for groin lymph node flap transfer and found MRA an accurate diagnostic tool for identifying the lymph nodes [9]. Furthermore, reconstruction of MRA can potentially give a vascular map regarding the relationship between the lymph nodes and donor vessels.

Flap Selection

First introduced by Oberline and Chen in a canine model, vascularized groin lymph node transfer was proved to be effective for drainage of lymphatic fluid from the edematous extremities in canines with effective reduction of limb circumference [10]. Groin lymph node was also the very first one that was used in human. After being used for a long period of time, flaps other than groin lymph nodes with different vascular pedicles, such as the submental flap, TCA flap, and lateral thoracic flaps, were introduced with a better hidden donor site scar and explored for different possibilities of using vascularized lymph node flaps for treatment of lymphedema in different locations [11–14]. Table 25.1 gives a comparison of lymph node transfer flaps.

Vascularized Groin Lymph Node Flap

Through an anatomical study by Cheng et al. involving ten groin dissections in five cadaveric studies, vascularized groin lymph node flap can be transferred basing on superficial circumflex iliac artery or a medial branch from the femoral artery [3]. There are two groups of lymph nodes that could be transferred, including the superficial row and the medial column, basing on either the superficial circumflex iliac artery or the medial branch of the femoral artery. In average, a total of 6.2 ± 1.3 lymph nodes could be identified in the groin area with 3.4 ± 0.3 nodes in the superior row and 2.8 ± 1.5 in the medial column. The length and diameter of the arteries were 2.5 cm and 1.5 mm in the superficial iliac artery and the medial branch of the femoral artery.

Before preoperative marking, the selection between the superior row and the medial column of the lymph nodes can be based on preoperative Doppler study as well as the Doppler signal of the artery. However, the medial artery is preferred due to better perfusion from it to the skin flap. The dissection can be started with a lateral incision and the dissection can be made all the way down to the Sartorius fascia. The flap can be elevated once the pedicle has been found. It is not necessary to identify the lymph nodes.

Table 25.1 Comparison of lymph node transfer flaps

	Pedicle	Pedicle size	Pedicle length	Flap thickness	Dissection difficulty	Advantage	Disadvantage
VGLN	Superficial circumflex iliac artery or medial branch from superficial femoral artery	++++	++	+	++++	Hidden scar	Donor site lymphedema
VSLN	Submental artery	+++	+++	+++	++	Hidden scar, thin flap	Dissection difficulty
TCALN	Transverse cervical artery	+++	++++	++++	+++	Thin flap, less donor site morbidity	Obvious scar
LTALN	Lateral thoracic artery	++++	++++	++	+++	Hidden scar	Potential upper extremity lymphedema

VGLN vascularized groin lymph node, *VSLN* vascularized submental lymph node, *TCALN* transverse cervical artery lymph node, *LTALN* lateral thoracic artery lymph node
++++ excellent, +++ good, ++ fair, + poor

Vascularized Submental Lymph Node Flap

Trying to explore more donor vascularized lymph node flap, Cheng and colleagues did a cadaveric anatomical study to confirm the presentation of lymph nodes inside the flap and applied the vascularized submental lymph node flap for treatment of lower extremity lymphedema after uterine cancer staging with pelvis lymph node dissection [13]. The VSLN flap is nourished by submental artery, which arises from the facial artery. After branching from the facial artery, the submental artery passes through the submandibular gland and runs medially across the mylohyoid muscle. After the mylohyoid muscle, it goes either superficial or deep to the digastric muscle and gives 1–4 skin perforators through the platysma muscle to the overlying skin. From a cadaveric study, an average of 3.3 ± 1.5 lymph nodes can be identified in the flap. Including the facial artery, the pedicle length is as long as 6 cm, which is more than adequate for safe flap transfer and anastomosis.

Before surgery, the facial artery can be palpated along the mandible angle and should be marked. An elliptical skin paddle of about 4×9 cm can be designed in the submental area. Incision is first made along the mandible margin. The distal facial artery and vein around the mandible angle should be first explored and marked. The marginal mandibular nerve, which is usually close to the distal facial artery and vein, is then identified and carefully preserved. The flap is then dissected with inclusion of the subcutaneous tissue as much as possible. In order to preserve the skin perforators, the anterior belly of the digastric muscle can be included in the flap. After the submental artery and vein are identified, the flap can be elevated. It is recommended to preserve the soft tissue around the junction of the facial artery and submental artery as much as possible to include the lymph nodes as many as possible.

Transverse Cervical Artery Lymph Node Flap

Transverse cervical artery based lymph node flap was applied for lymphedema surgery by Chang and Chen [12, 15]. Located on the lower neck, transverse cervical artery based lymph node flap has the advantages of being soft, easy to be dissected, thin with better recipient site cosmesis. However, compared to the submental lymph node flap, the donor site scar is relatively more obvious and the width of the flap taken is limited for primary donor site wound closure. In rat model, six lymph nodes could be identified over the transverse cervical artery nourished area. However, there is no large series study using TCA flap for surgical treatment of lymphedema so far.

Lymph Fasciocutaneous Lateral Thoracic Artery Flap

Lateral thoracic area is a donor site rich in donor arteries and has been used as a flap donor site since 1970s. It contains the skin between the anterior and posterior axillary line. The cutaneous pedicle was from thoracodorsal pedicle or lateral thoracic artery. Due to the anatomical variation, the lateral thoracic flap was not popular. However, in recent years, due to the high interest on lymph nodes, surgeons started exploring more donor sites that could provide vascular lymph nodes for transferring without affecting the donor site, and the lateral thoracic area has been considered a good one because the axillary lymph nodes are actually separated into two groups, draining the upper extremity and thorax. The group of lymph nodes draining the thorax is considered a good donor site for vascular lymph nodes without causing lymphedema on the upper extremity.

According to an anatomical study by Barreiro, the lateral thoracic artery arises from the axillary and takes a straight course deep in the subcutaneous tissue between the anterior axillary line and mid-axillary line. It takes about 2.7 cm from its origin to reach lymph nodes nourished by it. There is usually one vein accompanying the artery, and the average size of the artery and vein is 1.3 mm and 2.6 mm, respectively. The lateral thoracic artery contains 3–7 lymph nodes along its course and a skin flap of about 7×14 cm nourished by it.

Recipient Site Selection and Preparation

Preparation of the recipient sites starts with incision of the selected recipient site. Before approaching the recipient vessels, there are usually a lot of fibrotic tissues around and it is recommended to remove part of the fibrotic tissues and create a pocket that is large enough for flap inset. After flap transfer, the lymph node flap will start to suck the lymphatic fluid immediately and soon become swollen. A tight pocket will result in larger tension and compress the vascular pedicle, which further compromises flap perfusion and causes functional loss on the flap.

The recipient artery and vein are selected based on preoperative study. Once the recipient artery and vein are identified, they are commonly found embedded with fibrotic tissue. The fibrotic tissue should be removed as much as possible as these fibrotic bands may limit the flow and result in poor postoperative outcome.

Upper Extremity

Based on preoperative evaluation and patient's preference, the wrist or the elbow is selected as the recipient site for flap transfer. The author prefers a distal recipient site, namely, the wrist; however, if cosmetic appearance concerns the patient and he/she has relatively mild swelling on the forearm, the flap can be transferred to the elbow, instead.

An S-shaped incision is made along the medial border of the elbow below the elbow joint when the elbow is selected as the recipient site. When approaching the subcutaneous tissue there are usually venous branches from the basilica vein that could be used as a recipient vein. A subcutaneous pocket should be created for flap inset, and part of the dense fibrotic tissue should be removed. The anterior recurrent ulnar artery, which locates between the muscles flexor digitorum superficialis and flexor carpi ulnaris, is used as a recipient artery. Because of the long-term subcutaneous inflammation resulting from lymphedema, there is usually a dense fibrotic tissue around the recipient artery. The fibrotic tissue

should be removed as much as possible. Besides, the arterial flow is commonly restricted by the inflamed tissue. Ensuring good spurting from the artery is important before dividing the flap pedicle and getting ready for flap transfer.

If the wrist is used as the recipient site for vascularized lymph node flap transfer, the dorsal branch of the radial artery is the most commonly used recipient artery. An S-shaped incision is made along the dorsal wrist crease and dissection on the subcutaneous plane to create a subcutaneous pocket for flap inset is performed. The cephalic vein locates just above the fascia layer and can be dissected out to be a recipient vein. The dorsal branch of the radial artery locates in the snuffbox. It is under the extensor pollicis longus tendon and the abductor pollicis longus tendon. The artery is dissected and transposed above the tendon to prevent it from being compressed by the tendon and compromise the flap perfusion. Again, strong spurting from the artery should be confirmed before the flap transfer.

Lower Extremity

Based on preoperative study, either the dorsalis pedis artery or the posterior tibial artery is selected as the recipient artery, and the great saphenous vein or the concomitant vein along the recipient artery is selected as the recipient vein.

An S-shaped incision is made along the anterior-medial surface of the ankle. Again, the skin flap is elevated and part of the subcutaneous tissue is removed for two purposes. Removing the subcutaneous tissue can create a space for transferring the flap. It also allows for a tension-free wound closure without compression on the flap by the dense fibrotic tissue. Any sizable subcutaneous vein should be carefully preserved until a healthy recipient vein is identified.

The great saphenous vein can be identified at the level just above the fascia. There is usually a dense fibrotic tissue around the vein and the advantita is usually becoming very thick because of prolonged inflammation. All the fibrotic band or dense advantita should be removed to prevent any tethering on the vein that may compromise the venous flow.

The dorsalis pedis artery or the posterior tibial artery can be used as a recipient artery. The dorsalis pedis artery runs under the extensor retinaculum and between the extensor digitorum longus and extensor halluces longus tendons. Exploration of the dorsalis pedis artery starts with palpation of the artery and opening the retinaculum. However, due to the long-term lymphedema and its subsequent fibrosis, the dorsalis pedis artery is sometimes hard to be detected. The retinaculum should be opened and partially removed to reduce postoperative compression on the artery. After identification of the artery between the EDL and EHL, the artery is then brought to surface for anastomosis.

The posterior tibial artery can be felt posterior to the medial malleolar. Again, due to the long-term fibrotic change of the subcutaneous tissue, the palpation can be difficult. It runs between the flexor digitorum longus and flexor halluces longus tendons. There are two concomitant veins and posterior tibial nerve running along the artery and should be carefully identified and preserved. The veins can also be used as recipient veins if indicated. By opening the overlying fascia, the artery can be identified. The artery is usually embedded under fibrotic tissue, and all the fibrotic tissue should be removed. The fascia should be totally opened for well exposure of the artery for anastomosis.

Flap Inset and Microvascular Anastomosis

The flap is transferred to the recipient site with three or four temporary sutures. It is recommended to do the arterial anastomosis first. If the posterior tibial artery, the ulnar artery, or the radial artery is used as the recipient artery, the author suggests doing the arterial anastomosis in an end-to-side manner to preserve some of the perfusion to the distal limb since the limb is already in relatively ischemic status due to the lymphedema. After confirmation with good venous backflow, the venous anastomosis can be done. The flap inset can be finished after the microvascular anastomosis. During wound closure, it is very important to achieve a tension-free closure since the whole tissue will be swollen the second day after surgery. If there is any subcutaneous tissue exposure after wound closure, it is recommended to cover it with skin graft since exposure of the soft tissue increases postoperative infection rate.

Postoperative Care

The patient is kept in micro ICU (intensive care unit) for 1 week. During their stay in ICU, the flap is monitored every 2 h. The color, temperature, capillary refilling, and puncture bleeding are carefully evaluated. The perforated artery and vein are monitored by a handheld Doppler. Anticoagulative agents such as heparin are not routinely used unless the patient shows high tendency of clot formation during surgery. The patient is kept in bed for 1 week and then allowed for ambulation slowly.

Due to the high infection rate of lymph-containing flaps, parenteral prophylactic antibiotics are given for 1 week and then oral antibiotics for another 1 week.

Donor Site Morbidities

The major concern in raising vascularized lymph node flap is the cause of donor site lymphedema. There are very few literatures discussing about the detailed postoperative change after harvesting lymph node flap. Pons reported one case with donor site swelling after superficial groin lymph node transfer in a series of 42 cases [16]. Two cases of donor site chronic swelling were identified in Vignes's experiences out of 26 cases. By doing postoperative lymphoscintigraphy in patients receiving simultaneous abdominal flap breast reconstruction and lymph node transfer, Viitanen reported no cases with symptomatic lymphedema on the donor site after surgery but found two out of the ten donor sites with slightly abnormal fining on the study [17]. Azuma commented on the possibility of subclinical lymphedema and suggested the use of ICG study to show a more real-time, higher sensitivity lymphatic function [18]. Besides diagnostic tools, a more careful donor site selection and accurate flap dissection are required to reduce donor site lymphedema.

The groin area has superficial and deep lymph nodes. Superficial lymph nodes drain lymphatic fluid from the abdominal wall. The use of only superficial lymph nodes with meticulous flap dissection prevents damage to the underlying lymphatic tissues and thus prevents donor site lymphedema. During dissection of submental lymph node flap, the dissection of distal facial artery and vein is inevitable. The marginal mandibular nerve branch runs very close to the distal facial artery and vein and should be carefully identified and preserved. The use of microscope during preservation of the nerve is sometimes required.

Outcome and Conclusion

The axilla was the first recipient site for vascularized lymph node transfer in order to treat postmastectomy upper extremity lymphedema. Due to the uncertain result, Lin and Cheng started to transfer groin lymph node to the distal extremity for upper extremity lymphedema, namely, the wrist. With the preliminary report of 13 cases with a follow-up time of 56.31 ± 27.12 months, the reduction of arm circumference was 50.5 ± 19.26 % [5]. The incidence of postoperative infection also reduced a lot. In advance, Cheng compared different recipient sites for vascularized groin lymph node transfer for upper extremity lymphedema [3]. Either wrist or the elbow was used as the recipient site. Both groups show similar reduction of arm circumference on the upper arm. However, the reduction rate of arm circumference on forearm is significantly higher in the group using the wrist as the recipient site. The concluded distal recipient site presented with better overall outcome. The use of wrist as recipient site is suggested in patients with lymphedema involving the forearm. The use of elbow is restricted to patients who have a lot of concern regarding cosmesis and present with lymphedema only on the upper arm.

Similarly, the same group used ankle as the recipient site in vascularized submental lymph node flap transfer for lower extremity lymphedema. With a mean follow-up of 8.7 ± 4.2 months, the reduction rate of the leg circumference was 64 ± 11.5 % in the thigh above knee and 63.7 ± 19.2 % in the lower leg below knee [13].

The use of proximal recipient sites requires dissection of the recipient vessels and creating a pocket for lymph node flap around scar area. The previous lymph node dissection and radiotherapy usually cause a lot of scarring and the dissection becomes difficult and the recipient vessels can be damaged during previous surgery. Using a distal recipient site, on the other hand, avoids dissection on the scar area, and the recipient vessels are usually relatively healthier. Besides, considering the "catchment" effect of the vascularized lymph node transfer in lymphedema patients and the natural gravity that brings the fluid distally, a distal recipient site is a better choice for vascularized lymph node flap transfer for treating lymphedema (Figs. 25.1, 25.2, 25.3, 25.4, 25.5, and 25.6).

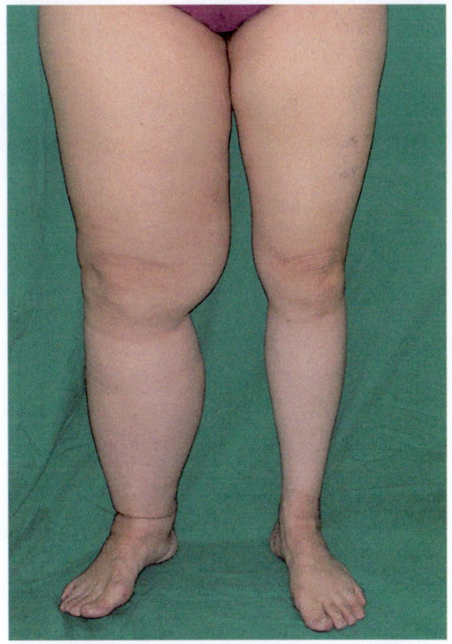

Fig. 25.1 A 58-year-old female patient with a history of cervical cancer postsurgical treatment. She presented with lymphedema on her right lower leg for 16 years. The volume differentiation between bilateral lower extremity was 28.7 % 15 cm above knee, 44.6 % 15 cm below knee, and 69 % 10 cm above ankle

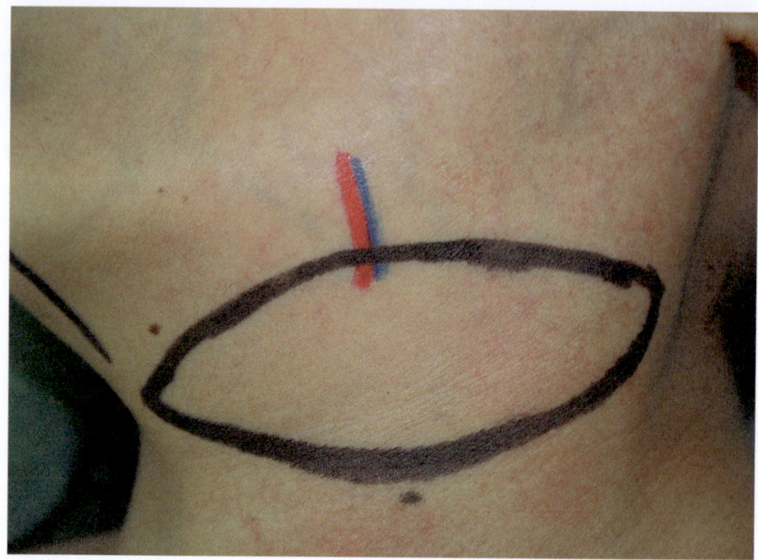

Fig. 25.2 Vascularized submental lymph node flap was designed and harvested from her left submental area with the flap sized 3.5×9 cm

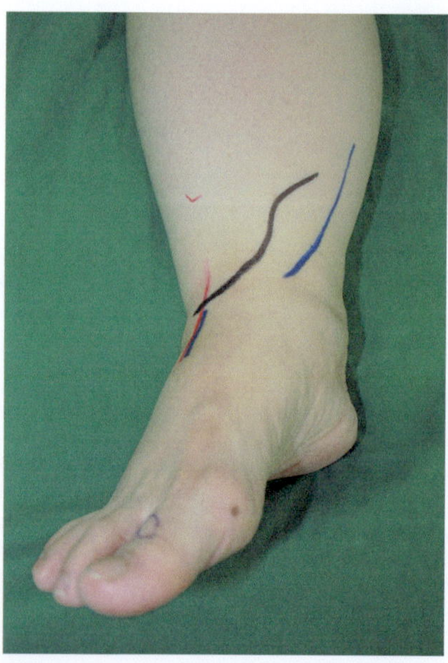

Fig. 25.3 The dorsalis pedis artery and great saphenous vein were selected as the recipient artery and vein, respectively

Fig. 25.4 During flap dissection, the marginal mandibular branch was carefully preserved (looped with white loop)

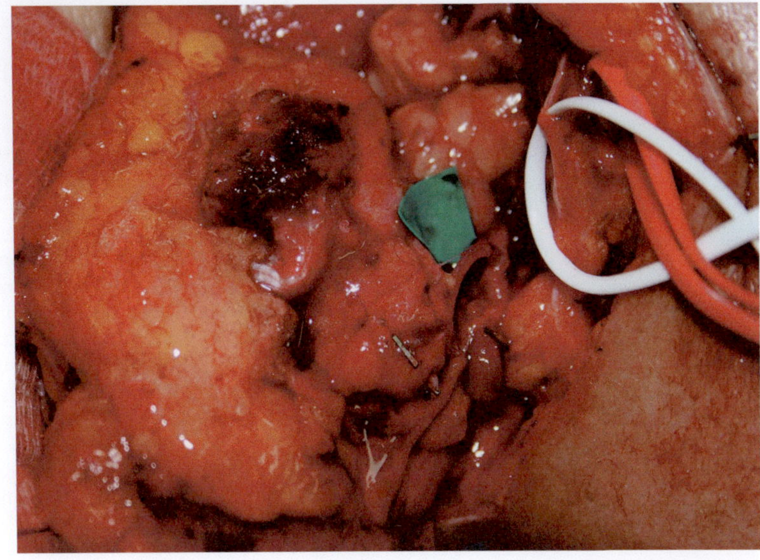

Fig. 25.5 The flap is ready for transfer

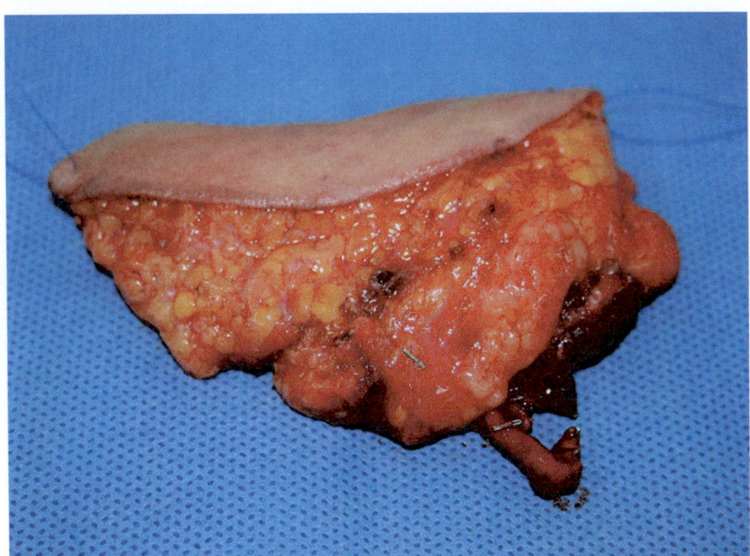

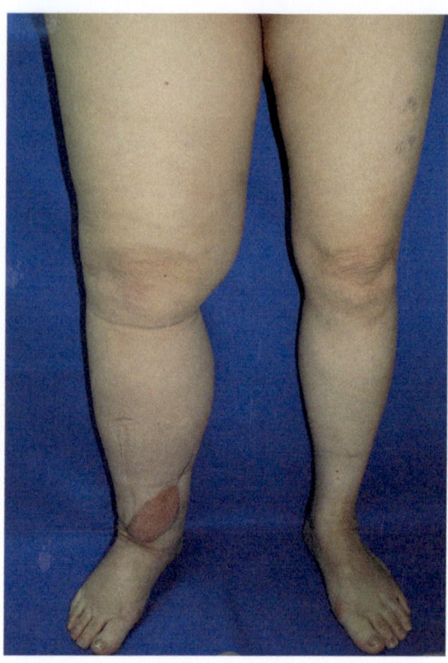

Fig. 25.6 With a follow-up of 14 months, the reduction rate of the limb circumference was 8 % 15 cm above ankle, 41.4 % 15 cm below knee, and 31 % 10 cm above ankle

References

1. Becker C, Hidden G, Godart S, et al. Free lymphatic transfer. Eur J Lymphol Rel Prob. 1991;6:25–77.
2. Saaristo AM, Niemi TS, Viitanen TP, Tervala TV, Hartiala P, Suominen EA. Microvascular breast reconstruction and lymph node transfer for postmastectomy lymphedema patients. Ann Surg. 2012; 255(3):468–73.
3. Cheng MH, Chen SC, Henry SL, Tan BK, Lin MC, Huang JJ. Vascularized groin lymph node flap transfer for postmastectomy upper limb lymphedema: flap anatomy, recipient sites and outcomes. Plast Reconstr Surg. 2013;131(6):1286–98.
4. Becker C, Assouad J, Riquet M, Hidden G. Postmastectomy lymphedema: long-term results following microsurgical lymph node transplantation. Ann Surg. 2006;243(3):313–5.
5. Lin CH, Ali R, Chen SC, Wallace C, Chang YC, Chen HC, et al. Vascularized groin lymph node transfer using the wrist as a recipient site for management of postmastectomy upper extremity lymphedema. Plast Reconstr Surg. 2009;123(4):1265–75.
6. Cheng MH, Huang JJ, Wu CW, Yang CY, Lin CY, Henry SL, et al. The mechanism of vascularized lymph node transfer for lymphedema; natural lymphaticovenous drainage. Plast Reconstr Surg. 2014;133(2):192e–8.
7. Aschen SZ, Farias-Eisner G, Cuzzone DA, Albano NJ, Ghanta S, Weitman ES, et al. Lymph node transplantation results in spontaneous lymphatic reconnection and restoration of lymphatic flow. Plast Reconstr Surg. 2014;133(2):301–10.
8. Patel KM, Chu SY, Huang JJ, Lin CY, Cheng MH. Pre-planning vascularized lymph node transfer with duplex ultrasonography: a prospective evaluation of three common donor sites. Plast Reconstr Surg. 2014;134(4 Suppl 1):32.
9. Dayan JH, Dayan E, Kagen A, Cheng MH, Sultan M, Samson W, et al. The use of magnetic resonance angiography in vascularized groin lymph node transfer: an anatomic study. J Reconstr Microsurg. 2014;30(1):41–5.
10. Chen HC, O'Brien BM, Rogers IW, Pribaz JJ, Eaton CJ. Lymph node transfer for the treatment of obstructive lymphedema in the canine model. Br J Plast Surg. 1990;43(5):578–86.
11. Uygur S, Ozturk C, Bozkurt M, Kwiecien G, Madajka M, Siemionow M. A new vascularized cervical lymph node transplantation model. Ann Plast Surg. 2013;71(6):671–4.
12. Sapountzis S, Singhal D, Rashid A, Ciudad P, Meo D, Chen HC. Lymph node flap based on tight transverse cervical artery as a donor site for lymph node transfer. Ann Plast Surg. 2014;73(4):398–401.
13. Cheng MH, Huang JJ, Nguyen DH, Saint-Cyr M, Zenn MR, Tan BK, et al. A novel approach to the treatment of lower extremity lymphedema by transferring a vascularized submental lymph node flap to the ankle. Gynecol Oncol. 2012;126(1):93–8.
14. Barreiro GC, Baptista RR, Kasai KE, dos Anjos DM, Busnardo Fde F, Modolin M, et al. Lymph fasciocutaneous lateral thoracic artery flap: anatomical study and clinical use. J Reconstr Microsurg. 2014;30(6):389–96.
15. Althubaiti GA, Crosby MA, Chang DW. Vascularized supraclavicular lymph node transfer for lower extremity lymphedema treatment. Plast Reconstr Surg. 2013;131(1):133e–5.
16. Pons G, Masia J, Loschi P, Nardulli ML, Duch J. A case of donor site lymphedema after lymph node superficial circumflex iliac artery perforator flap transfer. J Plast Reconstr Aesthet Surg. 2014;67(1):119–23.
17. Viitanen TP, Mäki MT, Seppänen MP, Suominen EA, Saaristo AM. Donor-site lymphatic function after microvascular lymph node transfer. Plast Reconstr Surg. 2012;130(6):1246–53.
18. Azuma S, Yamamoto T, Koshima I. Donor site lymphatic function after microvascular lymph node transfer should be followed using indocyanine green lymphography. Plast Reconstr Surg. 2013;131(3):443e–4.

Modified Charles' Procedure and Its Combination with Lymph Node Flap Transfer for Advanced Lymphedema

Michele Maruccia, Hung-Chi Chen, and Shih-Heng Chen

Key Points

- Treatment of advanced lymphedema remains a challenge in reconstructive surgery and Charles' procedure is one of the excisional techniques that can be useful in selected cases.
- In the treatment of advanced lymphedema of the lower extremity, the toes are the major determinant of future infection after surgery.
- HCC-modified Charles' procedure consists in the association of the traditional Charles technique with the lymph node flap.
- HCC-modified Charles' procedure seems to be a reliable method for treatment of advanced stage of limb lymphedema.
- HCC-modified Charles' procedure prevents potential complications of the traditional technique such as recurrence, infection, and aggravation of the lymphedema.

Introduction

The Charles' procedure, named for Sir Richard Henry Havelock Charles, is an eponym for a surgical treatment of advanced lymphedema. Sir Havelock Charles was an adventurous man that he

M. Maruccia, M.D.
H.-C. Chen, M.D., Ph.D., F.A.C.S. (✉) • S.-H. Chen
Department of Plastic Surgery,
China Medical University Hospital,
2 Yuh-Der Road, Taichung 40447, Taiwan
e-mail: D19722@mail.cmuh.org.tw;
shihheng@icloud.com

led a fascinating life. He traveled from the wilds of the Afghan territories as chief medical officer in a military mission, to Calcutta as professor of anatomy and surgery where he published a series of 140 consecutive patients treated successfully for scrotal lymphedema [1]. In 1912, he wrote a chapter entitled "Elephantiasis Scroti" that was the source for references made to Charles concerning the treatment of leg lymphedema [2]. For one-half of one page of this 13-page article he described the treatment of leg lymphedema. He wrote that when radical treatment was required, the leg was decorticated down to, but without injury of, the deep fascia. Skin grafting was to be performed at once, covering as large a surface as was deemed possible and arrangement for skin graft to be previously made [1]. This definition of more than 100 years ago is the base for the description of the Charles' procedure and other modified techniques.

In advanced lymphedema the excisional approach has been a reliable treatment strategy that provides satisfactory long-term results. Chronic inflammation and repeated episodes of infection leads to gradual fibrosis of subcutaneous tissue, making lymphatic channels amenable to microsurgical anastomosis due to occlusion. The most important goal of treatment is the control or eradication of infection. In particular, prevention of toe infection has proven to be an important step in controlling infections in general [3].

A variety of excisional procedures have been described for this stage of lymphedema, notably by Charles [1], Sistrunk [4], Macey [5], and

A.K. Greene et al. (eds.), *Lymphedema: Presentation, Diagnosis, and Treatment*,
DOI 10.1007/978-3-319-14493-1_26, © Springer International Publishing Switzerland 2015

Auchincloss [6]. Actually, Charles' procedure is described as a radical circumferential excision of the subcutaneous tissue and part of the fibrotic fascia of the affected limb and resurfacing with split-thickness skin grafts (STSG) [7].

The Charles' procedure has been the only treatment that decreases lymphatic load, whilst aiming to control infection. In patients with primary or secondary advanced lower limb lymphoedema, with induration, fibrosis, brawny leather-like skin, "squared-off" toes, hyperkeratosis and multiple fistulas can be treated most effectively using the Charles' procedure [3]. O'Brien et al. state that in primary and secondary advanced lymphedema, there is no place for microlymphatic surgery, as there are no suitable lymphatics for anastomoses. They also stated that venous hypertension in obstructive lymphoedema is an absolute contraindication to microlymphaticovenous anastomoses because venous hypertension results in blood flow from the vein to the lymphatics (Fig. 26.1) [8].

Campisi et al. described successful outcomes of micro-lymphaticovenous anastomoses (LVA) for moderate-stage lymphedema. However, this procedure is not favored for Campisi stage IV (fibrotic and column-shaped limb) and Campisi stage V (elephantiasis with severe limb deformation, scleroindurative pachidermatitis and widespread lymphstatic verrucosis) advanced lymphoedema. They also support microlymphatic surgery only for the obstructive type of lymphoedema characterized by lymphadenodysplasia, but not for lymphatic-lymphonodal aplasia [9, 10]. On the other hand, Koshima et al. have recommended microsurgical lymphaticovenous anastomoses for primary and secondary lymphoedema, even in advanced stages IV and V. They base this recommendation on the ultrastructural observations of human lymphatics in edematous limbs [11, 12].

We, however, have not been successful in performing lymphaticovenous anastomoses in advanced lymphoedema and we think this is because the lymphatic trunks are neither patent nor functional. Recurrent episodes of infection and cellulitis lead to subcutaneous fibrosis, thereby occluding any remaining functional lymphatic channels. A vicious cycle develops in which the edema worsens, causing further damage to the subcutaneous tissue, rendering it unreliable for LVA. In anaplastic and hypoplastic types of primary lymphoedema, there are only a few or no lymphatics. Microsurgery, therefore, has little role to play in the treatment of these patients. Infection, with recurrent cellulitis and lymphangitis, is an undesirable complication and upgrades the stage of the disease, adding to the patient's frustration and lack of well-being. Control of infection is therefore paramount in advanced disease. The excisional technique of the Charles' procedure can produce good long-term results and is a realistic approach in advanced lymphedema [3, 7].

Recent evidence suggests that the Charles' procedure can result in a 30 % reduction of the circumference, which can be maintained over a 3-year period, resulting in a 90 % reduction in cellulitis [3].

Potential complications of the procedure are wound breakdown, hyperkeratosis, ulceration, and aggravation of foot lymphedema (Fig. 26.2).

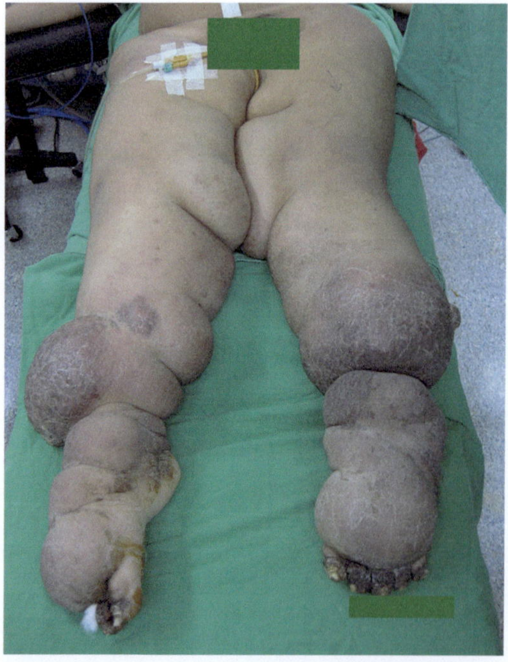

Fig. 26.1 Patients with chronic bilateral advanced lymphedema

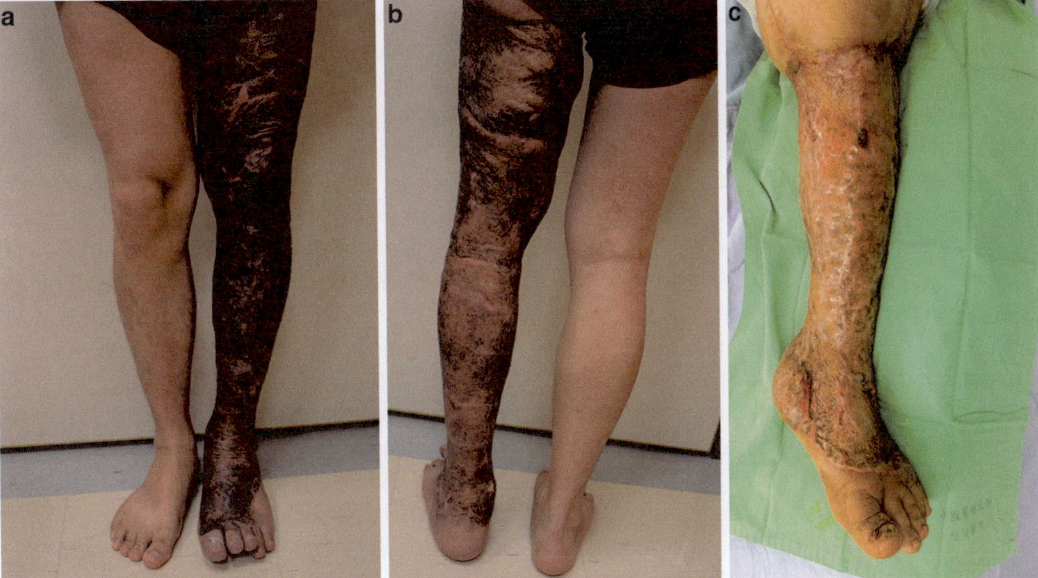

Fig. 26.2 Poor aesthetic result due to hyperpigmentation following the conventional Charles' procedure but with good quality of the skin. (**a**) Anterior view; (**b**) Posterior view; (**c**) Hypertrophic scaring with fibrosis and history of ulcerations

To prevent these problems many authors described a modified Charles' procedure. Van der Walt et al. presented a modified Charles' procedure, applying negative-dressing after the initial debulking surgery and then they delayed the skin grafting by 5–7 days [13].

Hung-Chi Chen (HCC)-modified Charles' procedure combined the excisional procedure with lymph node flap transfer.

Charles' Procedure: Surgical Technique

Preoperative Treatment

One week prior to surgery the patient is encouraged to optimize foot hygiene, have regular baths and bed rest with leg elevation. On hospital admission, a plastic surgery specialist nurse records the circumference of the affected limb. Measurements are taken at four levels: midfoot, ankle (between medial and lateral malleoli), mid-calf (15 cm below knee joint), and mid-thigh (15 cm above knee joint). Routine preoperative investigations are performed and anesthetic consultation undertaken. Antibiotics (usually cephalosporin) are administered 1 h before surgery and continued postoperatively for 3 days.

Operative Technique

Only one limb is operated at a time and the procedure is performed in one stage. The patient is positioned supine and incisions are marked. Proximally at the thigh, a circumferential incision is marked with two wedge incisions at the proximal thigh, one at the medial aspect and the other at the lateral. Excision can be limited to below knee if the thigh is relatively unaffected or on the patient's request. Distally, at the foot and toes, markings are placed at the mid-lateral and medial aspect of the foot, above the heel and at the dorsum of the toes and web spaces, preserving the clefts between the toes. The leg will be circumferentially denuded down to fascia. Split thickness skin grafts are harvested from the entire circumference of the affected limb in a proximal to distal (axial) direction with an air-powered dermatome set at 12/1,000 of an inch. It is imperative that the lengths of the harvested STSG are as long as possible. The STSG can thus be "wrapped" around the limb in a circular fashion, so that the ends meet on the lateral aspect rather than inner aspect of the limb. Consequently, the risk of hypertrophic scar formation on the inner aspect of the limb is minimized. Furthermore, using long strips reduces the number of seams between STSG and risk of excessive hypertrophic scarring. Using long strips of STSG also avoids a patchwork appearance. The harvested STSGs can be fenestrated (but not meshed) for drainage of hematoma if necessary. A pneumatic tourniquet is placed on the proximal thigh and inflated to 375 mmHg following exsanguination. An ordinary pneumatic tourniquet cannot be used when the thigh is so large. Then a rubber tourniquet can be applied at the proximal thigh after exsanguination.

To access the posterior surface of the limb, a 3 mm pin is drilled through the distal tibia and the limb is suspended from a stand. This pin can also help elevate the leg postoperatively and is usually removed 5 days postoperatively at the bedside, before the patient is discharged.

The fibrosclerotic lymphedematous tissue is then separated from the deep fascia using blunt and sharp dissection, removing all of the soft tissue superficial to the deep fascia. The thickened deep fascia is also trimmed to its normal size.

Toes are amputated if there are recurrent infections, verrucous hyperkeratosis, or osteomyelitis, as indicated in HCC-Stage IVB. Otherwise, nails and nail beds are removed, and the defect is closed using C-V/rotation-advancement flaps, to preserve length. The tip of the distal phalanx of the toe can be shortened by 0.5 cm if there is any tension during wound closure.

Once the leg has been denuded, adrenaline soaked gauze and compressive bandaging is applied and the tourniquet is deflated. All tissue excision and control of the major bleeders should be completed within 2 h of tourniquet ischemia time. Therefore, a team of surgeons is necessary.

Whilst waiting for the adrenaline to act, the proximal thigh can be debulked. Two wedge excisions are made starting at the medial and lateral mid-axial lines. The skin is undermined circumferentially and proximally to about 10 cm. The resultant flaps at anterior and posterior thigh are thinned tangentially to 2 cm and sutured together to the deep fascia to allow a smoother transition from the distal grafted thigh to the proximal thigh. Suction drains are left in situ. A full-thickness skin graft is taken from the wedge-excised tissues and used for grafting of the dorsum of the foot. FTSG on the dorsum of the foot results in more resistant skin with less hypertrophic scarring and verrucous hyperkeratosis.

The adrenaline-soaked compressive bandages are then sequentially removed in a proximal to distal direction and meticulous haemostasis is performed. The tourniquet is reinflated and the split thickness skin graft is applied circumferentially with 1 cm edge overlap. This is to prevent gap formation between the STSGs that may arise because of swelling, minimizing hypertrophic scarring. The skin grafts are applied around the ankles and knees in such a way that the seams lie on the lateral aspect of the joints.

Finally, non-adherent dressings, bulky gauze, ACE wrap, and a posterior plaster is applied. The tourniquet is then deflated. Elevation of the limb and thus avoidance of shearing force ensures STSG take on the posterior surface of the leg and thigh (Fig. 26.2).

Postoperative Treatment

During inpatient stay (5–7 days) the patient is strongly encouraged to keep the leg elevated. Deep vein thrombosis prophylaxis is administered postoperatively for Caucasian patients. Due to the low incidence of deep vein thrombosis in the Chinese population, prophylaxis of deep vein thrombosis is not needed for them [14]. Leg elevation is encouraged for the next 2 weeks and compression stocking is worn after 2 weeks. Physiotherapy and long-term limb compression are commenced subsequently (Fig. 26.3).

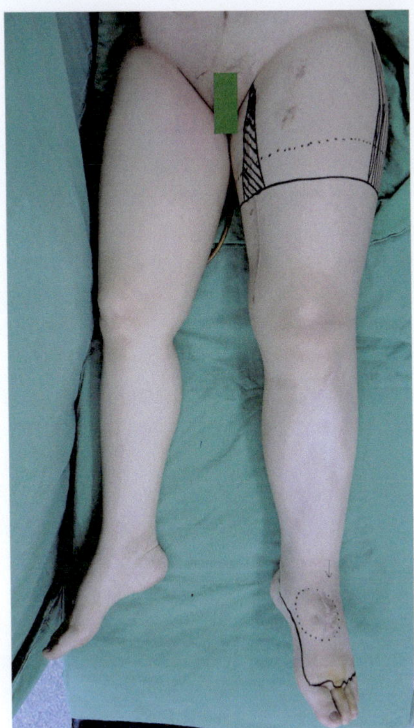

Fig. 26.3 Markings

Preservation or Amputation of Toes in Advanced Lymphedema

In advanced lymphedema, the most important goal of treatment is control or eradication of infection. The repeated episodes of infection and cellulites lead to chronic inflammation and fibrosis, resulting in occlusion of the lymphatic channels, which therefore are not amenable to any microsurgical anastomosis [3].

Toes are the major source of infection, especially in older patients [15]. Toe crowding, nail infections, skin changes such as verrucous hyperkeratosis and poor hygiene can all contribute to infection of the toes, which may ascend to involve the foot or even the proximal leg. If the toes are affected but left untreated, the patient will invariably have recurrent infections and a compromised result. Control of infection is therefore paramount. For preservation of the toes different conditions must be met in advanced stage lymphedema (HCC-Stage IVA).

(a) The toes are swollen, but there is no history of recurrent episodes of cellulitis or appearance of verrucous hyperkeratosis.

(b) The toes are not deformed.

(c) There is no evidence of osteomyelitis of the toes.

The surgical technique to treat the toes includes:

(a) Excision of the soft tissue at the dorsum of the toes with preservation of the extensor tendon and its paratenon, which can support a skin graft take. After surgery, the skin graft at the dorsum of the toes should be compressed to achieve a flat and smooth surface.

(b) The skin flaps in the web spaces should be preserved to avoid contracture at the web spaces with resultant crowding of the toes. This can improve foot hygiene and prevent infection.

(c) Removal of the toe nails and closure using C-V rotation advancement flaps in order to preserve length.

(d) Amputation of toes when there is recurrent infection of the toes, verrucous hyperkeratosis, or osteomyelitis.

If the toes are affected but left untreated, the patient will have recurrent infection after performing Charles' procedure. A recent prospective study showed that only 20 % of patients who underwent Charles' procedure with toe amputation suffered from recurrent infections, compared to 83 % of patients who had Charles' procedure without toes amputation. Moreover, 88 % of the latter group eventually needed toe amputation [3, 16].

Our management algorithm for treating the toes in patients with advanced lymphedema includes:

(a) removal of nail beds (HCC-Stage IVA—with infection of nail)

(b) removal of second and fourth toes (HCC-Stage IVB—with infection of web spaces, who want to preserve some toes)

(c) removal of all toes (HCC-Stage IVB—with infection, who do not want to preserve toes)

In Hung-Chi Chen (HCC) Staging, in stage IVA a fibrovascular proliferation is seen with brawny leather-like skin, crypts, and cutaneous ulcers. IVB stage is stage IVA + severely affected toes with notably swelling with repeated episodes of cellulitis, verrucous hyperkeratosis, deformity, or osteomyelitis.

Removal of the nails is performed when the patient has no infection. When recurrent infections occur in patients with HCC-Stage IVA, the nails and nail beds are removed and the defect closed with a C-V rotation-advancement flap. The patient's second and fourth toes are removed when patients are in stage IVB, have recurrent infections, but refuse to have all their toes amputated. Ideally, patients who are in this advanced stage should have all toes removed.

Advantages

- One-stage procedure.
- The incidence of postoperative cellulitis is reduced or eliminated.
- Heaviness is reduced.
- Limb circumference is much improved.
- Functional and long-lasting result.
- Satisfactory aesthetic result, taking into consideration the stage of the disease.
- Improved quality of life.

Disadvantages

- The patient may still have occasional episodes of infection (although less frequent).
- Hypertrophic scarring, particularly at the junctions between the sheets of skin grafts.
- Recurrent ulcers.
- Skin crypts.
- Lymphorrhea.
- Pigmentation.
- Skin dryness due to loss of sweat glands and sebaceous glands.
- Unsatisfactory aesthetic result if scarring is excessive or verrucous hyperkeratosis develops on the dorsum of the foot.

However, most of the complications can be prevented by primary take of all skin grafts (such as using VAC therapy) and good hygiene through education of postoperative care.

HCC-Modified Charles' Procedure: Charles + Lymph Node Flap

Lymphedema is a chronic, progressive, and debilitating condition, which negatively affects the quality of life. Treatment of advanced lymphedema remains a challenge in reconstructive surgery. Surgical procedures are indicated when previous conservative methods fail to improve the lymphedema. They can be categorized as excisional, in which the diseased soft tissue is removed, or physiologic, in which an attempt is made to improve the lymphatic flow. Among the physiologic procedures that have been used for the treatment of lymphedema, the lymphaticovenous by-pass using transferring vascularized lymph node flap is gaining popularity [7].

Felmerer et al. [17] proposed the microsurgical lymphatic vessel transplantation as a method for bypassing the obstructed lymph pathway with satisfactory results in 14 patients with secondary lymphedema of the limb, face, and genitalia. On the other hand, the mechanism of the lymph node flap transfer is based on the spontaneous generation of lymphatic channels between the transferred lymph nodes and the surrounding tissues. The lymph is absorbed by the vascularized lymph nodes and drained to the venous system through the lympaticovenous connections inside the flap.

In 1990, Chen et al. [18] investigated the efficacy of transferring lymph node flap into lympoedematous limbs. The medical literature is limited regarding the efficacy of the vascularized lymph node flap transfer in lower extremity lymphedema.

Cheng et al. [19] reported reduction of the limb circumference after transferring submental lymph node flap at the ankle. Similarly, Althubaiti et al. [20], using also vascularized supraclavicular lymph node flap transfer for lower extremity lymphedema, presented satisfactory postoperative results. Our previous experience using either inguinal or supraclavicular lymph node flap transfer for lower extremity lymphedema agree with the above studies that the lymph node flap

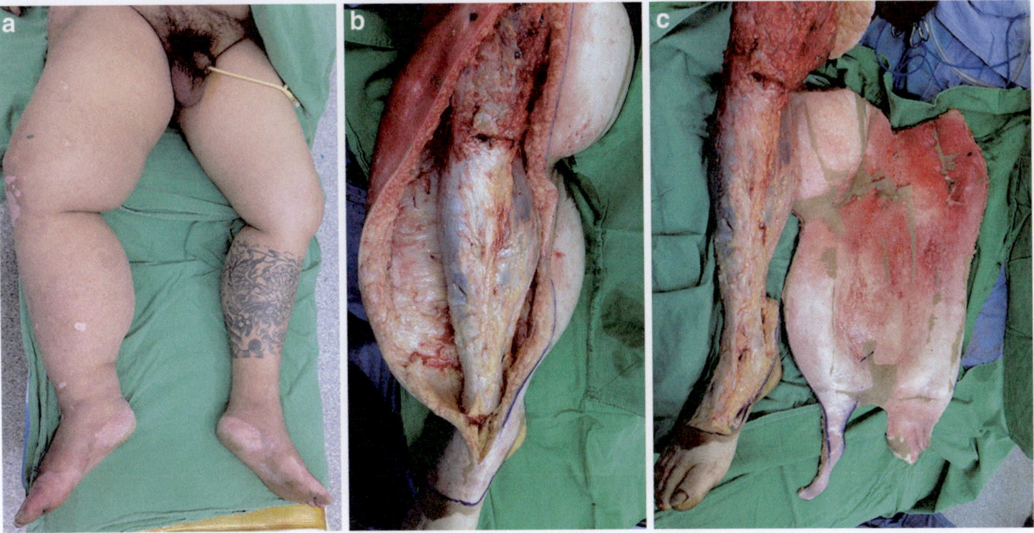

Fig. 26.4 (**a**) Patient with right lower limb lymphedema; (**b**) The fibrosclerotic lymphedematous tissue is separated from the deep fascia (**c**) The resected tissue is this case was 15 kg

transfer is able to reduce the circumference of the lymphedematous limb and relieve the subjective symptoms at the early stages of disease.

When the disease is long-lasting, and permanent changes of the limb has been established such as extensive fibrosis and skin changes with hyperkeratosis, the role of lymph node flap transfer is not well established and can offer only limited improvement.

In the cases, with advanced lymphedema, significant improvement can be achieved with excisional procedures, in which the lymphedematous tissues are partially or totally removed.

Radical reduction of the lymphedematous limb can be achieved with Charles' procedure, which involves radical excision of the skin, subcutaneous tissue, and fascia, and then resurfacing of the limb with STSG. Potential complications of the procedure are wound breakdown, hyperkeratosis, ulceration, and aggravation of foot lymphedema (Fig. 26.4) [7].

On the basis of our previous experience in Charles' procedure, it is possible to improve the postoperative results eliminating the risk of recurrence and the need for secondary operations combining this procedure with lymph node flap.

The modification of the Charles' procedure consists of preserving the lesser saphenous vein along with its superficial branch on the dorsum of the foot. The superficial venous system is preserved to be used for the second venous anastomosis with the lymph node flap. The main mechanism of the lymph node flap transfer is the lymphaticovenous bypass. After the implantation of the lymph nodes spontaneous regeneration of lymphatic channel between the lymph nodes and the surrounding lymphedematous tissue occurs and then the lymph is drained to the venous system through the normal lymphaticovenous connections inside the lymph node flap. On the basis of this mechanism, we supercharged the lymph node flap with two venous anastomoses maximizing the lymph drainage into the venous system. In our practice, none of the patients experienced aggravation of the lymphedema on the foot as the transferred lymph node flap had protective role. In addition, in our cases we had low incidence of postoperative infection. The transferred lymph node flap contains macrophages and lymphocytes, which have the ability to capture, phagocytes, and destroy pathogens draining from sites of infection.

This immunological mechanism of the lymph nodes can explain the reduction of the infection rate of the diseased limb after lymph node flap transfer [7].

Surgical Technique

With the patient under general anesthesia, two teams worked simultaneously, performing the Charles' procedure and harvesting the lymph node flap. The Charles' procedure was performed as it previously has been described.

The same team that performs the modified Charles' procedure also prepared the recipient artery and the deep vein. Either the dorsalis pedis or the medial plantar artery with their concomitant veins could be used for anastomosis with the lymph node flap.

At the same time, the second team harvested the lymph node flap. For the inguinal lymph node flap, the common femoral artery was palpated and then a skin paddle was designed about 2 cm below the inguinal ligament, and lateral to the femoral artery. In cases, that we harvested the flap without skin paddle a lazy "S"-shape incision, 6–8 cm in length was made 2 cm below the inguinal ligament. The flap can be harvested either from medial to lateral, identifying first the SCIA and vein, or from lateral to medial. Of note, a "patch" of the femoral artery can be harvested to increase the diameter of the arterial distal end. The femoral artery is then repaired with 5-0 prolene (Fig. 26.5).

Harvesting of the right side supraclavicular lymph node flap has been described in our previously published article [21]. In brief, an incision was made 1.5 cm above the clavicle, and a free style lymph node flap was harvested based on the transverse cervical artery (TCA). The anatomical landmarks of the flap were the sternocleidomastoid muscle anteriorly, the trapezius muscle posteriorly, the clavicle inferiorly, and the external jugular vein, which was also included with the flap and used for the second venous anastomosis. The main lymph nodes are deep to the omohyoid muscle, and careful dissection should

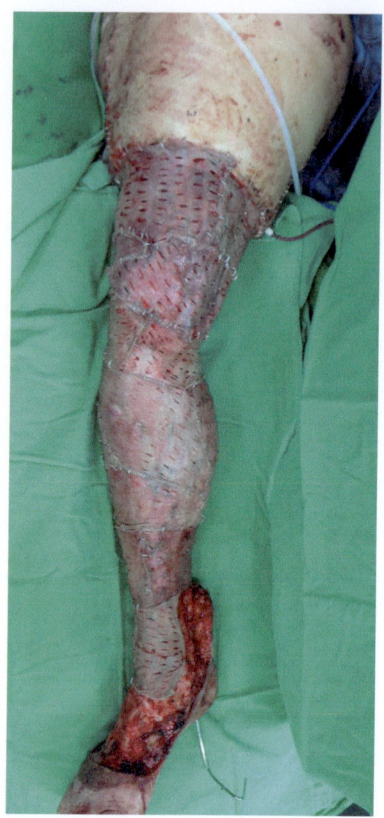

Fig. 26.5 Circumferential application of slit-thickness skin graft

be performed not to separate the lymph node from the underlying TCA. The concomitant vein was also identified and included with the flap. The skin paddle could be harvested with safety, unless careless dissection separate the skin from the underlying soft tissue when it is possible identify the direct perforator from the TCA to the skin (Fig. 26.6).

After the Charles' procedure was completed and the lymph node was harvested, one arterial and two venous anastomoses were performed at the recipient site (Fig. 26.7). A piece of split skin graft or local flap is used to cover the lymph node flap. For venous anastomoses, one deep and one superficial vein (branch of the lesser saphenous vein) were used. The method of lymph node flap transfer was similar to our previously published paper [22].

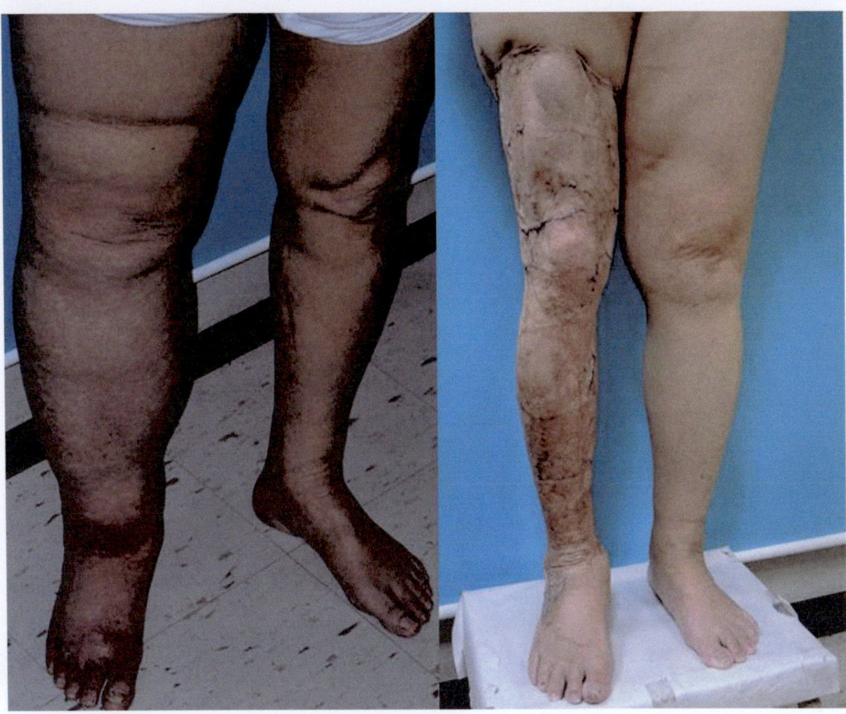

Fig. 26.6 Patient with right lower limb lymphedema treated with Charles' procedure. *Right* preoperative view, *Left* postoperative view after 1 year

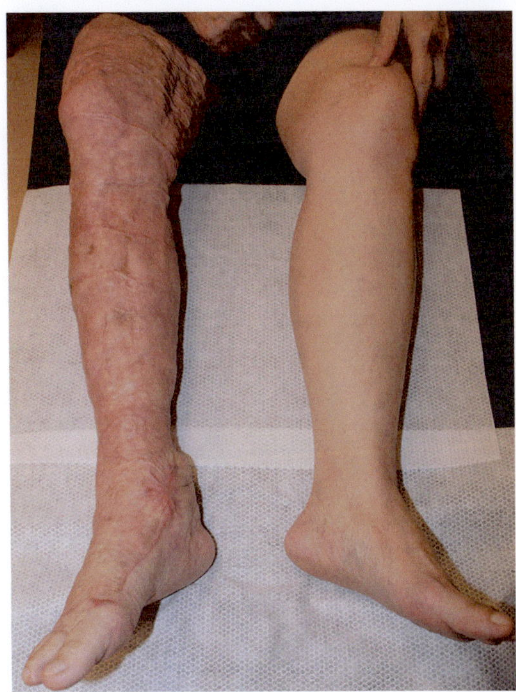

Fig. 26.7 Good aesthetic result after Modified Charles' Procedure (Charles' + Supraclavicular Lymph node flap) (follow-up 18 months)

Postoperative the patients remained inpatient for 5–7 days with the leg elevated and then discharged. Compression garment for the foot, leg, and thigh, was used 1 month later, when the skin graft was stabilized.

The HCC-Modified Charles' Procedure can be performed in one stage or in two stages (Fig. 26.8). In the latter case, the lymph node transfer can be performed before or after the Charles' procedure. The advantage of the two-stage technique is that it increases the flap survival because it does not require the compression for the STSG after Charles' procedure. The disadvantage is that it requires two surgical procedures. Further studies are required to clarify which it is the most effective.

In our experience the lymph node flaps used in HCC-modified Charles' procedure are the inguinal and supraclavicular lymph node flap, but each lymph node flap can be used. Recently we used intraabdominal lymph node flap (right gastroepiploic lymph node flap) with laparoscopic harvest to minimize the morbidity of the donor site.

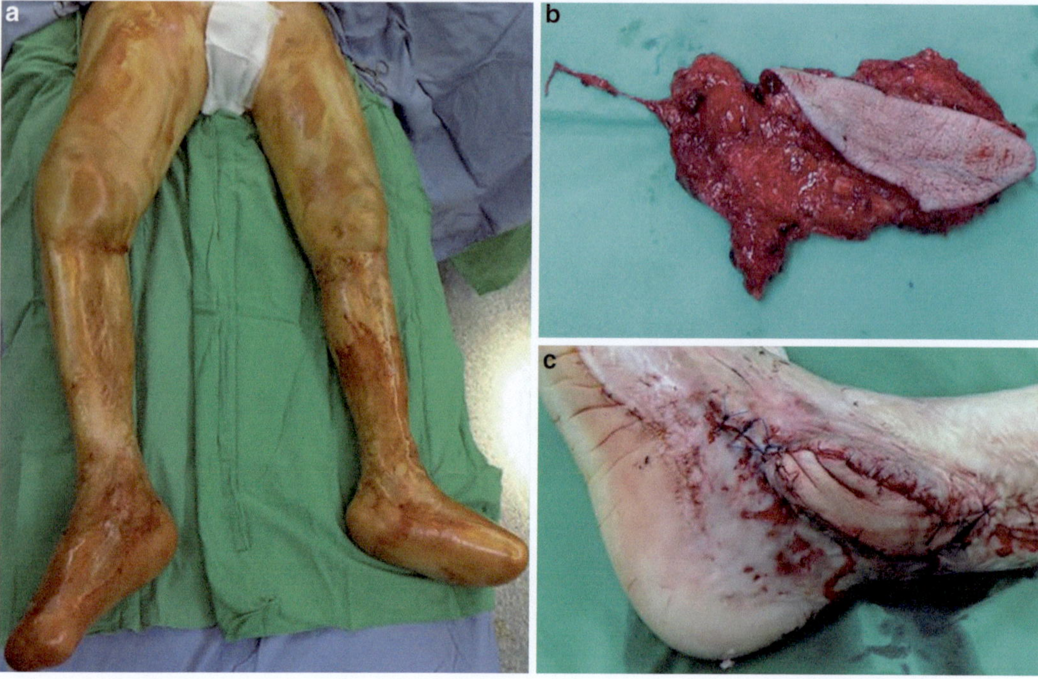

Fig. 26.8 Modified Charles' procedure in two stages. (**a**) Patient with previous bilateral lymphedema treated with bilateral Charles' procedure. (**b**) Groin lymph node flap (**c**) *Inset*

Ten Suggestions to Improve the Charles' Procedure

1. Have the patient on bed rest 1 week preoperatively for leg elevation, skin hygiene, and intermittent positive pressure pumping (IPPPP) to minimize the edema prior to surgery.
2. Before excising the lymphedematous tissue in the leg, apply the tourniquet at the proximal thigh following exsanguination (to minimize blood loss during harvesting of skin graft).
3. Extensive resection of the fibrotic skin and subcutaneous tissue down to the fascia. Wedge resections of the proximal thigh (medially and laterally) achieve sufficient reduction of lymphatic load. This can also avoid a sharp step between the skin graft in the distal half of the thigh and the skin flap of the proximal thigh. Avoid exposure of tendons. Leave a layer of fascia over the Achilles tendon as well as extensors of the ankles and toes to ensure good skin graft takes over the tendons.
4. Trim the thickened fascia to 1 mm in thickness (just enough to prevent herniation of muscle)
5. Obtain a smooth surface at the junction between the raw surface and the intact skin.
6. Obtain good hemostasis prior to application of skin graft. STSG can be done on the next day if necessary.
7. Skin grafts are applied in a circular or spiral fashion, instead of longitudinal fashion. The skin grafts are overlapped for 1 cm to prevent raw surface after swelling in the next few days.
8. Full-thickness skin graft for the dorsum of the foot and around the ankle but split-thickness skin graft for the leg, knee, and thigh.
9. Insert a pin through distal tibia for suspension of the leg from the bed to prevent shifting of the skin graft and subsequent skin graft loss at the posterior surface of the leg

10. Apply VAC (if available) to improve skin graft take and continue antibiotics for 3 days postoperatively. The key to success is to minimize the residual soft tissue beneath the skin graft, and perfect skin graft take.

Conclusions

Many authors consider Charles' procedure as old and outdated because of its complications and unsatisfactory aesthetic results. We believe that in selected cases and in advanced lymphedema this technique can be considered especially if some changes are made to avoid from potential complications such as recurrence, infection, and aggravation of the disease. HCC-Modified Charles' procedure is a novel approach combining excisional procedure with lymph node flap transfer to the distal limb, and it seems to be a reliable method for treating advanced stage of limb lymphedema.

References

1. Dumanian GA, Futrell JW. The Charles procedure: misquoted and misunderstood since 1950. Plast Reconstr Surg. 1996;98(7):1258–63.
2. Charles RH. Elephantiasis scroti. In: Latham AC, English TC, editors. A system of treatment, vol. 3. London: J & A Churcill; 1912. p. 504.
3. Karonidis A, Chen HC. Preservation of toes in advanced lymphedema: an important step in the control of infection. Ann Plast Surg. 2010;64(4):446–50.
4. Sistrunk WE. Further experience with the Kondoleon operation for elephantiasis. JAMA. 1918;1:800–5.
5. Macey HB. A surgical procedure for lymphoedema of the extremities: a follow-up report. J Bone Joint Surg Am. 1948;30:339–46.
6. Auchincloss H. A new operation for elephantiasis. Porto Rico J Pub Health Trop Med. 1930;6:149–50.
7. Sapountzis S, Ciudad P, Lim SY, Chilgar RM, Kiranantawat K, Nicoli F, Constantinides J, Wei MY, Sönmez TT, Singhal D, Chen HC. Modified Charles procedure and lymph node flap transfer for advanced lower extremity lymphedema. Microsurgery. 2014; 34:439.
8. O'Brien BM, Mellow CG, Khazanchi RK, Dvir E, Kumar V, Pederson WC. Long-Term Results after Microlymphaticovenous Anastomoses for the Treatment of Obstructive Lymphedema. Plast Reconstr Surg. 1990;85(4):562–72.
9. Campisi C, Eretta C, Pertile D, Da Rin E, Campisi C, Maccio A, Campisi M, Accogli S, Bellini C, Bonioli E, Boccardo F. Microsurgery for treatment of peripheral lymphedema: long-term outcome and future perspectives. Microsurgery. 2007;27:333–8.
10. Campisi C, Boccardo F, Zilli A, Maccio A, Napoli F. Long-term results after lymphatic-venous anastomoses for the treatment of obstructive lymphedema. Microsurgery. 2001;21:135–9.
11. Koshima I, Nanba Y, Tsutsui T, Takahashi Y, Itoh S. Long-term follow-up after lymphaticovenular anastomosis for lymphedema in the leg. J Reconstr Microsurg. 2003;19(4):209–15.
12. Koshima I, Kawada S, Moriguchi T, Kajiwara Y. Ultrastructural observations of lymphatic vessels in lymphedema in human extremities. Plast Reconstr Surg. 1996;97(2):397–405.
13. Van der Walt JC, Perks TJ, Zeeman BJ, Bruce-Chwatt AJ, Graewe FR. Modified Charles procedure using negative pressure dressings for primary lymphedema: a functional assessment. Ann Plast Surg. 2009;62: 669–75.
14. Nandi P, Wong KP, Wei WI, Ngan H, Ong GB. Incidence of postoperative deep vein thrombosis in Hong Kong Chinese. Br J Surg. 1980;67:251–3.
15. Badger C, Preston N, Seers K, Mortimer P. Antibiotics/anti-inflammatories for reducing acute episodes in lymphoedema of the limb (review). Cochrane Collab. 2008;2:1–15.
16. Chen HC, Garb BB, et al. Elective amputation of the toes in severe lymphoedema of the lower leg: rational and indications. Ann Plast Surg. 2009;63(2):193–7.
17. Felmerer G, Sattler T, Lohrmann C, Tobbia D. Treatment of various secondary lymphedemas by microsurgical lymph vessel transplantation. Microsurgery. 2012;32:171–7.
18. Chen HC, O'Brien BM, Rogers IW, et al. Lymph node transfer for the treatment of obstructive lymphoedema in the canine model. Br J Plast Surg. 1990;43(5): 578–86.
19. Cheng MH, Huang JJ, Nguyen DH, Saint-Cyr M, Zenn MR, Tan BK, Lee CL. A novel approach to the treatment of lower extremity lymphedema by transferring a vascularized submental lymph node flap to the ankle. Gynecol Oncol. 2012;126(1):93–8.
20. Althubaiti GA, Crosby MA, Chang DW. Vascularized supraclavicular lymph node transfer for lower extremity lymphedema treatment. Plast Reconstr Surg. 2013;131(1):133e–5.
21. Sapountzis S, Singha D, Rashid A, Ciudad P, Meo D, Chen HC. Lymph node flap based on the right transverse cervical artery as a donor site for lymph node transfer. Ann Plast Surg. 2014;73:398.
22. Feng GM, Yang WG, Huang CH, Wang SY, Chen HC. Lymph nodes transfer for treating mild to moderate lymphedema—A preliminary result. J Plast Surg Asso ROC. 2003;12(2):95–104.

Neil R. Feins and Sigrid Bairdain

N.R. Feins, M.D. (✉)
Department of Pediatric Surgery, Boston Children's
Hospital, Harvard Medical School, Fegan Building,
3rd Floor, Boston, MA 02115, USA
e-mail: neil.feins@childrens.harvard.edu

S. Bairdain, M.D., M.P.H.
Department of Pediatric Surgery,
Boston Children's Hospital, Boston, MA USA

Key Points

- Lymphedema is a relatively rare disorder, but it is caused by the abnormal collection of lymphatic fluid in the interstitial tissues.
- Lymphedema must be differentiated first from venous edema, hemihypertrophy, and/or lipedema (painful fat syndrome).
- Staged excision of the subcutaneous tissue provides for the best resolve of the proteinaceous fluid the collects in this tissue.

Introduction

Lymphedema is a relatively rare problem. Lymphedema results from abnormal and inappropriate collection of lymphatic fluid in the subcutaneous tissues. The etiologies underlying this abnormal collection of proteinaceous fluid may be from congenital anomalies, functional overload of the superficial draining system, or a combination of both entities. There have been a variety of surgical approaches to manage this condition; however, staged skin and subcutaneous excision has provided the most durable results to this chronic condition [1].

Operative Therapy

Indications

There are two relative indications for an operative procedure, regardless of the patient's age. The first is an extremity which is too heavy and cumbersome to permit daily activities despite compliance with conservative measures. These patients may not be able to wear normal clothing or shoes. The second indication for surgical intervention is recurrent cellulitis and lymphangitis. This complication can be crippling. One of the patients needed bed rest and antibiotics for approximately 10 days monthly because of high fevers, lymphangitis, and pain. Since resection over 30 years ago, this patient has not had an attack of cellulitis or lymphangitis. Most patients with an infection respond well to bed rest and antibiotics. Positive blood cultures are rare in the patients with infection. The organism is presumed to be *Streptococcus* and treatment is penicillin, if there is no allergy.

Patients, females and are interested in cosmetic improvement. Extensive resection for minor to moderate lymphedema is not indicated for appearance only, there is considerable scarring, and the contour achieved rarely satisfies these patients.

A.K. Greene et al. (eds.), *Lymphedema: Presentation, Diagnosis, and Treatment*,
DOI 10.1007/978-3-319-14493-1_27, © Springer International Publishing Switzerland 2015

History of Staged Skin and Subcutaneous Excision

Lanz in 1911 was the first to recommend excision of skin and subcutaneous tissue along the entire length of the leg [2]. A year later in 1912, Kondoleon described excision of the deep fascia in the extremity to allow the superficial lymphatics to connect and drain into the deep lymphatics [3]. Three years later, he admitted unsatisfactory results of fasciectomy [3]. In 1927, Sistrunk modified the Kondoleon procedure by excising extensive amounts of tissue and fascia [4]. He reasoned that the more tissue removed, the better the result, and reported that 75 % of patients were improved by this treatment. Ghormley and Overton reported that about half of their patients were improved by a procedure quite similar to Sistrunk's operation [5].

In 1912, Charles described a method for treatment of tropical elephantiasis of the lower extremities. This involved resection of all edematous tissues down to the muscle and covering the denuded surface with split thickness skin grafts obtained from other areas of the body (see Fig. 27.1) [6]. The Charles procedure, or modifications thereof, is the most consistently successful procedure for permanent reduction in the size of a lymphedematous limb and its major disadvantage is the bizarre configuration of the limb (see Figs. 27.2 and 27.3a, b) [7]. Furthermore, the grafts are susceptible to trauma with chronic ulceration and infections (see Fig. 27.4). Other problems are hyperkeratinization, papillomatosis, and eczema of the grafted extremity. One patient, who had a Charles procedure in the distant past, suffered numerous breakdowns of the grafts and developed squamous cell carcinoma in the grafted sites of the extremity (see Fig. 27.5).

Epstein, in 1984, reported a case of squamous carcinoma developing in a patient's foot arising in association with long standing verrucous hyperplasia of congenital lymphedema [8]. Some authors still advocate Charles procedure for very severe lymphedema [8, 9]. There is no doubt that the procedure is the most effective for reduction in size of the extremity, but the secondary problems are too formidable to justify this operation, except as a last resort.

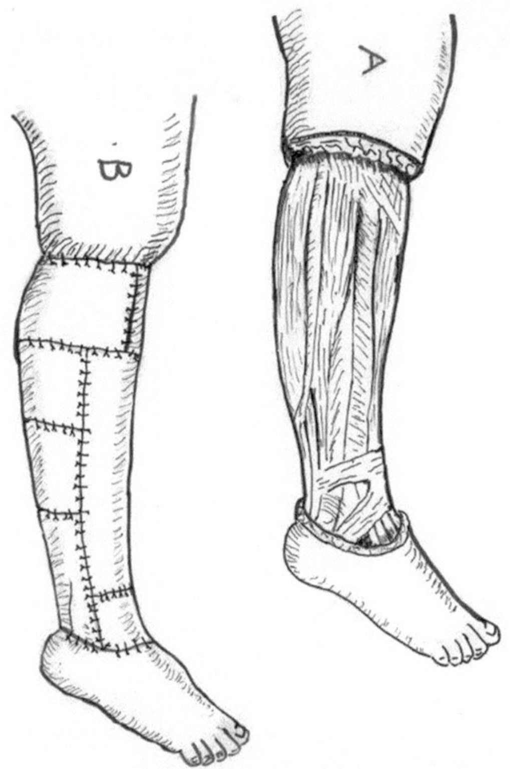

Fig. 27.1 The Charles Procedure

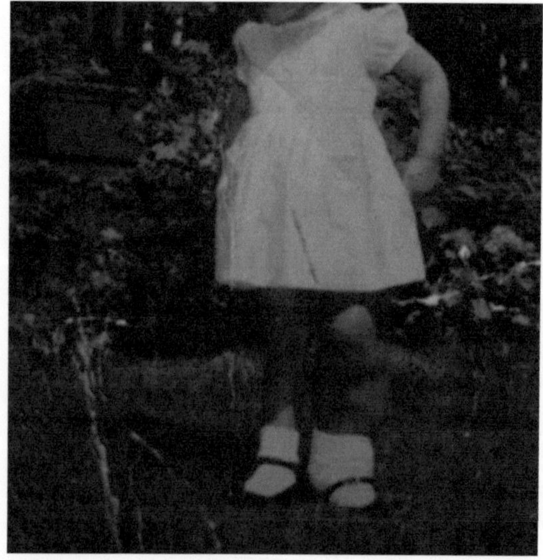

Fig. 27.2 This patient had a Charles procedure in childhood given her lymphedema present in the left lower extremity. "Mulliken and Young's Vascular Anomalies: Hemangiomas and Malformations" edited by Mulliken, J.B., Burrows, P. E. & Fishman, S.J. (2013) by permission of Oxford University Press, USA

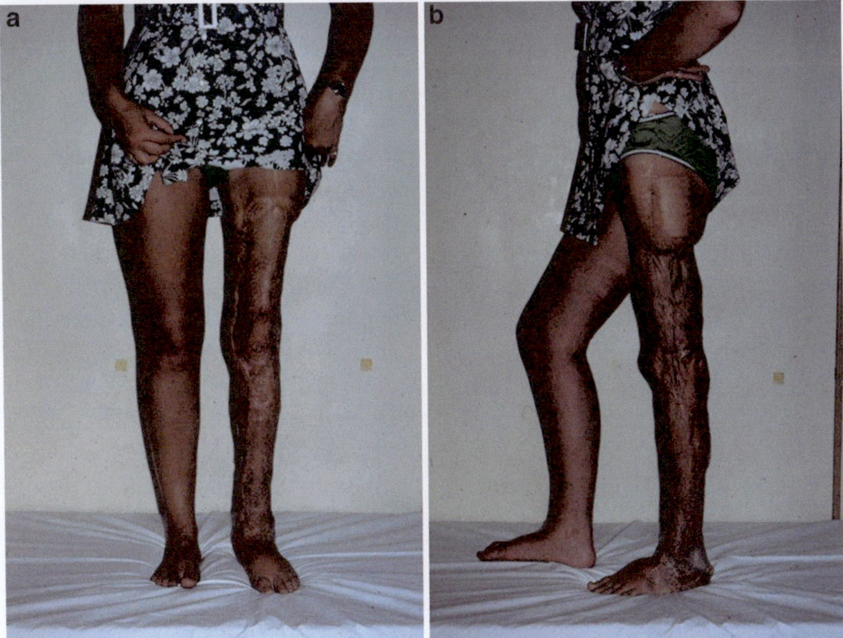

Fig. 27.3 (**a**) This is the same patient who had the Charles procedure in childhood (see Fig. 27.2). Lymphedema is gone, but removing all subcutaneous tissue and applying split thickness skin grafts to the underlying muscle results in an abnormal configuration of the extremity. (**b**) This is the same patient who had the Charles procedure in childhood (see Fig. 27.2). Lymphedema is gone, but removing all subcutaneous tissue and applying split thickness skin grafts to the underlying muscle results in an abnormal configuration of the extremity. "Mulliken and Young's Vascular Anomalies: Hemangiomas and Malformations" edited by Mulliken, J.B., Burrows, P. E. & Fishman, S.J. (2013) by permission of Oxford University Press, USA

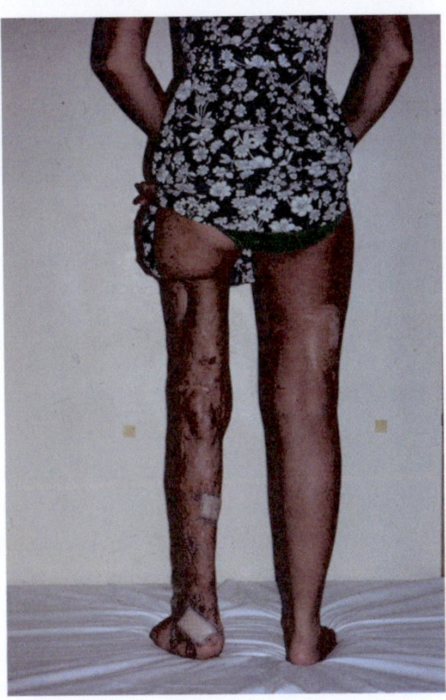

Fig. 27.4 This is the same patient who had the Charles procedure in childhood (see Fig. 27.2). Note the multiple Band-Aids® covering the areas of chronic breakdown, a common late sequelae of the Charles procedure. "Mulliken and Young's Vascular Anomalies: Hemangiomas and Malformations" edited by Mulliken, J.B., Burrows, P. E. & Fishman, S.J. (2013) by permission of Oxford University Press, USA

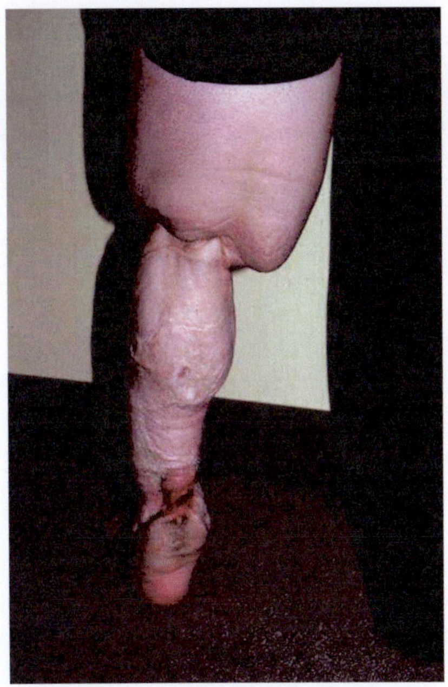

Fig. 27.5 Long-term results of the Charles's procedure. There can be concern for cutaneous breakdown, disfigurement of the extremity, and concern for squamous cell carcinoma of the grafted site. "Mulliken and Young's Vascular Anomalies: Hemangiomas and Malformations" edited by Mulliken, J.B., Burrows, P. E. & Fishman, S.J. (2013) by permission of Oxford University Press, USA

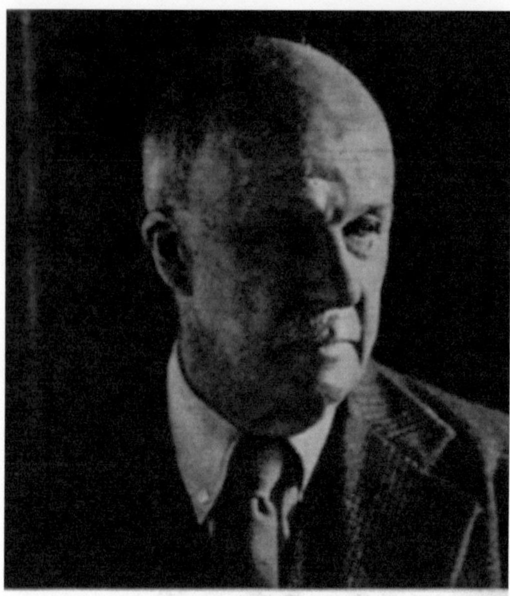

Fig. 27.6 John Homans (1877–1954): Born and bred in Boston he was educated at Harvard College and Harvard Medical School and served as surgical "House Pupil" at the Massachusetts General Hospital. While a staff member at the Peter Bent Brigham Hospital he wrote a textbook, *Circulatory Diseases of the Extremities* (*date*). His name is remembered for the sign of pain in the calf on active or passive dorsiflexion of the foot in patients with deep venous thrombosis of the calf. Homans once remarked (with a slight lisp) "If they had to name a sign after me; why didn't they pick one that was damn good?" Courtesy of Harvard Medical School Alumni Assoc. Arch Surg 134:1019, 1999

Homans extended Sistrunk's operation, as suggested by Auchincloss [10, 11] (see Figs. 27.6 and 27.7). He excised the subcutaneous tissue and the deep fascia and created thin cutaneous flaps to cover the excised areas. The operation was done in four stages. The medial and lateral sides were done within weeks of each other. The subsequent procedures were carried out 2 months later [12]. Homans reported on eight cases: four patients needed only two or three excisional procedures, and the others had all four procedures. All patients were said to have a satisfactory result. Thus, the ablative principle, i.e., excision of large amount of edematous tissue, was established [10].

In 1967, Fonkalsrud was the first to advocate staged subcutaneous lymphangiectomy for congenital lymphedema in infants and children and a follow-up report in 1973 confirmed his earlier impressions [13]. Miller et al. presented excellent results using staged subcutaneous excisions in adults with lymphedema [14]. Lymphatic function was estimated using radioiodinated human serum albumin injections before and after staged excision. Their patients cleared 39 % in 24 h preoperatively, 43 % in 24 h 1 month postoperatively, but averaged 80 % per 24 h at 1 year postoperatively. These findings provided the first objective evidence that staged resection significantly increased clearance at 1 year.

Suction-assisted lipectomy (SAL) can be a first line operative intervention for extremity lymphedema because of its superior efficacy, consistent results, and low morbidity [15]. Excellent results are achieved using modern liposuction techniques (circumferential suctioning, tumescence, and power-assisted cannulas), with minimal morbidity and short recovery. This technique removes the excess, subcutaneous adipose tissue present in chronic lymphedema. The ideal candidate for SAL has moderate disease. Patients with minor disease do not require operative intervention. If major skin excess is predicted after (SAL) (as in severe lymphedema), the patient may be better managed by staged skin/subcutaneous excision [15].

Personal Surgical Protocol

Preoperative Preparation

We use a modified Homan's procedure, or a modified staged subcutaneous excision, for lymphedema of the lower extremities [16]. The patient is placed on strict bed rest at home for 3–14 days before the procedure. One patient lost 54 lb by mobilization of lymphedematous fluid, without a diuretic. I do not routinely use a diuretic. The extremity is painted with povidone–iodine ointment every 8 h and wrapped with Kerlix™. A Jobst™ air splint is placed around the extremity; this is the simple model used for emergency

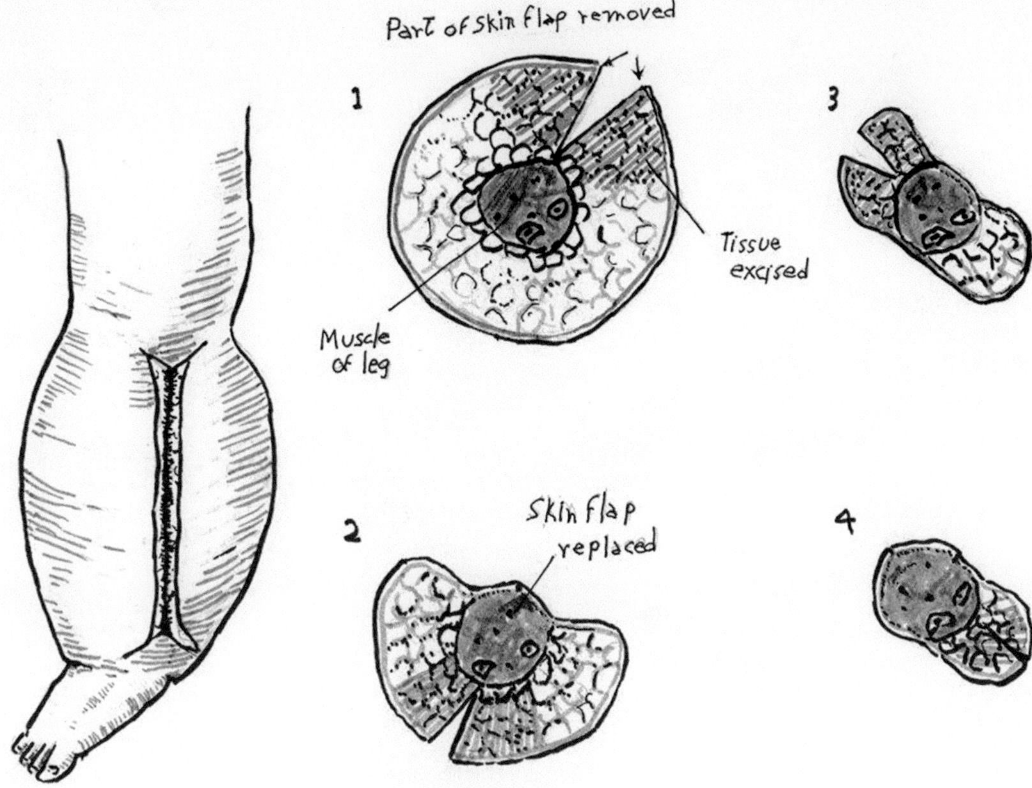

Fig. 27.7 John Homans procedure

treatment of fractures. The pressure is set at 30 mmHg and the splint is released every 4 h for 15 min, or as is necessary. A plastic margarine cup is stuffed with cotton and placed over the toes to prevent painful compression of the distal foot. This regimen results in a rapid shrinking of the edematous extremity in preparation for resection. Penicillin or erythromycin, if there a history of allergy to penicillin, is given 1 h preoperatively and continued for 7 days postoperatively or as long as drains are in place.

Technique

The first operation is on the medial aspect of the leg, as this incision is less visible. In patients with moderate and even severe edema, only one excisional procedure may suffice. If the lymphedema involves the foot and extends above the knee, we mark the incision on the medial aspect of the foot, continue behind the malleolus up the medial aspect of the knee, and proceed up the thigh (see Fig. 27.8). If the edema does not involve the thigh, the incision is gently curved and ends at the medial aspect of the popliteal fossa. The flaps are full thickness, but as thin as possible (see Fig. 27.9). The skin flaps are developed 1/6th the circumference of the leg medially and 1/6th laterally for a total of 1/3rd the circumference of the leg. The total length of the skin flaps is not made beyond 1/3rd the circumference of the leg to minimize the chance of necrosis (see Fig. 27.8). Using a Kelly clamp, a tunnel is developed beneath the subcutaneous tissue and removal of most of the edematous tissue is done by blunt finger dissection. The greater saphenous venous system invariably is removed and/or interrupted during the excision. Intradermal silk sutures are placed along the entire incision: there are used

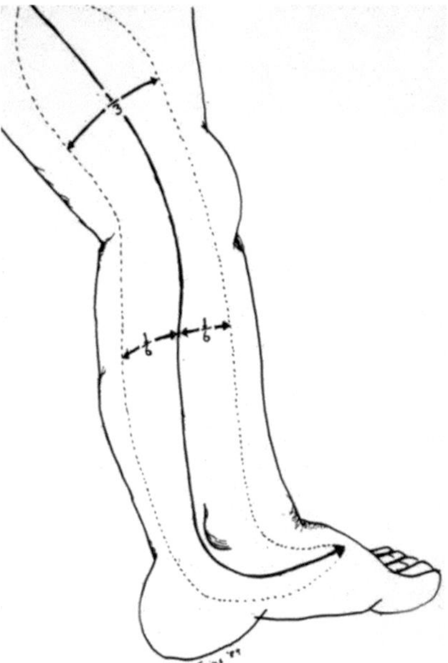

Fig. 27.8 Incision on the medical aspect of the foot. The *vertical arrow* indicates length. The *horizontal arrows* indicate the width of the skin flaps. Each flap developed for one-sixth the circumference of the leg for a total exposure of one-third of the extremity. "Mulliken and Young's Vascular Anomalies: Hemangiomas and Malformations" edited by Mulliken, J.B., Burrows, P. E. & Fishman, S.J. (2013) by permission of Oxford University Press, USA

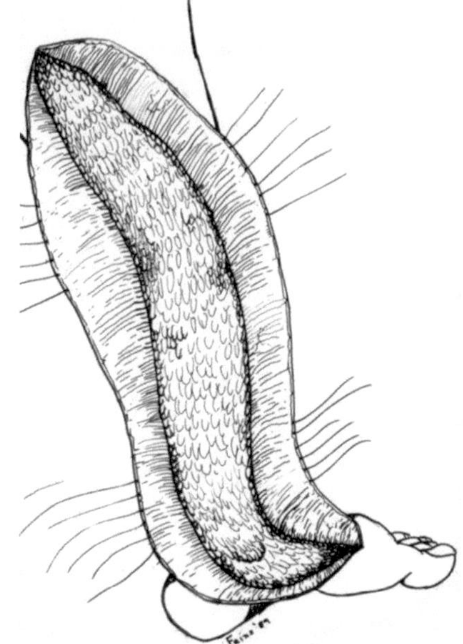

Fig. 27.9 Flaps are full-thickness, but very thin. Holding sutures are placed in the dermal layer and used for traction to minimize manipulation of the skin. The exposed subcutaneous tissue and underlying fascia are removed entirely. "Mulliken and Young's Vascular Anomalies: Hemangiomas and Malformations" edited by Mulliken, J.B., Burrows, P. E. & Fishman, S.J. (2013) by permission of Oxford University Press, USA

for traction during development of the cutaneous flaps (see Fig. 27.10a) [17].

It is imperative that the presence of a competent deep venous system is documented preoperatively by preoperative MRI, CT, or ultrasound. The fascia is removed from the muscles by sharp dissection (see Fig. 27.10b, c). The pneumatic cuff is released and meticulous hemostasis is secured. One large round suction drain with extra holes is placed beneath each flap and brought out via separate incisions above the knee or higher in the thigh and the skin is closed in one layer with staples (see Fig. 27.11). Rarely is there redundant skin to trim; however if the skin edge is cyanotic, it is excised. The suture line is covered with povidone–iodine ointment, fluff gauze and wrapped with Kerlix™. The air splint is placed and expanded to 30 mmHg pressure (see Fig. 27.12). The drainage tube is placed to wall suction for 24 h and is attached to canister suction for 7 days.

The patient is kept at complete bed rest with elevation of the operated extremity. Pressure in the air splint is released every 4 h for 15 min and as necessary. With the splint decompressed, the suture line is painted every 8 h with povidone–iodine ointment. The combination of the suction drainage and the air splint prevents collection of fluid under the flaps, and circumferential compression allows for adherence of the flaps to the underlying muscle.

Seven days postoperatively the suction drains are removed and the patient is measured for a Jobst™ stocking set at 50 mmHg pressure. Careful non-weight bearing ambulation with crutches is begun while tight elastic bandages are worn. Weight-bearing ambulation is allowed about 3 weeks postoperatively. The custom-made stocking is usually available by that time. Every second or third staple is removed at about 2 weeks postoperatively. The suture line is continually covered with povidone–iodine ointment until all the staples are removed and the incision is completely healed. This process can last for more than 1 month. The patient or parents are taught to dress the incision early during hospitalization.

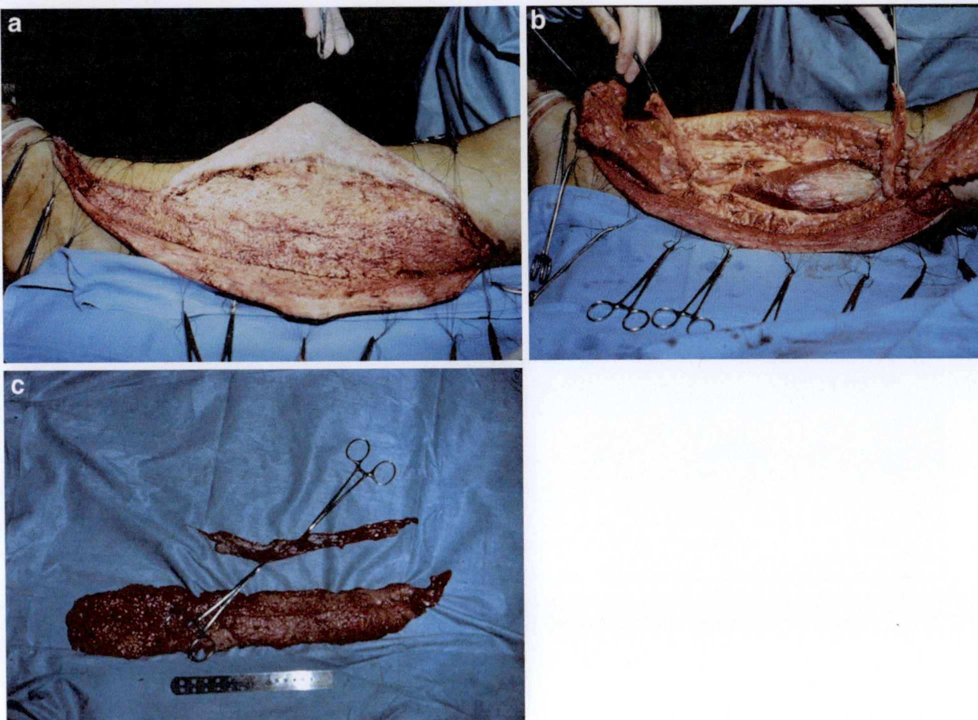

Fig. 27.10 (a) Flaps are full-thickness, but very thin. Holding sutures are placed in the dermal layer and used for traction to minimize manipulation of the skin. (b) Subcutaneous tissue and fascia to be removed. Here they are opened in the middle for demonstration purposes. (c) The subcutaneous tissue and fascia are removed separately each in one section. "Mulliken and Young's Vascular Anomalies: Hemangiomas and Malformations" edited by Mulliken, J.B., Burrows, P. E. & Fishman, S.J. (2013) by permission of Oxford University Press, USA

Steri-Strips are not used as too often they cause maceration of the desquamating skin.

For a patient with bilateral lymphedema, we prefer to address one extremity at a time. If the initial procedure is uncomplicated, the operation on the opposite leg is scheduled 10 days after the first operation. With over 10 days of bed rest, the unoperated leg is soft, pliable, and ideally prepared. About 30 % of my patients have a satisfactory result after a single operation, and need no further procedures.

The majority of patients, because of persistent enlargement of the extremity, return for staged or serial excision. We perform the second procedure

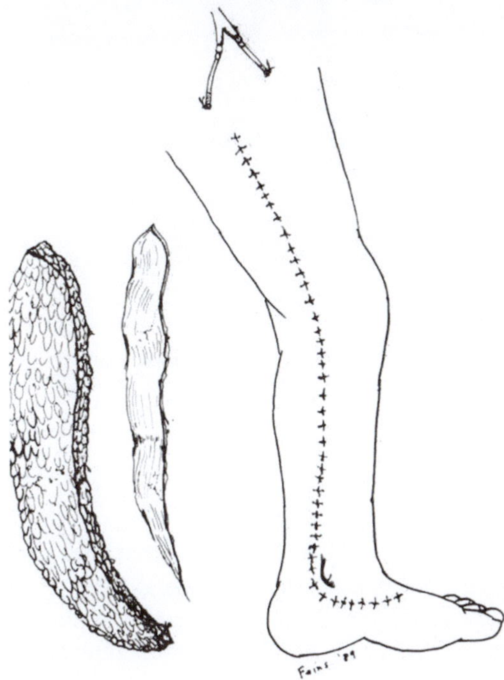

Fig. 27.11 Incision closed with staples after two large suction drains are placed beneath flaps. The drains are usually placed above the knee. "Mulliken and Young's Vascular Anomalies: Hemangiomas and Malformations" edited by Mulliken, J.B., Burrows, P. E. & Fishman, S.J. (2013) by permission of Oxford University Press, USA

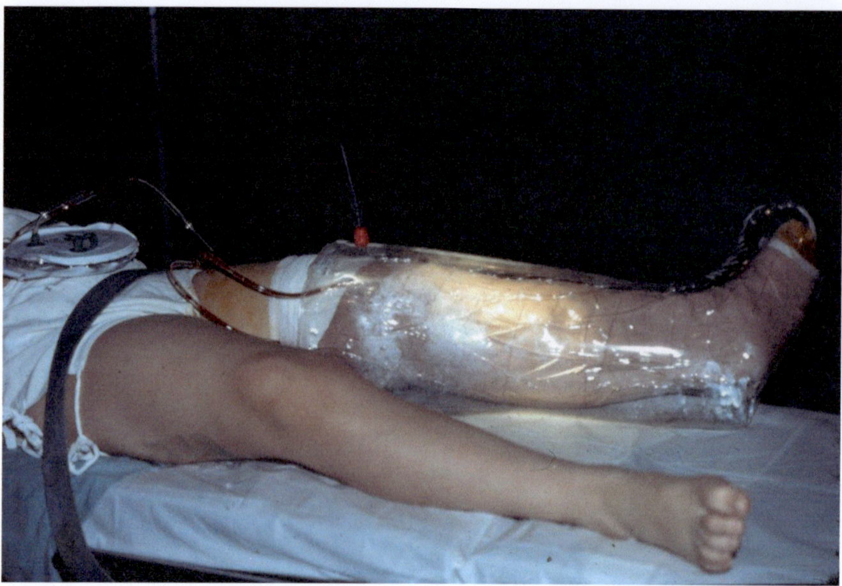

Fig. 27.12 Air splint in place following staged excision

on the lateral aspect of the extremity. The technique is the same as on the medial side. Originally, we identified the peroneal nerve to keep it from harm's way. However, this step is unnecessary if the fascia is not penetrated near the head of the fibula since the nerve is deep to the fascia. Early in the series, we also attempted to identify and spare the sural nerve, which was a time-consuming step. We often noticed that the distal branches of the sural nerve were difficult to preserve in the excised subcutaneous tissue even if the main trunk was identified higher in the leg. In some of the patients the nerve was inadvertently transected without any obvious signs. Therefore, we no longer identify the sural nerve. If minor hypoesthesia occurs, it usually disappears.

In 1936, Homans suggested the second operation on the involved extremity be undertaken after 1 week [10]. Several authors agree that lymphatic function, as studied by clearance of radio-iodinated human serum albumin, increases with time and is greater at 1 year than at a few months after excision [14, 18, 19]. Because of these findings, we do not do the second lateral operation during the first postoperative year. If lymphatic function improves, there may be no need to do serial excision. Usually, the initial size of the extremity indicates the number of serial stages

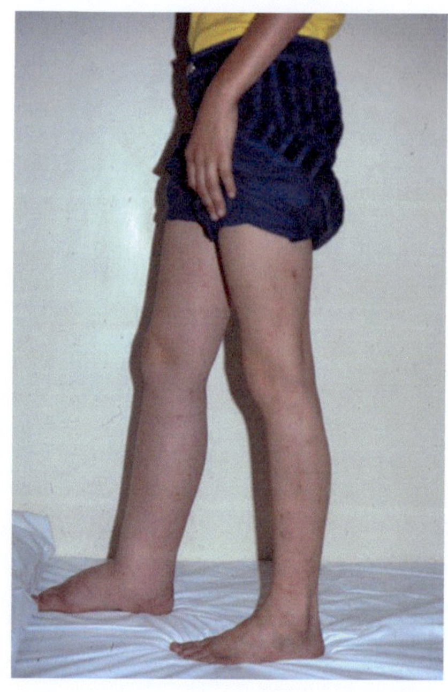

Fig. 27.13 Young girl with lymphedema of the right lower extremity preoperatively

needed. About 10 % of patients need three excisional procedures. The third operation, if necessary, is done on the posterior aspect of the calf. (see Figs. 27.13 and 27.14a, b) Following the procedure the patient must wear support hose

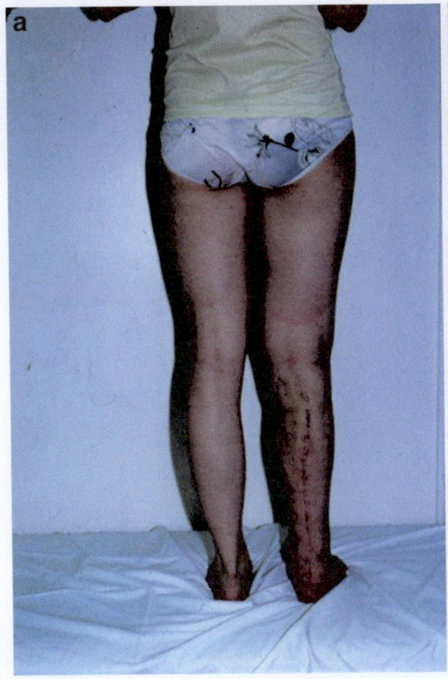
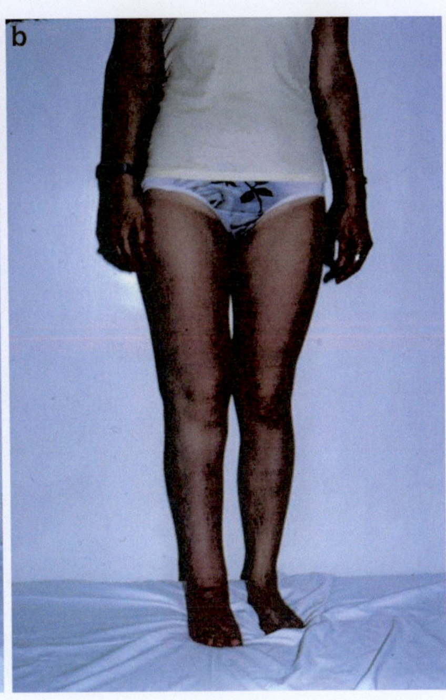

Fig. 27.14 (**a**) The posterior view following the third serial excision. The third operation, if necessary, is done on the posterior aspect of the calf. "Mulliken and Young's Vascular Anomalies: Hemangiomas and Malformations" edited by Mulliken, J.B., Burrows, P. E. & Fishman, S.J. (2013) by permission of Oxford University Press, USA. (**b**) The anterior view following the third serial excision. "Mulliken and Young's Vascular Anomalies: Hemangiomas and Malformations" edited by Mulliken, J.B., Burrows, P. E. & Fishman, S.J. (2013) by permission of Oxford University Press, USA

indefinitely to help control swelling. Many patients continue to use the Jobst™ air splint at home to minimize the edema and maintain contour of the extremity. This splint is an adequate substitute for the expensive and bulky pump machines (see Fig. 27.15a–c).

In the author's experience, three patients with lymphedema had chylous reflux into their legs, and two patients had severe chylous fistulas of the scrotum. Computed tomographic (CT) scans showed dilated latero-aortic and iliac lymphatic vessels in two patients, and the third patient had diffuse pelvic changes, including bony involvement. The patients with chylous reflux were treated with a two-stage retroperitoneal resection of the large incompetent latero-aortic lymphatic vessels, from the level of the first lumbar vertebrae to the aortic bifurcation and iliac vessels. The procedure was performed 4 h after ingestion of 40 g of butter melted into milk to help display the lymphatics. The abdominal incision was a lateral "J" type, similar to the incision used for renal transplantation. A midline incision does not allow adequate access. The opposite side was managed 3 weeks later. The leg size was reduced in two patients and chylous fistulas closed. The third patient had no specific lymphatics that could be resected and he remained unchanged.

Results

Over 100 children, young adults, and a few older patients underwent staged excision for lymphedema. The female-to-male ratio was 5:3. All had primary lymphedema, except one whom had secondary lymphedema due to a radical groin operation followed by radiation. All procedures were in the lower limbs; 4 had excision in the upper extremity; 14 had procedures related to the genitalia.

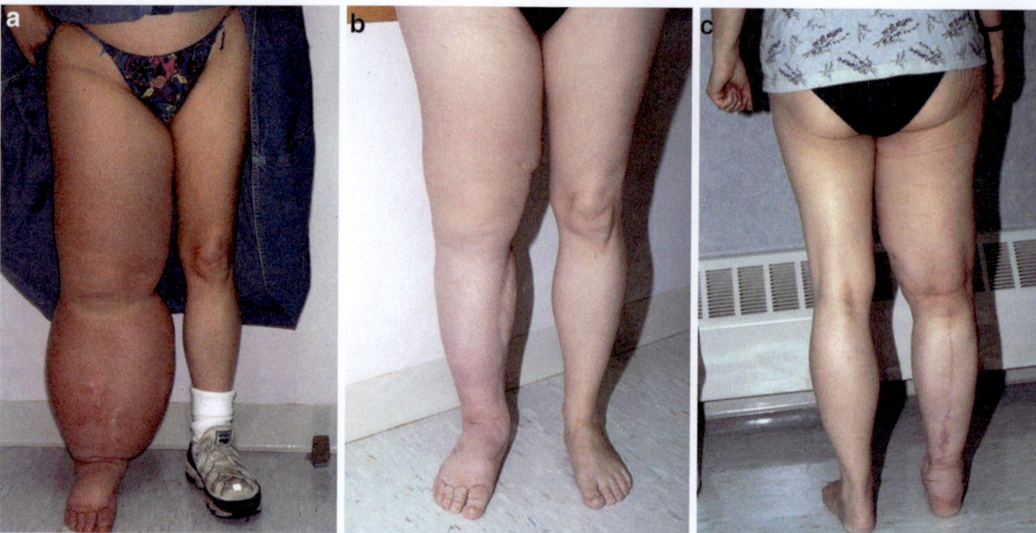

Fig. 27.15 (**a**) 44-year-old female with massive lymphedema of the left lower extremity. She could not find clothes that fit her properly and was unable to conduct daily activities. (**b**) Anterior view following three serial excisions. (**c**) Posterior view displaying reduction 3 years later. She uses support hose daily and air splint during evenings

Over 100 patients are being followed and treated with conservative measures.

All patients were improved by following excision as evidenced by decreased swelling. The longest follow-up of a patient is over 30 years. Some patients have improved remarkably after one procedure. Other patients required 2–3 three excisional operations, and improved only moderately, but the cycle of increasing edema had definitely been controlled. Episodes of lymphangitis and cellulitis noted preoperatively in 21 patients have not recurred. Excisional therapy appears to enhance drainage or at least diminish stasis.

Overall Complications

Two-percent of patients developed seroma under the flaps, which required drainage. One patient's leg was still too large to be placed into the air splint immediately after the first operation, and despite the use of elastic bandages, evenly distributed compression was impossible. Another patient produced a huge volume of lymph; larger suction drains were placed beneath the flaps for 3 weeks.

The patients' assessment of outcome was determined by follow-up telephone interview, photos, and questioning during postoperative visits. Ninety-percent of the patients were pleased with the results of resection; 10 % were not satisfied. Early in our experience, we found that patients with minor to moderate lymphedema who desired cosmetic improvement were rarely pleased with the scarring and contour.

No patients had a full-thickness flap loss requiring a skin graft. There were two wound separations related to premature removal of staples. One healed spontaneously and the other had episodic lymphangitis in the granulating wound and required secondary closure. Once the wound closed, no further attacks occurred. Four patients, including one of the above, needed revision for hypertrophic scarring. Five benefited from injection of corticosteroid into the heavy scars. Only one patient developed a seroma or lymphocele under the flaps that needed drainage. The patient's leg after surgery could not be placed into an air splint and adequate compression was not applied.

Studies done postoperatively with labeled serum albumin revealed significant increased clearance after 1 year in the operated extremity [20]. This finding could be an evidence of utilization of new pathways of lymph drainage. Early appearance of the radioactive albumin in the groin after injection into the foot may be due to acquired lympho-venous connections.

Most patients can wear normal shoes and clothing. No limitations on activities are necessary. All patients need a custom-made support hose set at 50 mmHg pressure, and this usually needs to be replaced every 3 months. Liberal use of the air splint at home helps to control swelling. Meticulous care and cleansing of the involved areas is always necessary. The involved extremity should be elevated frequently. Any injury or cut to the involved area must be cleaned and dressed with topical antibiotic to prevent infection and cellulitis.

Many patients have delivered babies without any significant problems. Swelling in the lower extremities usually increases in the later stages of pregnancy but diminishes after delivery and weight loss. Approximately 50 % of the patients who have had two excisional procedures; about 10 % needed three staged serial operations. To date, about 40 % of our patients have had one procedure, but later analysis is necessary to determine whether further operations are needed.

Conclusions

Lymphedema is a rare disease; however, the patient population that it affects as well as the surgical intervention is well described. Through a thoughtful approach to these patients, functional activity can be restored, infections can be reduced, and psychological functioning can be restored.

Most young patients with lymphedema of the lower limbs are managed conservatively with elastic support, elevation, hygiene, and massage. Non-operative measures should be exhausted before an operation is contemplated, since no procedure is curative. All patients with lymphedema must be followed annually, or more often as necessary. They will require support stockings for life regardless of whether or not they have an ablative procedure. Full activity should be encouraged. Infections, bacterial and fungal, should be avoided if possible by daily hygienic care. Vigorous therapy should be instituted at early signs of inflammation of an involved area to prevent further damage to the lymphatics.

All the operated patients have been improved and have a more normal appearance. Staged subcutaneous excision remains the procedure of choice in moderate to severe lymphedema in children and adults regardless of etiology nevertheless an ablative procedure is not curative. Studies done postoperatively with labeled serum albumin demonstrate significantly increased clearance after 1 year in the operated extremity. This finding could be evidence of utilization of new pathways of lymph drainage. Early appearance of the radioactive albumin in the groin after injection into the foot may be due to traumatic lympho-venous anastomosis.

References

1. Feins NR. Surgical management of patients with lymphedema. Surg Rounds. 1997;20(2):63–72.
2. Lanz O. Eröffnung neuer Abfuhrwege bei Stauung in Bauch und unteren Extremitäten. Zentralbl Chir. 1911;38:153.
3. Kondoleon E. Die Dauerresulate der chirurgischen Behandlung der elefantiastischen Lymphodeme. Munch Med Wochenschr. 1915;62:541.
4. Sistrunk WE. Contribution to plastic surgery. Certain modifications of the Kondoleon operation for elephantiasis. Ann Surg. 1927;85:185.
5. Ghormley RK, Overton LM. Surgical treatment of severe forms of lymphedema of the extremities. Surg Gynecol Obstret. 1935;61:83.
6. Charles RH, Latham A, English TC, editors. A system of treatment. London: Churchill; 1912.
7. Pratt GH. Surgical correction of lymphedema; application of a new operative technique in lymph stasis and allied conditions. J Am Med Assoc. 1953;151(11): 888–91.
8. Epstein J, Mendelsohn G. Squamous carcinoma of the foot arising in association with long-standing verrucous hyperplasia in a patient with congenital lymphedema. Cancer. 1984;54:943.
9. Dale WA. The swollen leg. Curr Prob Surg Chicago: Gen Med Pub Inc; 1973.
10. Homans J. The treatment of elephantiasis of the legs, preliminary report. N Engl J Med. 1936;215:1099.
11. Auchincloss H. New operation for elephantiasis. Puerto Rico J Publ Health Trop Med. 1930;6:149.

12. Feins NR, Rubin R, Crais T, et al. Surgical management of thirthy-nine children with lymphedema. J Pediatr Surg. 1977;12:471.
13. Fonkalsrud EW, Coulson WF. Management of congenital lymphedema in infants and children. Ann Surg. 1973;177:280.
14. Miller TA, Harper J, Longmire Jr WP. The management of lymphedema by staged subcutaneous excision. Surg Gynecol Obstet. 1973;136:586.
15. Eryilmaz T, Kaya B, Ozmen S, Kandal S. Suction-assisted lipectomy for treatment of lower-extremity lymphedema. Aesthetic Plast Surg. 2009;4:671.
16. Feins NR, Greene AK. Primary lymphedema. In: Mulliken JB, Burrows PE, Fishman SJ, editors. Vascular anomalies: hemangiomas and malformations. 2nd ed. New York: Oxford University Press; 2013. p. 1056–76.
17. Kinmonth JB, Taylor GW, Tracy GD, Marsh JD. Primary lymphedema: clinical and lymphangiographic studies of a series of 107 patients in which the lower limbs were affected. Br J Surg. 1957;45:1–9.
18. Thompson N. Surgical treatment of chronic lymphodema of the lower limb with preliminary report of new operation. Br Med J. 1962;2:1566–73.
19. Harvey RF. The use of I131 labeled human serum albumin in the assessment of improved lymph flow following buried dermis flap operation in cases of post-mastectomy lymphoedema of the arm. Br J Radiol. 1969;42:260.
20. Miller TA, Wyatt LE, Rudkin GH. Staged skin and subcutaneous excision for lymphedema: a favorable report of long-term results. Plast Reconstr Surg. 1998;102:1486.

Håkan Brorson, Barbro Svensson, and Karin Ohlin

Key Points

- Excess arm or leg volume without pitting implies that excess adipose tissue is present.
- Excess adipose tissue can be removed by the use of liposuction. Conservative treatment and microsurgical reconstructions cannot remove adipose tissue.
- As in conservative treatment, the lifelong use (24 h a day) of custom made, flat knitted compression garments is mandatory for maintaining the effect of surgery.
- Patients that are happy with an excess volume in the arm or leg are not candidates for liposuction.
- Liposuction is a potent therapeutical modality for special indications in persistent primary and secondary lymphedema. The treatment is embedded within a multidisciplinary team and centralized in an expert center.

H. Brorson, M.D., Ph.D. (✉)
B. Svensson, B.S., P.T., L.T. • K. Ohlin, B.S., O.T.
The Lymphedema Unit, Department of Clinical Sciences, Lund University, Plastic and Reconstructive Surgery, Jan Waldenströms gata 18, 2nd floor, Skåne University Hospital, SE-205 02 Malmo, Sweden
e-mail: hakan.brorson@med.lu.se
http://www.plasticsurg.nu

Introduction

The various types of treatment of lymphedema are under discussion, and there has been some controversy regarding liposuction for lymphedema. Although it is clear that conservative therapies such as complex decongestive therapy (CDT) and controlled compression therapy (CCT) should be tried in the first instance, options for the treatment of late-stage lymphedema that is not responding to such treatment is not so clear. Improvements in technique, patient preparation, and patient follow-up have led to a greater and a wider acceptance of liposuction as a treatment for lymphedema. This chapter outlines the benefits of using liposuction and presents the evidence to support its use.

There is an increasing body of evidence, based on well-controlled clinical trials and long-term follow-up, that liposuction can result in significant objective and subjective benefit to patients who have long-term chronic lymphedema [1, 2]. There are, however, different views on the immediate, short-term, and long-term benefits of liposuction for treating lymphedema, with a strong dichotomy between those who support surgical and conservative treatments.

A.K. Greene et al. (eds.), *Lymphedema: Presentation, Diagnosis, and Treatment*,
DOI 10.1007/978-3-319-14493-1_28, © Springer International Publishing Switzerland 2015

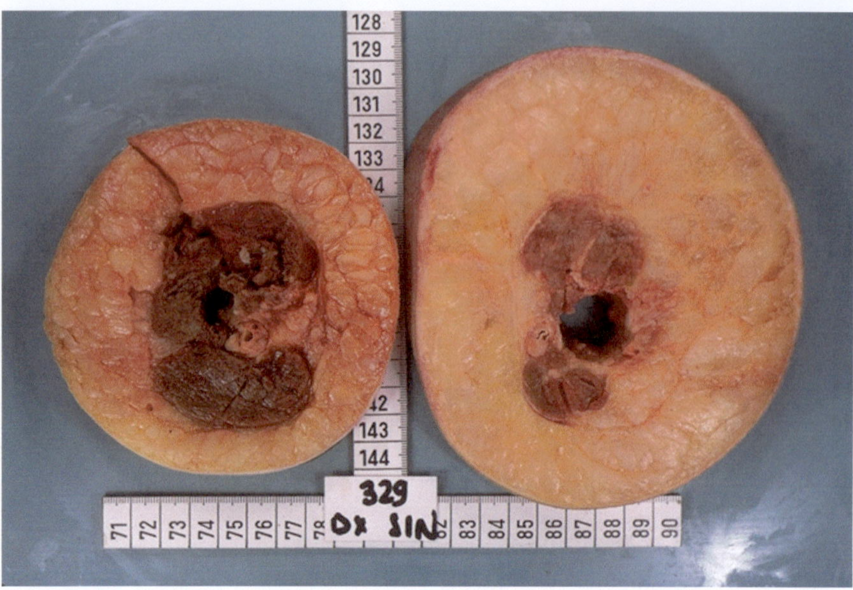

Fig. 28.1 Cross sections of a lymphedematous (*right*) and a normal arm (*left*) showing abundance of excess adipose tissue in the affected arm. Courtesy of Dr. C.H. Håkansson, Department of Oncology, Skåne University Hospital, Lund (the author has rights to use image with permission)

Excess Subcutaneous Adiposity and Chronic Lymphedema

The incidence of post-mastectomy arm lymphedema varies between 6 and 49 %, depending on the combination of therapy, including mastectomy, sentinel node biopsy, standard axillary lymph node dissection, and/or postoperative irradiation [3–5].

The outcome of the surgical procedure as well as of the irradiation of the tissue often results in the destruction of lymphatic vessels. When this is combined with the removal of lymph nodes and tissue scarring, the lymphatic vessels that remain are likely to be unable to remove the load of lymph. The remaining lymph collectors become dilated and overloaded and their valves become incompetent, preventing the lymphatics from performing their function. This failure spreads distally until even the most peripheral lymph vessels, draining into the affected system, also become dilated [6].

The enlargement of the arm leads to discomfort and complaints in the form of heaviness, weakness [7], pain, tension, and a sensory deficit of the limb, as well as anxiety, psychological morbidity, maladjustment, and social isolation [8, 9], and increasing hardness of the limb [10]. In time, there is also an increase in the adipose tissue content of the swollen arm. We have observed this clinically since 1987, when the first lymphedema patient was operated on [11, 12]. Figure 28.1 shows a picture of excess fat volume in the lymphedematous arm taken in the 1960s; still this phenomenon was never brought up in the literature.

Presently there is no cure for lymphedema. With early diagnosis, the majority of patients can be treated by conservative treatment, such as complex decongestive therapy (CDT) [13], which comprises manual lymph drainage, compression therapy, physical exercise, skin care and self-management, followed by wearing flat knitted compression garments. The effect of CDT on long-standing massive edema with excess adipose tissue is poor, since adipose tissue does not disappear by means of compression alone. In addition, surgical intervention is reserved for patients with excess volume and heaviness causing severe strain in the shoulder and neck, functional impairment, recurrent attacks of erysipelas, and problems with clothing fit.

For the treatment of late-stage lymphedema that does not respond to conservative treatment, liposuction combined with postoperative, life-long effective compression therapy has become a viable alternative. Postoperative follow-up and regular adjustment of the compression technology is mandatory.

There are various possible explanations for the adipose tissue hypertrophy. There is a physiological imbalance of blood flow and lymphatic drainage, resulting in the impaired clearance of lipids and their uptake by macrophages [14]. However, there is increasing support, for the view that the fat cell is not simply a container of fat, but is an endocrine organ and a cytokine-activated cell [15, 16] and that chronic inflammation plays a role here [15, 17]. The same pathophysiology applies for primary and secondary leg lymphedema. Recent research showed a relationship between slow lymph flow and adiposity, as well as that between structural changes in the lymphatic system and adiposity [18, 19].

From a more clinical view, other indications for adipose tissue hypertrophy have been found:

- Consecutive analyses of the content of the aspirate by the author, removed under bloodless conditions using a tourniquet, showed a very high content of adipose tissue in 44 women with post-mastectomy arm lymphedema (mean 90 %, range 58–100) [20]. This has been confirmed by Damstra et al.'s [21] study of 37 patients with end-stage breast cancer related lymphedema where the proportion of fat in the aspirate (when a tourniquet was used) was 93 % (range 59–100 %). The same outcome was shown in a study by Schaverien et al. in 12 patients with arm lymphedema following breast cancer treatment with 92 % (range, 75–100) of fat in the aspirate [22].

- Analyses with dual X-ray absorptiometry (DXA) in 18 women with arm lymphedema following a mastectomy showed a significant increase of adipose (73 %) and muscle tissue (47 %), and even bone mineral content (7 %) in the non-pitting swollen arm before surgery. The greater weight of the affected arm leads to a higher mechanical load on both the muscle and the skeleton, resulting in increased muscle and bone mass. There was no correlation between the duration of lymphedema and the amount of excess adipose, muscle, or bone tissue. This indicates that the increase in soft tissue volume develops when the lymphedema appears or soon thereafter [23].

- Preoperative investigation with volume-rendered computer tomography (VRCT) in 11 women showed a significant preoperative increase of adipose tissue in the swollen arm, the excess volume consisting of 81 % (range 68–96) fat [24].

- Tonometry findings in 20 women with post-mastectomy arm lymphedema showed postoperative changes in the upper arm, but not in the forearm, which also showed significantly higher absolute values than in the upper arm. This is probably caused by the high adipose tissue content with little or no free fluid, as in the normal arm. The thinner subcutaneous tissue in the forearm may also play a part [25].

- The findings of increased adipose tissue in intestinal segments in patients with Crohn's disease, known as "fat wrapping," have clearly shown that inflammation plays an important role [17, 26, 27].

- A major problem in Graves's ophthalmopathy is an increase in the intraorbital adipose tissue volume leading to exophthalmos. Overexpression of adipocyte-related immediate early genes in active ophthalmopathy and cysteine-rich, angiogenic inducer 61 (CYR61) may have a role in both orbital inflammation and adipogenesis and serve as a marker of disease activity [28].

- Recent research had showed that adipogenesis in response to lymphatic fluid stasis was associated with a marked mononuclear cell inflammatory response [29], and that lymphatic fluid stasis potently upregulates the expression of fat differentiation markers both spatially and temporally [30].

The common understanding among clinicians is that the swelling of a lymphedematous extremity is due purely to the accumulation of lymph fluid, which can be removed by use of noninvasive conservative regimens such as CDT.

Microsurgery and lympho-venous anastomosis (LVA) have been studied for a long time without convincing results [31]. Although the LVA has been performed and studied for more than three decades, this method still has not had a breakthrough and will never become a treatment of choice in daily practice. In a large overview article by Campisi et al. [32], a positive effect was described in early stages of lymphedema. However, for later, more irreversible stages, this therapeutic option was not suitable. Moreover, a recent study showed that the net effect of LVA was minor and that the outcome was due to the CDT performed preoperatively and postoperatively [33].

Brorson et al. [12] concluded that when the excess volume is dominated by adipose tissue, supra-facial clearance by liposuction is the only method to achieve up to 100 % excess volume reduction.

Today, chronic non-pitting arm lymphedema of up to 4 l in excess can be effectively removed by use of liposuction and compression therapy, without any further reduction in lymph transport [34]. Long-term results, up to 15 years, have not shown any recurrence of the arm swelling. Complete reduction is mostly achieved in between 3 and 6 months, often earlier (see Figs. 28.2 and 28.3) [12, 35].

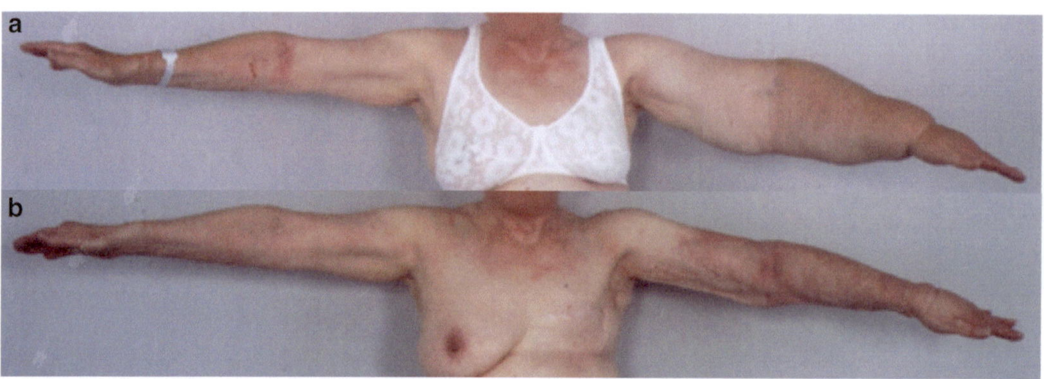

Fig. 28.2 (**a**) A 74-year-old woman with a non-pitting arm lymphedema for 15 years. Preoperative excess volume was 3,090 ml. © *Håkan Brorson*. (**b**) Postoperative result. © *Håkan Brorson*

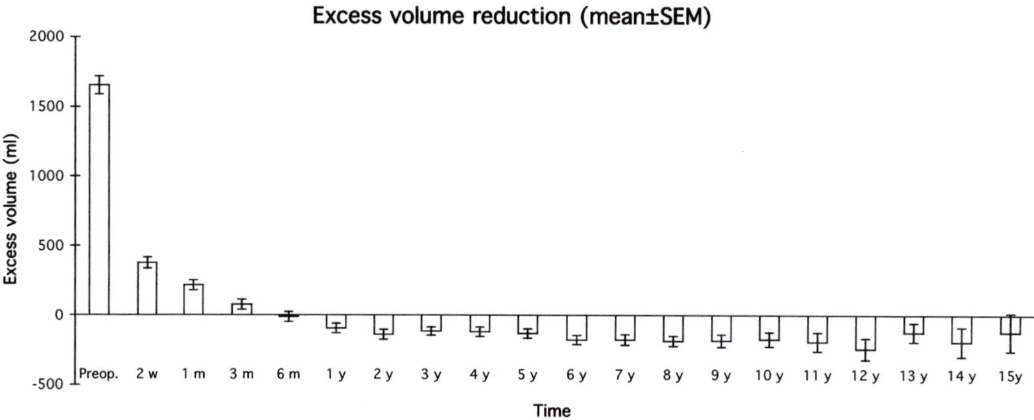

Fig. 28.3 Mean (±SEM) postoperative excess volume reduction in 116 women with arm lymphedema following breast cancer. © *Håkan Brorson*

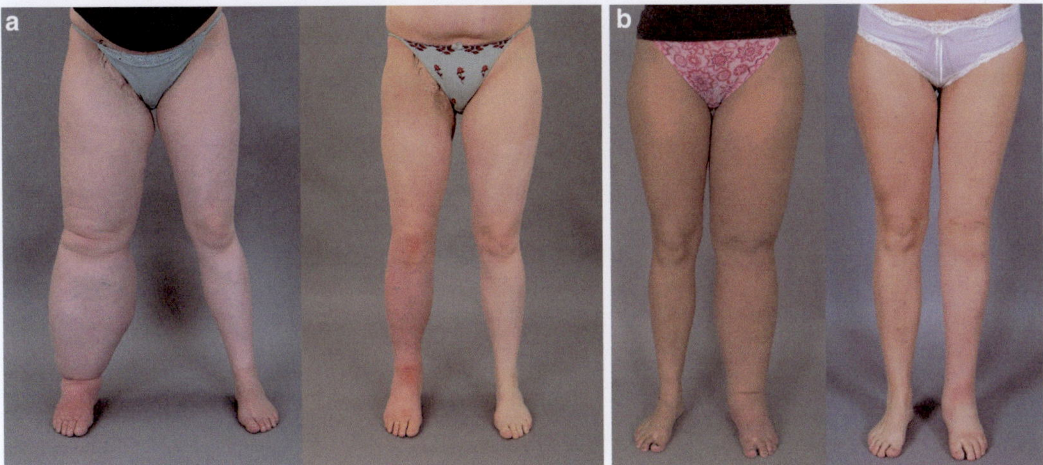

Fig. 28.4 (**a**) Secondary lymphedema: Preoperative excess volume 7,070 ml (*left*). Postoperative result after 6 months where excess volume is –445 ml, i.e., the treated leg is somewhat smaller than the normal one (*right*).

© *Håkan Brorson*. (**b**) Primary lymphedema: Preoperative excess volume 6,630 ml (*left*). Postoperative result after 2 years where excess volume is 30 ml (*right*). © *Håkan Brorson*

In 2009 Damstra et al. [21] reproduced these results in a large study with 37 breast cancer-related lymphedema patients. A recent publication from 2012 with a 5-year follow-up in 12 patients with breast cancer related lymphedema confirmed no recurrence with this technique [22]. Promising results can also be achieved for leg lymphedema, for which complete reduction is usually reached at around 6 months (see Figs. 28.4a, b) [36, 37].

Liposuction

Surgical Technique

Made-to-measure compression garments (two sleeves and two gloves) are measured and ordered 2 weeks before surgery, using the healthy arm and hand as a template. Nowadays we use power-assisted liposuction because the vibrating cannula facilitates the liposuction, especially in the leg, which is more demanding to treat. Initially the "dry technique" was used [38]. Later, to minimize blood loss, a tourniquet was utilized in combination with tumescence, which involves infiltration of 1–2 l of saline containing low-dose adrenaline and lignocaine [39, 40].

Through approximately 10–15, 3-mm-long incisions, liposuction is performed using 15- and 25-cm-long cannulas with diameters of 3 and 4 mm (see Figs. 28.5 and 28.6). Liposuction is executed circumferentially, step-by-step from wrist to shoulder, and the hypertrophied fat is removed as completely as possible (see Figs. 28.5, 28.6, and 28.7).

When the arm distal to the tourniquet has been treated, a sterilized made-to-measure compression sleeve is applied (Jobst¨ Elvarex BSN medical, compression class 2) to the arm to stem bleeding and reduce postoperative edema. A sterilized, standard interim glove (Cicatrex interim, Thuasne¨, France) in which the tips of the fingers have been cut to facilitate gripping, is put on the hand. The tourniquet is removed and the most proximal part of the upper arm is treated using the tumescent technique [39, 40]. Finally, the proximal part of the compression sleeve is pulled up to compress the proximal part of the upper arm. The incisions are left open to drain through the sleeve. The arm is lightly wrapped with a large absorbent compress covering the whole arm (60×60 cm, Cover-Dri, www.attends.co.uk). The arm is kept at heart level on a large pillow. The compress is changed when needed.

The following day, a standard gauntlet (i.e., a glove without fingers, but with a thumb; Jobst Elvarex compression class 2) is put over the interim glove after the thumb of the gauntlet has been cut off to ease the pressure on the thumb.

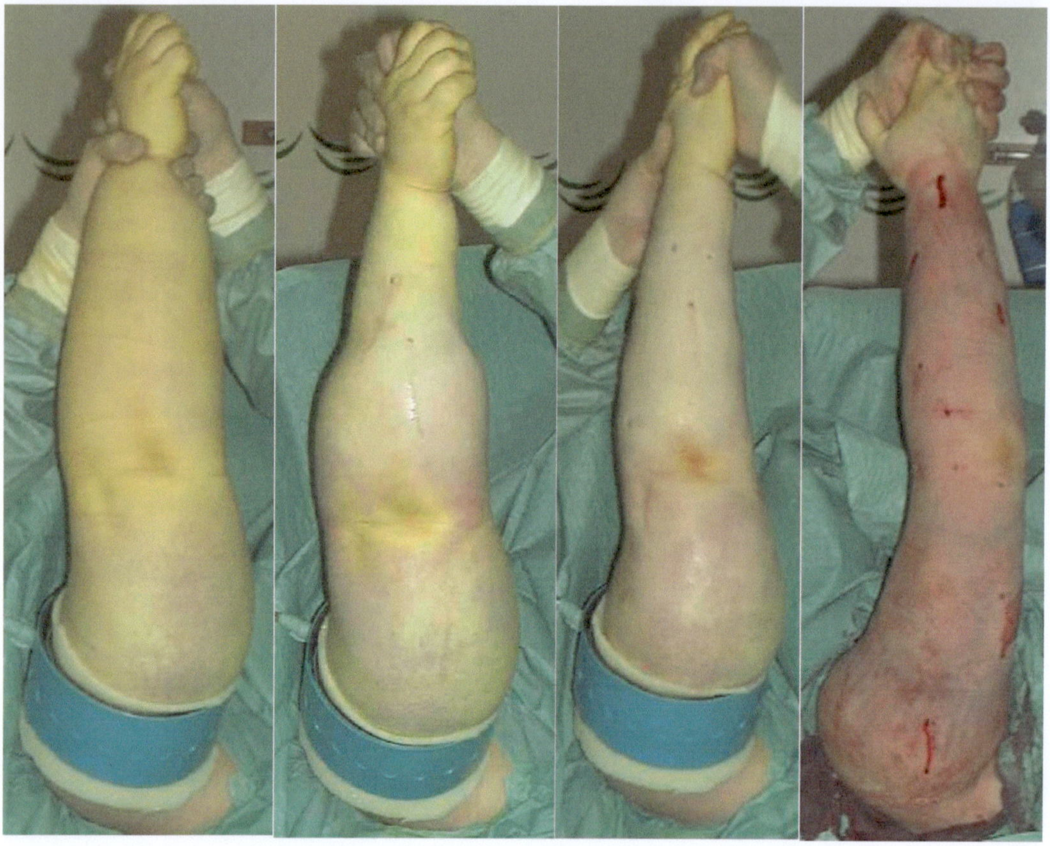

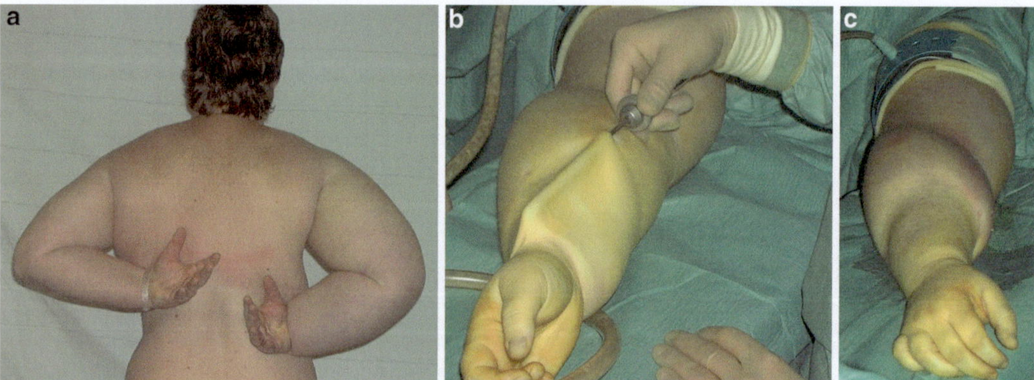

Fig. 28.5 Liposuction of arm lymphedema. The procedure takes about 2 h. From preoperative to postoperative state (*left* to *right*). Note the tourniquet, which has been removed at the right, and the concomitant reactive hyperemia. © *Håkan Brorson*

Fig. 28.6 (**a**) Preoperative picture showing a patient with a large lymphedema (2,865 ml) and decreased mobility of the right arm. © *Håkan Brorson*. (**b**) The cannula lifts the loose skin of the treated forearm. (**c**) The distal half of the forearm has been treated. Note the sharp border between treated (distal forearm) and untreated (proximal arm) area. © *Håkan Brorson*

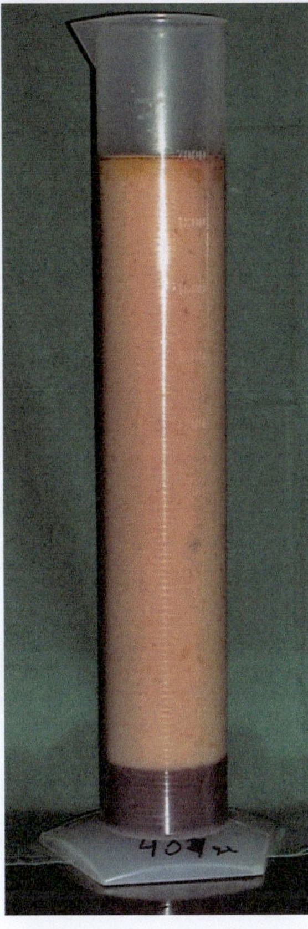

Fig. 28.7 The aspirate contains 90–100 % adipose tissue in general. This picture shows the aspirate collected from the lymphedematous arm of the patient shown in Figs. 28.4, 28.5, and 28.7 before removal of the tourniquet. The aspirate sediments into an upper adipose fraction (90 %) and a lower fluid (lymph) fraction (10 %). © *Håkan Brorson*

If the gauntlet is put on straight after surgery, it can exert too much pressure on the hand when the patient is still not able to move the fingers after the anesthesia. Operating time is, on average, 2 h. An isoxazolylpenicillin or a cephalosporin is given intravenously for the first 24 h and then in tablet form until incisions are healed, about 10–14 days after surgery. Liposuction technique for leg lymphedema is similar to that for the arm.

Postoperative Care

Garments are removed 2 days postoperatively so that the patient can take a shower. Then, the other set of garments is put on and the used set is

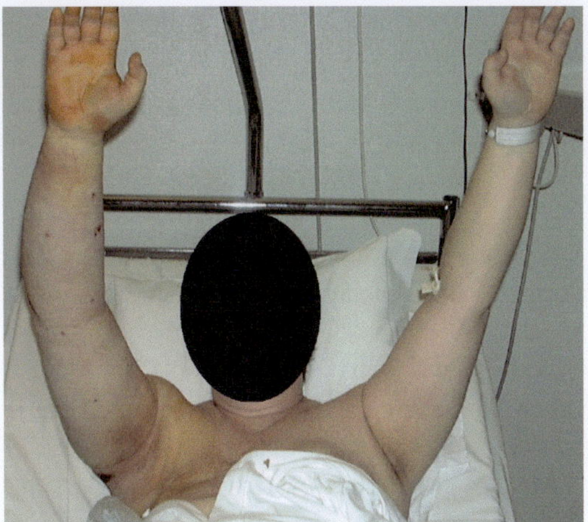

Fig. 28.8 The compression garment is removed two days after surgery so that the patient can take a shower. When bandages are used, at the first bandage change, made-to-measure, flat knitted garment are measured and ordered. Then, the other set of garments is put on and the used set is washed and dried or the arm is re-bandaged. A significant reduction of the right arm has been achieved, as compared with the preoperative condition seen in Fig. 28.6a. © *Håkan Brorson*

washed and dried. The patient repeats this after another 2 days before discharge. The standard glove and gauntlet is usually changed to the made-to-measure glove at the end of the hospital stay (Fig. 28.8).

The patient alternates between the two sets of garments (1 set = 1 sleeve and 1 glove) during the 2 weeks postoperatively, changing them daily or every other day so that a clean set is always put on after showering and lubricating the arm. After the 2-week control, the garments are changed every day after being washed. Washing "activates" the garment by increasing the compression due to shrinkage.

Controlled Compression Therapy (CCT)

A prerequisite to maintaining the effect of liposuction and, for that matter, conservative treatment, is the continuous use of a compression garment [12]. Compression therapy is crucial, and its application is therefore thoroughly described and discussed at the first clinical evaluation. If the patient has any doubts about continued CCT, she is not accepted for treatment. After initiating compression therapy, the custom-made garment is taken in, when needed, at each visit using a sewing machine, to compensate for reduced elasticity and reduced arm volume.

This is most important during the first 3 months when the most notable changes in volume occur. At the 1- and 3-month visits, the arm is measured for new custom-made garments (two sets). This procedure is repeated at 6, (9), and 12 months. If complete reduction has been achieved at 6 months, the 9-month control may be omitted. If this is the case, remember to prescribe garments for 6 months, which normally means double the amount than would be needed for 3 months. It is important, however, to take in the garment repeatedly to compensate for wear and tear.

This may require additional visits in some instances, although the patient can often make such adjustments herself. When the excess volume has decreased as much as possible and a steady state is achieved, new garments can be prescribed using the latest measurements. In this way, the garments are renewed three or four times during the first year. Two sets of sleeve-and-glove garments are always at the patient's disposal; one being worn while the other is washed. Thus, a garment is worn permanently, and treatment is interrupted only briefly when showering and, possibly, for formal social occasions. The patient is informed about the importance of hygiene and skin care, as all patients with lymphedema are susceptible to infections, and keeping the skin clean and soft is a prophylactic measure [11, 12].

The life span of two garments worn alternately is usually 4–6 months. Complete reduction is usually achieved after 3–6 months, often earlier. After the first year, the patient is seen again after 6 months (1.5 years after surgery) and then at 2 years after surgery. Then the patient is seen once a year only, when new garments are prescribed for the coming year, usually four garments and four gloves (or four gauntlets). For very active patients, six to eight garments and the same amount of gauntlets/gloves a year are needed. Patients without preoperative swelling of the hand can usually stop using the glove/gauntlet after 6–12 months postoperatively.

For legs, the author's team often uses up to two, sometimes three compression garments, on top of each other, depending on what is needed to prevent pitting. A typical example is Elvarex˘ compression class 3 (or 3 Forte), and Elvarex˘ compression class 2 (BSN Medical); the latter being a below-the-knee garment. Sometimes a leg-long Jobst Bellavar˘ compression class 2 (or Elvarex˘ compression class 2) is added when needed. Thus, such a patient needs two sets of two to three garments/set. One set is worn while the other is washed. Depending on the age and activity of the patient, two such sets usually lasts for (2–)4 months. That means that they must be prescribed 3(–6) times during the first year. After complete reduction has been achieved, usually at around 6 months, the patient is seen once a year when all new garments are prescribed for the coming year. During night only one leg-long garment is used.

CCT can also be used primarily to effectively treat a pitting edema as an alternative to CDT, which, in contrast to CCT, comprises daily interventions [12] (see Chap. 18).

Arm Volume Measurements

Arm volumes are recorded for each patient using the water displacement technique. The displaced water is weighed on a balance to the nearest 5 g, corresponding to 5 mL. Both arms are always measured at each visit, and the difference in arm volumes is designated as the edema volume. The decrease in the edema volume is calculated in a percentage of the preoperative value [11].

The Lymphedema Team

To investigate and treat patients with lymphedema, a team comprising a plastic surgeon, an occupational therapist, a physiotherapist, and a social welfare officer is needed. An hour is reserved for each scheduled visit to the team when arm volumes are measured, garments are adjusted or renewed, the social circumstances are assessed, and other matters of concern are discussed.

The patient is also encouraged to contact the team whenever any unexpected problems arise, so that these can be tackled without delay. In retrospect, a working group such as this one seems to be a prerequisite both for thorough preoperative consideration and informing patients and for successful maintenance of immediate postoperative improvements. The team also monitors the long-term outcome, and the authors' experience so far indicates that a visit once a year is necessary, in most cases, to maintain a good functional and cosmetic result after complete reduction.

Why Does Liposuction Help?

If the lymphedema is treated immediately by conservative regimens, the swelling can disappear. If not, or improperly treated, the swelling increases in time and can end up in an even larger pitting edema with concomitant adipose tissue formation, which starts early when the lymphedema appears or soon thereafter [23].

For many patients with lymphedema conservative treatment does not work well or come up to their expectations, and no matter what therapy they receive, neither conservative treatment nor microsurgical procedures can remove excess adipose tissue [31–33, 41–44]. Subcutaneous tissue debulking seems the only option to reduce the limb volume and lead to an improvement in the patient's quality of life [10].

Lymph Transport System and Liposuction

To investigate the effect of liposuction on lymph transport, the authors conducted an investigation using indirect lymphoscintigraphy in 20 patients with post-mastectomy arm lymphedema. Scintigraphies were performed before liposuction, with and without wearing a garment. This was repeated after 3 and 12 months. In conclusion, it was found that the already decreased lymph transport was not further reduced after liposuction [34].

When to Use Liposuction to Treat Lymphedema

Especially for more extended stages of lymphedema with irreversible changes; nonoperative treatment will give inappropriate reduction of volume and complaints. For these people conservative treatment does not work well or come up to their expectations, and no matter what therapy they receive, neither conservative treatment nor microsurgical procedures can remove excess adipose tissue [31–33, 41–44]. Subcutaneous tissue debulking seems the only option to reduce the limb volume and to lead to an improvement in the patient's quality of life. As patients treated by conservative treatment also need a life garment, this issue is the same for both groups.

A surgical approach, with the intention of removing the hypertrophied adipose tissue, seems logic when conservative treatment has not achieved satisfactory edema reduction and the patient has subjective discomfort of a heavy arm. This condition is especially seen in chronic, large arm lymphedema around 1 l in volume, or when the volume ratio (edematous arm/healthy arm) is 1.3.

Contraindications for Liposuction

Liposuction should never be performed in a patient who is not maximal conservatively treated. Clinical features show pits on pressure (Fig. 28.9a). In a patient with an arm lymphedema, the author accepts around 4–5 mm of pitting, and in a leg lymphedema 6–7 mm. Patients with more pitting should be treated conservatively until the pitting has been reduced. The reason for not doing liposuction in a pitting edema is that liposuction is a method to remove fat, not fluid, even if theoretically it could remove all the accumulated fluid in a pitting lymphedema without excess adipose tissue formation.

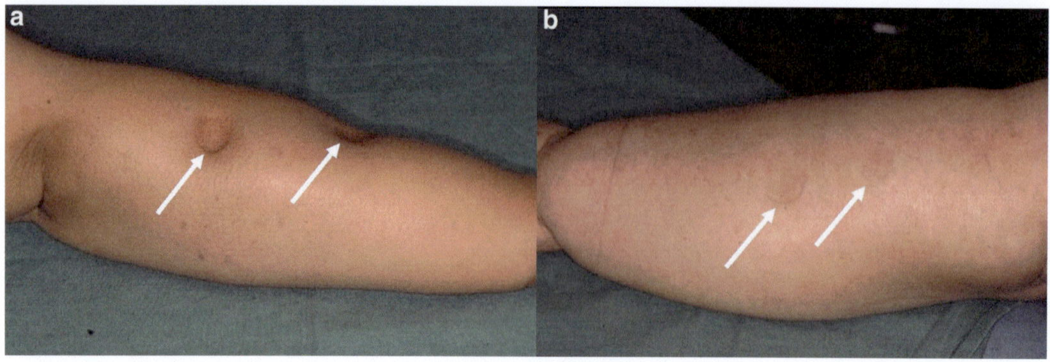

Fig. 28.9 (**a**) Marked lymphedema of the arm after breast cancer treatment, showing pitting several centimeters in depth (grade I edema). The arm swelling is dominated by the presence of fluid, i.e., the accumulation of lymph. © *Håkan Brorson.* (**b**) Pronounced arm lymphedema after breast cancer treatment (grade II edema). There is no pitting in spite of hard pressure by the thumb for 1 min. A slight reddening is seen at the two spots where pressure has been exerted. The "edema" is completely dominated by adipose tissue. The term "edema" is improper at this stage since the swelling is dominated by hypertrophied adipose tissue and not by lymph. At this stage, the aspirate contains either no, or a minimal amount of lymph. © *Håkan Brorson*

Other contraindications for liposuction are:
- Metastatic disease or open wounds
- Medical or family history of coagulation disorders or intake of drugs that affect coagulation
- Physically not fit for surgery
- Patient reluctant to wear compression garments continuously after surgery

The first and most important goal is to transform a pitting edema into a non-pitting one by conservative regimens such as CDT or CCT. "Pitting" means that a depression is formed after pressure on the edematous tissue by the fingertip, resulting in lymph being squeezed into the surroundings (see Fig. 28.9a). To standardize the pitting test, one presses *as hard as possible* with the thumb on the region to be investigated for 1 min, the amount of depression being estimated in millimeters. A swelling that is dominated by hypertrophied adipose tissue shows little or no pitting (see Fig. 28.9b) [45].

Stemmer's sign implies that you can pinch the skin at the base of the toes or fingers with difficulty or not at all. This is due to increased fibrosis and is characteristic for chronic lymphedema. On the other hand, a negative sign does not exclude lymphedema. The author has not seen any relationship between either a positive or negative sign and the occurrence of adipose tissue.

When a patient has been treated conservatively and shows no pitting, liposuction can be performed. If quality of life is low, this can be especially effective. The cancer itself is a worry, but the swollen and heavy arm introduces an additional handicap for the patient from a physical, psychosocial, and psychological point of view. Physical problems include pain, limited limb movement, and physical mobility and problems with clothing, thus interfering with everyday activities. Also, the heavy and swollen arm is impractical and cosmetically unappealing, all of which contribute to emotional distress [10].

Benefits to the Patient

Liposuction improves patients' quality of life, particularly qualities associated with everyday activities, and hence those that can be directly related to the complete arm edema reduction [10]. CCT is also beneficial, but the effect is less obvious than when combined with surgery, conceivably because the reduction of excess volume is less [12].

Skin blood flow and cellulitis after liposuction reduces the incidence of erysipelas; the annual incidence of cellulitis was 0.4 before liposuction and 0.1 after. Improved local skin blood flow may be an important contributing factor to the reduced episodes of arm infection [46]. The point of bacterial entry may be a minor injury to the edematous skin, and impaired skin blood flow may respond inadequately to counteract impending infection. Reducing the excess volume by liposuction increases skin blood flow in the arm, and decreases the reservoir of adipose tissue, which may enhance bacterial overgrowth.

Potential Negative Effects to the Patient

Liposuction typically leads to numbness in the skin, which disappears within 3–6 months. Continuous, that is, lifelong wearing of compression garments is a prerequisite of maintaining the effect of any lymphedema treatment and should not be considered as a negative effect.

Conclusion

Liposuction combined with permanent compression therapy is a proven effective treatment. The technique can be a potent therapeutic modality within an integrated, multidisciplinary lymphological care program. Accumulated lymph should be initially removed using the well-documented conservative regimens until minimal or no pitting is seen. If there is still a significant excess volume, this can be removed by the use of liposuction. In some patients increased fibrous tissue can be present, especially in male patients and in women with a male distribution of body fat. When seen, fibrous tissue is more common in leg than in arm lymphedema, and more common in men than in women. Continuous wearing of a compression garment prevents recurrence.

References

1. Brorson H, Ohlin K, Olsson G, Svensson B. Liposuction of leg lymphedema: preliminary 2 year results. Lymphology. 2007;40(Suppl):250–2.
2. Brorson H, Ohlin K, Olsson G, Svensson B. Long term cosmetic and functional results following liposuction for arm lymphedema: an eleven year study. Lymphology. 2007;40(Suppl):253–5.
3. Segerstrom K, Bjerle P, Graffman S, Nystrom A. Factors that influence the incidence of brachial oedema after treatment of breast cancer. Scand J Plast Reconstr Surg Hand Surg. 1992;26(2):223–7.
4. Petrek JA, Senie RT, Peters M, Rosen PP. Lymphedema in a cohort of breast carcinoma survivors 20 years after diagnosis. Cancer. 2001;92(6):1368–77.
5. Mansel RE, Fallowfield L, Kissin M, Goyal A, Newcombe RG, Dixon JM, et al. Randomized multicenter trial of sentinel node biopsy versus standard axillary treatment in operable breast cancer: the ALMANAC Trial. J Natl Cancer Inst. 2006;98(9): 599–609.
6. Olszewski WL. Lymph stasis: pathophysiology, diagnosis and treatment. 1st ed. Boca Raton: CRC; 1991. p. 648.
7. Johansson K, Piller N. Weight-bearing exercise and its impact on arm lymphoedema. J Lymphoedema. 2007;2(1):15–22.
8. Ridner SH. Quality of life and a symptom cluster associated with breast cancer treatment-related lymphedema. Support Care Cancer. 2005;13(11):904–11.
9. Piller NB, Thelander A. Treatment of chronic postmastectomy lymphedema with low level laser therapy: a 2.5 year follow-up. Lymphology. 1998;31(2):74–86.
10. Brorson H, Ohlin K, Olsson G, Långström G, Wiklund I, Svensson H. Quality of life following liposuction and conservative treatment of arm lymphedema. Lymphology. 2006;39(1):8–25.
11. Brorson H, Svensson H. Complete reduction of lymphoedema of the arm by liposuction after breast cancer. Scand J Plast Reconstr Surg Hand Surg. 1997;31(2):137–43.
12. Brorson H, Svensson H. Liposuction combined with controlled compression therapy reduces arm lymphedema more effectively than controlled compression therapy alone. Plast Reconstr Surg. 1998;102(4):1058–67. discussion 68.
13. Rockson SG, Miller LT, Senie R, Brennan MJ, Casley-Smith JR, Foldi E, et al. American Cancer Society Lymphedema Workshop. Workgroup III: diagnosis and management of lymphedema. Cancer. 1998;83(12):2882–5.
14. Ryan TJ. Lymphatics and adipose tissue. Clin Dermatol. 1995;13(5):493–8.
15. Sadler D, Mattacks CA, Pond CM. Changes in adipocytes and dendritic cells in lymph node containing adipose depots during and after many weeks of mild inflammation. J Anat. 2005;207(6):769–81.
16. Pond CM. Adipose tissue and the immune system. Prostaglandins Leukot Essent Fatty Acids. 2005; 73(1):17–30.
17. Borley NR, Mortensen NJ, Jewell DP, Warren BF. The relationship between inflammatory and serosal connective tissue changes in ileal Crohn's disease: evidence for a possible causative link. J Pathol. 2000; 190(2):196–202.
18. Harvey NL, Srinivasan RS, Dillard ME, Johnson NC, Witte MH, Boyd K, et al. Lymphatic vascular defects promoted by Prox1 haploinsufficiency cause adult-onset obesity. Nat Genet. 2005;37(10):1072–81.

19. Schneider M, Conway EM, Carmeliet P. Lymph makes you fat. Nat Genet. 2005;37(10):1023–4.
20. Brorson H, Åberg M, Svensson H. Chronic lymphedema and adipocyte proliferation: clinical therapeutic implications. Lymphology. 2004;37(Suppl):153–5.
21. Damstra RJ, Voesten HG, Klinkert P, Brorson H. Circumferential suction-assisted lipectomy for lymphoedema after surgery for breast cancer. Br J Surg. 2009;96(8):859–64.
22. Schaverien MV, Munro KJ, Baker PA, Munnoch DA. Liposuction for chronic lymphoedema of the upper limb: 5 years of experience. J Plast Reconstr Aesthet Surg. 2012;65(7):935–42.
23. Brorson H, Ohlin K, Olsson G, Karlsson MK. Breast cancer-related chronic arm lymphedema is associated with excess adipose and muscle tissue. Lymphat Res Biol. 2009;7(1):3–10.
24. Brorson H, Ohlin K, Olsson G, Nilsson M. Adipose tissue dominates chronic arm lymphedema following breast cancer: an analysis using volume rendered CT images. Lymphat Res Biol. 2006;4(4):199–210.
25. Bagheri S, Ohlin K, Olsson G, Brorson H. Tissue tonometry before and after liposuction of arm lymphedema following breast cancer. Lymphat Res Biol. 2005;3(2):66–80.
26. Jones B, Fishman EK, Hamilton SR, Rubesin SE, Bayless TM, Cameron JC, et al. Submucosal accumulation of fat in inflammatory bowel disease: CT/pathologic correlation. J Comput Assist Tomogr. 1986;10:759–63.
27. Sheehan AL, Warren BF, Gear MW, Shepherd NA. Fat-wrapping in Crohn's disease: pathological basis and relevance to surgical practice. Br J Surg. 1992;79(9):955–8.
28. Lantz M, Vondrichova T, Parikh H, Frenander C, Ridderstrale M, Asman P, et al. Overexpression of immediate early genes in active Graves' ophthalmopathy. J Clin Endocrinol Metab. 2005;90(8):4784–91.
29. Zampell JC, Aschen S, Weitman ES, Yan A, Elhadad S, De Brot M, et al. Regulation of adipogenesis by lymphatic fluid stasis: part I. Adipogenesis, fibrosis, and inflammation. Plast Reconstr Surg. 2012;129(4):825–34.
30. Aschen S, Zampell JC, Elhadad S, Weitman E, De Brot M, Mehrara BJ. Regulation of adipogenesis by lymphatic fluid stasis: part II. Expression of adipose differentiation genes. Plast Reconstr Surg. 2012;129(4):838–47.
31. Damstra RJ, Voesten HG, van Schelven WD, van der Lei B. Lymphatic venous anastomosis (LVA) for treatment of secondary arm lymphedema. A prospective study of 11 LVA procedures in 10 patients with breast cancer related lymphedema and a critical review of the literature. Breast Cancer Res Treat. 2009;113(2):199–206.
32. Campisi C, Bellini C, Campisi C, Accogli S, Bonioli E, Boccardo F. Microsurgery for lymphedema: clinical research and long-term results. Microsurgery. 2010;30(4):256–60.
33. Maegawa J, Hosono M, Tomoeda H, Tosaki A, Kobayashi S, Iwai T. Net effect of lymphaticovenous anastomosis on volume reduction of peripheral lymphoedema after complex decongestive physiotherapy. Eur J Vasc Endovasc Surg. 2012;43(5):602–8.
34. Brorson H, Svensson H, Norrgren K, Thorsson O. Liposuction reduces arm lymphedema without significantly altering the already impaired lymph transport. Lymphology. 1998;31(4):156–72.
35. Brorson H. From lymph to fat: liposuction as a treatment for complete reduction of lymphedema. Int J Low Extrem Wounds. 2012;11(1):10–9.
36. Brorson H, Ohlin K, Olsson G, Svensson B, Svensson H. Controlled compression and liposuction treatment for lower extremity lymphedema. Lymphology. 2008;41(2):52–63.
37. Brorson HFC, Ohlin K, Svensson B, Åberg M, Svensson H. Liposuction normalizes elephantiasis of the leg—a prospective study with an eight-year follow-up. Lymphology. 2012;45(Suppl):292–5.
38. Clayton DN, Clayton JN, Lindley TS, Clayton JL. Large volume lipoplasty. Clin Plast Surg. 1989;16(2):305–12.
39. Klein JA. The tumescent technique for lipo-suction surgery. Am J Cosmet Surg. 1987;4(4):263–7.
40. Wojnikow S, Malm J, Brorson H. Use of a tourniquet with and without adrenaline reduces blood loss during liposuction for lymphoedema of the arm. Scand J Plast Reconstr Surg Hand Surg. 2007;43(5):1–7.
41. Baumeister RG, Siuda S. Treatment of lymphedemas by microsurgical lymphatic grafting: what is proved? Plast Reconstr Surg. 1990;85(1):64–74. discussion 5–6.
42. Andersen L, Hojris I, Erlandsen M, Andersen J. Treatment of breast-cancer-related lymphedema with or without manual lymphatic drainage—a randomized study. Acta Oncol. 2000;39(3):399–405.
43. Campisi C, Davini D, Bellini C, Taddei G, Villa G, Fulcheri E, et al. Lymphatic microsurgery for the treatment of lymphedema. Microsurgery. 2006;26(1):65–9.
44. Baumeister RG, Frick A. [The microsurgical lymph vessel transplantation]. Handchir Mikrochir Plast Chir. 2003;35(4):202–9.
45. Brorson H. Liposuction in arm lymphedema treatment. Scand J Surg. 2003;92(4):287–95.
46. Brorson H, Svensson H. Skin blood flow of the lymphedematous arm before and after liposuction. Lymphology. 1997;30(4):165–72.

Sumner A. Slavin

S.A. Slavin, M.D. (✉)
Lymphedema Program, Division of Plastic Surgery,
Beth Israel Deaconess Medical Center, Boston
Children's Hospital, Harvard Medical School,
Boston, MA, USA
e-mail: ssbsj@aol.com

Key Points

- Lymphocele occurs following procedures that surgically disrupt channels imbedded within the subcutaneous tissues, most commonly in the extremities.
- These fluid collections contain an increased concentration of lymph and are associated with painful swelling, prolonged drainage, and infection.
- Recent advancements in the management of lymphocele include recognition of high-risk patients, preoperative and intraoperative identification of lymphatic channels using radiopharmaceuticals, and newer, improved surgical treatments that utilize a variety of muscle flap transpositions, sometimes prophylactically, to fill dead space and promote wound healing.
- The increasing popularity of bariatric procedures for obesity has concomitantly led to a larger number of patients seeking thigh lift and brachioplasty enhancements of redundant skin folds.
- These procedures are particularly prone to causing damage to existing subcutaneous lymphatics.

Introduction

Lymphocele is a lymph-filled space without a distinct epithelial lining. It occurs most commonly after surgical disruption of lymphatic vessels leading to the leakage of lymph into the soft tissues or a body cavity. These collections of fluid may be contained, creating a well-defined lymphocele, or can exit through an open wound, changing its name to a lymphatic fistula. They can occur in a number of situations following procedures in the groin after lymph node dissection for gynecologic tumors, where they were first described, after radical prostatectomy, vascular reconstruction, renal transplantation, medial thigh lift, and following body contouring surgery for patients with massive weight loss. Lymphoceles tend to develop more often in extraperitoneal sites as compared to intraabdominal ones where serosal surfaces of the peritoneum can absorb lymphatic fluid [1]. Often refractory to simple compression maneuvers or percutaneous aspiration, these collections of lymphatic fluid lead to significant morbidity, including infection, chronic drainage, and prolonged hospitalization. An absence of platelets and a low concentration of clotting factors within lymph potentiate a tendency toward prolonged drainage.

A.K. Greene et al. (eds.), *Lymphedema: Presentation, Diagnosis, and Treatment*,
DOI 10.1007/978-3-319-14493-1_29, © Springer International Publishing Switzerland 2015

Pathogenesis and Diagnosis of Lymphocele

Numerous types of swelling and fluid collection can mimic lymphocele and delay formulation of a correct diagnosis and treatment plan. Postoperative edema that is well localized, along with seroma, imitates a lymphocele. Whereas seroma is a general term denoting a fluid filled space that is primarily composed of serum, lymphocele is distinguishable on the basis of its content of lymph. Lymphoceles, like a chronic seroma, can become loculated collections in a space that lacks a true epithelial lining. Similar to pseudocyst formation, the lymphocele can become a permanent mass-like collection that deforms adjacent soft tissue structures and promotes local sear tissue through inflammatory mechanisms. Because the pathogenesis invariably involves division of lymphatics, and the types of procedures encompass areas where major vascular structures are present, the frequency of lymphocele formations has been reported from 3 to 49 % for groin and pelvic lymphadenectomy.

Physical examination will usually disclose a mobile, non-pulsatile, non-tender mass when a lymphocele is in its initial stage. After a lymphocele becomes infected—most likely by staphylococcus—it becomes painful, sometimes accompanied by erythema of the overlying skin. Open drainage or needle aspiration can be instituted during its inception, but the lymphocele cavity may require packing and compression, or closed treatment with drainage catheters.

Technique of Lymphatic Mapping

Groin lymphoceles can be both diagnosed and resected using a technique of lymphatic mapping [2, 3] which identifies the boundaries of the lymphocele cavity and its disrupted afferent lymphatic feeding channels. Lower extremity ultrasound examination, alone or combined with magnetic resonance imaging can be used to visualize a subcutaneous soft tissue mass and its surrounding fibrous capsule, but lymphoscintigraphy is more specific for lymphatic channels. A preoperative lymphoscintigram not only confirms the diagnosis but also can be helpful in delineating crucial lymph flow patterns that perpetuate the fluid accumulation.

Lymphangiography was formerly used for this purpose, but it has been largely supplanted by lymphoscintigraphy utilizing a technetium-antimony sulfide radiopharmaceutical. The former technique utilized a lipiodol contrast medium that has been shown to be toxic to the endothelial lining of lymphatic vessels. In such circumstances, the lymphangiogram demonstrated the existing channels while damaging normal contiguous lymphatic structures, thus worsening the functioning channels but not obliterating the leaking ones.

In the case of mapping a groin lymphocele, an injection of isosulfan blue dye (Lymphazurin 1 %; Ben Venue Labs, Inc., Bedord, Ohio) can be injected in the area of the knee of the involved leg; massage of adjacent lymphatics is performed for 10–15 min until filling is observed. Similarly for a lower extremity lymphocele, lymphatic mapping is conducted by a series of injections of isosulfan blue around the ankle [3]. Following elevation of the limb for approximately 10 min, the lymphocele is incised. At this point it is possible to visualize the entire extent of the lymphocele cavity, along with the location of feeding vessels which are to be serially ligated. Without such thorough identification, the leakage of lymph via unidentified feeders will continue, resulting in reaccumulation. Failure to identify feeding lymphatics is a major cause of the reoccurrence that characterizes simple excisional approaches. Incomplete treatment has serious consequences of wound morbidity: wound infections can occur in up to 57 % of patients, and increased wound dehiscence is a common comorbidity. For a successful surgical result it is usually necessary to combine preoperative lymphoscintigraphy with the isosulfan blue dye injection technique.

Unfortunately, there is little data available on the efficacy of either lymphoscintigraphy or injectional mapping because of the low frequency of this type of lesion. Furthermore, lymphoscintigraphy provides a low-resolution image of

Fig. 29.1 Injection of lymphazurin blue or other dyes can visualize dermal and subcutaneous lymphatics. This method of mapping assists in the identification of feeding lymphatics which sustain and increase the volume of a lymphocele

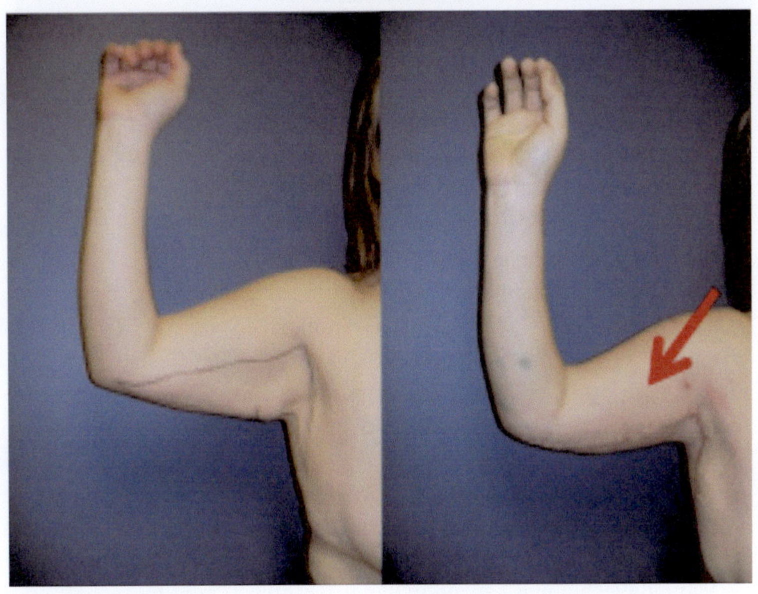

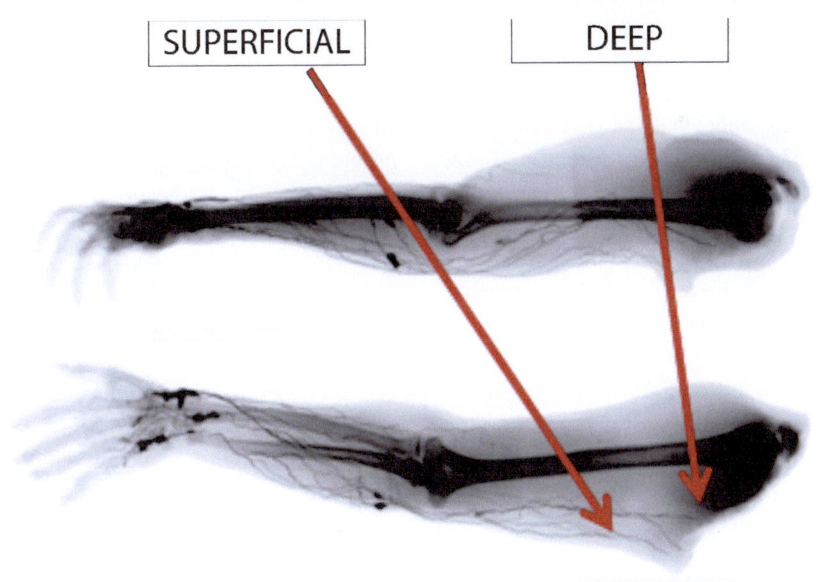

Fig. 29.2 Cadaver lymphangiographic research has increased our knowledge of the anatomy of the lymphatic system. Lymphatics actually travel at multiple levels within the subcutaneous tissues

functioning normal lymphatics, much less so of leaking structures. It does, however, provide a broad picture of the entire lymphatic system of the involved anatomical area, and when combined with dye injection (Figs. 29.1 and 29.2) can reasonably assure a complete surgical treatment.

It is important to note that excessive excision—beyond the confines of the lymphocele—combined with injury to functioning lymphatic channels in proximity to the cavity can result in lymphedema that is localized to the groin or involves the entire affected extremity. It is not known whether adjunctive therapy, such as microsurgical lymphatico-venous anastomosis can be used to bypass leaking lymphatics or redirect it toward nodal basins. In one series of 19 groin lymphoceles [4], the identification and ligation of leaking lymphatics yielded no recurrences. Other benefits of the isosulfan blue dye technique have been manifested by diminished hospital stay (4–17 days instead of 30), decreased infections by 50 %, and decreased duration of all therapies being used. This reduction of wound morbidity is particularly notable, as is the safety record of isosulfan blue, which appears to be safe with the exceptions of skin pigmentation and serious hypotension in 0.75 % of patients.

Mapping techniques can aid in the differentiation between a seroma and a lymphocele, but sometimes the results are inconclusive. Treatment approaches are generally the same for both types of complication. Just as elevated body mass index, extensive subcutaneous dissection, large dead space, and local shearing forces are known factors contributing to seroma formation, this constellation plus division of afferent lymphatics is likely to result in a lymphocele. Additional preventive strategies besides avoiding lymphatic injury have included decreasing dead space with early external compression and internal suturing methods such as quilting sutures. A meta-analysis [5] investigating both compression and quilting sutures in the management of seroma found quilting sutures to be effective, but not so compression. Unfortunately, the infrequency of lymphocele has meant that randomized studies of these maneuvers are neither feasible nor statistically valid. Similarly, another meta-analysis confirmed a minimal benefit of fibrin glue in the management of seroma but lymphocele was not studied. Sclerotherapy employing agents such as doxycycline, alcohol, or bleomycin has been used with varying success in both seroma and lymphocele collections [6, 7].

Obesity, Bariatric Surgery, and Lymphocele Formation

Recent attention has been drawn to an epidemic of overweight problems in the US adult population [8]. Current studies [9] indicate that 68.5 % of American adults are overweight and 34.9 % or 78.6 million [9] are obese; for children, 31.8 % are overweight and 16.9 % are obese. Given the severity of these statistics, the development of procedures that abet weight loss by limiting stomach capacity, such as gastric stapling and banding techniques has been strikingly successful. In 2009, over 200,000 such operations were performed. Because this figure represents only 1 % of the population eligible for weight loss therapy, a significant increase in the number of these procedures performed is anticipated [8]. Following bariatric surgery, massive weight loss is a pleasing result but it can often be accompanied by severely redundant folds of skin located all over the body. The medial thighs, in particular, graphically demonstrate the aesthetic hazards of extreme weight loss often surpassing 150 lbs. This growing population of patients post massive weight loss suffers a variety of body contouring problems secondary to redundant skin. When redundant skin folds of the extremities are treated, it is necessary to excise extensive areas. The wide elevation of flaps of skin in the subcutaneous plane of the inner thighs is particularly prone to injure the numerous lymphatic structures traversing the medial thigh which can occupy different levels within the subcutaneous space and are easily injured. More recent cadaveric studies [10] utilizing a radiopaque lead oxide mixture have clearly illustrated the vulnerability of these channels.

Lymphocele Following Medial Thigh Lift

Just as groin wound complications following arterial revascularization—estimated to have an incidence of 1.8–5 % [11]—can create serious consequences for the patient in the context of

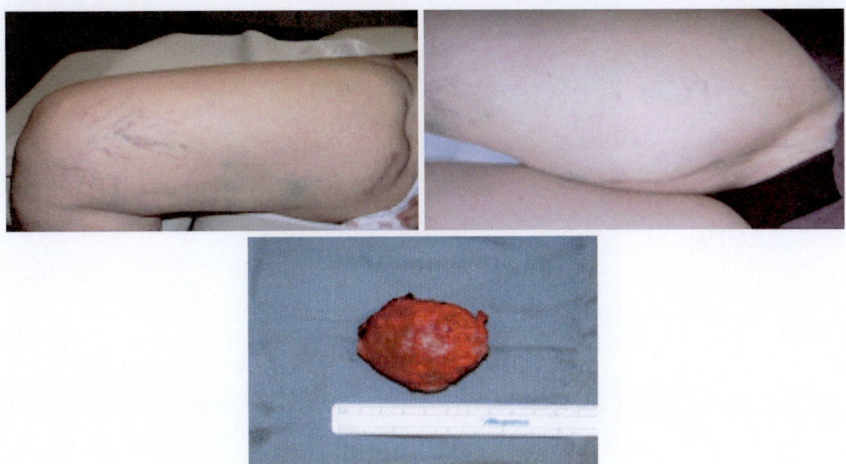

Fig. 29.3 Recurrent lymphocele after thigh lift. Lymphocele is known to occur following injury to the lymphatics traversing the thigh during a medial thigh lift procedure. Such lesions occur when there is a chronic accumulation of lymph, which develops into a pseudo-cyst-like structure known as a lymphocele. If bandaging and aspiration fail, excision is recommended. The lymphocele structure is depicted in the *bottom* figure

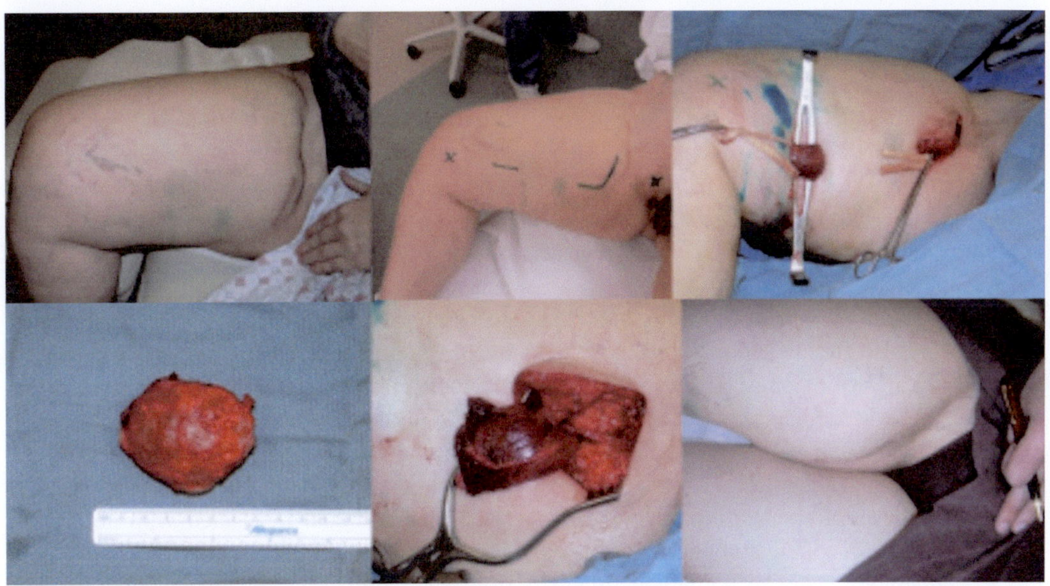

Fig. 29.4 Treatment of recurrent lymphocele after thigh lift. Operative steps involved in excision of a recurrent lymphocele and reconstruction with a muscle flap of gracilis muscle. After demarcation of the lesion (*upper left* and *center*) the lesion is dissected from its surroundings (*upper right*). The lymphocele mass is shown in the *lower left* photo. A gracilis muscle flap has been elevated (*lower-center*). In the *lower right* photo, patient's thigh is healed and there has been no recurrence. With permission from [12]

infection or even loss of limb, accumulations of lymph (lymphocele) or prolonged lymph drainage (lymphorrea) following medial thigh lift (Figs. 29.3 and 29.4) can also cause prolonged wound morbidity [12]. From wound drainage to cyst or lymphocele formation, these conditions are difficult to diagnose and eradicate. Although an incidence of 3–49 % has been observed after

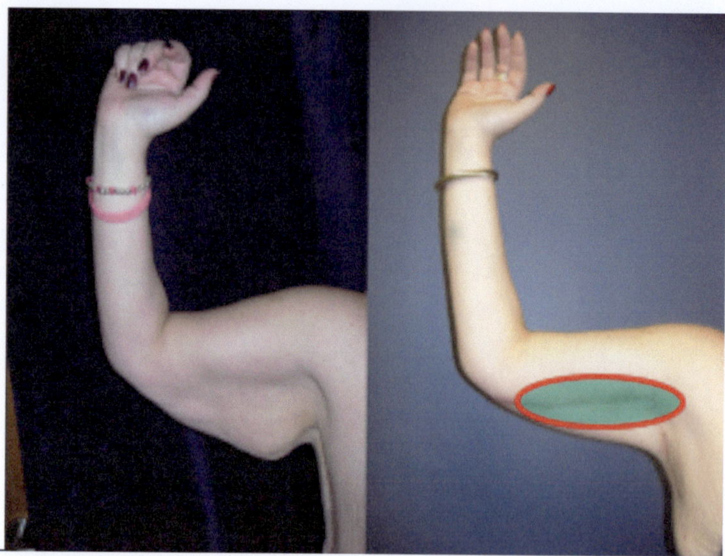

Fig. 29.5 Brachioplasty. Small lymphoceles from superficial injury. Multiple small lymphoceles occurring after brachioplasty. These lesions can be opened and drained repeatedly because of their size. They are more amenable to incision and drainage than thigh lymphoceles and a muscle flap is usually not needed

groin and pelvic lymphadenectomies, the exact incidence of lymphocele after medial thigh lift is not well established, but thought to be low, below 10 %. The dissection in the subcutaneous plane that is routinely done during the elevation of medial skin flaps has the potential to injure afferent lymphatics traveling subcutaneously toward the inguinal nodal basin.

Lymphocele development following a medial thigh lift, and also after brachioplasty (Fig. 29.5), is usually clinically manifest at about 2 weeks postoperative, when it appears as a subtle asymmetry or more obvious bulge. Most patients with a refractory lymphocele relate a history of multiple percutaneous aspirations followed by reaccumulation. Cellulitis often complicates an area that has undergone many such attempts, requiring intravenous antibiotics. Once resolved, the usual approach is to attempt a complete excision and intraoperative ligation of leaking lymphatic channels that are identifiable during the procedure. The success of such an undertaking is known within a few weeks to months, either when complete resolution and contraction of the original site is evident or when a new swelling becomes apparent.

An additional recurrence in this sequence of events calls for preoperative evaluation with a lymphoscintigram and MRI examination. Our preferred operative technique has included injection of isosulfan blue into the area of the knee of the involved leg, waiting for filling of adjacent dermal lymphatics. Incisions can then be planned to include the borders of the lesion, but also to provide access to sites of lymphatic leakage. Surgical site planning should include access to sites of lymphatic leakage. Surgical site planning should include access to adjacent muscles when a muscle flap is anticipated for filling and closure of the excised lymphocele's cavity. It is important to both insure completeness of the excision and elimination of lymphatic drainage sites, which should be ligated with absorbable suture. After careful inspection for any evidence of leakage, fibrin glue can be applied to seal any area suspected or demonstrated to contain leaking lymphatics.

Role of Muscle Flap Transposition in the Treatment of Recurrent Lymphocele

Elimination of dead space left over after a definitive excision is treated by muscle flap transposition. The gracilis muscle is well suited and situated in the circumstance of an upper thigh lymphocele, and in most situations can be rotated easily into the defect. Maximal apposition of the muscle to the surrounding tissues of the excised lymphocele promotes healing and may play a role in prevention of a seroma. Patients with no evidence of recurrence 6–12 months after operation can usually be considered cured. Similarly, it is reasonable to wait 6 months before performing a muscle slap closure for a failed excisional ablatement. In our series [12] of muscle flap treatment of the refractory lymphocele, all healed uneventfully. The failure of nonoperative therapies, including aspiration and compression bandaging, have contributed to an anecdotally high apparent recurrence rate following lymphocele formation.

A successful treatment of lymphocele should firstly embrace a studious plan of avoidance of injury to lymphatic structures occupying the surgical field of thigh lift and brachioplasty procedures. Although drainage catheters can be helpful in the intraoperative management of a lymphocele, different surgical approaches are needed to maximize the safety and preservation of lymph channels. An ideal technical modification, now widely advocated, is to perform suction lipectomy of the medial thigh, for thighplasty or arm subcutaneous tissues for brachioplasty. This approach minimizes risk by avoiding direct injury to lymphatics, as has been shown in longitudinal studies of patients following liposuctioning for lymphedema [13]. After suction lipectomy, performed at the time of the medial thighplasty or as a staged procedure, the lymphatics are not damaged and the excess skin can be excised in a superficial plane. Other technical modifications aimed at minimizing lymphatic disturbance include careful orientation of skin incisions, undermining the anteromedial thigh flap lateral to the femoral triangle, and limited subcutaneous dissection of the medial thigh. Improved intraoperative visualization of lymphatic channels using isocyanine green lymphography represents a newer, more advanced method of avoiding injury to the lymphatic drainage system.

Role of Prophylactic Muscle Flaps in the Prevention of Postoperative Lymphocele and Lymphatic Complications

The known efficacy of muscle flaps [5, 14–16] in achieving closure of chronic wounds, including those characterized by radionecrosis and infection, has inspired their widespread application on a prophylactic basis. High-risk patients undergoing difficult vascular procedures prone to complications of lymphocele and seroma appear to be excellent candidates for this approach. Groin complications in particular, arising from open vascular procedures involving the femoral vessels, have posed serious threats and potentially catastrophic outcomes when arterial vessels are involved. Infection and necrosis, along with fluid collections that abet delayed healing and wound disruption, can lead to more reoperation and vascular or prosthetic reconstruction. Performing prophylactic muscle flaps—gracilis, sartorius, rectus femoris, and rectus abdominis being among the most commonly selected—has led to lower overall rates of complications, including lymphocele and seroma and decreased incidence of infection. Lymphocele occurred in 1.5 % of patients receiving a flap as compared to 15.4 % in those who did not; no seromas appeared in the prophylactic muscle flap population. Clearly, covering the femoral vessels and eliminating dead space—both benefits of a muscle flap—produced dramatic improvement in healing following reoperative, high-risk vascular procedures, mostly conducted on the femoral vessels. Safety and efficacy of prophylactic muscle flaps, with minimal donor site morbidity, was the conclusion that emerged from a retrospective review of 248 patients. Whether all patients having operations on the femoral vessels should have a prophylactic muscle flap done concomitantly has not been established, but high-risk, reoperative cases demonstrate major benefit. In the Penn Groin Assessment Scale [17], the authors presented an evidence-based algorithm and comprehensive cost analysis in their determination of a system that accurately predicts groin complications, noting that the principal risk factors were obesity, reoperative surgery, smoking, and prosthetic graft reconstruction.

Nonoperative Treatment of Lymphocele

In addition to the surgical advances in the treatment of lymphocele—exemplified by appreciation of the lymphatic anatomy of any given region, recent developments in the field of Negative Pressure Wound Therapy [18] may someday provide effective nonoperative management of lymphocele that is superior to current bandaging and compression methods. Negative wound pressure techniques gained traction in the 1990s. These devices [19] are comprised of an adhesive, semi-occlusive dressing, tubing, a collection canister, a vacuum source, and an interface material, which distributes the vacuum throughout a wound. As a result of the occlusive dressing and the vacuum, fluid can be removed and tissues—skin and wound components—are drawn together.

Wounds with excess fluid become edematous, a situation that is present in lymphedema when clinical pitting of a limb is evident. Not only does the fluid in lymphedematous extremities appear to stimulate hyperplasia in the fat of the subcutaneous compartment through presumed but undefined growth factors, but the fluid can also impede blood supply to the skin and interfere with the transport of various nutrients. Negative pressure devices have shown an ability to remove fluid volume in patients with lymphedema by means of the pressure gradient that is generated, but the exact mechanism by which this is achieved is unknown. Still, it may be effective for newly formed accumulations but less likely in an established, chronic type of lymphocele or seroma. Since lymphocele appears in approximately 1–4 % of patients following femoral vessel dissection, causing severe comorbidity, application of negative pressure in such circumstances has been borne out by case studies showing resolution of drainage for both femoral lymphocele and lymphatic fistula in a mean of 14–18 days.

Although unproven, negative pressure wound therapy, if successful, would compare favorably to the longer periods of persistent lymphatic drainage, estimated at 47 days [20]. These devices, however, have been associated with bleeding and infection, and in 2009 the FDA reported that there had been 12 deaths and 174 injuries following negative pressure wound therapy [21].

Lymphocele Conclusion

Lymphocele, an accumulation of lymph bearing fluid that occurs after procedures that disrupt lymphatic channels, leading to drainage within a wound, or externally (lymph fistula) is traditionally treated with conservative measures such as repeated aspiration and compression. When these measures fail, more aggressive steps, both diagnostically and surgically are necessary. Preoperative imaging with lymphoscintigraphy identifies lymphatic drainage patterns and assists in the identification of leaking channels. When combined with excision, the lymphocele can be eradicated, but some cases are still refractory and will require an adjacent muscle transfer to eliminate dead space and promote wound healing. Prophylactic use of muscle flaps appears to prevent lymphocele and seroma in high-risk situations. Nonoperative therapy utilizing negative pressure wound therapy has shown promise in a limited number of patients. The best management is, of course, recognition of how this lesion occurs and its avoidance.

References

1. Mori N. Clinical and experimental studies on the so called lymphocyst, which develops after radical hysterectomy in cancer of uterine cervix. J Jpn Obstet Gynecol Soc. 1995;2:178–203.
2. Clouse ME, Wallace S. Lymphatic imaging. 2nd ed. Baltimore: Williams and Wilkins; 1985.
3. Canders CP, Nguyen PD, Festekjian JH, Rudkin GH. Treatment of a lower extremity lymphocele with intraoperative lymphatic mapping. Eplasty. 2013;13:489–94.
4. Stadelman WK, Tobin GR. Successful treatment of 19 groin lymphoceles with the assistance of intraopera-

tive lymphatic mapping. Plast Reconstr Surg. 2002; 109(4):1274–80.

5. Shermak MA, Rotellini Coltvet LA, Chang D. Seroma development following body contouring surgery for massive weight loss. Plast Reconstr Surg. 2008;122(1):280–8.

6. Caliendo MV, Lee DE, Quieroz R, Waldman DL. Sclerotherapy with the use of doxycycline after percutaneous drainage of postoperative lymphocele. J Vasc Interv Radiol. 2001;12:73.

7. Sawhney R, D'Agostino HB, Zinck S. Treatment of postoperative lymphoceles with percutaneous drainage and alcohol sclerotherapy. J Vasc Interv Radiol. 1996;7(2):241–5.

8. American Society for Metabolic and Bariatric Surgery. 2010. www.asmbs.org.

9. Ogden CL, Carroll MD, Kit BK, Flegal KM. Prevalence of childhood and adult obesity in the United States, 2011–2012. JAMA. 2014;311(8):806–14.

10. Suami H, Taylor GI. The lymphatic territories of the upper limb: anatomical study and clinical implications. Plast Reconstr Surg. 2007;119(6):1813–22.

11. Tyndall SH, Shepard AD, Wilczewski JM, Reddy DJ, Elliott JP, Ernst CB. Groin lymphatic complications. J Vasc Surg. 1994;19(5):858–63.

12. Borud LJ, Cooper JS, Slavin SA. New management algorithm for lymphocele following medial thigh lift. Plast Reconstr Surg. 2008;121(4): 1450–5.

13. Brorson H, Svensson H, Norrgren K, Thorsson O. Liposuction reduces arm lymphedema without significantly altering the already impaired lymph transport. Lymphology. 1998;31:156.

14. Yee K, Wong L, Wong J, Shermak MA, Jones CE. Surgical management of groin lymphatic complications after arterial bypass surgery. Plast Reconstr Surg. 2005;115(7):1954–62.

15. Fischer JP, Nelson JA, Mirzabeigi MN, Wang GJ, Foley PJ, Wu LC, Woo EY, Kanchwala S. Prophylactic muscle flaps in vascular surgery. J Vasc Surg. 2012;55(4):1081–6.

16. Shermak MA, Yee K, Wong L, Jones CE, Wong J. Surgical management of groin lymphatic complications after arterial bypass surgery. Plast Reconstr Surg. 2005;115(7):1954–62.

17. Fischer JP, Nelson JA, Rohrbach JI, Wu LC, Woo EY, Kovach SJ, Low DW, Serletti JM, Kanchwala S. Prophylactic muscle flaps in vascular surgery: the penn groin assessment scale. Plast Reconstr Surg. 2012;129(6):e940–8.

18. Orgill DP, Bayer LR. Update on negative-pressure wound therapy. Plast Reconstr Surg. 2011;127(1S): 105S–15.

19. Argenta LC, Morykwas MJ. Vacuum-assisted closure: a new method for wound control and treatment: Clinical experience. Ann Plast Surg. 1997;38:563–76.

20. Schwartz MA, Schanzer H, Skladany M, Haimoy M, Stein J. A comparison of conservative therapy and early selective ligation in the treatment of lymphatic complications following vascular procedures. Am J Surg. 1995;170(2):206–8.

21. FDA Report, Medical Devices and Medical Device Safety, February 24, 2011, US Department of Health and Human Services.

Genital Lymphedema

Rudy Murillo and Steven J. Fishman

Definition and Classification

Progressive and chronic swelling of tissue due to poor lymphatic drainage causes lymphedema. Lymphedema is classified as either primary (from anomalous lymphatic development) or secondary/acquired (from injury to lymphatic nodes or vessels) [1]. Affected tissue initially swells from accumulation of subcutaneous lymph, and resultant inflammation then stimulates adipose deposition and fibrosis, causing further enlargement over time [1, 2]. Lymphedema can also be classified by the age of onset: developing during infancy, childhood, adolescence, or adulthood [2]. Primary lymphedema is uncommon; it affects 1.2 per 100,000 persons less than 20 years of age [3]. Secondary lymphedema affects the majority of patients worldwide (90 %), but is uncommon in the developed world. Its most common cause is parasitic infection with *Wuchereria bancrofti*, *Brugia malayi*, or *Brugia timori* [4]. Other causes of secondary lymphedema in the developed world include radiation treatment, surgical removal of lymphatic tissue, penetrating trauma, and bacterial infection. Complications of lymphedema include infection, functional disability, and chronic cutaneous changes.

Genital lymphedema is often associated with lower extremity disease and occurs when swelling from inadequate lymphatic drainage involves the male or female genitalia. Genital lymphedema is rare. Existing reports on genital lymphedema in the pediatric population have been limited by the small numbers of patients [1, 5, 6] studied and/or are comprised largely of adults [7, 8]. Males and females are affected equally [9]. This chapter reviews the known causes of genital

R. Murillo, M.D.
Department of Surgery, Boston Children's Hospital, Boston, MA, USA

S.J. Fishman, M.D. (✉)
Department of Surgery, Vascular Anomalies Center, Boston Children's Hospital, Harvard Medical School, 300 Longwood Avenue, Fegan, 3rd Floor, Boston, MA 02115, USA
e-mail: Steven.Fishman@childrens.harvard.edu

A.K. Greene et al. (eds.), *Lymphedema: Presentation, Diagnosis, and Treatment*, DOI 10.1007/978-3-319-14493-1_30, © Springer International Publishing Switzerland 2015

lymphedema, the clinical findings patients commonly present with, as well as the workup and treatment options currently available to patients.

Pathogenesis

The cause of primary genital lymphedema is currently unknown but is thought to be due to a developmental defect in the regional lymphatic system that leads to lymph stasis and accumulation. Lymphedema can extend to the genitalia in hereditary lymphedemas. These include Milroy disease, where lymphedema of the lower extremities is present at birth, and there is also a family history of the lymphedema [10]; Meige disease, where patients develop lower extremity lymphedema during adolescence (OMIM 153200); and lymphedema–distichiasis, where the lymphedema is associated with an extra row of eyelashes. Nonsense mutations in the vascular endothelial growth factor receptor 3 (*VEGFR3*) have been linked to primary lymphedemas [11]. VEGFR3 expression is restricted to the lymphatic endothelium after early angiogenesis [12], and has been shown to induce cell proliferation, migration, and survival, via activation of the ERK, AKT, and JNK pathways [13]. Lymphedema with distichiasis is caused by splice site mutations in forkhead box protein C2 (FOXC2), a transcription factor involved in lymphatic development [14]. The genetic cause of Meige disease is currently unknown.

Scrotal and vaginal swelling can also be caused by lymphatic malformations and by obstruction or malfunction of central conducting lymphatic channels. Both of these disorders have been linked to activating somatic mutations in the *PIK3CA* gene, which encodes the catalytic subunit of the enzyme phosphatidylinositol 3-kinase, and is involved in regulating the AKT pathway [15]. Though not fully understood, it is thought that post-zygotic *PIK3CA* mutations drive overgrowth of lymphatic tissue within affected tissues. To our knowledge, no form of familial or syndromic lymphedema has been uniquely linked to the genitalia.

Clinical Findings

In all forms of lymphedema, the lower extremities are often concurrently involved, although isolated genital disease does occur. In a recent review of primary lymphedema patients, 91.7 % had lower extremity involvement, eighteen percent had genital lymphedema (most commonly associated with lower extremity disease), and 4 % had isolated genital involvement [1]. In males the scrotum is involved in almost all patients (Fig. 30.1a). Combined peno-scrotal disease is seen commonly (Fig. 30.1b, c), while isolated penile enlargement is rarely seen (Fig. 30.1d). Lymphedema can also involve the labia (Fig. 30.2). Pitting edema and minimal cutaneous changes are present in early disease; non-pitting overgrowth occurs over time from adipose deposition and fibrosis. Hyperkeratosis, lymphatic leakage from skin, and bleeding from vesicles is commonly seen. Cutaneous lymphatic vesicles can also be seen in patients with lymphedema (Fig. 30.3) [16]. Disfigurement from lymphedema, particularly of the genitalia, can cause considerable psychosocial distress.

Obstruction, malformation, or dysfunction of the central conducting lymphatic channels (cisterni chili, thoracic duct, and accessory thoracic duct) can lead to lymph reflux and manifest as pulmonary and pericardial effusions, ascites, and sometimes vaginal or scrotal lymphedema. Patients may even present with leakage of chylous fluid from the genitalia [9, 17]. Isolated lymphatic malformations are most commonly located in the neck, axilla, chest wall, and pelvis [18], but can also be found within the genitalia. Lymphatic malformations are classified as macrocystic, microcystic, or combined [19, 20].

Complications associated with primary genital lymphedema include lymphorrhea, chyluria, hematuria, and cellulitis. Cellulitis has the potential to be life threatening and should be treated aggressively. Patients with scrotal or vaginal cutaneous lymphatic malformations are also at an increased risk of developing cellulitis, as the abnormal lymphatic channels act as a portal of entry for bacteria. Another common complication

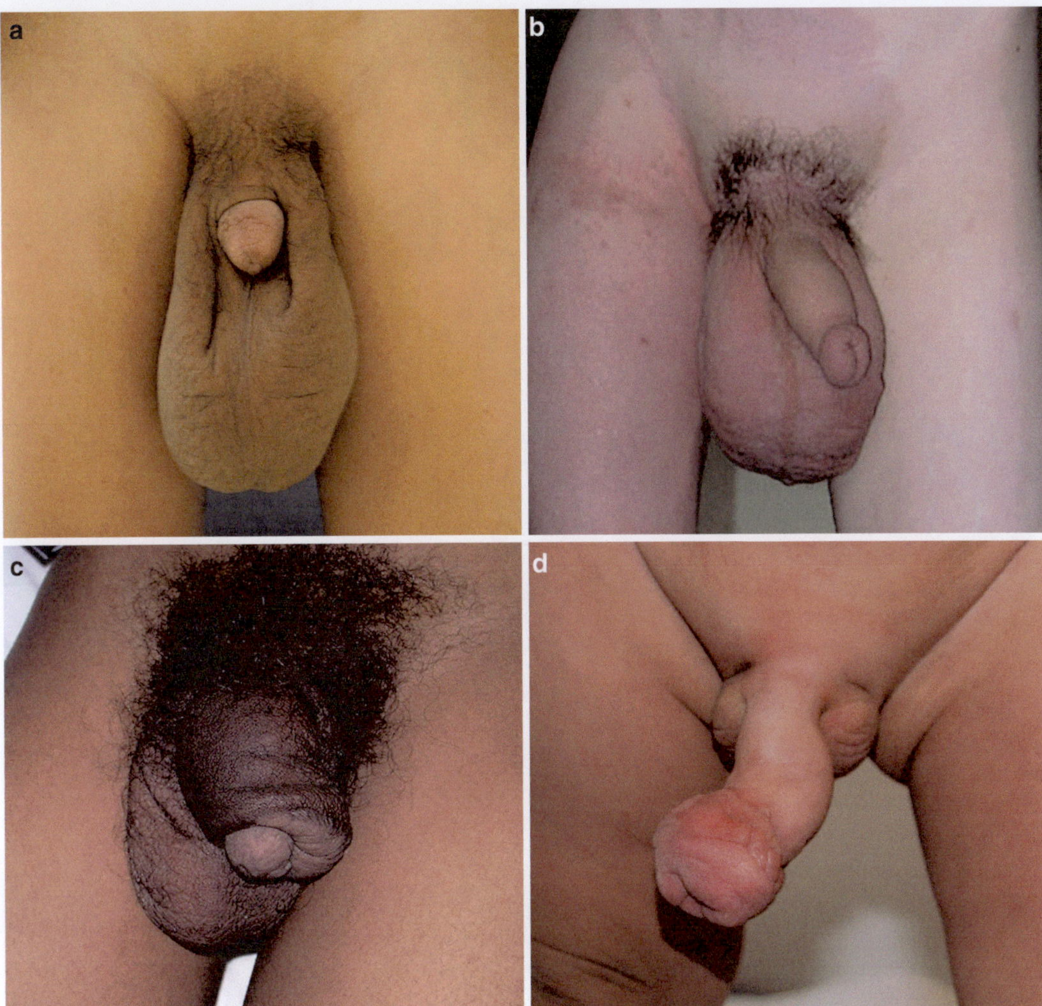

Fig. 30.1 Penile and scrotal lymphedema (**a**) 14-year-old male with isolated scrotal lymphedema. (**b**) 15-year-old male with combined penile and scrotal lymphedema. (**c**) 17-year-old male with a central conducting lymphatic anomaly and associated penile and scrotal lymphedema. (**d**) 15-month-old male with congenital lymphedema–distichiasis involving his penis

of lymphatic malformations is intralesional bleeding. This typically presents with the acute development of swelling and pain. Hematuria or chyluria can be seen in patients with lymphatic malformations along the urethra or bladder wall.

Diagnosis

Genital lymphedema is an uncommon but troubling cause of deformity of the male and female genitalia. While most patients develop symptoms in infancy or early childhood, the diagnosis is often delayed for several years. Lymphedema is most commonly confused with other vascular anomalies, particularly if the lower extremities are also affected. An accurate diagnosis is imperative in providing appropriate counseling and treatment. History and physical examination are the primary mode of diagnosis, followed by imaging in limited cases. A detailed history should document when the lymphedema first developed and also rule out causes of secondary lymphedema such as infection, trauma, prior

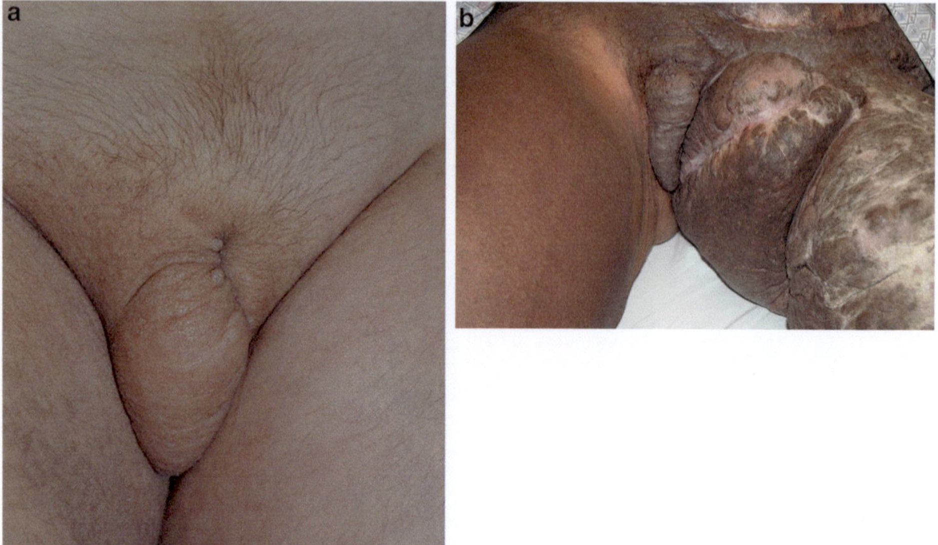

Fig. 30.2 Labial lymphedema. (**a**) 7-year-old female with a generalized lymphatic anomaly and associated right lower extremity and right labial lymphedema. (**b**) 29-year-old female with left-sided lymphedema and bilateral labial involvement

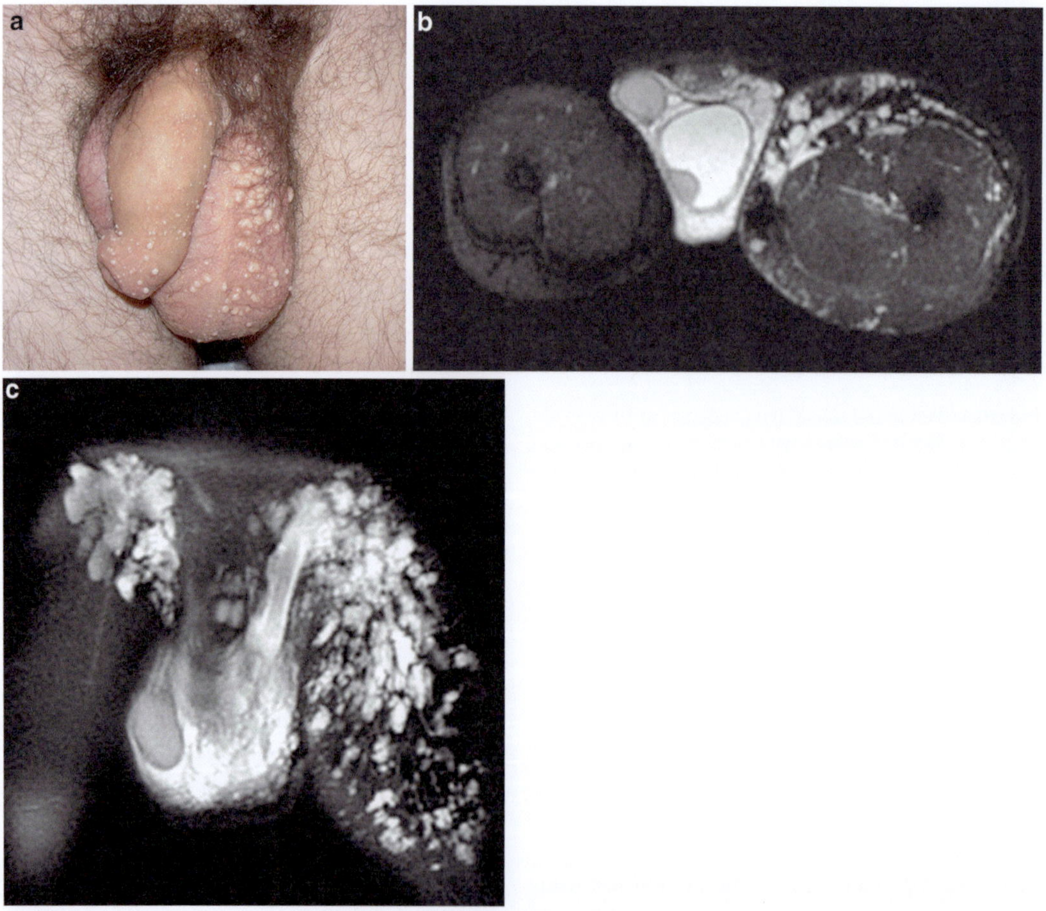

Fig. 30.3 (**a**) 27-year-old male with a central conducting lymphatic anomaly and associated combined penile and scrotal lymphedema as well as cutaneous lymphatic malformations. This patient had chyle leakage from the cutaneous penile and scrotal vesicles and had experienced numerous bouts of scrotal cellulitis. (**b**) T2-weighted fat/sat axial and (**c**) coronal MRI images depicting lower extremity and scrotal lymphatic malformations

radiation, or prior surgical procedures. A family history should also be obtained, as genital lymphedema can be part of inherited diseases such as Noonan syndrome, lymphedema–distichiasis, or Milroy disease [11, 14]. Some patients with concomitant lower extremity manifestations will have had confirmatory lymphoscintigraphy prior to referral. Delayed transport and/or dermal backflow of radiolabeled colloid indicate lymphatic dysfunction with 92 % sensitivity and 100 % specificity [21]. Ultrasonography is less specific and CT exposes the reproductive organs to radiation and should therefore be avoided. MRI can help distinguish lymphedema from other vascular anomalies, such as venous or lymphatic malformations, and can also be of value in operative planning. Patients with a central conducting anomaly may benefit from lymphangiography as this study may localize the lymphatic blockage or abnormality. Biopsy should be utilized only if malignancy or other conditions, such as noninfectious granulomatous disease, are suspected.

Treatment

Once the diagnosis of genital lymphatic disease is made, treatment should be initiated. Genital lymphatic disease can adversely influence a patient's quality of life, affecting both their functional and emotional well-being. While many patients do not have symptoms beyond enlargement of the genitalia, the psychosocial consequences of disfigurement should not be underestimated, particularly as a child becomes aware of genital anatomic differences in adolescence. Emotional health should be routinely screened in all patients as referral for a formal psychiatric assessment may be indicated in some patients.

Conservative Management

Patient education is key in managing genital lymphedema. Infection prevention is of great importance. Daily washing of the genitalia and application of a moisturizing agent to prevent skin breakdown should be emphasized. The patient and family should be taught to recognize signs or symptoms of cellulitis as this complication can be life threatening. Treatment with oral or intravenous antibiotics should be initiated promptly once cellulitis is diagnosed. Prophylactic low dose antibiotics should be considered in patients who have had three or more episodes of cellulitis in a year. Patients with lymphatic malformations also are at an increased risk of infection and should practice good hygiene. Patients with lymphatic malformations can develop intralesional bleeding, which is often painful, and difficult to manage. The bleeding is often self-limiting and is treated with compression and nonsteroidal anti-inflammatory medications. Lymph leakage from cutaneous lymphatic vesicles or from the genitalia of patients with central conducting anomalies should be kept dry. Patients can apply absorbent pads to affected areas. Cutaneous lymphatic vesicles, particularly on or near the genitalia, act as a portal for bacterial entry and can be aggressively treated with CO_2 laser ablation of the lesions [22] and or sclerosis of macrocystic lymphatic channels [23]. Often with CO_2 laser treatments, multiple sessions are required to create enough scar tissue to slow or stop lymphatic leakage. Sclerosis near the meatus or urethra runs the risk of causing a stricture and should only be attempted by experienced clinicians. Sclerotherapy within the scrotum may also risk damage to the testicles.

Initiation of compression therapy with compression garments, pneumatic devices, or fitted clothing is the mainstay of nonoperative treatment in patients with lower extremity and genital lymphedema [1, 23]. Patients with lymphatic malformations and central conducting anomalies affecting the genitalia may also benefit from compression therapy. Due to the shape and location of genital lymphedema, wrapping and stocking material can be difficult to apply and may require ingenuity on behalf of the patient and family (Fig. 30.4). Another consideration is that applying compression devices to a growing infant is challenging and often not feasible. Elastic shorts may be a good option for older patients. Some patients apply wedge under the pelvis to elevate the genitalia while sleeping to

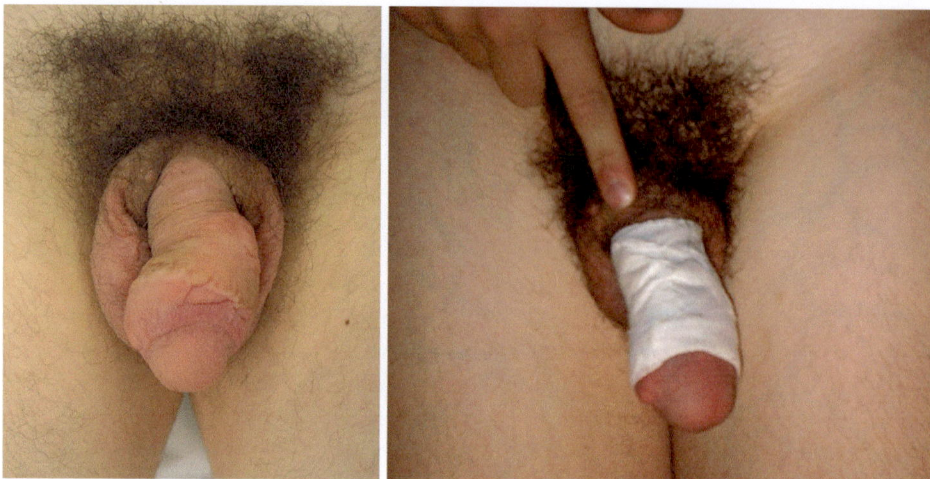

Fig. 30.4 13-year-old boy with congenital lymphedema involving his penis. (**a**) Penis is shown unwrapped (*Left*) and wrapped circumferentially (*Right*) with Kerlix gauze

improve lymphatic return. The benefits of compression therapy and elevation need to be weighed against the inconvenience this causes the patient. Our institutional experience has shown that when tolerated, compression therapy is useful in maintaining and at times reducing genital size. Postoperative penile wrapping is particularly effective at reducing the risk of recurrent swelling.

Operative Intervention

Surgical treatment of genital lymphedema is indicated for patients with significant disfigurement or morbidity that have failed nonoperative management. Operative indications include excessive mass, functional impairment, and/or disfigurement. Operative intervention for female genital lymphedema is rare. It is preferable to wait until the child has completed puberty and is fully developed before attempting to debulk excess tissue. For extreme cases of genital lymphedema, conservative early debulking can be performed, with the expectation of potential additional intervention when the child is older. Patients and their families should be counseled regarding expectations. While disfigurement can be greatly improved, the genitalia will likely never appear completely normal. The point that operative intervention will not impair function or reproductive capabilities if done correctly should be emphasized. At our center we employ excisional intervention for both penile and scrotal lymphedema. The goal of the procedures is to excise lymphedematous tissue as well as removal of the redundant overlying skin. Alternate surgical approaches have been previously described with different incisions without removing redundant skin [24–26]. We believe the smaller scars of these methods are outweighed by the likelihood of less satisfactory long-term outcomes. The residual redundant skin contains lymphedematous tissue, which is prone to re-expand. The greater surface area of skin and deeper tissue removed, the less remaining to re-enlarge.

Debulking of penile lymphedema is performed in the following manner (Fig. 30.5). A circumferential incision is made in the penile skin several millimeters proximal to the corona of the glans penis, using the scar from previous circumcision, if relevant (Fig. 30.5b). The skin, just below the dermis, is then dissected circumferentially off the shaft of the penis, to the base. The entirety of the shaft skin is unfolded proximally using blunt, sharp, and/or cautery dissection. Underlying lymphedematous and adipose tissue is then circumferentially dissected off

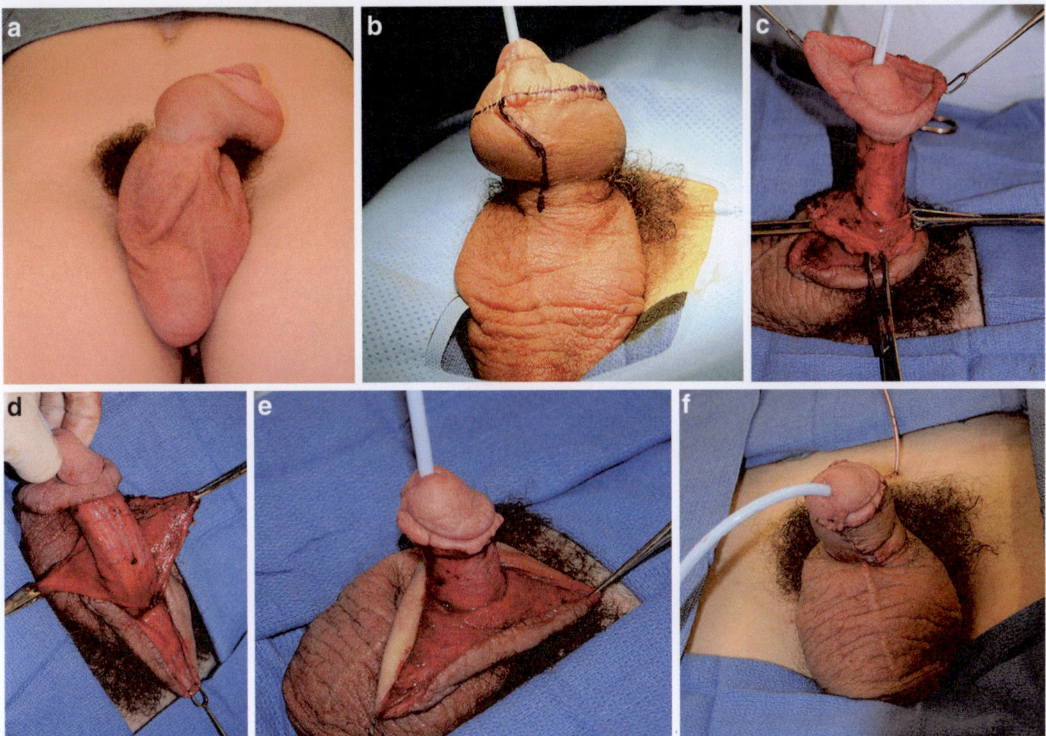

Fig. 30.5 Penile lymphedema debulking (**a**) 18-year-old male with penile lymphedema. (**b**) Markings showing the circumferential skin incision made just proximal to the corona of the glans penis as well as a line demarcating the midline raphe. (**c**) The penis following unfolding of the skin and dissection of lymphatic tissue off Buck's fascia. (**d**) This is followed by circumferential removal of lymphatic tissue. (**e**) Skin is advanced along the penile shaft and contoured so that it comfortably covers the shaft. (**f**) Penis following suturing of skin and drain placement

Buck's fascia (Fig. 30.5c). Care is taken to avoid injury to the neurovascular bundles, urethra, or skin. Once the lymphedematous tissue is removed (Fig. 30.5d, e), the redundant skin is advanced back down the penile shaft. Excess circumference of skin is resected to leave just enough to comfortably wrap the penile shaft. When possible, an attempt is made to remove as much abnormal skin (containing vesicles, dimples, or fibrosis) as possible while still allowing for comfortable penile coverage. The skin is approximated to create a longitudinal scar at the ventral midline (Fig. 30.5f). The excess length of skin is excised to facilitate re-approximation at the distal pre-coronal incisional location. A small round closed-suction drain is placed under the skin flap, positioned dorsally away from the urethra and brought out in a suprapubic position. Interrupted intradermal absorbable sutures followed by a running subcuticular suture are used for closure. A penile block with 0.25 % bupivacaine is performed prior to dressing the wound. The penis is gently wrapped with circumferential gauze, and a urinary catheter is left in place for 24 h. Figure 30.6 shows patients following excision of lymphedematous tissue.

Scrotal debulking of lymphedema or lymphatic malformations occurs in the following fashion (Fig. 30.7): An incision is made either transversely (Fig. 30.7a) at the most dependent portion of the scrotum, or vertically (Fig. 30.7b) encompassing the median raphe. The testes and spermatic cord are identified and protected. A full thickness wedge of scrotal tissue—encompassing skin, adipose tissue, and dartos fascia—is excised. If hydroceles are present, the tunica vaginalis is also excised. The excess scrotal septum is resected and the testes are secured with non-absorbable

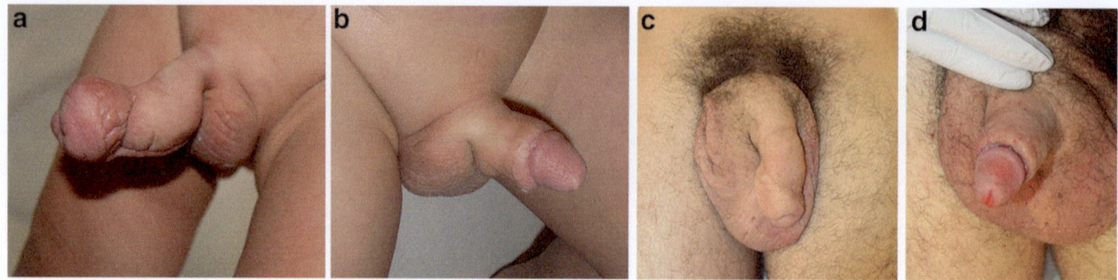

Fig. 30.6 Preoperative and postoperative photos of penile debulking. (**a**) 14-month-old male with congenital lymphedema–distichiasis involving his penis, shown prior to debulking. (**b**) At 24 months of age following debulking and circumcision. (**c**) 21-year-old male with congenital penile, scrotal, and lower extremity lymphedema, prior to resection and (**d**) following surgery

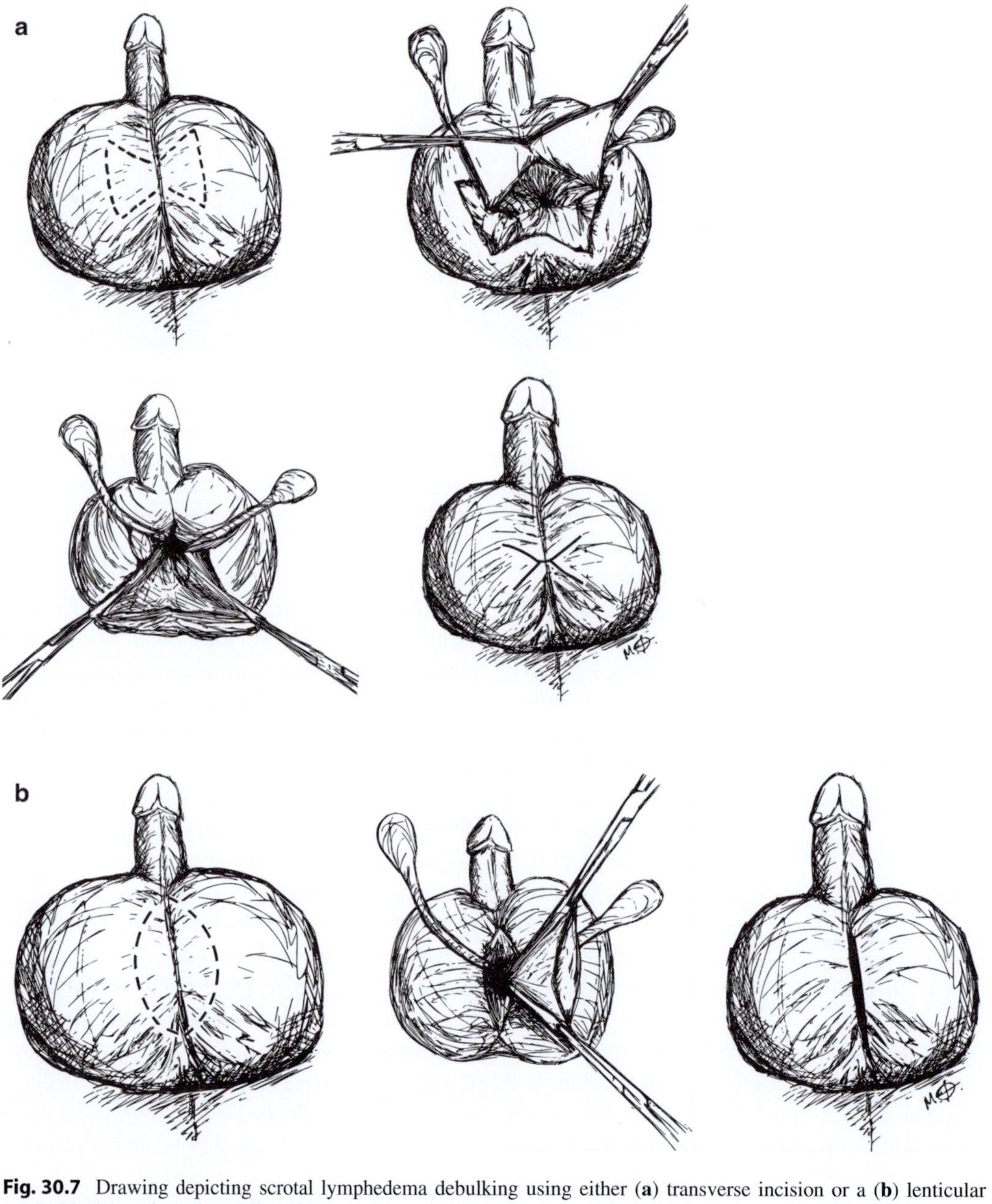

Fig. 30.7 Drawing depicting scrotal lymphedema debulking using either (**a**) transverse incision or a (**b**) lenticular vertical incision along the midline raphe

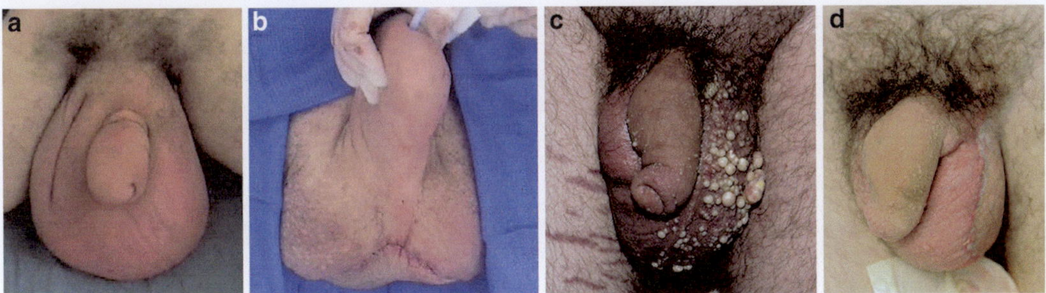

Fig. 30.8 Scrotal Debulking: (**a**) 20-year-old male with combined peno-scrotal lymphedema prior to surgery. (**b**) The same male following scrotal debulking via a transverse incision. (**c**) 27-year-old male with a central conducting lymphatic anomaly prior to debulking. Note the presence of cellulitis and the numerous cutaneous lymphatic vesicles along the left scrotum. (**d**) The same male following debulking using a vertical lenticular incision. The incision was made laterally instead of along the midline raphe to maximize removal of cutaneous lymphatic vesicles

sutures to the reduced septum. Scrotoplasty is performed to facilitate either a transverse closure parallel to the rugae or vertically to create a new midline raphe. For patients with extreme scrotal enlargement, additional redundant tissue can be resected from the lateral aspect of each hemiscrotum and closed in a V-Y advancement fashion. Closure is accomplished with multiple layers of absorbable suture in the tunica vaginalis, dartos, subcutaneous tissue, and skin. Postoperatively, bedrest with scrotal elevation is employed for 1 week (allowing limited ambulation for showers, bathroom activities and meals) and patients are encouraged to wear a compression undergarment thereafter. Figure 30.8 shows patients following scrotal debulking.

Labial lymphedema rarely requires surgery. Lymphatic malformations involving the labia can be sclerosed or debulked. As with male patients, resections should be conservative in younger females to allow for development of the labia during puberty. It is essential with either sclerosis or debulking of the labia, to avoid damaging either the clitoris or its innervation. Patients with central conducting lymphatic anomalies who experience leakage of chyle from the vagina or scrotum can be treated with either sclerotherapy or CO_2 laser ablation [16]. These patients may also benefit from ligation or excision of the refluxing chylous channels. A subset of patients with central conducting lymphatic anomalies has benefited from thoracic duct bypass. This surgical approach is actively being investigated at our institution.

References

1. Schook CC, Mulliken JB, Fishman SJ, Grant FD, Zurakowski D, Greene AK. Primary lymphedema: clinical features and management in 138 pediatric patients. Plast Reconstr Surg. 2011;127:2419–31.
2. Greene AK, Schook CC. Primary lymphedema: definition of onset based on developmental age. Plast Reconstr Surg. 2012;129:221e–2e.
3. Smeltzer DM, Stickler GB, Schirger A. Primary lymphedema in children and adolescents: a follow-up study and review. Pediatrics. 1985;76:206–18.
4. Addiss DG, Brady MA. Morbidity management in the global programme to eliminate lymphatic filariasis: a review of the scientific literature. Filaria J. 2007;6:2.
5. Bolt RJ, Peelen W, Nikkels PG, de Jong TP. Congenital lymphoedema of the genitalia. Eur J Pediatr. 1998;157:943–6.
6. Ross JH, Kay R, Yetman RJ, Angermeier K. Primary lymphedema of the genitalia in children and adolescents. J Urol. 1998;160:1485–9.
7. Morey AF, Meng MV, McAninch JW. Skin graft reconstruction of chronic genital lymphedema. Urology. 1997;50:423–6.
8. McDougal WS. Lymphedema of the external genitalia. J Urol. 2003;170:711–6.
9. Mulliken JB, Burrows PE, Fishman SJ, Mulliken JB. Mulliken and Young's vascular anomalies: hemangiomas and malformations. 2nd ed. Oxford: Oxford University Press; 2013.
10. William Forsyth Milroy (1855–1942): hereditary edema of the lower legs. JAMA. 1968;204:166.
11. Connell FC, Ostergaard P, Carver C, Brice G, Williams N, Mansour S, et al. Analysis of the coding regions of VEGFR3 and VEGFC in Milroy disease and other primary lymphoedemas. Hum Genet. 2009;124:625–31.
12. Kaipainen A, Korhonen J, Mustonen T, van Hinsbergh VW, Fang GH, Dumont D, et al. Expression of the fms-like tyrosine kinase 4 gene becomes restricted to

lymphatic endothelium during development. Proc Natl Acad Sci U S A. 1995;92:3566–70.

13. Salameh A, Galvagni F, Bardelli M, Bussolino F, Oliviero S. Direct recruitment of CRK and GRB2 to VEGFR-3 induces proliferation, migration, and survival of endothelial cells through the activation of ERK, AKT, and JNK pathways. Blood. 2005;106:3423–31.

14. Fang J, Dagenais SL, Erickson RP, Arlt MF, Glynn MW, Gorski JL, et al. Mutations in FOXC2 (MFH-1), a forkhead family transcription factor, are responsible for the hereditary lymphedema-distichiasis syndrome. Am J Hum Genet. 2000;67:1382–8.

15. Luks VL, Kamitaki N, Vivero MP, Uller W, Rab R, Bovee JV et al. Lymphatic and other vascular malformative/overgrowth disorders are caused by somatic mutations in PIK3CA. In Press.

16. Vogel AM, Alesbury JM, Burrows PE, Fishman SJ. Vascular anomalies of the female external genitalia. J Pediatr Surg. 2006;41:993–9.

17. Noel AA, Gloviczki P, Bender CE, Whitley D, Stanson AW, Deschamps C. Treatment of symptomatic primary chylous disorders. J Vasc Surg. 2001;34:785–91.

18. Borecky N, Gudinchet F, Laurini R, Duvoisin B, Hohlfeld J, Schnyder P. Imaging of cervico-thoracic lymphangiomas in children. Pediatr Radiol. 1995;25: 127–30.

19. Mulliken JB, Glowacki J. Hemangiomas and vascular malformations in infants and children: a classification based on endothelial characteristics. Plast Reconstr Surg. 1982;69:412–22.

20. Greene AK, Perlyn CA, Alomari AI. Management of lymphatic malformations. Clin Plast Surg. 2011;38: 75–82.

21. Richards TB, McBiles M, Collins PS. An easy method for diagnosis of lymphedema. Ann Vasc Surg. 1990;4:255–9.

22. Haas AF, Narurkar VA. Recalcitrant breast lymphangioma circumscriptum treated by UltraPulse carbon dioxide laser. Dermatol Surg. 1998;24:893–5.

23. Kulungowski AM, Schook CC, Alomari AI, Vogel AM, Mulliken JB, Fishman SJ. Vascular anomalies of the male genitalia. J Pediatr Surg. 2011;46: 1214–21.

24. Feins NR. A new surgical technique for lymphedema of the penis and scrotum. J Pediatr Surg. 1980;15: 787–9.

25. Feins NR. A new incision for penile surgery. J Pediatr Surg. 1981;16:817–9.

26. Modolin M, Mitre AI, da Silva JC, Cintra W, Quagliano AP, Arap S, et al. Surgical treatment of lymphedema of the penis and scrotum. Clinics. 2006;61:289–94.

Index

A.K. Greene et al. (eds.), *Lymphedema: Presentation, Diagnosis, and Treatment,*
DOI 10.1007/978-3-319-14493-1, © Springer International Publishing Switzerland 2015